ATHEROSCLEROSIS V
THE FIFTH SARATOGA INTERNATIONAL CONFERENCE

ANNALS OF
THE NEW YORK ACADEMY
OF SCIENCES

Volume 902

EDITORIAL STAFF

Executive Editor
BARBARA M. GOLDMAN

Managing Editor
JUSTINE CULLINAN

Associate Editor
MARY KATHERINE BRENNAN

The New York Academy of Sciences
2 East 63rd Street
New York, New York 10021

THE NEW YORK ACADEMY OF SCIENCES
(Founded in 1817)

BOARD OF GOVERNORS, September 15, 1999 – September 15, 2000

BILL GREEN, *Chairman of the Board*
TORSTEN WIESEL, *Vice Chairman of the Board*
RODNEY W. NICHOLS, *President and CEO* [ex officio]

Honorary Life Governors
WILLIAM T. GOLDEN   JOSHUA LEDERBERG

JOHN T. MORGAN, *Treasurer*

Governors

D. ALLAN BROMLEY	LAWRENCE B. BUTTENWIESER	PRAVEEN CHAUDHARI
JOHN H. GIBBONS	RONALD L. GRAHAM	HENRY M. GREENBERG
ROBERT G. LAHITA	MARTIN L. LEIBOWITZ	JACQUELINE LEO
WILLIAM J. McDONOUGH	KATHLEEN P. MULLINIX	JOHN F. NIBLACK
SANDRA PANEM	RICHARD RAVITCH	RICHARD A. RIFKIND

SARA LEE SCHUPF   JAMES H. SIMONS

ELEANOR BAUM, *Past Chairman of the Board*
HELENE L. KAPLAN, *Counsel* [ex officio]   PETER H. KOHN, *Secretary* [ex officio]

ANNALS OF THE NEW YORK ACADEMY OF SCIENCES
Volume 902

ATHEROSCLEROSIS V
THE FIFTH SARATOGA INTERNATIONAL CONFERENCE

Edited by Fujio Numano and Michael A. Gimbrone, Jr.

The New York Academy of Sciences
New York, New York
2000

Copyright © 2000 by the New York Academy of Sciences. All rights reserved. Under the provisions of the United States Copyright Act of 1976, individual readers of the Annals are permitted to make fair use of the material in them for teaching or research. Permission is granted to quote from the Annals provided that the customary acknowledgment is made of the source. Material in the Annals may be republished only by permission of the Academy. Address inquiries to the Permissions Department (editorial@nyas.org) at the New York Academy of Sciences.

Copying fees: For each copy of an article made beyond the free copying permitted under Section 107 or 108 of the 1976 Copyright Act, a fee should be paid through the Copyright Clearance Center, Inc., 222 Rosewood Drive, Danvers, MA 01923. (www.copyright.com).

∞The paper used in this publication meets the minimum requirements of the American National Standard for Information Sciences—Permanence of Paper for Printed Library Materials, ANSI Z39.48-1984.

Library of Congress Cataloging-in-Publication Data

Saratoga International Conference on Atherosclerosis (5th : 1999 Barcelona, Spain)
   Atherosclerosis V: the fifth Saratoga International Conference / edited by Fujio Numano and Michael A. Gimbrone.
      p. cm. — (Annals of the New York Academy of Sciences, ISSN 0077-8923 ; v. 902)
   "This volume is the result of a conference entitled The Fifth Saratoga International Conference on Atherosclerosis held on May 18–20, 1999, in Barcelona, Spain"—Contents p.
   Includes bibliographical references and index.
   ISBN 1-57331-246-0 (cloth: alk. paper) — ISBN 1-57331-247-9 (pbk: alk. paper).
    1. Atherosclerosis—Congresses. I. Title: Atherosclerosis 5. II. Title: Atherosclerosis five. III. Numano, Fujio. IV. Gimbrone, Michael A. V. Title. VI. Series.

Q11 .N5 vol. 902
[RC692]
500 s—dc21
[616.1'36]
                                                                                                                00-036154

GYAT / PCP
Printed in the United States of America
ISBN 1-57331-246-0 (cloth)
ISBN 1-57331-247-9 (paper)
ISSN 0077-8923

ANNALS OF THE NEW YORK ACADEMY OF SCIENCES
Volume 902
May 2000

ATHEROSCLEROSIS V
THE FIFTH SARATOGA INTERNATIONAL CONFERENCE[a]

Editors and Conference Chairs
FUJIO NUMANO AND MICHAEL A. GIMBRONE, JR.

Conference Organizers
VALENTINE FUSTER, MICHAEL A. GIMBRONE, JR., YOSHIYA HATA,
PETER LIBBY, CHIKAYUKI NAITO, FUJIO NUMANO, RUSSELL ROSS,
AKIO SUZUKI, AKIRA TANAKA, KENZO TANAKA,
ROBERT W. WISSLER, AND YOSHIO YAZAKI

CONTENTS

In Memoriam: Russell Ross, Ph.D. By FUJIO NUMANO AND MICHAEL A. GIMBRONE, JR.	xiii
Introductory Remarks. By FUJIO NUMANO	xv
Genomic Searches for Genes That Influence Atherosclerosis and Its Risk Factors. By JAMES E. HIXSON AND JOHN BLANGERO	1
Genetic Analysis of Essential Hypertension in Japanese Populations. By TOSHIO OGIHARA, TOMOHIRO KATSUYA, AND JITSUO HIGAKI	8
Tailored Therapy to Fit Individual Profiles: Genetics and Coronary Artery Disease. By J.WOUTER JUKEMA AND JOHN J.P. KASTELEIN	17
Genetic Diversity in the Matrix Metalloproteinase Family: Effects on Function and Disease Progression. By ADRIANO M. HENNEY, SHU YE, BAIPING ZHANG, SOPHIA JORMSJÖ, CARL WHATLING, PER ERIKSSON, AND ANDERS HAMSTEN	27
The Extracellular Matrix Dynamically Regulates Smooth Muscle Cell Responsiveness to PDGF. By ELAINE W. RAINES, HIDENORI KOYAMA, AND NEIL O. CARRAGHER	39

[a]This volume is the result of a conference entitled **The Fifth Saratoga International Conference on Atherosclerosis** held on May 18–20, 1999 in Barcelona, Spain.

The Role of Adaptive Immunity in Atherosclerosis. *By* GÖRAN K. HANSSON, XINGHUA ZHOU, ELISABETH TÖRNQUIST, AND GABRIELLE PAULSSON 53

Inflammation and Atherosclerosis: Atherosclerotic Lesions in Takayasu Arteritis. *By* FUJIO NUMANO, YUKIO KISHI, AKIRA TANAKA, MIHO OHKAWARA, TSUNEKAZU KAKUTA, AND YASUSHI KOBAYASHI 65

Gene Therapy for Heart Transplantation-Associated Coronary Arteriosclerosis. *By* MITSUAKI ISOBE, JUN-ICHI SUZUKI, RYUICHI MORISHITA, YASUFUMI KANEDA, AND JUN AMANO 77

Role of Endothelin-1 in Atherosclerosis. *By* JIANGLIN FAN, HIROYUKI UNOKI, SATOSHI IWASA, AND TERUO WATANABE 84

Oxidized-LDL and Atherosclerosis: Role of LOX-1. *By* TORU KITA, NORIAKI KUME, MASAYUKI YOKODE, KENJI ISHII, HIDENORI ARAI, HISANORI HORIUCHI, HIDEAKI MORIWAKI, MANABU MINAMI, HIROHARU KATAOKA, YOSHIO WAKATSUKI 95

Receptors and Lipid Transfer Proteins in HDL Metabolism. *By* DAVID L. SILVER, XIAN-CHENG JIANG, TAKESHI ARAI, CAN BRUCE, AND ALAN R. TALL 103

Scavenger Receptor Classes A and B: Their Roles in Atherogenesis and the Metabolism of Modified LDL and HDL. *By* THEO J.C. VAN BERKEL, MIRANDA VAN ECK, NICOLE HERIJGERS, KEES FLUITER, AND S. NION 113

CD36 in Atherosclerosis: The Role of a Class B Macrophage Scavenger Receptor. *By* ANDREW C. NICHOLSON, MARIA FEBBRAIO, JIHONG HAN, RAY L. SILVERSTEIN, AND DAVID P. HAJJAR 128

Animal Models for Hyperinsulinemia and Insulin Resistance. *By* HIDEKI ABE AND NOBUHIRO YAMADA 134

Lipid Lowering Reduces Proteolytic and Prothrombotic Potential in Rabbit Atheroma. *By* MASANORI AIKAWA AND PETER LIBBY 140

Mechanisms of Vascular Atrophy and Fibrous Cap Disruption. *By* ALEXANDER W. CLOWES AND SCOTT A. BERCELI 153

Roles of the AGE-RAGE System in Vascular Injury in Diabetes. *By* YASUHIKO YAMAMOTO, SHO-ICHI YAMAGISHI, HIDETO YONEKURA, TOSHIO DOI, HIROKO TSUJI, ICHIRO KATO, SHIN TAKASAWA, HIROSHI OKAMOTO, JOYNAL ABEDIN, NOBUSHIGE TANAKA, SHIGERU SAKURAI, HIDEYUKI MIGITA, HIROYUKI UNOK, HUA WANG, TAKAHIRO ZENDA, PING-SHENG WU, YASUNORI SEGAWA, TOMOMI HIGASHIDE, KAZUO KAWASAKI, AND HIROSHI YAMAMOTO 163

Characterization of Atherosclerotic Plaques by Magnetic Resonance Imaging. *By* ZAHI A. FAYAD AND VALENTIN FUSTER 173

Signaling Angiogenesis via p42/p44 MAP Kinase Cascade. *By* GILLES PAGÈS, JULIE MILANINI, DARREN E. RICHARD, EDURNE BERRA, EMMANUEL GOTHIÉ, FRANCESC VIÑALS, AND JACQUES POUYSSÉGUR 187

Properties of Two VEGF Receptors, Flt-1 and KDR, in Signal Transduction. *By* YASUFUMI SATO, SHINICHI KANNO, NOBUYUKI ODA, MAYUMI ABE, MIKITO ITO, KENYA SHITARA, AND MASABUMI SHIBUYA 201

Regulation of Angiogenesis by Controlling VEGF Receptor. *By* SEI-ITSU MUROTA, MITSUE ONODERA, AND IKUO MORITA 208

Transcriptional Regulation of Smooth Muscle Phenotypic Modulation. *By* RYOZO NAGAI, KEIKO KOWASE, AND MASAHIKO KURABAYASHI 214

Blood Vessels from Bone Marrow. *By* JULIE H. CAMPBELL, JOHNNY L. EFENDY, C.-L. HAN, AND GORDON R. CAMPBELL 224

Endothelial Dysfunction, Hemodynamic Forces, and Atherogenesis. *By* MICHAEL A. GIMBRONE, JR., JAMES N. TOPPER, TOBI NAGEL, KEITH R. ANDERSON, AND GUILLERMO GARCIA-CARDEÑA 230

Role of the Vascular NADH/NADPH Oxidase System in Atherosclerosis. *By* MITSUHIRO YOKOYAMA, NOBUTAKA INOUE, AND SEINOSUKE KAWASHIMA 241

Molecular Basis of Angiogenesis: Role of VEGF and VE-Cadherin. *By* PETER CARMELIET AND DESIRE COLLEN 249

Annexin II and Regulation of Cell Surface Fibrinolysis. *By* KATHERINE A. HAJJAR AND SUCHITRA S. ACHARYA 265

The Fat Mouse: A Powerful Genetic Model to Study Hemostatic Gene Expression in Obesity/NIDDM. *By* DAVID J. LOSKUTOFF, KAZUHIKO FUJISAWA, AND FAHUMIYA SAMAD 272

Participation of Reactive Oxygen Intermediates in the Angiotensin II–Activated Signaling Pathways in Vascular Smooth Muscle Cells. *By* TOMOSABURO TAKAHASHI, TAKAHIRO TANIGUCHI, MASANORI OKUDA, AKIHIRO TAKAHASHI, SATORU KAWASAKI, KOJI DOMOTO, MASAKO TAGUCHI, YUICHI ISHIKAWA, AND MITSUHIRO YOKOYAMA . 283

C–C and C–X–C Chemokines Trigger Firm Adhesion of Monocytes to Vascular Endothelium under Flow Conditions. *By* FRANCIS W. LUSCINSKAS, ROBERT E. GERSZTEN, EDUARDO A. GARCIA-ZEPEDA, YAW-CHYN LIM, MASAYUKI YOSHIDA, HAN A. DING, MICHAEL A. GIMBRONE, JR., ANDREW D. LUSTER, AND ANTHONY ROSENZWEIG .. 288

Distinct Mechanical Stimuli Differentially Regulate the PI3K/Akt Survival Pathway in Endothelial Cells. *By* GUILLERMO GARCÍA-CARDEÑA, KEITH R. ANDERSON, LAURA MAURI, AND MICHAEL A. GIMBRONE, JR. 294

Mechanical Stress Modulates Glutathione Peroxidase Expression in Cultured Bovine Aortic Endothelial Cells. *By* SAORI TAKESHITA, NOBUTAKA INOUE, YOSHIYUKI RIKITAKE, SEINOSUKE KAWASHIMA, AND MITSUHIRO YOKOYAMA 298

Estrogen Receptor Deficiency Leads to Impaired Endothelial Nitric Oxide Production and Premature Coronary Arteriosclerosis. *By* GABOR M. RUBANYI 302

Differentiation-Induced Transmigration of HL60 Cells across Activated HUVEC Monolayer Involves E-selectin–Dependent Mechanism. *By* MASAYUKI YOSHIDA, LEE-JUNG CHIEN, YUKIO YASUKOCHI, AND FUJIO NUMANO 307

Construction of Recombinant Adenoviral Vector of Annexin II. *By* HIDETO ISHII, MASAYUKI YOSHIDA, KATHERINE A. HAJJAR, YUKIO YASUKOCHI, AND FUJIO NUMANO 311

Effect of Leptin in Platelet and Endothelial Cells: Obesity and Arterial Thrombosis. *By* IKURO MARUYAMA, MASANORI NAKATA, AND KAZUYO YAMAJI 315

Cytokines and Soluble Cell Adhesion Molecules: Possible Markers of Inflammatory Response in Atherosclerosis. *By* A.I. TEPLYAKOV, E.V. PRYSCHEPOVA, N.G. KRUCHINSKY, AND T.I. CHEGEROVA 320

Inducible Expression of LOX-1, a Novel Receptor for Oxidized LDL, in Macrophages and Vascular Smooth Muscle Cells. *By* NORIAKI KUME, HIDEAKI MORIWAKI, HIROHARU KATAOKA, MANABU MINAMI, TAKATOSHI MURASE, TATSUYA SAWAMURA, TOMOH MASAKI, AND TORU KITA 323

Expression of Lectin-like Oxidized LDL Receptor-1 in Human Atherosclerotic Lesions. *By* HIROHARU KATAOKA, NORIAKI KUME, MANABU MINAMI, HIDEAKI MORIWAKI, TATSUYA SAWAMURA, TOMOH MASAKI, AND TORU KITA 328

Chylomicron Remnant Induces Apoptosis in Vascular Endothelial Cells. *By* SATORU KAWASAKI, TAKAHIRO TANIGUCHI, YOSHIO FUJIOKA, AKIHIRO TAKAHASHI, TOMOSABURO TAKAHASHI, KOJI DOMOTO, MASAKO TAGUCHI, YUICHI ISHIKAWA, AND MITSUHIRO YOKOYAMA ... 336

Granulocyte Macrophage Colony-Stimulating Factor Plays a Priming Role in Murine Macrophage Growth Induced by Oxidized Low Density Lipoprotein. *By* AKIRA MIYAZAKI, TAKESHI BIWA, HIDEKI HAKAMATA, MASAKAZU SAKAI, YUICHIRO SAKAMOTO, KYU KYU MAUNG, MEHTAP YUKSEL, AND SEIKOH HORIUCHI 342

Transgenic Rabbits Expressing Human Apolipoprotein(a) as a Useful Model for the Study of Lipoprotein(a). *By* JIANGLIN FAN, MIREILLE CHALLAH, HIROAKI SHIMOYAMADA, AND TERUO WATANABE 347

The Role of Remnant Lipoproteins in Atherosclerosis. *By* AKIO KAWAKAMI, AKIRA TANAKA, TAKAMITSU NAKANO, KATSUYUKI NAKAJIMA, AND FUJIO NUMANO 352

Enhanced Expression of Osteopontin by High Glucose: Involvement of Osteopontin in Diabetic Macroangiopathy. *By* MINORU TAKEMOTO, KOUTARO YOKOTE, MASASHI YAMAZAKI, AMY L. RIDALL, WILLIAM T. BUTLER, TARO MATSUMOTO, KEN TAMURA, YASUSHI SAITO, AND SEIJIRO MORI 357

The Second Nationwide Study of Atherosclerosis in Infants, Children, and Young Adults in Japan: Comparison with the First Study Carried Out 13 Years Ago. *By* MASAMI IMAKITA, CHIKAO YUTANI, ISAMU SAKURAI, AKINOBU SUMIYOSHI, TERUO WATANABE, MASAKO MITSUMATA, YOSHIAKI KUSUMI, SHOICHI KATAYAMA, MASAYUKI MANO, SHUNROKU BABA, TOSHIFUMI MANNAMI, KATSUO SUEISHI, AND KENZO TANAKA .. 364

Gene Therapy for Cardiovascular Disease Using Hepatocyte Growth Factor. *By* RYUICHI MORISHITA, MOTOKUNI AOKI, SHIGEFUMI NAKAMURA, JITSUO HIGAKI, YASUFUMI KANEDA, AND TOSHIO OGIHARA 369

INDEX OF CONTRIBUTORS 377

Financial assistance was received from:
- JAPAN ARTERIOSCLEROSIS RESEARCH FOUNDATION
- JAPAN ATHEROSCLEROSIS SOCIETY
- JAPAN CIRCULATION SOCIETY
- JAPANESE COLLEGE OF ANGIOLOGY

The New York Academy of Sciences believes it has a responsibility to provide an open forum for discussion of scientific questions. The positions taken by the participants in the reported conferences are their own and not necessarily those of the Academy. The Academy has no intent to influence legislation by providing such forums.

ATHEROSCLEROSIS V
THE FIFTH SARATOGA INTERNATIONAL CONFERENCE

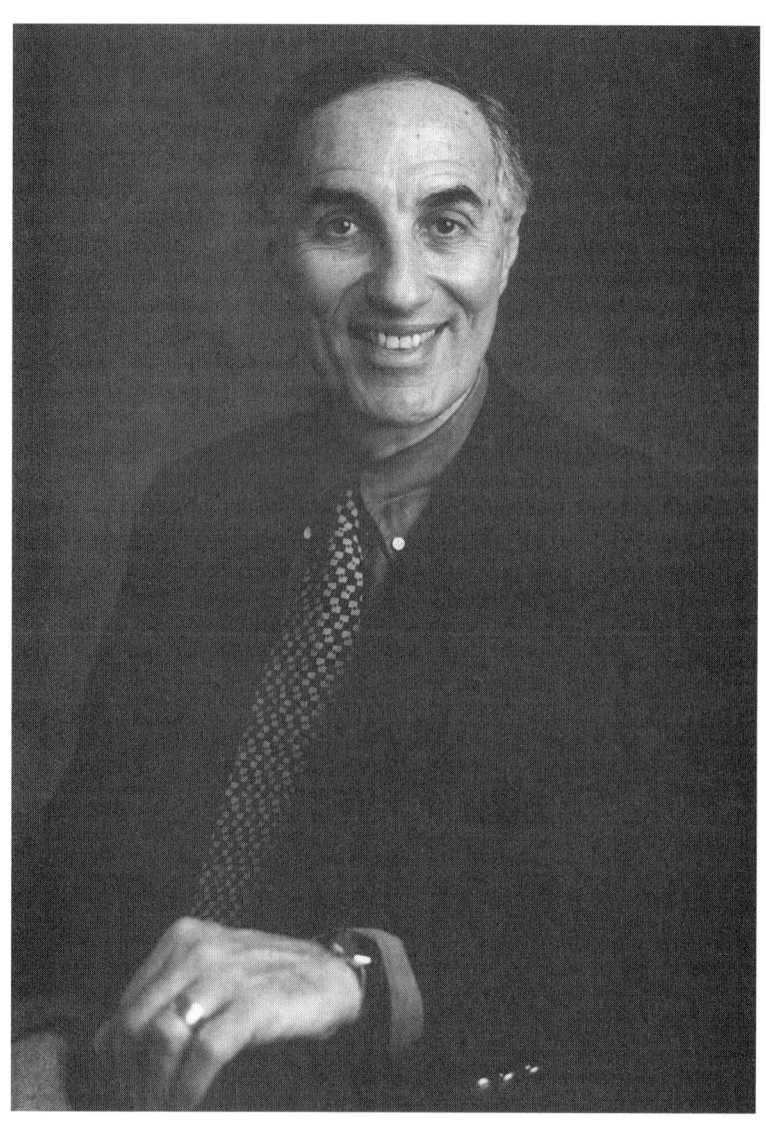

Russell Ross, Ph.D. 1929–1999

In Memoriam
Russell Ross, Ph.D.

Times flies like an arrow and life is so short

Who would have thought that our Russ would leave us so soon at the age of 69? Professor Russell Ross, our dear friend passed away on March 18, 1999. He was Director of the Center for Vascular Biology, Professor of Pathology, University of Washington, and Organizing Committee member of the Saratoga International Conference on Atherosclerosis. Words cannot express our deep sorrow.

I need not describe his scientific career and brilliant achievements in the field of atherosclerosis research, because everyone who joined this Saratoga meeting knows these very well. I would like, however, to mention only two of his numerous contributions. He played a key role in establishing the field of vascular biology. His "response to injury hypothesis" and the subsequent discovery of PDGF have led to the application of molecular biology to this field. He was an excellent scientist and a wonderful teacher. More that 50 young students and fellows worked in his laboratory and are now among the leading investigators in vascular biology.

In 1981, I sent K. Shimokado to his laboratory and he succeeded in elucidating the monocyte-macrophage–derived growth factor (MDGF). Since then, more than ten Japanese fellows have studied in Russ's laboratory and are now active in vascular biology research in Japan.

Russ came to Japan many times and lectured enthusiastically and joyfully about his work. He was in Tokyo last fall as the special guest of a symposium organized by *Nature*. We enjoyed a sushi dinner together on his last night in Tokyo. He departed saying, "Good-bye, see you in Barcelona." His not being here saddens me deeply. Again, I appreciate his contribution to the development of vascular biology research in Japan.

Thank you Russ and good-bye.

— Fujio Numano

We mourn the loss of a major figure in the field of cardiovascular research, Dr. Russell Ross, Professor and Past-Chair of the Department of Pathology at the University of Washington, School of Medicine. He died suddenly on March 18, 1999, after a brief illness. He was 69 years old.

In an extraordinary career that spanned four decades, Dr. Ross was a leader in the crusade to understand the cellular and molecular mechanisms of atherosclerotic vascular disease, the primary cause of heart attack and stroke in the industrialized world. His response-to-injury hypothesis, first detailed in a *New England Journal of Medicine* article in 1976, provided a conceptual framework for much of the subsequent research on the contributions of vascular cells, endothelium and smooth muscle, and their interactions with monocyte-macrophages, in the initiation and progression of atherosclerotic lesions. His early work focused on the identification and characterization of the platelet-derived growth factor as a key mediator in the response of the arterial wall to injury; subsequent studies explored the contributions of monocyte-macrophages (foam cells) to the local cytokine/growth factor milieu of developing lesions. His group's most recent contributions focused on the role of extracellular matrix in the modulation of vascular smooth muscle phenotype.

Dr. Ross's groundbreaking research and dedication to understanding a major human disease won him the respect and recognition of academic colleagues worldwide. He was the recipient of numerous prestigious awards and played a leadership role in the biomedical research community in the United States and abroad.

Since their inception more than a decade ago, Dr. Ross played an active role in the planning of these Saratoga conferences. He was very committed to the concept of creating an international forum for exchange of information in the field of atherosclerosis and, in particular, of fostering the participation of young investigators. It is therefore especially fitting that we dedicate the Fifth Saratoga International Conference on Atherosclerosis to his memory.

— MICHAEL A. GIMBRONE, JR.

Introductory Remarks

FUJIO NUMANO

Chairman of the Fifth Saratoga International, Conference on Atherosclerosis
Professor of Internal Medicine, Tokyo Medical and Dental University

Atherosclerosis V is the proceedings of the Fifth Saratoga International Conference on Atherosclerosis held on May 18–20, 1999 in Barcelona, Spain.

The conference was initially established to promote the exchange of up-to-date information in the field of atherosclerosis research among prominent invited scientists from three continents: North America, Europe, and Asia.

Just as the previous four conferences in Saratoga Springs, New York (Atherosclerosis I, 1985); Towada, Japan (Atherosclerosis II, 1989); Nekoma, Japan (Atherosclerosis III, 1993); and Kona, Hawaii (Atherosclerosis IV, 1997), the Barcelona Conference was held in the luxurious atmosphere of the Hotel "Art" and included excellent presentations, followed by many spirited discussions.

All of these are included in "Atherosclerosis V" and were published within a year after the conference to make it available to members of the New York Academy of Sciences.

This conference was held also in the memory of Professor Russell Ross, a member of the Organizing Committee and my dear friend, who passed away suddenly in March, 1999. I would like to dedicate this volume to the late Russ, his wife Jeannie, and his family.

Lastly, I would like to express my sincere appreciation to the Organizing Committee members, Drs. Michael A. Gimbrone Jr., Robert W. Wissler, the late Russell Ross, Valentine Fuster, Peter Libby, Kenzo Tanaka, Akio Suzuki, Chikayuki Naito, Yoshio Yazaki, Yoshiya Hata, and Akira Tanaka. I offer special appreciation to Dr. Michael A. Gimbrone, who always supported me warmheartedly as co-chairman; Dr. Akira Tanaka, who worked vigorously as the general secretary; and Mrs. Seishu Matsumura, who created the wonderful book cover for us.

Genomic Searches for Genes That Influence Atherosclerosis and Its Risk Factors

JAMES E. HIXSON[a] AND JOHN BLANGERO

Department of Genetics, Southwest Foundation for Biomedical Research, San Antonio, Texas 78245, USA

ABSTRACT: We are performing genomic searches in randomly ascertained families to identify new quantitative trait loci (QTLs) that influence atherosclerosis and its risk factors. The genetic markers used for genomic searches are random microsatellite markers distributed throughout the human chromosomes. These markers are used for linkage analysis with variance component methods to identify QTLs for measured phenotypes related to lipid metabolism and atherosclerosis. We conducted such a genomic search in 477 participants of the San Antonio Family Heart Study. This genomic search identified QTLs on chromosomes 3 and 4 that influence LDL size class, an important risk factor of atherosclerosis. In addition to lipid risk factors, we measured a variety of gene products involved in atherogenesis in the arterial wall (such as adhesion molecules and components of hemostasis). We found QTLs for serum levels of soluble P-selectin on chromosome 15 (LOD = 3.8) and chromosome 12 (LOD = 2.6).

INTRODUCTION

In the last twenty years, human genetic research has made great progress in identifying new genes that cause rare, single-gene disorders using genomic technologies. For many such monogenic diseases, an important part of the gene identification process was linkage analysis in affected families using polymorphisms as genetic markers. These studies were greatly facilitated by the development of the human genetic map, which has now mapped thousands of genetic markers at high density throughout the chromosomes. The next great challenge for human genetics is the identification of genes that influence predisposition to common diseases, such as atherosclerosis, diabetes, hypertension, and obesity, which represent the largest health burdens for human populations. In general, genetic studies of common diseases have focused on candidate genes that are known to be involved in relevant metabolic processes, such as cholesterol metabolism (heart disease) or glucose metabolism (diabetes). Surprisingly, many years of such studies have yielded only a few candidate genes that significantly affect common diseases or associated risk factors. Moreover, the few candidate genes that are associated with disease phenotypes typically have small effects, accounting for only a small proportion of the variation in the population. We and others have turned to the genomic technologies that proved successful for identification of genes for monogenic disorders. We are performing

[a]Address for correspondence: James E. Hixson, Department of Genetics, Southwest Foundation for Biomedical Research, P.O. Box 760549, San Antonio, TX 78245. Voice: 210-258-9443; fax: 210-670-3337.
jhixson@darwin.sfbr.org

genomic searches using linkage analysis with hundreds of microsatellite markers distributed evenly across the genome in extended pedigrees that have been measured for many disease-related phenotypes.

SELECTION OF PEDIGREES

Our approach to genetic studies of atherosclerosis is to use large extended pedigrees that have not been ascertained by any particular disease or risk factor. In general, our goal is to identify genes that influence the normal quantitative variation of risk factors, such as serum cholesterol or lipoproteins. By nature, common diseases are well represented in unselected populations and are influenced by genes that are found in the general population, rather than only in rare individuals defined by extreme phenotypes. In this paper, we present the San Antonio Family Heart Study (SAFHS) as an example of this approach. SAFHS includes 1,400 Mexican-Americans in San Antonio who are members of 41 large extended pedigrees. Of these families, we have genotyped 477 individuals in the ten largest pedigrees for the genomic scan presented in this report. The families were ascertained without regard to disease or disease phenotypes, and probands were chosen on the basis of age (40–60 yr) and numbers of relatives (at least six first-degree relatives excluding parents living in San Antonio). Males and females were included in approximately equal numbers, and each participant visited the clinic for blood collection, physical exam, and questionnaires concerning demographic, socioeconomic, and lifestyle variables.[1]

QUANTITATIVE PHENOTYPES

Our studies in living populations are based on quantitative measures of known risk factors for atherosclerosis, rather than clinical endpoints of heart disease. In SAFHS, we have used blood samples to measure serum levels of a wide array of phenotypes related to lipid metabolism and atherosclerosis. For lipid measurements, we measured triglycerides, total serum cholesterol, HDL-C, V+LDL-C, as well as size fractions of HDL and LDL using gradient gel electrophoresis.[2,3] We also measured serum levels of apolipoproteins associated with lipoproteins, and distributions of apolipoproteins among lipoprotein size classes using immunoblotting of gradient gels.[4] More recently, we have measured serum levels of a variety of gene products involved in atherogenesis in the arterial wall, such as adhesion molecules (P-selectin, E-selectin, VCAM-1, ICAM-1) and hemostasis components (D-dimer, plasminogen, fibrinogen).

HIGH THROUGHPUT GENOTYPING AND LINKAGE ANALYSIS

The genomic screen for genes that influence atherosclerosis and its risk factors required typing each SAFHS family member for approximately 300 microsatellite markers distributed at 15-cM intervals along the human chromosomes. The microsatellite markers were typed using oligonucleotide primers labeled with fluorescent dyes (MapPairs version 6 Linkage Screening Set from Research Genetics, Inc.) for PCR amplification of DNA samples prepared from lymphocytes from each SAFHS participant as previously described.[5] The products of individual PCR reactions were pooled according to multiplexed panels (3–9 markers per lane) for electrophoresis on automated DNA sequencers (ABI Model 377), and genotypes were processed using associated software (GENESCAN, GENOTYPER programs). Multipoint linkage analysis was performed with the software package SOLAR using variance component methods as previously described.[6] Variance component linkage analysis can be classified as nonparametric in that no particular model of inheritance is specified. However, this approach provides greater statistical power to detect quantitative trait loci (QTLs) than standard sibpair-based methods because all of the individuals in the extended pedigrees are used for variance component linkage analysis.

IDENTIFICATION OF QTLS FOR LDL SIZE CLASSES

We performed a genomic search in SAFHS for QTLs that affect LDL size distributions as measured by gradient gel electrophoresis in serum samples from SAFHS participants.[7] LDL particles circulate as a heterogeneous array of sizes, and many studies have shown that the small, dense LDL particle phenotype is an important risk factor for cardiovascular disease.[8,9] We divided the LDL particles into four size classes that were measured by densitometry of gradient gels stained for cholesterol with Sudan Black B. All four LDL size classes had significant heritabilities (22–37%), and were significantly influenced by several covariates including age and sex. We performed a genomic search using variance component linkage analysis with microsatellite markers (15-cM intervals), and found two QTLs with LOD scores > 3 (nominal criterion for linkage) for LDL size fraction 3 (LDL-3), a fraction that contains only small LDL particles (24.2–25.5 nm). The highest multipoint LOD scores for LDL-3 were found on chromosome 3 (LOD = 4.1) at 244 cM, and chromosome 4 (LOD = 4.1) at 126 cM. We performed oligogenic linkage analyses to test whether these two QTLs comprise a true multiple locus system to influence LDL-3 variation. We repeated the genome screen fixing the location of the major QTL on chromosome 4 and found the highest LOD score on chromosome 3, identifying the other major QTL from the initial screen. Likelihood comparisons showed that a model including independent effects of both QTLs was significantly better than including only one QTL ($p = 0.0012$). This two-locus model showed that the chromosome 3 and 4 QTLs each explained 22.8% and 23.0% of the variation in LDL-3 concentrations, respectively. We are currently investigating positional candidate genes that are located in these chromosomal regions, particularly the gene for microsomal triglyceride transfer protein (MTP), which is required for assembly of VLDL particles in the liver and chylomicrons in the intestine. Mutations in the MTP gene abolish production of apoB-containing lipoproteins, resulting in the rare recessive genetic disorder abetalipoproteinemia.[10,11]

IDENTIFICATION OF QTLS FOR SOLUBLE P-SELECTIN

In addition to lipoprotein phenotypes, we are measuring serum levels of gene products involved in atherogenesis, such as the adhesion molecule, P-selectin. P-selectin is expressed in activated platelets and endothelial cells and mediates tethering and rolling of leukocytes along the endothelial cell lining of the artery via interactions with P-selectin glycoprotein ligand-1 (PSGL-1). Although P-selectin acts locally in the arterial wall, many recent studies have shown that increased serum levels of soluble P-selectin are associated with atherosclerosis, acute myocardial infarction, and hypertension.[12-14] Therefore, we measured serum levels of soluble P-selectin in 370 SAFHS family members using a colorimetric ELISA assay (R & D Systems, Inc., Minneapolis, MN). We found a substantial genetic component for variation in soluble P-selectin levels in the SAFHS families, with a heritability of 70%. We also performed a genomic scan to identify QTLs that influence this trait. As described above, we used microsatellite markers distributed at approximately 15-cM intervals for variance component linkage analysis in the 10 largest SAFHS families. FIGURE 1(A) shows the multipoint linkage curve for chromosome 15 that contained the QTL with the highest LOD score. The maximum LOD score reached 3.8, corresponding to a $p = 0.000014$. This region of chromosome 15 also contains a positional candidate gene, sialyltransferase X (STX), which regulates linkage of neural cell adhesion molecule (NCAM1) to polysialic acid (PSA).[15] FIGURE 1(B) shows a second QTL for soluble P-selectin on chromosome 12 (LOD = 2.59). The evidence for this second QTL remained even after controlling for the chromosome 15 QTL (conditional LOD = 2.12). The chromosome 12 QTL is of particular interest since this region also contains the gene for PSGL-1, the ligand for P-selectin expressed on leukocytes. The next step is to identify the causative variants in the genes that are truly responsible for these QTLs, which will require (1) evaluation of positional candidate genes like PSGL-1 or (2) positional cloning to identify novel genes in these chromosomal regions.

CONCLUSION

While great progress has been made in identifying risk factors and pathophysiological processes leading to atherosclerosis, little is known about the genes that influence predisposition to atherosclerosis in human populations. In recent years, genetic studies have focused on identification and evaluation of variation in candidate genes known to be involved in relevant physiological pathways. However, these candidate genes have not proven to play substantial roles in determining atherosclerosis risk. We and others have turned to an alternate strategy to search the entire genome to discover genes that influence atherosclerosis and its risk factors, rather than relying on prior hypotheses concerning specific candidate genes. We are performing genomic searches in randomly ascertained human pedigrees, using microsatellite polymorphisms and linkage analysis, to identify QTLs that influence quantitative phenotypes related to atherosclerosis. SAFHS represents one such study that has successfully identified QTLs for phenotypes such as LDL size class and serum levels of soluble P-selectin—important risk factors for atherosclerosis and clinical endpoints of heart disease. The next challenge is the identification of genes in these chromosomal regions that are responsible for the QTLs we have detected using random markers. One approach is the evaluation of variants in known positional candidate genes in chromosomal regions containing QTLs using linkage and association studies. For example, we investigated the gene for pro-opiomelanocortin (POMC), which is found in the region of chromosome 2 containing a major QTL for leptin lev-

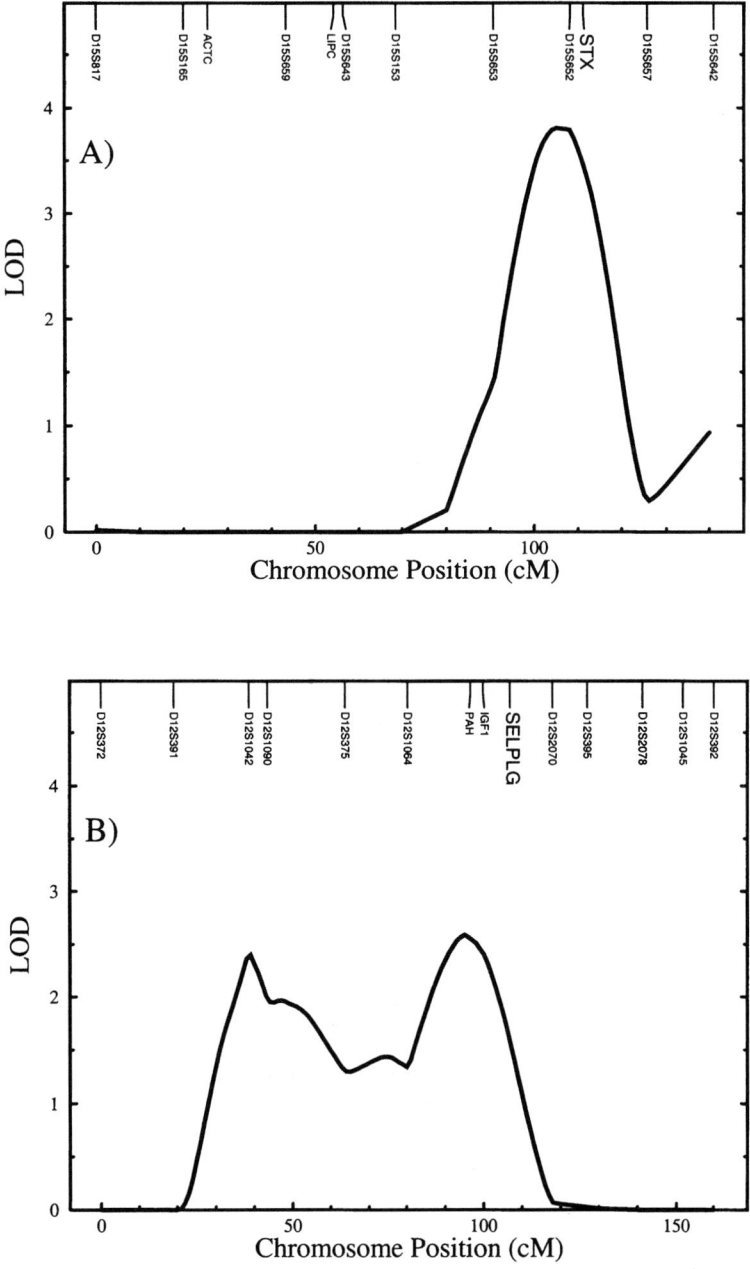

FIGURE 1. Multipoint linkage analysis of serum levels of soluble P-selectin on chromosome 15 (**A**) and chromosome 12 (**B**).

els in SAFHS families.[5] POMC encodes several hormones that are critical for regulation of energy homeostasis. Rare POMC mutations cause early onset obesity.[16] We identified polymorphisms in POMC and found that haplotypes are significantly associated with leptin levels, providing evidence that POMC may be responsible for the chromosome 2 QTL.[17] However, many chromosomal regions containing QTLs may not harbor strong positional candidate genes, and positional cloning strategies will be required to identify novel genes in such regions. At present, positional cloning is a formidable task that requires sequencing of large chromosomal regions to identify novel genes. However, the current private and public initiative to sequence the entire human genome may soon provide the identification of all expressed genes in such chromosomal regions. Similarly, private and public initiatives to identify single nucleotide polymorphisms (SNPs) distributed throughout the genome will greatly facilitate statistical analysis of novel genes for linkage and association studies. While the identification of common disease genes remains a daunting task, the application of new genomic search strategies and the availability of new information concerning the human genome should greatly accelerate the discovery of genes that underlie predisposition to atherosclerosis in human populations.

REFERENCES

1. MITCHELL, B.D., C.M. KAMMERER, J. BLANGERO, M.C. MAHANEY, D.L. RAINWATER, B. DYKE, J.E. HIXSON, R.D. HENKEL, M.R. SHARP, A.G. COMUZZIE & J.L. VANDEBERG. 1996. Genetic and environmental contributions to cardiovascular risk factors in Mexican Americans: the San Antonio family heart study. Circulation **94:** 2159–2170.
2. SINGH, A.T.K., D.L. RAINWATER, S.M. HAFFNER, J.L. VANDEBERG, W.R. SHELLEDY, P.H. MOORE, JR. & T.D. DYER. 1995. Effect of diabetes on lipoprotein size. Arterioscler. Thromb. Vasc. Biol. **15:** 1805–1811.
3. RAINWATER, D.L., D.W. ANDRES, A.L. FORD, W.F. LOWE, P.J. BLANCHE & R.M. KRAUSS. 1992. Production of polyacrylamide gradient gels for the electrophoretic resolution of lipoproteins. J. Lipid Res. **33:** 1876–1881.
4. RAINWATER, D.L., J. BLANGERO, P.H. MOORE, JR., W.R. SHELLEDY & T.D. DYER. 1995. Genetic control of apolipoprotein A-I distribution among HDL subclasses. Atherosclerosis **118:** 307–317.
5. COMUZZIE, A.G., J.E. HIXSON, L. ALMASY, B.D. MITCHELL, M.C. MAHANEY, T.D. DYER, M.P. STERN, J.W. MACCLUER & J. BLANGERO. 1997. A major quantitative trait locus determining serum leptin levels and fat mass is located on human chromosome 2. Nature Genet. **15:** 273–276.
6. ALMASY, L. & J. BLANGERO. 1998. Multipoint quantitative-trait linkage analysis in general pedigrees. Am. J. Hum. Genet. **62:** 1198–1211.
7. RAINWATER, D.L., L. ALMASY, J. BLANGERO, S.A. COLE, J.L. VANDEBERG, J.W. MACCLUER & J.E. HIXSON. 1999. A genome search identifies major quantitative trait loci on human chromosomes 3 and 4 that influence cholesterol concentrations in small LDL particles. Arterioscler. Thromb. Vasc. Biol. **19:** 777–783.
8. AUSTIN, M.A. 1992. Genetic epidemiology of low-density lipoprotein subclass phenotypes. Ann. Med. **24:** 477–481.
9. GARDNER, C.D., S.P FORTMANN & R.M. KRAUSS. 1996. Association of small low-density lipoprotein particles with the incidence of coronary artery disease in men and women. J. Am. Med. Assoc. **276:** 875–881.
10. SHARP, D., L. BLINDERMAN, K.A. COMBS, B. KIENZLE, B. RICCI, K. WAGER-SMITH, C.M. GIL, C.W. TURCK, M.-E. BOURMA, D.J. RADER, L.P. AGGERBECK, R.E. GREGG, D.A. GORDON & J.R. WETTERAU. 1993. Cloning and gene defects in microsomal triglyceride transfer protein associated with abetalipoproteinaemia. Nature **365:** 65–69.

11. NARCISI, T.M.E., C.C. SHOULDERS, S.A. CHESTER, J. READ, D.J. BRETT, G.B. HARRISON, T.T. GRANTHAM, M.F. FOX, S. POVEY, T.W.A. DE BRUIN, D.W. ERKELENS, D.P.R. MULLER, J.K. LLOYD & J. SCOTT. 1995. Mutation of the microsomal triglyceride-transfer-protein gene in abetalipoproteinemia. Am. J. Hum. Genet. **57:** 1298–1310.
12. GURBEL, P.A., V.L. SEREBRUANY, A.R. SHUSTOV, M. DALESANDRO, C.I. GUMBS, L.B. GRABLUTZ, R.D. BAHR, E.M. OHMAN & E.J. TOPOL. 1998. Increased baseline levels of platelet P-selectin, and platelet-endothelial cell adhesion molecule-1 in patients with acute myocardial infarction as predictors of unsuccessful thrombolysis. Coron. Artery Dis. **9:** 451–456.
13. BLANN, A.D., M. SEIGNEUR, M.R. BOISSEAU, D.A. TABERNER & C.N. MCCOLLUM. 1996. Soluble P-selectin in peripheral vascular disease: relationship to the location and extent of atherosclerotic disease and its risk factors. Blood Coagul. Fibrinolysis **7:** 789–793.
14. LIP, G.Y., A.D. BLANN, J. ZARIFIS, M. BEEVERS, P.L. LIP & D.G. BEEVERS. 1995. Soluble adhesion molecule P-selectin and endothelial dysfunction in essential hypertension: implications for atherogenesis? A preliminary report. J. Hypertens. **13:** 1674–1678.
15. ANGATA, K., J. NAKAYAMA, B. FREDETTE, K. CHONG, B. RANSCHT & M. FUKUDA. 1997. Human STX polysialyltransferase forms the embryonic form of the neural cell adhesion molecule: tissue-specific expression, neurite outgrowth, and chromosomal localization in comparison with another polysialyltransferase. J. Biol. Chem. **272:** 7182–7190.
16. KRUDE, H., H. BIEBERMANN, W. LUCK, R. HORN, G. BRABANT & A. GRUTERS. 1998. Severe early-onset obesity, adrenal insufficiency and red hair pigmentation caused by POMC mutations in humans. Nature Genet. **19:** 155–157.
17. HIXSON, J.E., L. ALMASY, S. COLE, S. BIRNBAUM, B.D. MITCHELL, M.C. MAHANEY, M.P. STERN, J.W. MACCLUER, J. BLANGERO & A.G. COMUZZIE. 1999. Normal variation in leptin levels is associated with polymorphisms in the proopiomelanocortin gene, *POMC*. J. Clin. Endocrinol. Metab. **84:** 3187–3191.

Genetic Analysis of Essential Hypertension in Japanese Populations

TOSHIO OGIHARA, TOMOHIRO KATSUYA,[a] AND JITSUO HIGAKI

Department of Geriatric Medicine, Osaka University Medical School, Suita, Osaka 565-0871, Japan

ABSTRACT: The reverse genetic approach, which examines genetic factors underlying the root of pathogenesis first, is a powerful tool to clarify the genetic cause of essential hypertension. Using the rat cross model, studies of the genetically hypertensive inbred rat model indicated several candidate loci on the rat chromosome responsible for blood pressure, but failed to identify the exact causal gene. Moreover, it was not certain that the rat data really reflect the human case. Thus, we shifted our focus to human genetics and carried out case control studies using the candidate gene approach. We mainly focused on gene components of the renin-angiotensin system as candidates, finding that angiotensinogen gene polymorphisms are genetic predisposing factors for hypertension. However, the results obtained from case-control studies using Japanese subjects were not consistent, suggesting that there was a problem in control sampling. In our recent study, we recruited more than 5,000 residents of an urban community as a general population and examined the association between genetic factors and their health status. Our results indicate that angiotensin-converting enzyme gene polymorphism is a male-specific genetic risk for essential hypertension. In light of our previous investigations, we present a discussion concerning the design of future studies of the genetics of hypertension.

Blood pressure has a continuous distribution and is influenced by multiple genes and multiple environmental factors.[1] Essential hypertension is defined as the upper end of the distribution and its pathogenesis has not been clarified yet. While excess salt intake, obesity, and stress are well known as environmental risk factors for hypertension, several genes have been considered as candidates for causative genes of essential hypertension, most of which are still controversial. To identify the genetic predisposing factor for essential hypertension, we have tried several kinds of reverse genetic approaches. In this paper, we review our previous investigations and propose the future directions for genetic research of hypertension.

[a]Address for correspondence: Tomohiro Katsuya, M.D., Ph.D., Department of Geriatric Medicine, Osaka University Medical School, 2-2 Yamada-oka, Suita, Osaka 565-0871, Japan. Voice: 81-6-6879-3852; fax: 81-6-6879-3859.
tkatsuya@yo.rim.or.jp

TABLE 1. Genetic approaches of hypertension

Animal models	Human samples
Genome screening	Genome screening
Rat cross model (hypertensive × normotensive) Congenic rat, Consomic rat	Linkage analysis Affected sib-pair analysis
Gene Function	Gene Function and Physical Mapping
Gene transfer technique (adenovirus, HVJ liposome)	Case control study, TDT (transmission disequilibrium test)
Gene targeting (knock out, transgenic)	

REVERSE GENETIC APPROACHES

Under classical strategy, scientists have tried first to find a physiological phenomenon specific for essential hypertension, then to identify the protein underlying the physiological abnormality, and finally to clarify the causative gene that encoded the protein. However, no one succeeded in getting to the third step. In contrast, using the reverse genetic approach, the correlation between hypertension and genetic abnormality is identified first and then the pathogenesis is clarified. Therefore, it is not extraordinary for unexpected results to be obtained in the correlation between a gene and a disease, suggesting that this approach might break through the chaos in hypertension research.

There are two major approaches to the genetic analysis of hypertension (TABLE 1): one that uses animal models and the other that uses humans.

RAT CROSS MODEL APPROACH

To use animal models, we must consider what kind of animal models to use. A knock-out mouse is a useful model to examine a gene function,[2] but the homeostasis of the knock-out mouse has been affected by disrupted gene since the fetal period, suggesting that it does not reflect the natural physiological state. In contrast, though the gene effect is mild in the rat cross model, it seems to be closer to the natural physiological state. Thus, we decided to use the rat cross model in our first investigation.

There are several advantages in using genetically hypertensive rats. First, every rat is genetically inbred. Second, if the rat has a hypertensive gene, the rat is sure to be affected with hypertension. Third, it is possible to carry out a cross experiment with rats but not with humans. Fourth, environmental conditions can be controlled. Lastly, the number of causative genes is relatively small. Accordingly, as the first approach to identify the hypertensive gene, we carried out a rat cross experiment.

Crosses were made between 3 male spontaneously hypertensive rats (SHR) (191.5 ± 1.9 mm Hg) and 3 female Wistar-Kyoto rats (WKY) (128.3 ± 0.8 mm Hg) in the Laboratory Animal Science and Toxicology Laboratories (Sankyo Co., Ltd., Shizuoka, Japan). We confirmed that these substrains were genetically inbred by fingerprint analysis.[3] The F1 hybrid was intercrossed for the study of F2 segregating generation. All

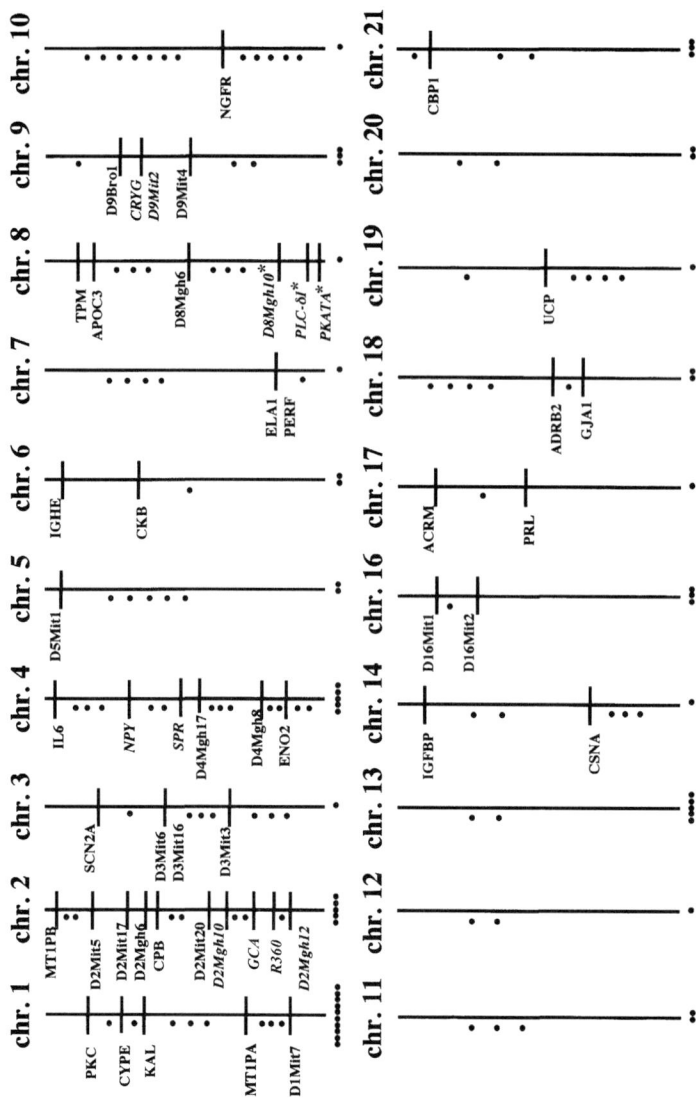

FIGURE 1. Rat linkage map using F2 rats derived from SHR and WKY. The dots indicate the loci of microsatellite markers and the horizontal line with locus name indicates the polymorphic site between SHR and WKY. At the name of loci shown in italic, the significant association between blood pressure and genotype was observed. An asterisk indicates that the locus showed the association with lower blood pressure.

rats were housed under normal conditions and were fed a normal salt diet, CE-2 (Japan Clea Co. Ltd.). A catheter was implanted into the abdominal aorta through a femoral artery under light ether anesthesia at 15 weeks of age. Systolic and diastolic blood pressure and heart rate were measured three times at 24-h intervals after catheterization, while the animals were at rest and in a freely mobile state. The measurements were carried out using a pressure transducer (TP-400T), monitors (AT-601G and AT-641G), and a recorder (RTA-1300), all from Nihon Koden Co. Ltd. During the measurements, animals were shielded from the observer. Blood pressure of F2 rats was close to normal distribution, because recombination occurred at random in meiosis. The genomic DNA samples were obtained from rat liver using phenol-chloroform extraction method. For the entire rat genome screening, we used 213 microsatellite markers. All genotype-phenotype (blood pressure) association was examined by analysis of variance (ANOVA) and significance was defined as $p < 0.05$.

According to the rat genome screening, we found several candidate loci responsible for high or low blood pressure (FIG. 1). The atrial natriuretic peptide receptor locus, GCA (guanylate cyclase A) on chromosome 2, neuropeptide Y locus[4] on chromosome 4, and gamma crystalin locus[5] on chromosome 9 were associated with high blood pressure. PKATA (peroxisomal ketoacyl-coA thiolase) locus[6] on chromosome 8 was associated with low blood pressure.

We succeeded in identifying several candidate loci for rat hypertension but failed to detect the exact causative gene. In reviewing rat genome screening approach, we noticed several problems. The first disadvantage is that there were few polymorphic sites between SHR and WKY. When SHR are crossbred with the distant relative Brown Norway strain, polymorphic sites are identified at ten times higher frequency and more than 30 candidate loci have been reported as positive (H. J. Jacob, personal communication). Another major problem is that there is a big difference in physiological state between rat and human, suggesting that rat results are not equal to human results.

CASE-CONTROL STUDY USING HUMAN SAMPLES

Given the reasons described above, the focus of our investigation moved on to humans. The case-control study using candidate gene approach is not suited for genome screening, but its statistical power is strong enough to examine the single-gene effect. Therefore, first of all, we focused our effort on the renin-angiotensin system because this system determines 15–20% of blood pressure variation.[7] Several gene polymorphisms in the renin-angiotensin system were already known and had just started to be examined as the candidate risk factor of cardiovascular disease. Recent progress of genetic studies in the renin-angiotensin system is summarized in TABLE 2.[8–18] The threonine allele of the angiotensinogen gene (AGT) at codon 235 is denoted as T235 and is considered to be associated with risk for hypertension and to increase plasma angiotensinogen concentration.[8] As the first candidate gene, we examined the genetic involvement of AGT in essential hypertension using a case-control study.

The subjects who had moderate-to-severe hypertension (>160/95 mm Hg or under antihypertensive medication) and a family history of hypertension were recruited from the outpatients of Osaka University Hospital for the present study. Subjects

TABLE 2. Association between gene polymorphism of renin-angiotensin system and cardiovascular disease

Gene	Polymorphism	Positive association	Reference
AGT	M235T	Hypertension	8
		Ischemic heart disease	9
		Plasma AGT concentration	8
ACE	Insertion/Deletion	Ischemic heart disease	10
		IgA nephropathy	11
		Diabetic nephropathy	12
		Hypertension*	13,14
		Plasma ACE concentration	15
AT1	C1166C	Hypertension	16
		Aortic stiffness	17
AT2	C3123A	?	18

Abbreviations: AGT, angiotensinogen; ACE, angiotensin-converting enzyme; AT1, angiotensin II type 1 receptor; and AT2, angiotensin II type 2 receptor.

with diabetes mellitus, stroke, ischemic heart disease, or family history of hypertension were excluded from controls. In the end, 180 cases and 195 control subjects were included in this study. Having identified two new polymorphisms, G-152A in promoter region and T+31C in intron 1, we examined whether eight biallelic polymorphisms, including G-1074T, G-152A, A-20C, C-18T, G-6A, T+31C, T174M and M235T, and one microsatellite marker, GT repeat in 3′ region, in AGT were associated with hypertension. Haplotype analysis revealed that G-6A, T+31C, and M235T polymorphisms were in the complete linkage disequilibrium, meaning that there is no recombination among them. This cluster of polymorphisms and the C-18T polymorphism were both associated with increased risk for hypertension. The calculated odds ratio is 1.6 in the subjects with T235 allele and 4.1 in those with C-18 allele. However, these polymorphisms were not associated with plasma angiotensinogen concentration. In contrast, G-1074T polymorphism was significantly associated with plasma angiotensinogen concentration but not with hypertension. These results suggest that the regulation of angiotensinogen gene expression should be discussed at the tissue level, but not at the systemic level.

At the same time, however, these investigations also revealed problems with case-control study. In case-control studies, it often happens that the results obtained at one institute could not be reconfirmed at another institute. We considered that this disagreement was due to differences in the background of controls (FIG. 2). In the case of hypertension, the criterion of hypertension is definite and clear and most of the cases were recruited from the medical institute. In contrast, controls are ascertained from various populations and its definition is based on exclusion criteria. Therefore, the results should be examined with the understanding that "controls" do not mean "healthy subjects." In order to avoid this problem, we decided to collect a large number of subjects from a general population.

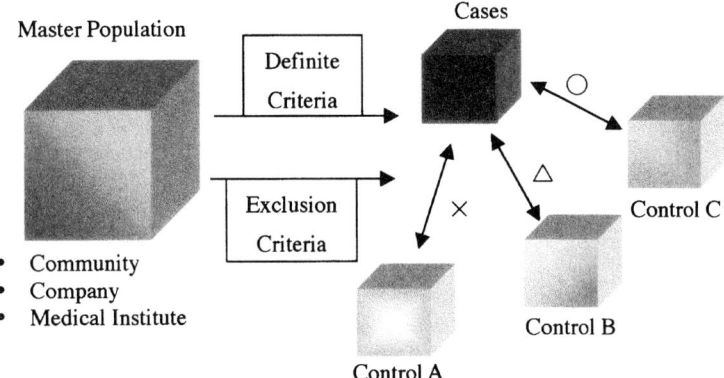

FIGURE 2. Problems in case-control study.

Genetic Epidemiological Survey using a General Population: The Suita Study

The Suita Study is a collaboration work with the National Cardiovascular Center.[19] Suita is a city located close to Osaka, the second biggest city in Japan. Participants between the ages of 30 and 79 were selected at random from the municipality population registry, stratified by sex and age groups of ten years. In addition to performing routine blood examinations, we extracted DNA from an extra 5 ml of blood withdrawn from those who visited the National Cardiovascular Center between May 1996 and February 1998. All participants were Japanese and only those who gave informed consent for genetic analysis were enrolled in the present study. Finally, we obtained 5,014 participants that were eligible for genetic analysis.

We examined the polymorphism of the angiotensinogen gene. To examine 5,000 samples, we applied a new method, TaqMan PCR.[20] TaqMan PCR is a unique method that combined TaqMan chemistry and allele-specific oligonucleotide hybridization. Since there is no suitable probe design to detect M235T in TaqMan PCR, T+31C polymorphism was examined instead. We simply divided a large general population of the Suita Study into two groups by criteria of hypertension, and compared the genotype frequency of T+31C polymorphism between them. We found that there was no significant association between angiotensinogen polymorphism and hypertension (unpublished data). However, the same polymorphism was significantly associated with the presence of a family history of hypertension. Similar results were obtained in the meta-analysis of Kunz and coworkers.[21] According to this meta-analysis, if cases were defined with family history of hypertension, positive association with T235 allele was frequently obtained. Consequently, our current conclusion is that angiotensinogen polymorphism indirectly increased risk for hypertension.

As the second candidate gene, we focused on ACE I/D polymorphism. Insertion-deletion polymorphism is famous as a genetic risk for ischemic heart disease. However, there is some evidence for an association between ACE gene and hypertension. In rat cross model, Jacob and colleagues[22] revealed that a quantitative trait locus

TABLE 3. Results of the associations between gene polymorphisms in renin-angiotensin system and cardiovascular risk[a]

	Hypertension	Stroke	IHD	LVH
AGT	+ (±[b])	±	+	−
ACE	− (+[c])	+	+	+
AT1	−	−	−	+
AT2	±	−	−	−

Abbreviations: +, the positive association with hypertension; −, negative results; ±, results that require further investigation and discussion. Symbols with parentheses indicate that the results were obtained from the study using a large general population.
[a]All results were based on our previous investigations.
[b]Polymorphism associated with family history of hypertension but not with hypertension.
[c]Positive association was obtained in male but not female.

(BP-SP1) responsible for high blood pressure is mapped nearby the ACE locus on rat chromosome 10.[22] Furthermore, recent reports in *Circulation*[13,14] showed a unique male-specific association between the ACE locus and hypertension. We examined the association and its sex specificity between ACE I/D polymorphism and hypertension using the Suita Study population. In total, 5,014 genotypes were determined. The basic genotype distribution of ACE gene in the Suita Study was compared with that in Copenhagen City Heart Study,[23] which was the biggest genetic epidemiological survey in a general Caucasian population. The frequency of DD genotype in Caucasians (26%) is twice that in Japanese (13%). The ACE I/D polymorphism was significantly associated with increase risk of hypertension in males but not in females. If a Japanese male had the DD genotype, his relative risk for hypertension is 1.75 times higher than a male with the II genotype, the effect of confounding factors being adjusted. The association with hypertension in males was compared between Suita and Framingham studies,[13] suggesting that DD was twice as frequent in Caucasians as in Japanese, while the male-specific hypertensive effect was quite similar in both studies. It seems important that a common gene variation plays the same role in different races.

FUTURE DIRECTIONS OF GENETIC STUDY OF ESSENTIAL HYPERTENSION

The results obtained from our previous investigations were summarized in TABLE 3. As was mentioned above, the population-based study made it possible to find a small but unique effect of ACE gene in hypertension, which was not detected by the case-control study. On the other hand, it did not show direct association between AGT polymorphism and hypertension as has been revealed by the case-control study. These results suggest that we have two directions to take in future genetic study. One way is to demonstrate the genome screening. The affected or discordant sib-pair method has been taken in the United States and European countries, and has recently revealed a candidate locus on chromosome 5.[24] Additionally, a large epidemiological survey with a cohort base would be very effective.

Another direction is to examine and to consider when, where, and on what the gene affects. In classical case-control study, sex and age should be matched between case and control, with the result that young healthy subjects were often recruited as controls in the study. However, the possibility that blood pressure of these young subjects will satisfy the criteria for hypertension in the future is not excluded. Thus, we would like to propose a different kind of case-control study: to consider early onset severe hypertensives with family history of hypertension as good model cases and to consider elderly subjects with normal blood pressure as good controls since they are normotensives without fail.

Since "genetics" is a theory based on statistics, the property of the object group and the method of the analysis decide whether the study will be a success or failure. The genetic heterogeneity in the Japanese population is considered to be relatively smaller than in Western populations. Even if the small genetic heterogeneity is a disadvantage for the survival from the natural selection, it should be an advantage for the positional cloning of the gene for polygenic disease. The genetic study using Japanese population must play an important role in the identification of genetic risk factors specific to Japanese but also in revealing common risks in humans regardless of race. We believe that the genetic information is useful not only for early diagnosis but also for patients' care and education.[25] The development of a particular therapy in accordance with the individual's genetic predisposition must be a future goal for medicine.

REFERENCES

1. PICKERING, G. 1978. Normotension and hypertension: the mysterious viability of the false. Am. J. Med. **65:** 561–563.
2. KIM, H.S. *et al.* 1995. Genetic control of blood pressure and the angiotensinogen locus. Proc. Natl. Acad. Sci. USA **92:** 2735–2739.
3. KATSUYA, T. *et al.* 1991. Substrain comparison of genetically hypertensive rats using DNA fingerprinting, and genetic analysis of blood pressure in the inbred rats. Tohoku J. Exp. Med. **165:** 253–260.
4. KATSUYA, T. *et al.* 1993. A neuropeptide Y locus on chromosome 4 cosegregates with blood pressure in the spontaneously hypertensive rat. Biochem. Biophys. Res. Commun. **192:** 261–267.
5. TAKAMI, S. *et al.* 1996. Analysis and comparison of new candidate loci for hypertension between genetic hypertensive rat strains. Hypertens. Res. **19:** 51–56.
6. KATSUYA, T. *et al.* 1992. Hypotensive effect associated with a phospholipase C-delta 1 gene mutation in the spontaneously hypertensive rat. Biochem. Biophys. Res. Commun. **187:** 1359–1366.
7. WALKER, W.G. *et al.* 1979. Relation between blood pressure and renin, renin substrate, angiotensin II, aldosterone and urinary sodium and potassium in 574 ambulatory subjects. Hypertension **1:** 287–291.
8. JEUNEMAITRE, X. *et al.* 1992. Molecular basis of human hypertension: role of angiotensinogen. Cell **71:** 169–180.
9. KATSUYA, T. *et al.* 1995. Association of angiotensinogen gene T235 variant with increased risk of coronary heart disease. Lancet **345:** 1600–1603.
10. CAMBIEN, F. *et al.* 1992. Deletion polymorphism in the gene for angiotensin-converting enzyme is a potent risk factor for myocardial infarction. Nature **359:** 641–644.
11. YOSHIDA, H. *et al.* 1995. Role of the deletion of polymorphism of the angiotensin converting enzyme gene in the progression and therapeutic responsiveness of IgA nephropathy. J. Clin. Invest. **96:** 2162–2169.

12. MARRE, M. et al. 1994. Relationships between angiotensin I converting enzyme gene polymorphism, plasma levels, and diabetic retinal and renal complications. Diabetes **43:** 384–388.
13. O'DONNELL, C.J. et al. 1998. Evidence for association and genetic linkage of the angiotensin-converting enzyme locus with hypertension and blood pressure in men but not women in the Framingham Heart Study. Circulation **97:** 1766–1772.
14. FORNAGE, M. et al. 1998. Variation in the region of the angiotensin-converting enzyme gene influences interindividual differences in blood pressure levels in young white males. Circulation **97:** 1773–1779.
15. CAMBIEN, F. 1994. The angiotensin-converting enzyme (ACE) genetic polymorphism: its relationship with plasma ACE level and myocardial infarction. Clin. Genet. **46:** 94–101.
16. BONNARDEAUX, A. et al. 1994. Angiotensin II type 1 receptor gene polymorphisms in human essential hypertension. Hypertension **24:** 63–69.
17. BENETOS, A. et al. 1995. Influence of angiotensin II type 1 receptor polymorphism on aortic stiffness in never-treated hypertensive patients. Hypertension **26:** 44–47.
18. KATSUYA, T. et al. 1997. Genomic organization and polymorphism of human angiotensin II type 2 receptor: No evidence for its gene mutation in two families of human premature ovarian failure syndrome. Mol. Cell. Endocrinol. **127:** 221–228.
19. MANNAMI, T., et al. 1997. Prevalence of asymptomatic carotid atherosclerotic lesions detected by high-resolution ultrasonography and its relation to cardiovascular risk factors in the general population of a Japanese city: the Suita study. Stroke **28:** 518–525.
20. KALININA, O. et al. 1997. Nanoliter scale PCR with TaqMan detection. Nucleic Acids Res. **25:** 1999–2004.
21. KUNZ, R. et al. 1997. Association between the angiotensinogen 235T-variant and essential hypertension in whites: a systematic review and methodological appraisal. Hypertension **30:** 1331–1337.
22. JACOB, H.J. et al. 1991. Genetic mapping of a gene causing hypertension in the stroke-prone spontaneously hypertensive rat. Cell **67:** 213–224.
23. AGERHOLM LARSEN, B. et al. 1997. ACE gene polymorphism: ischemic heart disease and longevity in 10,150 individuals. A case-referent and retrospective cohort study based on the Copenhagen City Heart Study. Circulation **95:** 2358–2367.
24. KRUSHKAL, J. et al. 1999. Genome-wide linkage analyses of systolic blood pressure using highly discordant siblings. Circulation **99:** 1407–1410.
25. HUNT, S.C. et al. 1998. Angiotensinogen genotype, sodium reduction, weight loss and prevention of hypertension—Trials of Hypertension Prevention, Phase II. Hypertension **32:** 393–401.

Questions and Answers

P. LIBBY (*Brigham and Women's Hospital, Boston, MA, USA*): Prospective surveys using large patient populations are very important in analyzing the effects of various polymorphisms and mutations because there has been a tendency to underestimate the incidence of polymorphisms in their control groups. For example, in Dr. Paul Ricker's analysis of the DD polymorphism in the more than 20,000 patients in the Physician's Health Study, he was unable to find, prospectively, the relationship between DD genotype and the expression of coronary heart disease. So I think you raised a very important point. When you compare the advantages and disadvantages in the human versus the rat, one of the problems with humans is that you cannot arrange the crosses, but you can take blood pressure in a human without anesthesia. When you were measuring central aortic blood pressure in rats, what kind of anesthesia did you use and does that affect the phenotype at all?

OGIHARA: For blood pressure measurement we used an indwelling catheter in unanesthetized rats.

Tailored Therapy to Fit Individual Profiles

Genetics and Coronary Artery Disease

J. WOUTER JUKEMA[a,b] AND JOHN J.P. KASTELEIN[c]

[b]*Department of Cardiology, C5-P, Leiden University Medical Center, Leiden, The Netherlands*

[c]*Department of Vascular Medicine, Academic Medical Center, Amsterdam, The Netherlands*

ABSTRACT: In the twentieth century, coronary artery disease (CAD) was the major cause of morbidity and mortality in western societies. Genetics and environmental influences clearly contribute to CAD. Our genetic makeup contributes to not only coronary risk factors, but also determines an individual's response to environmental challenges such as diet, drugs, and tobacco. Genetic testing is likely to be more predictive of our predisposition to CAD than current conventional testing of known risk factors. Therapy aimed at altering the regulation of genes or their transcribed proteins may prove appropriate in individual patients, depending on their genetic background. The understanding of our genetic predisposition to CAD may enable targeted environmental modification strategies aimed at individuals at greatest risk. Both in terms of the huge costs of drugs to society and in terms of needless medicalization, genotyping in order to tailor therapy might become a routine part of risk management earlier than we think.

INTRODUCTION

In the twentieth century, coronary artery disease (CAD) was the major cause of morbidity and mortality in western societies. Recent World Health Organization (WHO) statistics illustrate that this trend will continue well into the next millennium.[1]

Genetics and environmental influences clearly contribute to CAD. Our genetic makeup contributes to not only coronary risk factors, such as lipoprotein production and clearance, blood pressure dynamics, hemostatic variables, and glucose metabolism, but also determines an individual's response to environmental challenges, such as diet, drugs, and tobacco. For example, studies in humans demonstrate dietary hypo- and hyperresponders[2] and the presence of individuals at exaggerated risk of CAD from tobacco smoke due to underlying mutations in the nitric oxide synthase gene.[3] Genetic testing is likely to be more predictive of our predisposition to CAD than current conventional testing of known risk factors. Therapy aimed at altering

---

[a]Address for correspondence: J.W. Jukema, M.D., Ph.D., Department of Cardiology, C5-P, Leiden University Medical Center, P.O. Box 9600, 2300 RC Leiden, the Netherlands. Voice: 31-71-5262020; fax: 31-71-5266885.

j.w.jukema@lumc.nl

the regulation of genes or their transcribed proteins may prove to be more appropriate. The understanding of our genetic predisposition to CAD may enable targeted environmental modification strategies aimed at individuals at greatest risk.

The contribution of genetic factors to CAD is well illustrated by twin studies. In a study of monozygotic and dizygotic male and female twins, death from CAD at an early age of one's twin was a strong predictor of the risk of death for the other twin.[4] The fact that this risk was greatest in monozygotic compared to dizygotic twins indicates a strong contribution of genes to CAD. The genes that contribute to this common disease are undoubtedly many and they code for proteins involved in the multiple metabolic pathways associated with processes such as atherosclerosis, thrombosis, and restenosis. Such genes include those controlling lipoprotein metabolism, vascular tone and reactivity, macrophage structure and function, and hemostatic as well as fibrinolytic pathways, to name just a few.

However, the earlier the coronary event, the more likely it is that genetic influences will predominate. The most obvious example is seen in children who are homozygous for mutations on both alleles of the low density lipoprotein (LDL) receptor gene resulting in familial hypercholesterolemia (FH).[5] This receptor is crucial for removing cholesterol from the circulation. Such children manifest early in life with evidence of peripheral lipid deposition and many of these children will have coronary disease in their first or second decade of life. This defect in the LDL receptor gene results in massive elevations in LDL with cholesterol deposition in the coronary vasculature and very early CAD. These children have developed these problems solely because they have a mutation in a crucial gene involved in cholesterol metabolism. Environmental change cannot modify the outcome in this particular circumstance. In addition, these children illustrate an important principle, which is that the earlier the coronary event occurs the more likely that genetic factors make a predominant contribution to its causation.

THE CASE OF LIPOPROTEIN LIPASE

In most people, plasma triglycerides are in dynamic equilibrium, mediated by a balance between very low density lipoprotein (VLDL) and chylomicron (CM) synthesis, lipolysis of triglyceride (TG)–rich lipoproteins, and by uptake of remnant particles through appropriate receptors. However, with abnormalities involving synthesis, lipolysis, or remnant uptake, hypertriglyceridemia may ensue. Lipoprotein lipase (LPL) is a multi-functional protein.[6] After synthesis in parenchymal cells, primarily in adipose tissue and skeletal muscle, LPL is transported to the intimal surface of the vascular endothelium where it is anchored by the heparin sulfate side chains of membrane proteoglycans. LPL plays a pivotal role in the hydrolysis of lipoprotein triacylglycerols to monoacylglycerols and fatty acids. The enzyme has recently also been shown to have other important functions where it acts as a ligand for the LDL receptor related protein (LRP) and influences the secretion and uptake of LDL-cholesterol.

Chylomicronemia, in association with LPL deficiency, was the phenotype originally chosen to search for naturally occurring mutations in the LPL gene. Patients with this phenotype had severe clinical sequelae and often presented in infancy with abdominal pain, pancreatitis, hepatosplenomegaly, and failure to thrive. More recently, however, it has been clearly established that mutations of the LPL gene may, more frequently, be associated with partial LPL activity and a milder clinical phenotype. It is possible that these mutations might underlie mild-to-moderate hypertriglyceridemia, but that their phenotype will not be recognized until other environmental or genetic factors are present.

We have recently shown that a mutation in the human LPL gene, Asn291Ser, which results in a partial deficiency of lipolytic activity, is present with increased frequency in patients with certain lipid disorders and may also be associated with hypoalphalipoproteinemia in patients with coronary artery disease.[7] This Asn291Ser mutation is present in approximately 5% of individuals with angiographically proven premature CAD where it is associated with significantly decreased HDL cholesterol and increased TG levels. Even in the control population, significant reductions in HDL cholesterol and increases in TG levels were noted in persons with this mutation.[7]

In individuals with combined hyperlipidemia and CAD, another mutation, i.e., an aspartic acid to an asparagine residue at position 9 (Asp9Asn) in the mature LPL protein was also identified. This mutation, too, was accompanied by high-TG/low-HDL cholesterol phenotype.[8] In addition, we recently investigated whether the presence of this Asp9Asn mutation could confer increased susceptibility to atherosclerosis and therefore be associated with more progression of CAD. The mutation was identified in 4.8% of the patients who participated in the lipid-lowering angiographic clinical study REGRESS.[9,10] Carriers of this Asp9Asn mutation more frequently had a positive family history of CAD and exhibited lower HDL cholesterol levels than non-carriers. Indeed, it could be shown that these patients—with only subtle disturbances of lipoprotein metabolism due to the presence of this mutation—exhibited accelerated progression of coronary atherosclerosis and a diminished clinical event-free survival.[10] Also of specific interest was the observation that the carriers of this mutation seemed particularly sensitive to pravastatin therapy, in that on average progression was abolished in this group.

Recently, a third common mutation in the LPL gene was described. This mutation, a C-to-G substitution, results in a truncation of the C-terminal end of the LPL protein by two amino acids (Ser477Ter). This mutation was reported to be present at lower frequency in hypertriglyceridemic subjects. It was suggested that this mutation might, conversely, be protective against hypertriglyceridemia.

In confirmation, we recently found that in carefully selected and matched groups of healthy individuals with low (<0.87 mmol/l), normal (1.09–1.15 mmol/l), and high (>1.44 mmol/l) HDL cholesterol levels, the frequency of the Ser447Ter allele significantly increases when comparing individuals with the lowest to those with the highest HDL cholesterol levels.[11] Furthermore, within the REGRESS population, the Ser447Ter allele carriers exhibit significantly higher HDL-cholesterol levels than non-carriers.[12] When subdivided into quartiles, the presence of the Ser447Ter mutation increased significantly in those in the highest quartile of HDL cholesterol, pointing towards a positive association of this premature stop codon with elevated levels of HDL cholesterol and thus subsequently with protection against the development of CAD.[12] A recent meta-analysis of Wittrup and colleagues on the impact of lipoprotein lipase mutations on risk of CAD underscores the abovedescribed observations.[13]

GENETIC FACTORS ALSO INFLUENCE THE RESPONSE TO A PARTICULAR ENVIRONMENT

Response to a High Fat Diet

It is well documented that diet can play a significant role in the moderation or acceleration of atherosclerosis. This is probably mediated through an increase of total and LDL cholesterol. However, the response to a particular diet for a given individual is often variable and several genetic determinants have been identified in humans. These include alterations in intestinal absorption as well as variations in cholesterol biosynthesis and LDL receptor activity together with some variation in the degradation of cholesterol into bile acids in the liver.

An excellent example of resistance to an adverse environment concerned the report of an 88-year-old man who ate 25 eggs per day and had been doing this for approximately 15 years.[14] Despite this obvious environmental insult, his plasma lipid levels were normal, with a total cholesterol of 5.18, LDL of 3.68, and an HDL of 1.17 mmol/l. Interestingly, in this particular individual, the rate of absorption of cholesterol was markedly depressed.

Recently, genetic factors underlying cholesterol absorption from dietary fats were elucidated.[15] One candidate gene includes the human apolipoprotein A-IV gene, a 46 kD protein synthesized by the small intestine during fat absorption. Variation in this particular gene results in a common protein polymorphism at residue 360, changing a glutamine to a histidine. Patients who were heterozygous for this polymorphism were compared to patients who had only the wild-type allele in an out-patient dietary study. These groups were given initially a low-cholesterol diet and then consumed a total of four egg yolks per day. Interestingly, the increase in LDL cholesterol was significantly diminished in the group with the protein polymorphism. This suggested that the presence of histidine in place of glutamine in the ApoA-IV gene attenuated the hypercholesterolemic response to a high cholesterol diet. Clearly, many other genes will also effect dietary responsiveness, but this study indicated how genetic changes may moderate the response to environmental challenges.

Response to Smoking

Recently, it has also been suggested that genetic changes might modify the risk of coronary artery disease due to smoking. This might be mediated through endothelial-derived nitric oxide. Nitric oxide relaxes vascular smooth muscle and causes vasodilatation, which inhibits smooth muscle cell proliferation and platelet and monocyte adhesion—actions that prevent early atherogenesis.

In contrast, smoking is thought to induce endothelial cell dysfunction by diminishing nitric oxide–dependent vasodilation. Recently, polymorphisms in the gene for endothelial cell NOS (ecNOS) have been identified. Analysis of individuals with premature coronary artery disease has identified a significant association between the ecNOS polymorphism and CAD in persons who smoke.[3] Persons homozygous for this polymorphism were more likely to have one or more significantly diseased coronary vessels. These studies provide evidence for a gene-environment interaction between smoking and the ecNOS gene.

Response to Balloon Angioplasty

Identification of patients at high risk of restenosis after percutaneous transluminal coronary balloon angioplasty (PTCA) is important since these patients might particularly benefit from early treatment or a treatment modality other than PTCA, such as stenting or surgical revascularization. With regard to restenosis after PTCA, an association has been demonstrated between the insertion/deletion (I/D) polymorphism of the ACE gene and (in-stent) restenosis.[16,17] This concept is valid since tissue/smooth muscle cell proliferation is observed in recurrent lesions, ACE is an important factor in this process and plasma ACE levels are largely controlled by the I/D polymorphism in the ACE gene. Other candidate genes, associated with the process of restenosis, are to be found in genes that code for matrix metalloproteinases (MMPs), since these MMPs are involved in connective tissue turnover in the vessel wall and are active in wound healing processes, which are both features of the process of restenosis. For a polymorphic variant of the MMP-3 (stromelysin-1) gene we could recently establish such an association where clinical restenosis leading to repeat PTCA was the clinical phenotype.[18] The consequence of these findings might be that prior to PTCA the genotype of that patient could be determined, where results could guide therapy, for instance preferably no stent for patients with the ACE D/D genotype. It should be emphasized, however that we need trials to turn these basic concepts into evidence-based medicine before they can be accepted in clinical practice.

Response to Lipid-Lowering Drugs/Pharmacogenomics

Why do patients with a similar disorder respond differently to the same drug? Understanding this variation at the molecular level would be very valuable because it would allow therapy to be tailored to the individual's specific needs, as for example has been demonstrated for the variation in the LPL and the CETP gene.[10,19] A number of recent developments are responsible for renewed interest in pharmacogenomics. Firstly, systematic discovery of genetic variation can provide important opportunities for the development of new therapeutic and diagnostic products from genomic information. In addition, the emergence of high-throughput methods for analysis of genetic variation in human populations will greatly facilitate the elucidation of pharmacogenomic principles. Finally, the emergence of managed care and ever-tightening budgets in medicine provides an economic incentive for the use of pharmacogenomics by pharmaceutical companies, government, and healthcare providers. Furthermore, it is increasingly recognized that a DNA test to identify patients in which a given product will be safe and effective may provide such a product with a competitive advantage. Pharmacogenomics is not meant to unravel complex disease, such as CAD, but rather provide simple improvements in patient care. Pharmacogenomics is not similar to predictive testing, which provides risk estimates of a disease. Rather, pharmacogenomics concerns itself with genetic effects on drugs themselves and with the genetic variation affecting drugs in different human beings.

The Case of the CETP Gene

In another exemplary study from the REGRESS trial, we could recently demonstrate that variation at the cholesterylester-transfer protein (CETP) gene locus is associated with changes in CETP activity and changes in lipid and lipoprotein activity.[19] In the placebo arm of this lipid-lowering regression trial it became obvious that homozygosity for a certain genotype (B1B1) was associated with the highest CETP protein mass and activity and consequently with the lowest HDL cholesterol. In addition, this high activity CETP genotype led to a faster rate of progression of coronary atherosclerosis in this particular patient group. The notion that high CETP activity, particularly when genetically determined, confers a high risk for the development of atherosclerosis was very recently confirmed by the Framingham Offspring Study (FOS) research group.[20] In the FOS cohort, an affluent Caucasian population, B1B1 CETP genotype was again associated with low HDL cholesterol and a higher incidence of cardiovascular disease. These associations, both in a CAD and in the general population, suggest that variation at the CETP gene influences the risk for premature CAD, at least in Caucasians living in an affluent society.

Far more important, in the pravastatin arm of the REGRESS trial a different picture emerged. Patients carrying the B1B1 genotype reacted most favorably to statin therapy when compared to their counterparts with the B2B2 genotype. This pharmacogenomic observation led to the concept that lowering CETP activity that is already at low, i.e., in the case of a B2B2 genotype, is possibly unwanted and does not lead to regression of coronary atherosclerosis. This notion was strengthened by the observation that pravastatin influenced lipids and lipoproteins to a similar extent in all CETP genotypes and decreased CETP mass activity by approximately 20% in all REGRESS patients. If these data were confirmed in trials with clinical endpoints, CETP genotyping could become an important decision point in the prescription of statins. Variation in genes coding for microsomal triglyceride transfer protein (MTP), lecithin:cholesterol acyltransferase (LCAT), hepatic lipase (HL), and LPL is currently studied to enable extension of these pharmacogenomic observations in those patients eligible for statin therapy.

CONCLUSIONS

Frequent variants in genes coding for critical enzymes in lipid and lipoprotein metabolism such as LPL, HL, and CETP can be used to further define an individual's risk for premature CAD or for progression of already present coronary atherosclerosis. However, we are still very far from a "gene passport" that can reliably predict an individual's risk to develop CAD later in life. The genetic contribution to atherosclerosis is extremely complex and involves undoubtedly a myriad of genes influencing cholesterol and lipoprotein metabolism.

It is not likely that all the described associations reflect causal relations. This illustrates the complexity of polygenic, multifactorial diseases. In a strong editorial in *The New England Journal of Medicine*, Rosenthal and Schwartz have described some criteria to be met in establishing medically useful links between genetic variations and disease.[19] First, the change in the gene must cause a relevant alteration in the function or level of the gene product (which is always a protein), however this cannot always be achieved. Second, the beneficial and harmful phenotypes must have apparent clinical differences. Third, the hypothesis linking the genotype to disease must be convincing. Fourth, the number of cases linking a genotype to disease must be sufficient. Finding the specific genetic and environmental components that are of relevance in a gene-environment interaction causing disease is not an easy task, but we are clearly making progress. Hopefully, new technology such as microarrays and gene chips will help to unravel the complex expression patterns underlying the responses to environmental injury that determine the atherosclerotic process. More importantly and less complicated is the differential response to lipid-lowering therapy, which is increasingly unraveled at the molecular level. Here we do not need the insight into complex molecular pathways leading to atherosclerosis, but simple and incremental steps in understanding better ways to tailor therapy.

Both in terms of costs of lipid-lowering drugs, a major burden on the pharmacological budget of most western countries, and in terms of needless medicalization, genotyping in order to tailor preventive therapy might become a routine part of risk management earlier than we think.

REFERENCES

1. MURRAY, C.J. & A.D. LOPEZ. 1997. Alternative projections of mortality and disability by cause 1990–2020: Global Burden of Disease Study. Lancet **349:** 1498–1504.
2. KATAN, M.B., A.C. BEYNEN, J.H.M. DE VRIES & A. NOBELS. 1986. Existence of hypo- and hyperresponders to dietary cholesterol in man. Am. J. Epidemiol. **123:** 221–234.
3. WANG, X.L., A.S. SIM, R.F. BADENHOP, R.M. MCCREDIE & D.E.L. WILCKEN. 1996. A smoking-dependent risk of coronary artery disease associated with a polymorphism of the endothelial nitric oxide synthase gene. Nat. Med. **2:** 41–45.
4. HELLER, D.A., U. DE FAIRE, N.L. PEDERSEN, G. DAHLÉN & G.E. MCCLEAR. 1993. Genetic and environmental influences on serum lipid levels in twins. N. Engl. J. Med. **328:** 1150–1156.
5. HOBBS, H.H., M.S. BROWN & J.L. GOLDSTEIN. 1992 Molecular genetics of the LDL receptor gene in familial hypercholesterolemia. Hum. Mol. Genet. **1:** 445–466.
6. BRUNZELL, J.D. 1995. In The Molecular Basis of Inherited Disease. J.B. Stanbury & J.B. Wyngaardner, Eds. McGraw-Hill. New York.
7. REYMER, P.W.A., E. GAGNE, B.E. GROENEMEYER et al. 1995. A lipoprotein lipase mutation (Asn291Ser) is associated with reduced HDL cholesterol levels in premature atherosclerosis. Nat. Genet. **10:** 28–34.
8. MAILLY, F., Y. TUGRUL, P.W.A. REYMER et al. 1995 A common variant in the gene for lipoprotein lipase (Asp9Asn): functional implications and prevalence in normal and hyperlipidemic subjects. Arterioscler. Thromb. Vasc. Biol. **15:** 468–478.
9. JUKEMA, J.W., A.V.G. BRUSCHKE, A.J. VAN BOVEN et al. 1995. Effects of lipid lowering by pravastatin on progression and regression of coronary artery disease in symptomatic men with normal to moderately elevated serum cholesterol levels. The "regression growth evaluation statin study" (REGRESS). Circulation **91:** 2528–2540.
10. JUKEMA, J.W., A.J. VAN BOVEN, B. GROENEMEYER et al. 1996. The Asp9 Asn mutation in the lipoprotein lipase gene is associated with increased progression of coronary atherosclerosis. Circulation **94:** 1913–1918.
11. KUIVENHOVEN, J.A., B.E. GROENEMEIJER, J.M.A. BOER et al. 1997. Ser447-Stop mutation in lipoprotein lipase is associated with elevated HDL cholesterol levels in normolipidemic males. Arterioscler. Thromb. Vasc. Biol. **17:** 595–599.
12. GROENEMEIJER, B.E., M.D. HALLMAN, P.W. REYMER et al. 1997. Genetic variant showing a positive interaction with beta-blocking agents with a beneficial influence on lipoprotein lipase activity, HDL cholesterol, and triglyceride levels in coronary artery disease patients. The Ser447-stop substitution in the lipoprotein lipase gene. REGRESS Study Group. Circulation **95:** 2628–2635.
13. WITTRUP, H.H., A. TYBJRG-HANSEN & B.G. NORDESTGAARD. 1999. Lipoprotein lipase mutations, plasma lipids and lipoproteins, and risk of ischemic heart disease. A meta-analysis. Circulation **99:** 2901–2907.
14. KEARN, JR., F. 1991. Normal plasma cholesterol in an 88-year-old man who eats 25 eggs a day. N. Engl. J. Med. **324:** 896–899.

15. McCombs R.J., D.E. Marcadis, J. Ellis & R.B. Weinberg. 1994. Attenuated hypercholesterolemic response to a high-cholesterol diet in subjects heterozygous for the apolipoprotein A-VI-2 allele, N. Engl. J. Med. **331:** 706–710.
16. Amant, C., C. Bauters, J.C. Bodart et al. 1997. D allele of the angiotensin I-converting enzyme is a major risk factor for restenosis after coronary stenting. Circulation **96:** 56–60.
17. Ribichini, F., G. Steffenino, A. Dellavalle et al. 1998. Plasma activity and insertion/deletion polymorphism of angiotensin I-converting enzyme. A major risk factor and a marker of risk for coronary stent restenosis. Circulation **97:** 147–154.
18. de Maat, M.P., J.W. Jukema, S. Ye et al. 1999. Effect of the human stromelysin-1 gene promoter on pravastatin treatment and in coronary atherosclerosis and restenosis. Am. J. Cardiol. **83:** 852–856.
19. Kuivenhoven, J.A., J.W. Jukema, A.H. Zwinderman et al. 1998. The role of a common variant of the cholesteryl ester transfer protein gene in the progression of coronary atherosclerosis. N. Engl. J. Med. **338:** 86–93.
20. Ordovas, G. 1999. Oral presentation. 8th International Congress on Cardiovascular Pharmacotherapy. March 1999. Amsterdam.
21. Rosenthal, N. & R.S. Schwartz. 1998. In search of perverse polymorphisms. N. Engl. J. Med. **338:** 122–124.

Questions and Answers

A. Henney (*Zeneca Pharmaceuticals, Cheshire, UK*): If you have genotypes which are showing differences between treatment and/or interactions with treatment in the progressional disease, as a clinician would you then use these data to decide not to put a patient on a statin to reduce cholesterol levels on a basis that it's going to have no impact at all on disease progression?

Jukema: Of course, one study is no study. We have to clarify in other independent material, which is now being done. At the moment, the answer is "no," but I think in two years from now the answer will be "yes." Then, when we see a patient, instead of checking a blood test form for just cholesterol or those kinds of things, we will also check a few boxes for genetic studies. When the patient returns, you will have not only a report of a cholesterol level of 300 mg/dl but also information regarding sensitivity to certain kinds of therapy. For instance, when you have myocardial infarction, you can be treated with aspirin, beta-blocker, ACE inhibitor, and statin—I think that patients can't cope with all that. We must find which treatment is good for the individual patient, not which is good for a large group in a big study.

Henney: I think, this opens a huge ethical question especially in relation to lipid reduction. I tend to agree with you, but I think the tendency is to put the patient on a statin, because that's successful in reducing LDL cholesterol, even if it is not affecting disease progression.

Jukema: But, your LDL cholesterol possibly is not bothering you. There are a lot of patients with elevated cholesterols and they live to be 80 years old.

P. Libby (*Brigham and Women's Hospital, Boston, MA, USA*): The way the angiogram looks is not important: but it is events that count. Could you elaborate on what is in progress? There are at least two large studies with the same treatment regimen that you studied in the REGRESS Study. They did not use angiographic endpoints, but clinical events were scored very closely in both the Lipid Populations (a study done in Australia and New Zealand) and the CARE Study (coordinated from Boston). The DNA collected in these studies could be analyzed for some of the same polymorphisms for some of the same issues that you have examined in REGRESS to prospectively evaluate the relationship to the events. Is that underway?

JUKEMA: Yes. We are currently setting up cooperation with the CARE investigators to check the hypothesis I just stated. Of course, it is events that are clinically relevant. However, one of the first slides I showed indicates that indeed angiographic progression predicts first events.

J.E. HIXSON (*Southwest Foundation for Biomedical Research, San Antonio, TX, USA*): I have a related question. When you do these studies looking at candidate polymorphisms in population case control and get an association, it is very different from saying individual A has a certain genotype which exactly predicts his phenotype. This is true in all sorts of studies, for example the apo-E4 association with Alzheimer's disease is very strong, but nobody knows quite what to do with it because in a given individual it may not be predictive. What will your criteria be for clinical application given that genotype may only have a mild predictive value?

JUKEMA: This is a highly relevant question. I think, in the end "the proof of the pudding is in the eating." After having described these associations we need to conduct prospective studies to prove that a specific association might be causative. For instance, patients with the DD genotype should be stratified and randomized to having a stent or no stent. Then, in the end, we will know if it is really useful to determine your ACE polymorphism. As far as we now know, nobody in the world is really using ACE polymorphism for the purpose of giving a patient a stent or not. But I think we should do this as a prospective study.

P. GANZ (*Brigham and Women's Hospital, Boston, MA, USA*): My question may be a bit naive, but I want to ask you about the importance of the genetic component in restenosis. Do you have patients where you treat multiple stenoses with multivessel angioplasty? I would think the genetic component was the critical one because all the lesions within the same patient would tend to restenose. On the other hand, if a genetic component was not a factor, if it is all technical factors, then there would be some independence between restenosis in different sites being treated in the same patient. What, in fact, is the experience with restenosis? I thought, based on other studies, that there is some sort of independence in restenosis at different sites treated in the same patient and that one could not predict restenosis based on one region of restenosis—implying that perhaps technical factors may be of critical importance.

JUKEMA: I completely agree with you that genetics will not solve the problem entirely because genetics for sure are not the only factor. What we know thus far is that if you have a restenosis you can simply try to redilate, then you have more or less the same chance of restenosis as in the initial site: 30% or slightly higher, but not much higher. If you get two restenoses then you have a very high chance of getting a third restenosis. There is a genetic component, but how strong it is nobody knows. And, for sure, it will not explain everything.

A. CLOWES (*University of Washington, Seattle, WA, USA*): It is very well known now that the restenosis after coronary angioplasty is the sum of some adverse remodeling plus some injury response in the form of intimal hyperplasia. In the study that you did with Dr. Henney, did you actually look at that in more detail? Was the benefit obtained by the 5A/5A genotype a change in the remodeling or a change in intimal hyperplasia? Did you have the opportunity to do some studies to find this out?

JUKEMA: This was a two-year angiographic follow-up that was not specifically designed to look at restenosis, and certainly we have no material because all the patients who got a reangiogram are alive.

M.A. GIMBRONE (*Brigham and Women's Hospital, Boston, MA, USA*): I find this discussion fascinating. As neither a geneticist nor clinician, I would like to offer the following thoughts. It seems to me, one of the key issues is how precisely we can define phenotype and associate that with genotype in a given individual. The two previous questions have pointed to a very important fact. Atherosclerosis is a very heterogeneous disease and the restenosis that occurs after angioplasty also is a heterogeneous response with multiple pathophysiology components. When the Framingham Heart Study first started, the surrogate marker for coronary artery disease was someone clutching their chest in pain, i.e., the symptom of the heart attack. Many years later, the PDAY Study looked right at the vessel wall and began to correlate risk factors that were surrogates (e.g., plasma cholesterol) with vascular pathology at autopsy. I would submit, as we get better at interrogating multiple lesions in a given individual during life, the question will become whether the person is at risk because a single lesion is becoming a critical lesion, or whether a person is at risk for having multiple lesions that are potentially critical lesions. Stratification will again become one of precision of phenotype. I don't think we are quite at that point. We are still looking at surrogate markers in plasma, but I think we will soon be able to interrogate lesions one by one by one (e.g., by non-invasive imaging) and the correlation with an individual's genetic profile may then become more evident.

JUKEMA: I certainly hope that your prediction will come true.

HENNEY: I'd like to just pick up on what Dr. Gimbrone just said. If you go back to the triad that you showed, which was very impressive, both genetics and intermediate phenotypes in blood plasma are being actively studied, but their relationship to the vessel wall requires more work. As far as imaging is concerned, those candidate genes involved in matrix modeling in the vessel wall can only be evaluated once we have very accurate imaging of the composition and remodeling of the different forms of atherosclerotic lesions, not just looking at luminopathy.

JUKEMA: I cannot agree more with you. That is why there will be a presentation at this conference on MRI of atherosclerotic lesions. In our institution we are also working on Raman spectroscopy, that is, we are sending laser light into the vessel wall (which you can do *in vivo*) and then regaining the spectra and analyzing what precisely is in the plaque. Maybe that is going to predict plaque stability.

LIBBY: If you were designing the REGRESS Study, which was designed over a decade ago, it would now very likely contain an arm with intravascular ultrasound. In fact, there are now studies ongoing where we will use the intravascular ultrasound —including the newer high frequency methods, which can delineate some characteristics of the plaque. I think we are exactly right in concluding that we will be getting better phenotyping, which will then permit more precise correlation with genotypes at our next Saratoga Conference.

Genetic Diversity in the Matrix Metalloproteinase Family

Effects on Function and Disease Progression[a]

ADRIANO M. HENNEY,[b,c] SHU YE,[d] BAIPING ZHANG,[d] SOPHIA JORMSJÖ,[b] CARL WHATLING,[d] PER ERIKSSON,[b] AND ANDERS HAMSTEN[b]

[b]*King Gustav Vth Research Institute, Karolinska Institute, Stockholm, Sweden*

[d]*Department of Cardiovascular Medicine, University of Oxford, Oxford OX3 7BN, United Kingdom*

ABSTRACT: Atherosclerosis is an example of a complex trait, where the course of the disease is influenced by a combination of common variation in a constellation of genes and the effect of a wide range of environmental variables. Thus, the underlying disease mechanisms will be modulated by genetic diversity and the effect this diversity has on an individual's response to environmental challenges such as smoking, diet, and exercise. Unlike the consequences of mutations in severe single-gene disorders on protein function, the impact of individual common, functionally important sequence changes in genes contributing to multifactorial diseases is likely to be very small. The challenge is to dissect the contribution that each of these genes makes to the disease process. We have tackled this by identifying common genetic variants, studying their effects on function, and applying them to the analysis of association in appropriately structured and suitably powered studies. Even with our incomplete understanding of the disease, the list of potential candidate genes we could study is vast; but, we do know from pathological studies that a wide spectrum of structural architecture exists in atherosclerotic plaques, suggesting that remodeling of vascular connective tissue is fundamentally important. Matrix remodeling is controlled by a complex network of cell and matrix interactions, the net outcome of which is the product of a balance between synthetic and degradative processes. Our work has focused on the family of enzymes and inhibitors most directly associated with matrix turnover—the matrix metalloproteinases (MMPs) and their natural inhibitors (TIMPs, tissue inhibitors of MPs). We specifically searched for functionally relevant genetic variants that might modulate the delicate control of matrix turnover. Using these molecular genetic strategies to investigate the impact of natural genetic variation on vascular matrix remodeling has begun to shed new light on the importance of these genes in atherogenesis.

---

[a]All of the work of the Oxford Group was funded by very generous project and programme grants, as well as a personal Senior Research Fellowship to A.M.H., and an Intermediate Research Fellowship to S.Y. awarded by the British Heart Foundation.

[c]Address for correspondence: Adriano M. Henney, CV-GI Research Department AstraZeneca Alderley Park, Macclesfield, Cheshire SK10 4TG, UK. Voice: 44-0-1625-518138; fax: 44-0-1625-516667.

adriano.henney@astrazeneca.com

It is quite clear from studies on the growth and anatomy of atherosclerotic lesions that vascular matrix modeling is an integral part of the natural history of atherosclerosis. These studies also show that there is a wide spectrum of structural architecture amongst lesions, suggesting that modulation of the control of the matrix turnover process may contribute significantly to the connective tissue content of the plaque as well as the extent of the remodeling process.[1] It follows therefore, that small changes in the local pericellular environment may have a significant impact on individual lesion characteristics, including vulnerability to rupture. The relative abundance of smooth muscle cells and macrophages in lesion caps, in particular, is likely to affect connective tissue content and structure significantly. On the one hand, the smooth muscle cells, responsible for the major proportion of matrix synthesis in the vessel wall, are relatively abundant in thick fibrous caps; on the other, the lipid-laden macrophage, an arsenal of diverse proteolytic activity, is a key feature of the thin vulnerable caps seen in inflammatory lesions many of which are angiographically occult (FIG. 1).

Within the protease armory of the macrophage is a specialized group of enzymes whose principal role is to mediate the connective tissue remodeling process: the matrix metalloproteinases (MMPs).[2,3] Our long-standing interest in the role of MMPs in atherogenesis was stimulated initially by the work of Richardson, Davies, and Born, studying the biophysics of vulnerable lesions[4] and the importance of macrophages to this process.[5] This lead to studies where we described for the first time the expression of an MMP in advanced atherosclerotic lesions.[6] This has been confirmed by many elegant studies from Libby's group in particular, demonstrating the presence of MMPs and their natural inhibitors (the TIMPs) in advanced atherosclerotic lesions by immunohistochemistry, *in situ* hybridization, and *in situ* zymography.[7–9] However, these studies offer only evidence of "guilt by association" and do not provide any evidence of the direct impact that MMPs may have on the natural history of the disease itself. For this reason, we adopted molecular genetic strategies

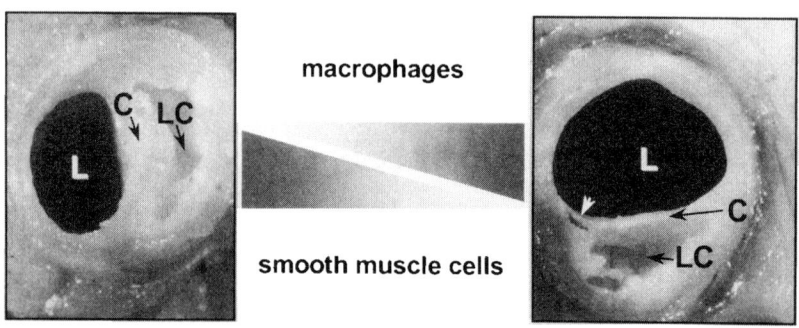

FIGURE 1. Plaque cap architecture is influenced by the relative abundance locally of macrophages and smooth muscle cells: vulnerable lesions tend to be characterized by an overabundance of macrophages over smooth muscle cells in caps (C) covering relatively large lipid cores (LC), but which do not necessarily encroach substantially into the lumen (L). Stable lesions, on the other hand, are characterized by thick caps, abundant smooth muscle cells covering relatively small cores. In contrast, these lesions often give rise to high-grade stenoses readily visible by angiography.

to identify associations between genetic polymorphisms in specific members of the MMP and TIMP families and a range of phenotypes representative of atherosclerotic lesion progression and rupture.[10] This approach involved the isolation of short segments of the genes of interest and the analysis for natural sequence variation in a panel of 40 to 60 randomly collected blood samples from unrelated individuals. Between 200 and 400 base-pair segments of the coding region, promoter, and 3′ untranslated region of these genes were systematically amplified by PCR and screened for sequence variation using the single-strand conformation polymorphism (SSCP) analytical technique.[11] Putative sequence variants identified by polyacrylamide gel electrophoresis were confirmed and characterized by sequencing and an estimate of the population frequency obtained. These markers were then used in case-control studies to assess the potential association with specific phenotypes. As the strategy specifically selected regions of the genes where genetic variation could reasonably be expected to affect expression or function, we undertook to investigate the potential allelic impact on function at the same time.

The working hypothesis for these studies was that events that interfere with the control of MMP or TIMP expression and activity would affect vascular matrix remodeling. The local effects of this in the vessel wall would be to modulate the rate of lesion progression and possibly destabilize plaque caps, resulting in their rupture.

TABLE 1 summarizes the classification of the MMPs and shows their distribution within the human genome. We extended our original work describing the expression of MMP-3 in advanced atherosclerotic lesions to adopt the molecular genetics strategies described above. The reasons for focusing our attentions on MMP-3 to begin with were predominantly because, at that time, (1) this enzyme apparently had the broadest substrate specificity within the MMP family and (2) it was also known to play a role in super-activating other members of the family from their latent state. This pointed to a potentially central role for this enzyme in vascular remodeling processes.

Information on the gene organization was limited, but data had been published on the MMP-3 promoter.[12] Focusing our attentions on this region, we identified a single base insertion-deletion polymorphism (5A/6A) at a position 1,612 bases 5′ of the start of transcription, estimated to have a population frequency of 0.49.[13] We observed that nuclear proteins bound to this stretch of the promoter and that one of these protein bands appeared to bind differentially depending on the allelic sequence.[14] *In vitro* transient transfection studies showed an approximately twofold difference in expression driven by the two alleles, with the 5A allele being the more active. Analysis of genetic association in two clinical trials (STARS and REGRESS) showed that this variant was not associated with myocardial infarction, but was associated with lesion progression as assessed by quantitative coronary angiography.[13,15] In the REGRESS trial we could also show a significant increased risk for development of angiographically visible new lesions in those homozygous for the 6A allele compared with other genotypes: relative risk 2.3 (1.14–4.68). More importantly, we also demonstrated a significant interaction between genotype and pravastatin medication on clinical event-free survival ($p = 0.002$).[15]

Thus, the allele which *in vitro* studies showed was associated with lower levels of transcription was associated with more rapid growth of angiographically visible lesions. We proposed the model outlined in FIGURE 2 to explain the difference in growth rates in those homozygous for the 6A allele: the synthesis and degradation of vascular matrix is necessary for the growth of all plaques, with the net effect re-

TABLE 1. The family of matrix metalloproteinases[a]

Subgroup	Name (alternative)	Number	Chromosomal location	Known substrates
Collagenases	Interstitial collagenase (Fibroblast-type collagenase)	MMP-1	11q22.3	Collagen I, II, III, VII, VIII, X, gelatin, aggrecan, versican, PLP, casein, α_1PI, α_2M, ovostatin, nidogen, myelin base protein, pro-TNFα, L-selectin, MMP-2, MMP-9
	Neutrophil collagenase (PMN-type collagenase)	MMP-8	11q21	Collagen I, II, III, V, VII, VIII, X, gelatin, aggrecan, α_1PI, α_2AP, fibronectin
	Collagenase-3	MMP-13	11q22.3	Collagen I, II, III, IV, gelatin, aggrecan, perlecan, tenascin, PAI-2
Gelatinases	Gelatinase A (72kD Type IV collagenase)	MMP-2	16q21	Gelatin, collagen I, IV, V, VII, X, XI, XIV, elastin, fibronectin, aggrecan, versican, PLP, myelin base protein, pro-TNFα, α_1PI, MMP-9, MMP-13, β amyloid
	Gelatinase B (92kD Type IV collagenase)	MMP-9	20q11.2–13.1	Gelatin, collagen IV, V, VII, X, XIV, elastin, aggrecan, versican, PLP, fibronectin, nidogen, α_1PI, myelin base protein, pro-TNFα
Stromelysins	Stromelysin-1	MMP-3	11q22.3	Collagen III, IV, IX and X, PLP, fibronectin, laminin, elastin, gelatin, aggrecan, perlecan, versican, casein, ovostatin, pro-TNFα, α_1PI, α_2M, myelin base protein, MMP-1, MMP-7, MMP-8, MMP-9, MMP-13
	Stromelysin-2	MMP-10	11q22.3	Collagen III, IV, V, gelatin, aggrecan, elastin, casein, fibronectin, PLP, MMP-1, MMP-8
	Stromelysin-3	MMP-11	22q11.2	α_1PI
		MMP-19	12q14	
Membrane type	MT-MMP-1	MMP-14	14q11–q12	Collagen I, II, III, gelatin, elastin, casein, fibronectin, aggrecan, vitronectin, MMP-2, MMP-13, pro-TNFα, laminin B chain, dermatan sulfate proteoglycan
	MT-MMP-2	MMP-15	16q13–q21	MMP-2, gelatin, tenascin, laminin, fibronectin, nidogen
	MT-MMP-3	MMP-16	8q21–q22.1	MMP-2
	MT-MMP-4	MMP-17	12q24.33	

— continued

TABLE 1. The family of matrix metalloproteinases[a]

Subgroup	Name (alternative)	Number	Chromosomal location	Known substrates
Not classified	Matrilysin (PUMP-1)	MMP-7	11q21–q22	Collagen IV, X, gelatin, elastin, aggrecan, PLP, fibronectin, laminin, casein, transferrin, pro-TNFα, α_1PI, MMP-1, MMP-2, MMP-9, myelin base protein, entactin
	Macrophage Metalloelastase	MMP-12	11q22.2–22.3	Collagen IV, gelatin, elastin, α_1PI, fibronectin, vitronectin, laminin, pro-TNFα, myelin base protein

Abbreviations: PLP, proteoglycan link protein; α_2M, $\alpha_2$macroglobulin; α_1PI, $\alpha_1$proteinase inhibitor.

flecting the balance that is struck between these two processes. However, in those homozygous for the 6A allele, the under-production of enzyme due to the lower promoter activity has the effect of allowing greater deposition of matrix compared with other genotypes. Whilst the differences in promoter strength may not be large in absolute terms, the impact locally in the plaque may be sufficient to contribute to more rapid expansion of the lesion. This relatively small effect associated with a single gene is consistent with the model of many genes of small effect contributing to a complex multifactorial process.

Looking at the promoter sequence surrounding the polymorphic site, there was no obvious consensus for any recognized transcription factor. Experiments were initiated

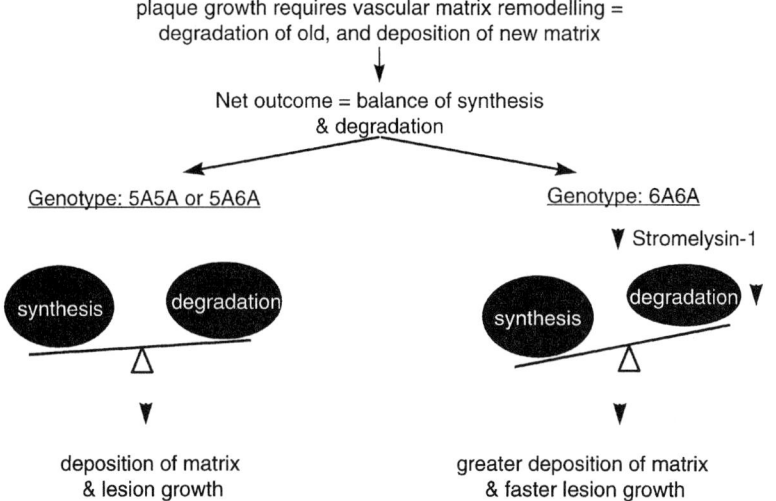

FIGURE 2. Contribution of the effect on gene regulation of the MMP-3 5A/6A promoter polymorphism to the dynamics of local vascular matrix remodeling.

to clone and identify the nuclear protein or proteins that were binding in this region of the human MMP-3 promoter. Using a yeast 1-hybrid approach, we isolated a cDNA encoding a nuclear protein, identified on sequencing as ZPB-89 (a member of the Krüppel-type zinc finger protein family).[16] Co-transfection of this cDNA with constructs containing the MMP-3 promoter alleles demonstrated that the recombinant nuclear factor significantly increased the MMP-3 promoter activity. Unfortunately, no allelic differences in binding could be shown with ZBP-89, suggesting that we probably had succeeded in cloning the protein that was responsible for the binding common to both alleles identified on our original electro-mobility shift assays.[14] New experiments are now underway to see if this protein can be used as a bait to isolate other members of the protein binding complex for this region of the MMP-3 promoter.

We decided that applying these molecular genetic techniques to other members of the MMP gene family was likely to give us novel insights into structure-and-function relationships that might not be so easily identified using conventional cell biological and biochemical approaches. For this reason we began to extend our studies to include other MMPs relevant to cardiovascular processes, beginning with MMP-9 and following on with MMP-12.

With MMP-9, we were fortunate in that substantially more information was available on the organization of the gene and its promoter than when we first started our experiments with MMP-3.[17] We had published previously on this gene, in the context of studies on abdominal aortic aneurysms, reporting a (CA)n repeat polymorphism in the promoter which we used to map the gene to human chromosome 20q12.2–13.1.[18] At that time we did not extend our studies to the remainder of the gene, preferring instead to concentrate on the early work with MMP-3. Building on these interesting data, we elected to extend our studies to the analysis of the MMP-9 promoter and also to undertake a systematic search, exon by exon, of the entire gene. As with our previous studies, the emphasis was on the identification of common, potentially functional genetic diversity. We have identified a number of variants in the MMP-9 gene, from the promoter through a variety of exons and also the 3′ untranslated region, with rare allele frequencies ranging from 0.01 to 0.35 (FIG. 3). Given that our expertise so far had been on the analysis of promoter function, we focused once again on the promoter variants to begin with, but analysis of the coding region polymorphisms is now well underway.

We have recently reported that the C-1562/T variant in the human MMP-9 gene binds nuclear proteins in an allele-specific manner.[19] As with our work with MMP-3, we were able to show that this was a specific DNA-protein interaction, to identify the specific binding sequence, and to demonstrate differences in transcription *in vitro* driven by allelic constructs of the human MMP-9 promoter. The rare allele, containing the T as opposed to the C base at position −1562, was estimated to have a population frequency of 0.14. Transient transfection assays in a range of cell types, including macrophage cell lines, showed that constructs containing the T-allele drove approximately twofold greater levels of transcription than those containing the C-allele. We have also been able to show a trend towards correlation between circulating levels of MMP-9, measured by ELISA, and individual genotypes, such that those homozygous for the C-allele had lower plasma levels of MMP-9 compared to those homozygous for the T-allele (TABLE 2). Whilst these data were consistent with the patterns of transcription observed *in vitro*, the small numbers were insufficient to achieve statistical significance.

TABLE 2. MMP-9 C-1562/T promoter polymorphism and plasma MMP-9 level

C-1562/T genotype	Levels ng/ml (± SD)
CC	6.18 (0.8)
CT	5.91 (0.8)
TT	8.22 (1.1)

Association studies conducted (1) in a large case controlled population of myocardial infarction and (2) in a placebo-controlled study of the effect of pravastatin on lesion regression showed that, unlike the MMP-3 promoter variant, this polymorphism was not associated with quantitative differences in the rates of angiographically measurable lesion growth. However, there was a significant association with the severity of disease in that 28% of those carrying the T-allele had stenoses of greater than 50% in three coronary arteries, compared with only 16% of C-allele carriers. It was also noticed that there was a significant interaction between age and genotype in determining the coronary artery stenosis score.

What do these data tell us about the role of MMP-9 in the vascular remodeling process? In these studies, we clearly showed that the T-allele, which is responsible for relatively higher expression of promoter constructs *in vitro* and appears to be associated with higher circulating levels of MMP-9 *in vivo*, is also associated with more severe disease. This is in direct contrast with the data for MMP-3, where the lower-expressing allele was associated with faster disease progression, but not lesion score, and where we proposed a "pro-fibrotic" model associated with chronic lesion growth[14] (FIG. 2). There are data to suggest that MMP-9 is associated with grossly

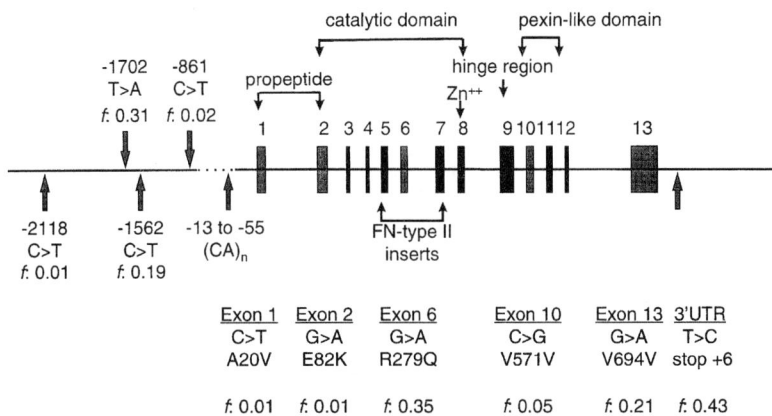

FIGURE 3. Schematic representation of the human MMP-9 gene. The location of promoter polymorphisms is indicated by base position 5' of the start of transcription, together with the nature of the base change and its estimated population frequency (f). Location of coding region variants is shown by exon and amino acid number, together with the base change and any consequent amino acid change. FN = fibronectin; Zn^{++} = location of Zinc-binding domain.

inflammatory lesions and unstable angina.[20] Our own unpublished observations as well as data presented by Davies[1] have shown that MMP-9 expression is consistently observed in macrophage-derived foam cells, which are a major constituent of advanced, inflammatory lesions and are known to accumulate at sites of plaque rupture.[1,21] We began our studies hoping to identify mechanisms that may contribute to excess local matrix degradation and a predisposition to plaque rupture. However, in none of the clinical cohorts we have used for our association studies has there been the possibility to assess plaque instability unequivocally; on the contrary, those lesions visible by angiography tended to be the stable, fibrotic type. It is known that the growth of atherosclerotic lesions occurs not only through episodes of primary expansion through smooth muscle cell proliferation, connective tissue deposition and lipid accumulation, eventually culminating in chronic obstruction, but also that "silent" plaque rupture may be a contributory factor. As outlined in FIGURE 4, the rupture of an angiographically occult lesion that does not result in the formation of an occlusive coronary thrombus leads to the formation of a contained, superficial clot, which eventually becomes organized as part of the repair process and leads to an episode of plaque growth and expansion. Such episodes of silent rupture are apparently relatively common: autopsy studies have shown that 70% of high-grade stenoses (>50% of the lumenal diameter by angiography) have had an episode of healed plaque disruption,[22] highlighting the importance of recurrent disruption and repair to the chronic progression of advanced stenoses.

Given that the MMP-9 C-1562/T variant was not associated with lesion growth, one possible explanation for the data is that a proportion of the lesions detected angiographically arose from sporadic episodes of repair following silent plaque rupture, rather than through chronic expansion through deposition of connective tissue, as was the proposed mechanism for the 6A allele in MMP-3. This hypothesis clearly would need to be verified, ideally in a case-controlled study of unstable angina,

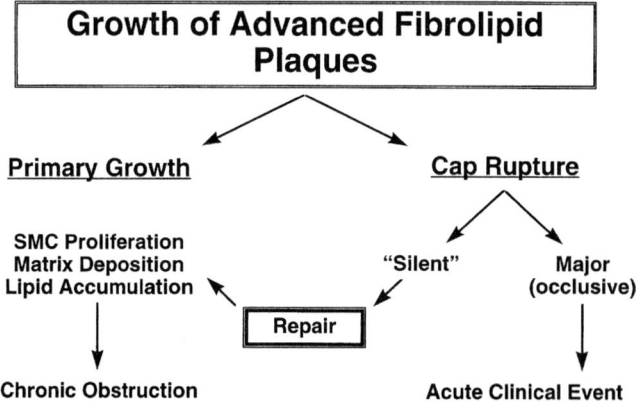

FIGURE 4. The contribution of asymptomatic plaque rupture to the growth of atherosclerotic lesions.

where the expectation would be that the T-allele would be enriched in unstable angina patients compared with those suffering from chronic stable disease.

Interestingly, a recent study has reported an association between the MMP-3 5A allele and myocardial infarction.[23] Our *in vitro* transfection studies showed that this allele drove higher levels of transcription than the 6A allele.[14] On first reading this study would seem to contradict our data showing no association with myocardial infarction; but an over-representation of the 5A allele in cases of plaque rupture, resulting in myocardial infarction, is consistent with our model as this higher-expressing allele could contribute to excess local matrix degradation. Our own unpublished observations in a large case-control study of myocardial infarction support these data and suggest that this might be the case, indicating the need for further investigation. Thus the general concept of MMP over-expression as a mechanism contributing to the burden of matrix degradation in vulnerable lesions remains plausible.

Finally, our most recent studies have focused on macrophage metalloelastase, also known as MMP-12. Recent work by Carmeliet and colleagues[24] has shown that this particular enzyme appears to be important in the formation of aortic aneurysms in mouse models of atherosclerosis. The enzyme is known primarily to degrade elastin, but it also degrades substrates, such as type IV collagen and fibronectin, and it is known to be expressed widely by macrophages in atherosclerotic lesions.

Once again, the same strategy has been adopted for MMP-12 as was used for MMP-9. This has resulted in the identification of a promoter variant, arising from a single nucleotide substitution and having an estimated population frequency of 0.16. Interestingly, this polymorphism is located very close to the consensus sequence for one of the *cis*-elements in the MMP-12 promoter critical to the gene-regulation apparatus. The presence of a relatively frequent variable base so close to such an element may have a significant impact on the binding of nuclear proteins and the subsequent transcription of the gene. Experimental evidence demonstrates that nuclear proteins do bind in this region and that there appears to be a difference in binding affinity between the two alleles. *In vitro* transcription assays in macrophage cell lines also demonstrate allele-specific differences. Further work on the characterization of this polymorphism, as well as the completion of the screening for variants in the coding region and 3' untranslated region of the gene continue. In addition, as with our previous studies, a range of case-control and other studies will be genotyped to investigate the potential impact on disease of this relatively common polymorphism apparently affecting promoter function.

ACKNOWLEDGMENTS

All of the work that has been presented in this talk is the result of close collaborations with a number of individuals, some of whom are listed as co-authors at the beginning of this paper. Others who are deserving of a special word of thanks are François Cambien and his group, with whom we have collaborated over a number of years on the ECTIM study, Wouter Joukema and Moniek deMaat, who were responsible for undertaking the analyses in the REGRESS trial, and especially to Michael Davies, whose interest in the pathophysiology of plaque rupture was the original stimulus prompting our investigations with MMPs in atherosclerosis.

REFERENCES

1. DAVIES, M.J. 1996. Stability and Instability: two faces of coronary atherosclerosis. The Paul Dudley White Lecture. 1995. Circulation **94:** 2013–2020.
2. BIRKEDAL-HANSEN, H. *et al.* 1993. Matrix Metalloproteinases: a review. Crit. Rev. Oral Biol. Med. **4:** 197–250.
3. DOLLERY, C.M., J. MCEWAN & A.M. HENNEY. 1995. Matrix metalloproteinases and cardiovascular disease. Circ. Res. **77**(5): 863–868.
4. RICHARDSON, P.D., M.J. DAVIES & G.V.R. BORN. 1989. Influence of plaque configuration and stress distribution on fissuring of coronary atherosclerotic plaques. Lancet **2:** 941–944.
5. LENDON, C.L. *et al.* 1991. Atherosclerotic plaque caps are locally weakened when macrophage density is increased. Atherosclerosis **87:** 87–90.
6. HENNEY, A.M. *et al.* 1991. Stromelysin gene expression in atherosclerotic plaques detected by *in situ* hybridization. Proc. Natl. Acad. Sci. USA **88:** 8154–8158.
7. GALIS, Z.S. *et al.* 1994. Increased expression of matrix metalloproteinases and matrix degrading activity in vulnerable lesions of human atherosclerotic plaques. J. Clin. Invest. **94:** 2493–2503.
8. GALIS, Z.S. *et al.* 1995. Macrophage foam cells from experimental atheroma constitutively produce matrix degrading proteinases. Proc. Natl. Acad. Sci. USA **92:** 402–406.
9. GALIS, Z.S. *et al.* 1995. Microscopic localization of active proteases by *in situ* zymography: detection of matrix metalloproteinase activity in vascular tissue. Methodol. Commun. **9:** 974–980.
10. HUMPHRIES, S.E., H. MONTGOMERY, S. YE & A.M. HENNEY. 1997. Genetic tests for coronary artery disease risk: the fibrinogen and stromelysin genes as examples. *In* Genetics of Common Diseases: Future Therapeutic and Diagnostic Possibilities I.N.M. Day & S.E. Humphries, Eds.: 151–170. Bios Scientific Publishers. Oxford.
11. YE, S. & A.M. HENNEY. 1999. Detection of mutations and DNA polymorphisms in genes involved in cardiovascular disease by polymerase chain reaction and single strand conformation polymorphism analysis. *In* Molecular Biology of Vascular Disease. A.H. Baker, Ed. Humana Press Inc. Totowa, NJ.
12. QUINONES, S. *et al.*1989. Transcriptional regulation of human stromelysin. J. Biol. Chem. **264:** 8339–8344.
13. YE, S.*et al.* 1995. Variation in the human stromelysin gene promoter is associated with progression of atherosclerosis. Brit. Heart J. **73:** 209–215.
14. YE, S. *et al.* 1996. Progression of coronary atherosclerosis is associated with a common genetic variant of the human stromelysin-1 promoter which results in reduced gene expression J. Biol. Chem. **271**(22): 13055–13060.
15. DE MAAT, M.P.M. *et al.* 1999. Risk of progression of coronary atherosclerosis is influenced by a common functional variant in the human stromelysin-1 gene promoter. Am. J. Cardiol. **83:** 852–856.
16. YE, S., C. WHATLING & A.M. HENNEY. 1999. Human stromelysin gene promoter activity is modulated by transcription factor ZBP-89. FEBS Lett. **450:** 268–272.
17. HUHTALA, P. *et al.* 1991. Complete structure of the human gene for 92-kDa type IV collagenase: divergent regulation of expression for the 92- and 72 kilodalton enzyme genes in HT-1080 cells. J. Biol. Chem. **266:** 16485–16490.
18. ST. JEAN, P.L. *et al.* 1995. Characterization of a dinucleotide repeat in the 92kDa type IV collagenase gene (CLG4B), localization of CLG4B to chromosome 20 and the role of CLG4B in aortic aneurysmal disease. Ann. Hum. Genet. **59:** 17–24.
19. ZHANG, B.P. *et al.* 1999. Functional polymorphism in the regulatory region of the gelatinase B gene in relation to severity of coronary atherosclerosis. Circulation **99:** 1788–1794.
20. BROWN, D. *et al.* 1995. Identification of 92kD gelatinase in human coronary atherosclerotic lesions: association of active enzyme synthesis with unstable angina. Circulation **91:** 2125–2131.
21. VAN DER WAL, A.C. *et al.* 1994. Site of intimal rupture or erosion of thrombosed coronary atherosclerotic plaques is characterised by an inflammatory process irrespective of the dominant plaque morphology. Circulation **89:** 36–44.

22. DAVIES, M.J. *et al.* 1989. Factors influencing the presence or absence of acute coronary artery thrombi in sudden ischemic death. Eur. Heart J. **10:** 203–208.
23. TERASHIMA, M. *et al.* 1999. Stromelysin promoter 5A/6A polymorphism is associated with acute myocardial infarction. Circulation **99:** 2717–2719.
24. CARMELIET, P. *et al.* 1997. Urokinase-generated plasmin activates matrix metalloproteinases during aneurysm formation. Nature Genetics **17:** 439–444.

Questions and Answers

UNIDENTIFIED: This is a very exciting study. This is the second time we hear about fluvastatin causing something bad if you have a 6A/6A genotype coming from the REGRESS Study. Have you any hypothesis to explain this? Is it simply due to cholesterol lowering, change in lipoprotein profile, or has it something to do with fluvastatin?

HENNEY: It is a very important question and an intriguing one. One of the prevalent issues with statins is to what extent other components of biology, in addition to cholesterol-lowering, are affected by HMG CoA-reductase inhibition. A lot of work is being done along these lines. The answer is we don't really know. One hypothesis is that some aspects of interference with the prenylation of proteins that function as nuclear transcription factors may be involved here.

J.W. JUKEMA (*Leiden University Medical Center, Leiden, the Netherlands*): Pravastatin is associated with stabilization of MMP3, which is not bad. In the placebo group you saw that a 5A/6A genotype was doing worse than a 5A/5A genotype. That difference was totally abolished when the patients were on pravastatin. So, in this case pravastatin was not doing something bad for you. It was abolishing the bad features of 6A in the pravastatin group.

P. LIBBY (*Brigham and Women's Hospital, Boston, MA, USA*): Before we leave this particular subject, let me interject an editorial comment. Regarding the pleiotropic effects of the statins, pravastatin is the one drug on the market, which I would expect to have the least pleiotropic effect because its permeability into non-hepatocytes is the least. Looking beyond the lipid lowering for an effect, pravastatin is quite a stretch at the doses that are used. It gets into liver by a bile acid transporter by stealth. It is really is so hydrophilic it does not get into peripheral cells. I don't want anybody to leave this room thinking that pravastatin does bad things, because the weight of the clinical evidence of 15,000 patients enrolled in randomized clinical trials with this drug shows an overwhelming benefit for the population groups studied.

HENNEY: I think that is a very important point. It goes back to the question that I asked earlier about the messages we are delivering at the genotypic level looking at progression compared with the major issues related to statin therapy.

A.R. TALL (*Columbia University, New York, NY, USA*): Is the stromelysin promoter variant with higher activity associated with progression of disease?

HENNEY: Yes.

TALL: That is counterintuitive to the idea that the metalloprotease should promote plaque rupture. Dr. Gene Damiento at Columbia has gotten somewhat surprising results with MMP-1 in transgenics he crossed into Apo-E knock-outs with actually less robust lesions. Some of the thinking we had as to the possible mechanism relates to the importance of collagen as a matrix element promoting LDL retention in lesions also possibly involved in the matrix that would allow macrophages to come in. Is that mechanistically plausible?

HENNEY: It makes a lot of sense. Another major component of the vessel wall, in terms of LDL retention in the matrix, is proteoglycan. Proteoglycan is something that also is degraded by MMP-3. It is a complex business, but what you suggest is entirely feasible.

The Extracellular Matrix Dynamically Regulates Smooth Muscle Cell Responsiveness to PDGF[a]

ELAINE W. RAINES,[b,c] HIDENORI KOYAMA,[b,d] AND NEIL O. CARRAGHER[b]

[b]*Department of Pathology, University of Washington, Seattle, Washington 98195, USA*

ABSTRACT: Focal accumulation of smooth muscle (SMC) within the arterial intima contributes to the formation of lesions of atherosclerosis. Platelet-derived growth factor (PDGF) is a potent stimulant of SMC migration and proliferation in culture that may play a role in the accumulation of SMC in atherogenesis. SMCs normally reside in the media of the artery wall surrounded by extracellular matrix (ECM), including type I collagen. In atherogenesis, the ECM is degraded, new ECM components, such as fibronectin, are synthesized and assembled, and these alterations in ECM components are associated with changes in SMC phenotype. To model the changes in ECM in normal and diseased arteries, we have analyzed SMCs cultured on different forms of type I collagen. Our studies demonstrate that integrin-mediated signals from various forms of type I collagen lead to specific and rapid modulation of the integrin signaling complex, including cytoskeletal connections, and of the responsiveness of SMC to PDGF stimulation.

INTRODUCTION

Occlusive lesions of atherosclerosis that result in myocardial infarction, stroke, and peripheral vascular disease are the consequence of focal accumulation within the innermost layer (intima) of the artery of monocytes and T-lymphocytes from the circulation and smooth muscle cells from the underlying media.[1,2] The intima becomes thickened due to this cell accumulation, connective tissue matrix formation by the smooth muscle cells, and an increase in intracellular and extracellular lipid. Defining the cellular and molecular mechanisms associated with development of lesions of atherosclerosis will help identify potential targets for interventional strategies.

The migration of SMCs from the media into the intima and SMC proliferation appear to be mediated by growth factors, such as the platelet-derived growth factor (PDGF), released by inflammatory cells.[3,4] However, the ECM surrounding SMCs can determine whether a SMC remains quiescent or whether it migrates and proliferates in

---

[a]This work was supported in part by National Institutes of Health grant HL18645 to E.W.R., and H.K. was a recipient of a visiting research scholarship awarded by the Department of Science and Technology of Japan.

[c]Address for correspondence: Elaine W. Raines, Department of Pathology, University of Washington School of Medicine, Box 357470, Seattle, WA 98195-7470. Voice: 206-685-7441; fax: 206-685-3018.
 ewraines@u.washington.edu
[d]Current address: Second Department of Internal Medicine, Osaka City University, Medical School, Asahi-machi, Abeno-ku, Osaka 545-8585, Japan.

response to growth factors.[5] This paper reviews our knowledge of the ECM in normal media and in developing lesions of atherosclerosis, as well as the molecular mechanisms involved in matrix regulation of SMC responsiveness to growth factors.

Extracellular Matrix Is Altered in Developing Lesions of Atherosclerosis and Is Associated with Phenotypic Changes in Smooth Muscle Cells

SMCs within the medial layer of normal arteries are described as "contractile" as they are arranged in concentric layers and are filled with myofilaments but contain a relatively poorly developed Golgi apparatus and rough endoplasmic reticulum.[6,7] Analysis of phenotypic markers of the medial SMCs demonstrates high levels of expression of smooth muscle myosin heavy chain isoforms SM1 and SM2 (TABLE 1). In contrast, SMCs found in intimal lesions of atherosclerosis (termed "synthetic") have decreased expression of many of these phenotypic markers (TABLE 1), contain an abundance of rough endoplasmic reticulum and Golgi bodies, but have few and sometimes no evident myofilaments.[6,7] Analysis of developing lesions of atherosclerosis in animal models and evaluation of the vascular response to acute injury (such as balloon-catheter injury) show reduced expression of SMC myosin heavy chain isoforms and upregulation of "synthetic" phenotype markers such as embryonic myosin (Smemb), embryonic myosin light chain kinase (MLCK-210 kD), and low molecular weight caldesmon (TABLE 1).

The ECM surrounding SMCs in the normal media and in developing lesions of atherosclerosis are also distinct. Normal medial SMCs are surrounded by a dense ECM network of interstitial collagen fibers, types I, III, IV, V and VI, and laminin (TABLE 1). The pathogenesis of atherosclerosis and restenosis includes the abnormal production of ECM proteins by "synthetic" SMCs combined with modification of newly synthesized and preexisting ECM (TABLE 1). Infiltrating macrophages and activated SMCs express increased levels of matrix metalloproteinases, which can significantly contribute to ECM breakdown during atherogenesis (TABLE 1). In addition, newly deposited fibronectin becomes assembled into a fibrillar network associated with the surface of "synthetic" SMC during the early stages of development of atherosclerotic and restenotic lesions.[26,27] Interestingly, laminin, a constituent of normal media, has been shown to inhibit the shift of cultured SMCs from the "contractile" phenotype, while fibronectin promotes the shift to the "synthetic" phenotype.[54] Five other matrix-associated glycoproteins—osteopontin, SPARC, thrombospondin, tenascin-C, and vitronectin—are present in lesions of atherosclerosis but not in surrounding normal medial SMCs (TABLE 1). SPARC, thrombospondin, and tenascin-C have been shown to exert common "anti-adhesive" functions involved in cell migration and proliferation[55] and osteopontin and vitronectin promote SMC adhesion and migration.[56,57] Thus, the ECM environment of the SMC in the developing lesion is quite distinct from that in the normal media, and this is associated with a change in the SMC phenotypic markers (TABLE 1).

Extracellular Matrix Surrounding Normal Medial SMCs May Be Non-Permissive for SMC Migration and Proliferation

The proliferative index of SMCs within the normal media is low (TABLE 1), but in developing lesions of atherosclerosis foci of SMC proliferation are often observed

TABLE 1. Comparison of SMC and ECM characteristics in normal media and in developing lesions of atherosclerosis

Characteristic	Normal media	Reference	Atherosclerotic lesion	Reference
Phenotype markers				
α-actin	high	8,9	low	8,9
h-caldesmon	high	10	low	10
l-caldesmon	low	11	high	12[a]
desmin	high	13,14	low	13,14
SM1-myosin	high	10	low	10
SM2-myosin	high	10	low	10
Smemb-myosin	low	15	high	15
MLCK-210 kD	low	16,17	high	18[a]
MLCK-160 kD	high	16,17	low	18[a]
SM22-α	high	19	low	19
tropomyosin	high	13	low	13
vimentin	low	13	high	13, 20[a]
meta-vinculin	high	9	low	9,21
Extracellular matrix				
	collagens type I, III, and V	22	collagens type I, III, and V	22
	collagen type IV	23	collagen type IV	23
	collagen type VI	24	collagen type VI	24
	laminin	23	collagen type VIII	25
			fibronectin fibrils	26–28
			osteopontin	29,30
			SPARC	31
			tenacin-C	32
			thrombospondin	33
			vitronectin	34–36
Matrix metalloproteinases				
	collagenase (MMP-1)	37	collagenase (MMP-1)	37,38
	tissue inhibitor of MMPs (TIMP-1, -2)	37	gelatinases (MMP-2)	37
			gelatinases (MMP-9)	37,39
			stromelysin (MMP-3)	37
			MMP-12	40
			MMP-13	41
			stromelysin-3	42
			MT1-MMP	43
			tissue inhibitor of MMPs (TIMP-1, -2, -3)	44,45
Other proteases and inhibitors				
			PAI-1	46–48
			tPA	49–52
			uPA	49–51
Proliferation				
	<0.05%	53	0.5%–1.0%	53

[a]In lesions induced by balloon or cuff injury of vessel.

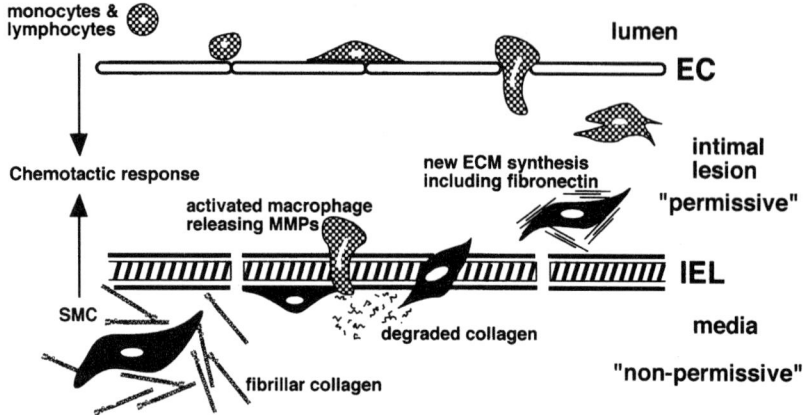

FIGURE 1. SMC migration and proliferation in developing lesions of atherosclerosis may require matrix alterations. Lesions of atherosclerosis result from the accumulation of leukocytes (*hatched*) from the circulation and SMC (*solid*) from the underlying media in response to growth factors and chemoattractants released during the inflammatory response. We hypothesize that (1) fibrillar collagen within the normal media may be "non-permissive" for SMC proliferation and migration in response to locally released growth factors and chemoattractants and (2) that degradation of the matrix by MMPs from activated macrophages and SMCs may be required to release SMC from "non-permissive" states. New ECM synthesis and assembly within the intima, for example fibronectin assembly, may further contribute to SMC migration and proliferation.

in the forming neointimas and the innermost part of the underlying media.[53] The capacity of polymerized collagen to inhibit cell proliferation has been appreciated for some time[58–60] and is consistent with the low proliferative index of SMCs in the media of the normal artery wall.[53] Interestingly, although cell proliferative activity and type-I collagen gene expression can occur simultaneously in the same cell in developing lesions, this is a rare event, and the vast majority of collagen-producing cells do not show proliferative activity.[61] It has also been observed that SMCs in aortic rings of normal vessels cultured in a physiologic bath will not proliferate in response to PDGF. However, if the same aortic rings are briefly treated with a combination of collagenase and elastase and then placed in the same bath, the SMCs in the aortic ring proliferate in response to exogenously added PDGF (F. Schaub, E.N. Olsen, and D.F. Bowen-Pope, unpublished observations). These observations have led us to hypothesize that the ECM of the normal media may be non-permissive to SMC proliferation, and that degradation of the ECM may be required to induce SMC migration and proliferation in developing lesions of atherosclerosis (FIG. 1).

SMC Cultured on Fibrillar Collagen Appear To Mimic Many of the Characteristics of Normal Medial SMC

When normal medial SMC are placed in culture, they lose their contractility and myofilaments within a few days and develop an extensive rough endoplasmic reticulum and a large Golgi complex,[62] similar to the features of SMC in developing le-

TABLE 2. Comparison of phenotypic markers and proliferative index of SMC cultured on monomer and fibrillar collagen with those of medial SMC[a]

Phenotype marker	Normal media	In culture on collagen type I	
		Monomer	Fibrillar
α-actin	+++++	++++	++++
h-caldesmon	+++	–	–
l-caldesmon	++	+++	+
Smemb-myosin	–	++++	++
SM1-myosin	++++	+	+
SM2-myosin	++++	–	–
MLCK-210 kD	+	+++	+
MLCK-160 kD	+++	++	++
tropomyosin	+++	++	+
meta-vinculin	+++	++	+
vinculin	++++	++++	++++
vimentin	++++	++++	++++
proliferative index	–	++++	+

[a]Very high, +++++; high, ++++; intermediate, +++; moderate, ++; low, +; none detected, –. Expression levels are based on a comparison of expression levels by Western blot analysis of extracts of normal non-human primate media and normal human smooth muscle cells cultured on monomer or fibrillar collagen as previously described by Koyama and colleagues.[5] Proliferative index is based on immunostaining of tissue sections with antibodies to the proliferating cell nuclear antigen[84] and evaluation of DNA synthesis, cell cycle analysis, and increase in cell numbers.[5]

sions.[7] This is accompanied by changes in SMC phenotypic markers, including a loss or total absence of expression of SMC myosin heavy chain isoforms SM1 and SM2 and upregulation of "synthetic" phenotype markers such as Smemb, MLCK-210 kD, and low molecular weight caldesmon (TABLE 2). However, modulation into this "synthetic" phenotype can be inhibited by growing the SMCs on a confluent layer of endothelial cells[63] and by growing them on particular ECM.[54]

To begin to model the differences that exist in the normal and diseased vessels (TABLE 1), we compared the culture of human SMCs on monomer and fibrillar type I collagen.[5] As shown in TABLE 2, many of the phenotypic markers of SMCs grown on fibrillar collagen more closely mimic those of medial SMCs. Interestingly, a recent report suggests that culture of SMCs on rigid gels of type IV collagen may reproduce even more closely the phenotype of medial SMCs.[64] In contrast, SMCs cultured on monomer collagen retain many of the characteristics of SMCs in developing lesions of atherosclerosis (TABLE 1). We have also shown that SMCs plated on fibrillar collagen are arrested in G1, while SMCs on monomer collagen proliferate in response to PDGF.[5] We have used this model system to examine the molecular mechanisms involved in the G1 arrest of SMC on fibrillar collagen that may reflect the regulation of SMC in the normal media.

A Cell cycle progression modulated by matrix

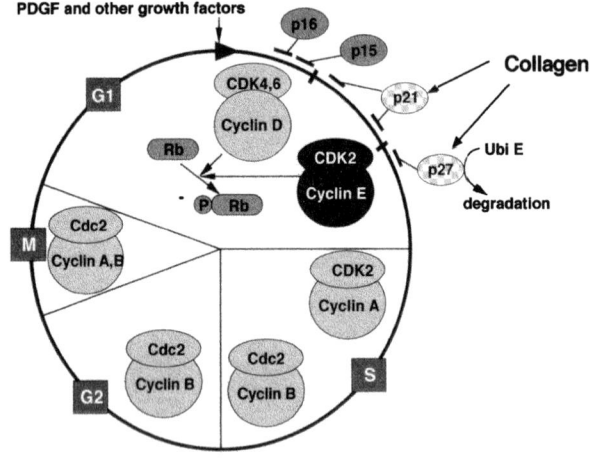

B Collagen regulates cyclin E-cdk2 complexes

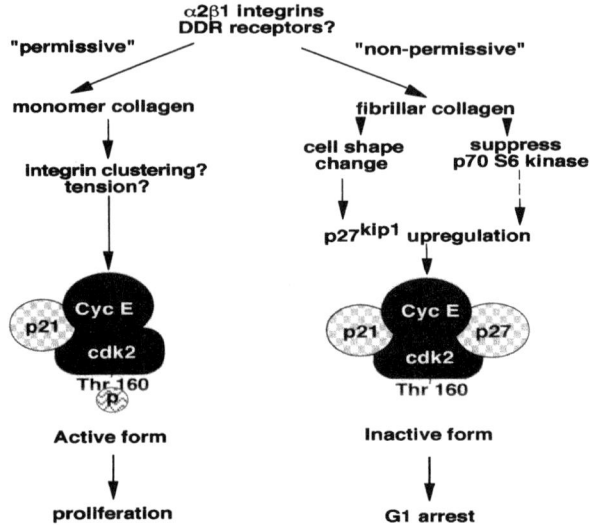

FIGURE 2. Different forms of collagen regulate SMC transition from G1 to S by targeting the cdk2 inhibitor p27^{Kip1}. (**A**) The cyclins and their associated kinases (cdks) have been proposed to control cell cycle transit in mammalian cells. Cyclin E and its associated kinase, cdk2, accumulate in late G1 and are critical for G1/S transition. The cdk inhibitors p21^{Cip1} and p27^{Kip1} can directly inhibit cdk2 activity and prevent its phosphorylation on Thr-160. (**B**) Our studies demonstrate that different forms of type I collagen regulate the ac-

Fibrillar Collagen Inhibits Arterial Smooth Muscle Proliferation through Regulation of Cell Cycle Inhibitors

It has been proposed that cyclin-dependent kinase activities control the G1/S transition in mammalian cells. Cyclin E and its associated kinase, cdk2, accumulate in late G1[65] (FIG. 2A), suggesting a role for this cyclin in regulating the transition to S phase. Since SMCs plated on fibrillar collagen are arrested in G1, we compared the effects of monomer and polymerized collagen on cyclin E, cdk2, and the cdk inhibitors, p21^{Cip1} and p27^{Kip1}, that directly inhibit cdk2 activity and prevent its phosphorylation on Thr-160 *in vitro*.[66,67] We have demonstrated that fibrillar collagen suppresses cyclin E–cdk2 activity and cdk2 phosphorylation by increasing the levels of the cdk2 inhibitors p21^{Cip1} and p27^{Kip1} associated with the cyclin E–cdk2–p21 complex (FIG. 2B).[5]

Monovalent blocking antibodies to α2 integrins, integrins that mediate adhesion to monomer and fibrillar collagen, are able to induce p27 and thus mimic the effects of polymerized collagen. Recently, native collagen was identified as the ligand for two related orphan tyrosine kinase receptors, discoidin domain receptors 1 and 2 (DDR1 and DDR2).[68–71] DDR1 and DDR2 are expressed in human SMC and their expression is increased in developing lesions of atherosclerosis (Carragher and colleagues, manuscript in preparation). It is therefore possible that the DDR receptors may also contribute to the regulation of SMC proliferation.

Our studies demonstrate that fibrillar collagen increases levels of the cdk2 inhibitors, p21^{Cip1} and p27^{Kip1}, which results in abrogation of cyclin E–cdk2 activity.[5] Fibrillar collagen rapidly suppresses a specific early signaling pathway, p70 S6 kinase, a possible regulator of p27^{Kip1}, without dramatic effects on MAP kinase pathway. Fibrillar collagen also modulates SMC shape (decreased formation of focal adhesion sites and delayed cell spreading) which is known to modulate cell proliferation[72,73] and levels of the cdk inhibitors.[74,75] The effects of polymerized collagen are also associated with decreased levels of α5β1 fibronectin receptor and the lack of fibronectin assembly on the cell surface.[76] On monomer collagen, blocking of fibronectin receptors by antibodies and/or cyclic RGD peptides leads to abrogation of fibronectin assembly, upregulation of p27^{Kip1}, suppression of cyclin E–cdk2 activity, and inhibition of DNA synthesis, suggesting that the fibronectin receptors are indispensable for regulation of the cell cycle molecules and SMC proliferation. Our studies are consistent with the report that treatment of vascular SMC *in vitro* with a recombinant fragment of fibronectin (III$_1$-C) or the anti-fibronectin antibody (mAB L8), both of which inhibit fibronectin assembly, results in inhibition of SMC proliferation by 75–90%.[77] Thus, our studies have identified the cyclin E–cdk2 complex as the molecular target of distinct signaling mechanisms from monomer and fibrillar collagen that regulate SMC proliferation (FIG. 2B). Consistent with our

---

tivity of cyclin E–cdk2 by regulating the composition of the cyclin E–cdk2 complex. Under "non-permissive" conditions on fibrillar type I collagen, it appears that both the induced change in cell shape and suppression of p70 S6 kinase contribute to the upregulation of p21^{Cip1} and p27^{Kip1} and their association with the cyclin E–cdk2 complex that prevent activation and cell cycle progression. Downregulation of p27^{Kip1} levels associated with cyclinE/cdk2 complexes on monomer collagen by fibronectin integrin-initiated signals may allow the cell to replicate in response to growth factors.

studies of cultured SMC, it has recently been shown that p27^{Kip1} is expressed in normal vessels *in vivo* and its expression is decreased following balloon injury coincident with SMC proliferation.[78]

Degraded Collagen May Be Required To Release SMC from Non-Permissive States

In vivo studies indicate that collagen fibers are degraded during atherogenesis as a result of increased MMP activity (TABLE 1) derived from either infiltrating macrophages or activated SMCs. *In vitro* studies suggest that denaturation or proteolysis of the type I collagen triple helix may reveal cryptic RGD integrin-binding motifs.[79,80] More recent studies demonstrate that MMP degradation of collagen modulates α2β1 binding to the collagen fragments[81] and reveals a cryptic β3 integrin binding site that induces specific integrin-signaling events in SMC, resulting in increased tenascin-C expression.[82] These studies raise the possibility that degraded collagen fragments generated within the atherosclerotic lesion may modulate SMC behavior by possessing specific integrin signaling properties distinct from those of intact native collagen present in the normal artery wall.

Our own studies have demonstrated that degraded collagen has unique signaling properties, primarily mediated through α2β1 and αvβ1, that rapidly promote focal adhesion disassembly and loss of substrate attachment.[83] Our studies show that treatment of vascular SMC with degraded collagen type I fragments induces calpain-mediated cleavage of two components of the focal adhesion complex, pp125^{FAK} and paxillin. Proteolytic cleavage of pp125^{FAK} and paxillin occurs in parallel with loss of focal adhesion structures, cell rounding, and loss of substrate attachment. This demonstration that degraded collagen fragments promote calpain-mediated disassembly of SMC focal adhesions suggests the possibility that during atherogenesis in areas of MMP-induced collagen degradation, SMC anchorage to the surrounding ECM may be disrupted, thereby promoting their release from that matrix and migration towards the neointima (FIG. 1).

EXTRACELLULAR MATRIX CAN DYNAMICALLY REGULATE SMC RESPONSIVENESS

In conclusion, our studies have defined molecular mechanisms whereby different forms of type I collagen can either prevent cell cycle traverse (fibrillar type I collagen), or promote cell rounding and release from other ECM (degraded type I collagen), or promote proliferation (monomer collagen). Analysis of developing lesions of atherosclerosis (TABLE 1) demonstrates that degraded collagen and monomeric collagen are present in lesions, as well as other ECM that can promote SMC migration and proliferation. In contrast, fibrillar collagen and other ECM constituents of the normal media (TABLE 1) have been shown to promote maintenance of SMC differentiated phenotype and SMC quiescence. Thus, the capacity of SMC to respond to growth factors can be dynamically regulated at a specific site by the surrounding ECM.

ACKNOWLEDGMENTS

We dedicate this chapter to the memory of Russell Ross, whose passion and dedication to scientific pursuits continue to inspire our own. We thank our other colleagues in the laboratory for continuing to question our hypotheses.

REFERENCES

1. Ross, R. 1993. The pathogenesis of atherosclerosis: a perspective for the 1990s. Nature **362:** 801–809.
2. Ross, R. 1999. Atherosclerosis—an inflammatory disease. N. Engl. J. Med. **340:** 115–126.
3. Ross, R., J. Masuda, E.W. Raines, A.M. Gown, S. Katsuda, M. Sasahara, L.T. Malden, H. Masuko & H. Sato. 1990. Localization of PDGF-B protein in macrophages in all phases of atherogenesis. Science **248:** 1009–1012.
4. Ferns, G.A., E.W. Raines, K.H. Sprugel, A.S. Motani, M.A. Reidy & R. Ross. 1991. Inhibition of neointimal smooth muscle accumulation after angioplasty by an antibody to PDGF. Science **253:** 1129–1132.
5. Koyama, H., E.W. Raines, K.E. Bornfeldt, J.M. Roberts & R. Ross. 1996. Fibrillar collagen inhibits arterial smooth muscle proliferation through regulation of Cdk2 inhibitors. Cell **87:** 1069–1078.
6. Campbell G.R. & J.H. Campbell. 1990. The phenotypes of smooth muscle expressed in human atheroma. Ann. N.Y. Acad. Sci. **598:** 143–158.
7. Thyberg, J., U. Hedin, M. Sjölund, L. Palmberg & B.A. Bottger. 1990. Regulation of differentiated properties and proliferation of arterial smooth muscle cells. Arteriosclerosis **10:** 966–990.
8. Gabbiani, G., O. Kocher, W.S. Bloom, J. Vandekerckhove & K. Weber. 1984. Actin expression in smooth muscle cells of rat aortic intimal thickening, human atheromatous plaque, and cultured rat aortic media. J. Clin. Invest. **73:** 148–152.
9. Glukhova, M.A., A.E. Kabakov, M.G. Frid, O.I. Ornatsky, A.M. Belkin, D.N. Mukhin, A.N. Orekhov, V.E. Koteliansky & V.N. Smirnov. 1988. Modulation of human aorta smooth muscle cell phenotype: a study of muscle-specific variants of vinculin, caldesmon, and actin expression. Proc. Natl. Acad. Sci. USA **85:** 9542–9546.
10. Aikawa, M., P.M. Sivam, M. Kuro-o, K. Kimura, K. Nakahara, S. Takewaki, M. Ueda, H. Yamaguchi, Y. Yazaki, M. Periasamy & R. Nagai. 1993. Human smooth muscle myosin heavy chain isoforms as molecular markers for vascular development and atherosclerosis. Circ. Res. **73:** 1000–1012.
11. Ueki, N., K. Sobue, K. Kanda, T. Hada & K. Higashino. 1987. Expression of high and low molecular weight caldesmons during phenotypic modulation of smooth muscle cells. Proc. Natl. Acad. Sci. USA **84:** 9049–9053.
12. Reckless, J., G. Fleetwood, L. Tilling, P.A. Huber, S.B. Marston & K. Pritchard. 1994. Changes in the caldesmon isoform content and intimal thickening in the rabbit carotid artery induced by a silicone elastomer collar. Arterioscler. Thromb. **14:** 1837–1845.
13. Kocher, O. & G. Gabbiani. 1986. Cytoskeletal features of normal and atheromatous human arterial smooth muscle cells. Hum. Pathol. **17:** 875–880.
14. Osborn, M., J. Caselitz, K. Puschel & K. Weber. 1987. Intermediate filament expression in human vascular smooth muscle and in arteriosclerotic plaques. Virchows Arch. A Pathol. Anat. Histopathol. **411:** 449–458.
15. Kuro-o, M., R. Nagai, K. Nakahara, H. Katoh, R.C. Tsai, H. Tsuchimochi, Y. Yazaki, A. Ohkubo & F. Takaku. 1991. cDNA cloning of a myosin heavy chain isoform in embryonic smooth muscle and its expression during vascular development and in arteriosclerosis. J. Biol. Chem. **266:** 3768–3773.
16. Gallagher, P.J., J.G. Garcia & B.P. Herring. 1995. Expression of a novel myosin light chain kinase in embryonic tissues and cultured cells. J. Biol. Chem. **270:** 29090–29095.

17. FISHER, S.A. & M. IKEBE. 1995. Developmental and tissue distribution of expression of nonmuscle and smooth muscle isoforms of myosin light chain kinase. Biochem. Biophys. Res. Commun. **217:** 696–703.
18. GALLAGHER, P.J., Y. JIN & V. LINDNER. 1998. Expression of myosin and myosin light chain kinase in response to vascular injury [abstract]. Presented at Keystone Symposium on Angiogenesis and Vascular Remodeling. Steamboat Springs, CO. No. 312.
19. SHANAHAN, C.M., N.R. CARY, J.C. METCALFE & P.L. WEISSBERG. 1994. High expression of genes for calcification-regulating proteins in human atherosclerotic plaques. J. Clin. Invest. **93:** 2393–2402.
20. KOCHER, O., F. GABBIANI, G. GABBIANI, M.A. REIDY, M.S. COKAY, H. PETERS & I. HUTTNER. 1991. Phenotypic features of smooth muscle cells during the evolution of experimental carotid artery intimal thickening. Biochemical and morphologic studies. Lab. Invest. **65:** 459–470.
21. MEYER, T., U. BRINK, C. UNTERBERG, S. STOHR, H. KREUZER & A.B. BUCHWALD. 1994. Expression of meta-vinculin in human coronary arteriosclerosis is related to the histological grade of plaque formation. Atherosclerosis **111:** 111–119.
22. MCCULLAGH, K.G., V.C. DUANCE & K.A. BISHOP. 1980. The distribution of collagen types I, III and V (AB) in normal and atherosclerotic human aorta. J. Pathol. **130:** 45–55.
23. VOSS, B. & J. RAUTERBERG. 1986. Localization of collagen types I, III, IV and V, fibronectin and laminin in human arteries by the indirect immunofluorescence method. Pathol. Res. Pract. **181:** 568–575.
24. KATSUDA, S., Y. OKADA, T. MINAMOTO, Y. ODA, Y. MATSUI & I. NAKANISHI. 1992. Collagens in human atherosclerosis. Immunohistochemical analysis using collagen type-specific antibodies. Arterioscler. Thromb. **12:** 494–502.
25. WEITKAMP, B., P. CULLEN, G. PLENZ, H. ROBENEK & J. RAUTERBERG. 1999. Human macrophages synthesize type VIII collagen *in vitro* and in the atherosclerotic plaque. FASEB J. **13:** 1445–1457.
26. KAKOLYRIS, S., P. KARAKITSOS, M. TZARDI & E. AGAPITOS. 1995. Immunohistochemical detection of fibronectin in early and advanced atherosclerosis. In Vivo **9:** 35–40.
27. THYBERG, J., K. BLOMGREN, J. ROY, P.K. TRAN & U. HEDIN. 1997. Phenotypic modulation of smooth muscle cells after arterial injury is associated with changes in the distribution of laminin and fibronectin. J. Histochem. Cytochem. **45:** 837–846.
28. STENMAN, S., K. VON SMITTEN & A. VAHERI. 1980. Fibronectin and atherosclerosis. Acta Med. Scand. Suppl. **642:** 165–170.
29. GIACHELLI, C.M., N. BAE, M. ALMEIDA, D.T. DENHARDT, C.E. ALPERS & S.M. SCHWARTZ. 1993. Osteopontin is elevated during neointima formation in rat arteries and is a novel component of human atherosclerotic plaques. J. Clin. Invest. **92:** 1686–1696.
30. IKEDA, T., T. SHIRASAWA, Y. ESAKI, S. YOSHIKI & K. HIROKAWA. 1993. Osteopontin mRNA is expressed by smooth muscle-derived foam cells in human atherosclerotic lesions of the aorta. J. Clin. Invest. **92:** 2814–2820.
31. RAINES, E.W., T.F. LANE, M.L. IRUELA-ARISPE, R. ROSS & E.H. SAGE. 1992. The extracellular glycoprotein SPARC interacts with platelet-derived growth factor (PDGF)-AB and -BB and inhibits the binding of PDGF to its receptors. Proc. Natl. Acad. Sci. USA **89:** 1281–1285.
32. WALLNER, K., C. LI, P.K. SHAH, M.C. FISHBEIN, J.S. FORRESTER, S. KAUL & B.G. SHARIFI. 1999. Tenascin-C is expressed in macrophage-rich human coronary atherosclerotic plaque. Circulation **99:** 1284–1289.
33. WIGHT, T.N., G.J. RAUGI, S.M. MUMBY & P. BORNSTEIN. 1985. Light microscopic immunolocation of thrombospondin in human tissues. J. Histochem. Cytochem. **33:** 295–302.
34. NICULESCU, F., H.G. RUS & R. VLAICU. 1987. Immunohistochemical localization of C5b-9, S-protein, C3d and apolipoprotein B in human arterial tissues with atherosclerosis. Atherosclerosis **65:** 1–11.
35. DUFOURCQ, P., H. LOUIS, C. MOREAU, D. DARET, M.R. BOISSEAU, J.M. LAMAZIERE & J. BONNET. 1998. Vitronectin expression and interaction with receptors in smooth muscle cells from human atheromatous plaque. Arterioscler. Thromb. Vasc. Biol. **18:** 168–176.

36. VAN AKEN, B.E., D. SEIFFERT, T. THINNES & D.J. LOSKUTOFF. 1997. Localization of vitronectin in the normal and atherosclerotic human vessel wall. Histochem. Cell Biol. **107:** 313–320.
37. GALIS, Z.S., G.K. SUKHOVA, M.W. LARK & P. LIBBY. 1994. Increased expression of matrix metalloproteinases and matrix degrading activity in vulnerable regions of human atherosclerotic plaques. J. Clin. Invest. **94:** 2493–2503.
38. NIKKARI, S.T., K.D. O'BRIEN, M. FERGUSON, T. HATSUKAMI, H.G. WELGUS, C.E. ALPERS & A.W. CLOWES. 1995. Interstitial collagenase (MMP-1) expression in human carotid atherosclerosis. Circulation **92:** 1393–1398.
39. BROWN, D.L., M.S. HIBBS, M. KEARNEY, C. LOUSHIN & J.M. ISNER. 1995. Identification of 92-kD gelatinase in human coronary atherosclerotic lesions. Association of active enzyme synthesis with unstable angina. Circulation **91:** 2125–2131.
40. CURCI, J.A., S. LIAO, M.D. HUFFMAN, S.D. SHAPIRO & R.W. THOMPSON. 1998. Expression and localization of macrophage elastase (matrix metalloproteinase-12) in abdominal aortic aneurysms. J. Clin. Invest. **102:** 1900–1910.
41. SUKHOVA, G.K., U. SCHONBECK, E. RABKIN, F.J. SCHOEN, A.R. POOLE, R.C. BILLINGHURST & P. LIBBY. 1999. Evidence for increased collagenolysis by interstitial collagenases-1 and -3 in vulnerable human atheromatous plaques. Circulation **99:** 2503–2509.
42. SCHONBECK, U., F. MACH, G.K. SUKHOVA, E. ATKINSON, E. LEVESQUE, M. HERMAN, P. GRABER, P. BASSET & P. LIBBY. 1999. Expression of stromelysin-3 in atherosclerotic lesions: regulation via CD40-CD40 ligand signaling *in vitro*. J. Exp. Med. **189:** 843–853.
43. RAJAVASHISTH, T.B., X.P. XU, S. JOVINGE, S. MEISEL, X.O. XU, N.N. CHAI, M.C. FISHBEIN, S. KAUL, B. CERCEK, B. SHARIFI & P.K. SHAH. 1999. Membrane type 1 matrix metalloproteinase expression in human atherosclerotic plaques: evidence for activation by proinflammatory mediators. Circulation **99:** 3103–3109.
44. FABUNMI, R.P., G.K. SUKHOVA, S. SUGIYAMA & P. LIBBY. 1998. Expression of tissue inhibitor of metalloproteinases-3 in human atheroma and regulation in lesion-associated cells: a potential protective mechanism in plaque stability. Circ. Res. **83:** 270–278.
45. NIKKARI, S.T., R.L. GEARY, T. HATSUKAMI, M. FERGUSON, R. FOROUGH, C.E. ALPERS & A.W. CLOWES. 1996. Expression of collagen, interstitial collagenase, and tissue inhibitor of metalloproteinases-1 in restenosis after carotid endarterectomy. Am. J. Pathol. **148:** 777–783.
46. SCHNEIDERMAN, J., M.S. SAWDEY, M.R. KEETON, G.M. BORDIN, E.F. BERNSTEIN, R.B. DILLEY & D.J. LOSKUTOFF. 1992. Increased type 1 plasminogen activator inhibitor gene expression in atherosclerotic human arteries. Proc. Natl. Acad. Sci. USA **89:** 6998–7002.
47. TIPPING, P.G., P. DAVENPORT, M. GALLICCHIO, E.L. FILONZI, J. APOSTOLOPOULOS & J. WOJTA. 1993. Atheromatous plaque macrophages produce plasminogen activator inhibitor type-1 and stimulate its production by endothelial cells and vascular smooth muscle cells. Am. J. Pathol. **143:** 875–885.
48. LUPU, F., G.E. BERGONZELLI, D.A. HEIM, E. COUSIN, C.Y. GENTON, F. BACHMANN & E.K. KRUITHOF. 1993. Localization and production of plasminogen activator inhibitor-1 in human healthy and atherosclerotic arteries. Arterioscler. Thromb. **13:** 1090–1000.
49. PADRO, T., J.J. EMEIS, M. STEINS, K.W. SCHMID & J. KIENAST. 1995. Quantification of plasminogen activators and their inhibitors in the aortic vessel wall in relation to the presence and severity of atherosclerotic disease. Arterioscler. Thromb. Vasc. Biol. **15:** 893–902.
50. RAGHUNATH, P.N., J.E. TOMASZEWSKI, S.T. BRADY, R.J. CARON, S.S. OKADA & E.S. BARNATHAN. 1995. Plasminogen activator system in human coronary atherosclerosis. Arterioscler. Thromb. Vasc. Biol. **15:** 1432–1443.
51. LUPU, F., D.A. HEIM, F. BACHMANN, M. HURNI, V.V. KAKKAR & E.K. KRUITHOF. 1995. Plasminogen activator expression in human atherosclerotic lesions. Arterioscler. Thromb. Vasc. Biol. **15:** 1444–1455.
52. ROBBIE, L.A., N.A. BOOTH, A.J. BROWN & B. BENNETT. 1996. Inhibitors of fibrinolysis are elevated in atherosclerotic plaque. Arterioscler. Thromb. Vasc. Biol. **16:** 539–545.
53. REKHTER, M.D. & D. GORDON. 1995. Active proliferation of different cell types, including lymphocytes, in human atherosclerotic plaques. Am. J. Pathol. **147:** 668–677.

54. HEDIN, U., B.A. BOTTGER, E. FORSBERG, S. JOHANSSON & J. THYBERG. 1988. Diverse effects of fibronectin and laminin on phenotypic properties of cultured arterial smooth muscle cells. J. Cell Biol. **107:** 307–319.
55. SAGE, E.H. & P. BORNSTEIN. 1991. Extracellular proteins that modulate cell-matrix interactions. SPARC, tenascin, and thrombospondin. J. Biol. Chem. **266:** 14831–14834.
56. LIAW, L., M.P. SKINNER, E.W. RAINES, R. ROSS, D.A. CHERESH, S.M. SCHWARTZ & C.M. GIACHELLI. 1995. The adhesive and migratory effects of osteopontin are mediated via distinct cell surface integrins. Role of alpha v beta 3 in smooth muscle cell migration to osteopontin *in vitro*. J. Clin. Invest. **95:** 713–724.
57. SLEPIAN, M.J., S.P. MASSIA, B. DEHDASHTI, A. FRITZ & L. WHITESELL. 1998. Beta3-integrins rather than beta1-integrins dominate integrin-matrix interactions involved in postinjury smooth muscle cell migration. Circulation **97:** 1818–1827.
58. SCHOR, S.L. 1980. Cell proliferation and migration on collagen substrata *in vitro*. J. Cell Sci. **41:** 159–175.
59. RHUDY, R.W. & J.M. MCPHERSON. 1988. Influence of the extracellular matrix on the proliferative response of human skin fibroblasts to serum and purified platelet-derived growth factor. J. Cell. Physiol. **137:** 185–191.
60. MARTIN, G.M. & A.C. SANK. 1990. Extracellular matrices, cells, and growth factors. *In* Peptide Growth Factors and Their Receptors II. M.B. Sporn & A.B. Roberts, Eds. Springer Verlag. Berlin.
61. REKHTER, M.D. & D. GORDON. 1994. Cell proliferation and collagen synthesis are two independent events in human atherosclerotic plaques. J. Vasc. Res. **31:** 280–286.
62. HULTGARDH-NILSSON, A., C. LOVDAHL, K. BLOMGREN, B. KALLIN & J. THYBERG. 1997. Expression of phenotype- and proliferation-related genes in rat aortic smooth muscle cells in primary culture. Cardiovasc. Res. **34:** 418–430.
63. VANE, J.R., E.E. ANGGARD & R.M. BOTTING. 1990. Regulatory functions of the vascular endothelium. N. Engl. J. Med. **323:** 27–36.
64. HIROSE, M., H. KOSUGI, K. NAKAZATO & T. HAYASHI. 1999. Restoration to a quiescent and contractile phenotype from a proliferative phenotype of myofibroblast-like human aortic smooth muscle cells by culture on type IV collagen gels. J. Biochem. (Tokyo) **125:** 991–1000.
65. SHERR, C.J. 1993. Mammalian G1 cyclins. Cell **73:** 1059–1065.
66. APRELIKOVA, O., Y. XIONG & E.T. LIU. 1995. Both p16 and p21 families of cyclin-dependent kinase (CDK) inhibitors block the phosphorylation of cyclin-dependent kinases by the CDK-activating kinase. J. Biol. Chem. **270:** 18195–18197.
67. SHERR, C.J. & J.M. ROBERTS. 1995. Inhibitors of mammalian G1 cyclin-dependent kinases. Genes Dev. **9:** 1149–1163.
68. VOGEL, W., G.D. GISH, F. ALVES & T. PAWSON. 1997. The discoidin domain receptor tyrosine kinases are activated by collagen. Molec. Cell **1:** 13–23.
69. SHRIVASTAVA, A., C. RADZIEJEWSKI, E. CAMPBELL, L. KOVAC, M. MCGLYNN, T.E. RYAN, S. DAVIS, M.P. GOLDFARB, D.J. GLASS, G. LEMKE & G.D. YANCOPOULOS. 1997. An orphan receptor tyrosine kinase family whose members serve as nonintegrin collagen receptors. Molec. Cell **1:** 25–34
70. SCHLESSINGER, J. 1997. Direct binding and activation of receptor tyrosine kinases by collagen. Cell **91:** 869–872.
71. VOGEL, W. 1999. Discoidin domain receptors: structural relations and functional implications. FASEB J. **13:** S77–82.
72. FOLKMAN J. & A. MOSCONA. 1978. Role of cell shape in growth control. Nature **273:** 345–349.
73. HANSEN, L.K., D.J. MOONEY, J.P. VACANTI & D.E. INGBER. 1994. Integrin binding and cell spreading on extracellular matrix act at different points in the cell cycle to promote hepatocyte growth. Mol. Biol. Cell **5:** 967–975.
74. FANG, F., G. OREND, N. WATANABE, T. HUNTER & E. RUOSLAHTI. 1996. Dependence of cyclin E-cdk2 kinase activity on cell anchorage. Science **271:** 499–502.
75. ZHU, S., M. OHTSUBO, R. BOHMER, J.M. ROBERTS & R.K. ASSOIAN. 1996. Adhesion dependent cell cycle progression linked to the expression of cyclin D1, activation of cyclin E-cdk2, and phosphorylation of the retinoblastoma protein. J. Cell Biol. **133:** 391–403.

76. KOYAMA, H., N.O. CARRAGHER, K.E. BORNFELDT, U. HEDIN, W.G. CARTER, R. ROSS & E.W. RAINES. 2000. Trans-dominant inhibition of fibronectin receptors by fibrillar collagen regulates arterial smooth muscle proliferation: p27^{Kip1} as the common target of integrin-mediated signals. Submitted for publication.
77. MERCURIUS, K.O. & A.O. MORLA. 1998. Inhibition of vascular smooth muscle cell growth by inhibition of fibronectin matrix assembly. Circ. Res. **82:** 548–556.
78. TANNER, F.C., Z.Y. YANG, E. DUCKERS, D. GORDON, G.J. NABEL & E.G. NABEL. 1998. Expression of cyclin-dependent kinase inhibitors in vascular disease. Circ. Res. **82:** 396–403.
79. DAVIS, G.E. 1992. Affinity of integrins for damaged extracellular matrix: alpha v beta 3 binds to denatured collagen type I through RGD sites. Biochem. Biophys. Res. Commun. **182:** 1025–1031.
80. MONTGOMERY, A.M., R.A. REISFELD & D.A. CHERESH. 1994. Integrin alpha v beta 3 rescues melanoma cells from apoptosis in three-dimensional dermal collagen. Proc. Natl. Acad. Sci. USA **91:** 8856–8860.
81. MESSENT, A.J., D.S. TUCKWELL, V. KNAUPER, M.J. HUMPHRIES, G. MURPHY & J. GAVRILOVIC. 1998. Effects of collagenase-cleavage of type I collagen on alpha2beta1 integrin-mediated cell adhesion. J. Cell Sci. **111:** 1127–1135.
82. JONES, P.L., J. CRACK & M. RABINOVITCH. 1997. Regulation of tenascin-C, a vascular smooth muscle cell survival factor that interacts with the alpha v beta 3 integrin to promote epidermal growth factor receptor phosphorylation and growth. J. Cell Biol. **139:** 279–293.
83. CARRAGHER N.O., B. LEVKAU, R. ROSS & E.W. RAINES. 1999. Degraded collagen fragments promote rapid disassembly of smooth muscle focal adhesions that correlates with cleavage of pp125^{FAK}, paxillin, and talin. J. Cell Biol. **147:** 619–629.
84. CHANG, M.Y., S. SASAHARA, A. CHAIT, E.W. RAINES & R. ROSS. 1995. Inhibition of hypercholesterolemia-induced atherosclerosis in the nonhuman primate by probucol. II. Cellular composition and proliferation. Arterioscler. Thromb. Vasc. Biol. **15:** 1631–1640.

Questions and Answers

K. SHIMOKADO (*National Cardiovascular Center Research Institute, Osaka, Japan*): I think there are focal adhesions on the surface and beneath the smooth muscle cells, but mainly beneath where the cells attach to the collagen. Where does the degraded collagen bind, on the upper surface or lower surface of the cell?

RAINES: We really don't know yet. We do know that there are free integrins on the surface of the cell that are presumably binding. However, other studies have shown that surface binding can affect the integrin focal adhesions. But, it is also possible that degraded collagen is much better able to get underneath the cell, as well.

H. YAMAMOTO (*Kanazawa University, Kanazawa, Japan*): You demonstrated the inhibitory effect of polymerized collagen on smooth muscle cells. My question is whether a similar effect occurs on smooth muscle covering microvascular cells, namely pericytes and mesangial cells in renal glomeruli?

RAINES: We have not done those experiments, but actually the observation that polymerized collagen was inhibitory to smooth muscle cells and fibroblasts is 20 years old. What was new was the comparison of structurally altered forms of collagen.

G.K. HANSSON (*Karolinska Hospital, Stockholm, Sweden*): Was the expression of PDGF or its receptors in the vessel wall by vascular cells themselves affected by the presence or absence of PDGF produced by the monocytes/macrophages?

RAINES: Unfortunately, some of our reagents really are not very good for those types of studies, but we have tried to evaluate the possibility by immunostaining and ELISA. So far, evaluation of tissue sections and isolated platelets and peritoneal macrophages from chimeric animals have not shown any differences in the level of PDGF-A expression. We have not looked at the receptors.

A.R. TALL (*Columbia University, New York, NY, USA*): I am also fascinated by these SMC-rich legions that get arrested at a certain stage of lesion development. Do they actually have an increase in the absolute number of macrophages? Do you have an impression about this? The absence of smooth muscle proliferative phenotype is a part of what you would expect from known biology, but is something else going on? It looks like you have more macrophages than you would expect.

RAINES: This is something that we are very actively pursuing in a number of different ways because I think that our knowledge of the potential role even of PDGF in macrophages is very limited. We are involved in doing some cDNA array screens that are unbiased to look at what differences may exist.

K. TANAKA (*Kyushu University, Fukuoka, Japan*): It is very interesting to know that the histological characteristics are different in the PDGF-deficient mice. If you keep the mice longer, how do they change histologically?

RAINES: It is a very important question. We thought that we were waiting a long time for the answer. Now we are waiting 50 weeks, almost a year. Part of this is because we have chosen to use chow-fed animals. The reason for that is that there is much less variability in cholesterol levels so that we have much a better matched set of animals.

R.W. WISSLER (*University of Chicago, Chicago, IL, USA*): I noticed at the beginning of your presentation that you talked a little bit about smooth muscle cell migration. I wonder whether your current work indicates that anything that stimulates proliferation also stimulates migration, or whether we still have two phenomena that should be looked at separately.

RAINES: Are you asking in relation to PDGF specifically or just in general?

WISSLER: In relation to the response to the stimuli that you did.

RAINES: If we look in the lesions either from the Apo-E null mice or some of our primates studies where we can look at early stages of lesion development, we see foci of both proliferating cells as well as cells that appear to be migrating. That is, their orientation is altered and they appear to be moving into the intima. In relation to PDGF we are looking at that as a part of this study. But, it is very hard to make correlations of the sort you are asking about because in atherosclerosis you don't have a huge wave of proliferation.

The Role of Adaptive Immunity in Atherosclerosis

GÖRAN K. HANSSON, XINGHUA ZHOU, ELISABETH TÖRNQUIST, AND GABRIELLE PAULSSON

Karolinska Institutet, Center for Molecular Medicine, Karolinska Hospital, SE- 17176 Stockholm, Sweden

ABSTRACT: Atherosclerosis is an inflammatory disease induced by a lipid metabolic disturbance at sites of hemodynamic strain in the vasculature. Studies in both man and experimental animal models show an involvement of innate and adaptive immune mechanisms in the disease process. Our recent studies in apoE-knockout mice show that the level of hypercholesterolemia affects the functional properties of the immune response. Modulating immune activity by injections of polyclonal immunoglobulins inhibits disease progression, suggesting that immunomodulation may be useful to treat atherosclerosis. Analysis of T cell receptor (TCR) mRNA in atherosclerotic lesions shows expansions of T cells expressing TCR-Vβ6, a receptor type that is also expressed by T cells recognizing oxidized low density lipoprotein (oxLDL). This suggests that oxLDL is an autoantigen that induces strong, local T cell responses in the plaque. Further characterization of this and other candidate antigens, such as heat shock proteins and macromolecular components of *Chlamydia pneumoniae*, may provide important information on which specific interference with the disease process could be based.

INTRODUCTION

Atherosclerosis is an inflammatory disease induced by a lipid metabolic disturbance at sites of hemodynamic strain in the vasculature. The inflammatory response manifests itself as infiltration and activation of mononuclear cells, activation of humoral cascade systems, cytokine secretion, cell death, and induction of fibroproliferative repair processes.[1,2]

The inflammatory response is controlled by the immune system, components of which are abundant in the atherosclerotic plaque.[1] Innate immunity, which carries the immunologically nonspecific responses elicited rapidly upon infection, is represented by macrophages, which are necessary for the initiation of atherosclerosis. Adaptive immunity, i.e., the immune responses initiated when T and B cells recognize specific antigens, is also involved in the disease process. Lesions contain significant numbers of T cells and there is also a systemic cellular and humoral immune response during disease development. The fact that T and B cell responses are detectable in atherosclerosis indicates that antigens, i.e., specific molecular signals associated with the disease induce immune reactions during its pathogenesis.

Adaptive immunity regulates inflammatory responses largely through cytokine secretion. Thus, cytokines produced by T cell subsets control macrophage activation, smooth muscle proliferation, collagen production, proteolysis, mast cell activation, and other aspects of inflammation and repair in the artery. Since adaptive immune responses are induced by highly specific molecular signals and its functional consequences include the regulation of inflammation and repair, key processes in atherogenesis, control of adaptive immunity may be an attractive approach to treating and/or preventing atherosclerosis.

IMMUNE DEFICIENCY, METABOLIC ABNORMALITIES, AND ATHEROSCLEROSIS

Research into immune mechanisms in atherosclerosis has been greatly facilitated by the construction of gene-targeted mouse models.[3] Two hypercholesterolemic mouse strains, the apolipoprotein E-knockout (apoE-KO) mouse[4,5] and the LDL receptor-KO (LDLR-KO) mouse,[6] have been particularly useful for this purpose. Both strains develop atherosclerosis when fed cholesterol and the apoE-KO mouse also exhibits spontaneous atherosclerosis.

Cross-breeding the apoE-KO mouse with RAG-1 mice that lack both T and B cells leads to a 40% reduction of the extent of atherosclerosis.[7] Interestingly, a lack of inflammatory immune activity, which is induced by targeting the interferon-γ receptor, causes an even more substantial reduction of atherosclerosis.[8] This suggests that interferon-γ is a particularly proatherogenic T cell cytokine. This cytokine is a key mediator of the so-called Th1 immune responses, which are dominated by inflammation and macrophage activation.[9] It is therefore possible that the Th1 pathway is an important driving force for atherosclerosis.[10] This idea is supported by the fact that the atherosclerosis-prone mouse strain C57BL/6J[11] is particularly prone to develop Th1 responses upon immune challenge.

With increasing cholesterol load and hypercholesterolemia, there is a switch from Th1- to Th2-dependent immune responses in the apoE-KO mouse.[10] This is reflected in increased circulating levels of Th2-dependent anti-oxLDL antibodies, increased interleukin-4– and interleukin-10–producing T cells in the spleen, as well as an infiltration of IL-4 producing cells into atherosclerotic plaques.[10] The observation that severely hypercholesterolemic, fat-fed apoE-KO mice are less sensitive to immune defects than moderately hypercholesterolemic ones could therefore reflect a switch to less atherogenic immune activity in the animal.

The situation in man is more complex: not only are clinical immune defects more complex than those induced in the mouse by gene targeting, the immune responses themselves are less polarized than those of the mice. Nevertheless, it is interesting to note that cardiovascular disease is becoming a major problem among individuals infected with the human immunodeficiency virus (HIV) now that the progression into the acquired immunodeficiency syndrome (AIDS) can be retarded by antiviral therapy.

IMMUNOMODULATION INHIBITS ATHEROSCLEROSIS

Since immunodeficient animals exhibit reduced atherosclerosis, it might be possible to reduce disease initiation or progression by inhibiting immune activity. We therefore evaluated the effects of immunomodulation in apoE-KO mice.[12] Polyclonal immunoglobulin preparations (intravenous immunoglobulins, ivIg) inhibit T cell activity and have been used to treat autoimmune diseases, both in man and experimental animals.[13] Five-week-old apoE-KO mice were injected with ivIg daily for five days.[12] They were then put on an atherogenic diet (0.15% cholesterol) for 2 or 4 months. Intravenous Ig treatment led to a long-lasting inhibition of proliferative T cell responses to antigen. This represented an inhibition or anergy rather than elimination of reactive T cells, since it could be overcome by adding a strong mitogen, such as concanavalin A.

Analysis of aortic lesions showed that ivIg treatment attenuated lesion development.[12] After two months, fatty streak lesions of ivIg-treated apoE-KO mice were significantly smaller than those of control apoE-KO mice injected with bovine serum albumin. The protective effect was no longer discernible after four months on the atherogenic diet but a significant reduction of fibrofatty plaques at 4 months could be accomplished if five ivIg injections were given again 2 months after the first series. A 50% reduction in fibrofatty plaques was also obtained if the mice were injected only at one time point two months after the initiation of a cholesterol-rich diet.

These findings indicate (1) that immunomodulation inhibits atherosclerosis; (2) that a short-term treatment is sufficient to inhibit disease development; and (3) that both the early fatty streak phase and the subsequent fibrofatty plaque phase are sensitive to immunomodulation. It remains to be determined whether the protective effect was due to inhibition of cellular immunity or to transfer of specific antibodies. Such investigations are presently underway in our laboratory.

The conclusion that immunomodulation inhibits atherosclerosis received support from an experiment performed by Mach and colleagues, who used LDLR-KO mice. They first studied the expression in atherosclerotic lesions of costimulatory factors for immune cell activation. The CD40 receptor and its counter-receptor, CD40 ligand (CD40L) are involved in T and B cell activation—both were detected on immune and vascular cells of atherosclerotic lesions, in man and experimental animals.[14] Mach and colleagues asked whether blocking the CD40-CD40L signaling could attenuate disease development and therefore injected LDLR-KO mice with anti-CD40L antibodies repeatedly while feeding the mice an atherogenic diet. This led to a very substantial reduction in lesion size as well as to a reduction in activated immune cells in the lesions.[15]

In conclusion, therefore, immunomodulation by two different protocols reduces atherosclerosis in two different mouse models. Although potentially useful for treatment of rapidly progressive atherosclerosis, neither of these protocols is likely to be suitable for preventing or treating slowly progressive, chronic atherosclerosis. There is, therefore, need for the development and evaluation of new antiatherosclerotic therapies based on immunomodulation.

SPECIFICITY OF IMMUNE RESPONSE IN ATHEROSCLEROSIS

The observation that adaptive immunity is involved in atherosclerosis and the demonstration that immunomodulation attenuates disease development, point to specific antigens, which are both initiators and targets for adaptive immune responses, as important in the disease process. Several putative antigens, both exogenous and endogenous, have been proposed to play a role. The strongest case is for oxidized LDL (oxLDL) but there are also interesting data supporting a role for microbial antigens.

When LDL accumulates extravascularly, it is prone to undergo oxidative modification.[16] This process starts when oxygen radicals attack unsaturated fatty acid residues of triglycerides and phospholipids of the lipoprotein particle. Oxidized lipids, such as PAPC, lyso-PC, 9- and 13-HODE, are proinflammatory and can activate both endothelial cells and macrophages.[17,18] Activation of endothelial cells by such lipid species causes expression of leukocyte adhesion molecules.[19] Finally, oxysterols derived from cholesterol can activate inflammatory cells[20] and also form aggregates that activate the complement cascade.[21]

Lipid peroxidation leads to release of aldehyde fragments such as malondialdehyde and 4-hydroxynonenal. These short aldehydes may react with the protein moiety of the lipoprotein, particularly by binding to ε-amino groups of lysine. This process generates new epitopes for which tolerance appears not to have developed; structures such as malondialdehyde-conjugated lysine are strongly immunogenic and induce high titer antibody production.[22] In addition, antibodies develop against oxidized phospholipids. In fact, many cardiolipin antibodies appear to be directed against oxidized structures of the cardiolipin molecule.[23]

Both the antigen, oxidized LDL, and anti-oxLDL antibodies are present in the artery wall during atherosclerosis.[24,25] It is likely that LDL–anti-oxLDL immune complexes are taken up by Fc receptors and thus contribute to foam cell formation.[26] In addition, they may activate the complement cascade and thereby enhance inflammation and the recruitment of mononuclear cells. However, it is also possible that systemic anti-oxLDL antibodies help remove oxLDL from the circulation before it reaches the artery wall.[27] The balance between oxidation and elimination of LDL may therefore at least in part depend on systemic elimination vis-à-vis local production in the artery wall.

Both IgM and IgG antibodies to oxLDL are produced during atherosclerosis.[10,28] The occurrence of the latter suggests that T cells as well as B cells may recognize oxLDL. This has been verified in cellular immunological studies. T cell clones were obtained from atherosclerotic plaques; when challenged with oxLDL, many of the CD4+ clones recognized it as a classical, HLA-DR dependent antigen.[29] Similarly, apoE-KO mice develop oxLDL-reactive T cells and T cell–dependent B cell responses to oxLDL.[10,30,31] The switch from Th1 to Th2 help for anti-oxLDL reactive B cells may be decisive both for the local cellular immune response to oxLDL in the plaque and for the effector properties of the systemic antibody response.

Since oxLDL is a major component of lesions, T cells reactive towards oxidation-induced epitopes should be activated, proliferate, and expand to represent a significant proportion of all T cells in the lesions. When we and others addressed this issue nearly ten years ago, no evidence was obtained for clonal expansions of T cells in advanced human plaques.[32,33] However, we thought it would be interesting to revisit the question using state-of-the-art molecular technology to analyze early lesions of apoE-KO mice.[30] mRNA was isolated from fatty streaks and fibrofatty plaques of such mice, reverse-transcribed to cDNA, and amplified using a set of primers covering more than 80% of the variable (Vα and β) domains of the T cell antigen receptors (TCR). This analysis showed restricted usage of variable domains in the lesions. Furthermore, a "spectratyping" analysis of the length of the V-D-J segments revealed expansions of certain rearranged TCR types; this is considered strong evidence for a clonal expansion. In particular, T cells carrying TCR-Vβ6 are expanded in atherosclerotic lesions, suggesting that such T cells are stimulated to proliferate during atherogenesis.[30] Interestingly, T cell clones reactive with oxLDL often express Vβ6 (A. Nicoletti, G. Paulsson, G. K. Hansson, unpublished observations). Processing of oxLDL for antigen presentation is partly dependent on uptake via SR-A scavenger receptors.[34] Together, these data suggest that Vβ6+ T cells recognizing oxLDL proliferate in response to antigen and form clonal populations in the atherosclerotic plaques of apoE-KO mice.

OxLDL antibodies are found in hypercholesterolemic, atherosclerotic experimental animals and they appear in humans with atherosclerotic disease. Their titers have been found to correlate with the progression of carotid artery atherosclerosis[35] and peripheral atherosclerosis[36] but not with coronary disease in hypercholesterolemia. The predictive value of such antibodies therefore remains controversial.

If oxLDL is an important autoantigen, one would expect immunization with it to affect disease development. This is actually the case: several experimental studies have shown substantial beneficial effects of oxLDL immunization on atherosclerosis in hypercholesterolemic rabbits and mice.[37–39] Although both the antigen preparations and adjuvants administered need to be improved, these findings are encouraging for future research aimed at preventing clinical disease.

In addition to oxLDL, heat shock protein 60 has also been proposed as an autoantigen in atherosclerosis.[40] Interestingly, this autologous protein exhibits sequence similarities and immunological crossreactions with related proteins of microorganisms such as *Chlamydia pneumoniae*.[41] The latter is a common airway pathogen that has also been linked to atherosclerosis on the basis of seroepidemiological studies.[34] *Chlamydia pneumoniae* can survive intracellularly in macrophages and has been detected in macrophages of atherosclerotic lesions,[42] where it is likely to undergo oxidative modifications. It is therefore possible that molecular mimicry between Chlamydia antigens and endogenous structures, such as heat shock proteins and oxidized lipoproteins, could play a role in atherosclerosis. Indeed, recent animal experiments support an aggravating role for *Chlamydia pneumoniae* infection in atherosclerosis.[43–45]

ATHEROSCLEROSIS AND MYOCARDIAL INFARCTION

Immune/inflammatory stimuli can act to initiate and/or aggravate atherosclerosis, as has been described above. In addition, such stimuli may play a role in the activation of plaques and precipitation of myocardial infarction. Recent research has shown that such active plaques are sites of intense inflammation with abundant, activated T cells, macrophages, and mast cells.[46–49] They show increased production of matrix metalloproteinases, which are collagenolytic and elastolytic enzymes, and of reactive radical species.[50,51] Since proinflammatory cytokines released by activated T cells and macrophages can induce metalloproteinase expression and radical production in macrophages, mast cells, smooth muscle, and endothelial cells, it appears likely that an immune/inflammatory activation in the plaque leads to tissue proteolysis and cytotoxicity.[52]

Such an activity would be expected to reduce the tensile strength of the tissue. Interestingly, plaque fissures and ruptures are found in the majority of culprit lesions in coronary arteries.[53] Thus, immune/inflammatory activation results in proteolysis, which in turn causes plaque rupture.

Plaque rupture does not usually lead to complete rupture of the artery. Instead, it exposes a small nidus of subendothelial tissue to the circulating blood. Since the extracellular matrix is highly thrombogenic, this will result in the formation of a thrombus. The process is enhanced if tissue factor, the initiator of the external pathway of coagulation, is expressed by cells in the vicinity. Interestingly, proinflammatory cytokines induce tissue factor in endothelial cells, smooth muscle cells, and macrophages.[54–56]

Similar to plaque fissures and ruptures, endothelial desquamation can cause thrombosis.[47,57] This process could be elicited, e.g., by local proteolysis that dissociates endothelial cells from their substratum or by vasospastic events that mechanically damage the endothelium in such a way that the cells detach. Such endothelial desquamation is also observed in many cases of coronary thrombosis.

Plaque inflammation leads to release of proinflammatory cytokines into the circulation. This, in turn, induces acute phase reactants in a similar manner to other types of inflammation. Therefore, the acute coronary syndrome is characterized by high levels of acute phase reactants such as IL-6, CRP, and fibrinogen, which are useful in the clinical diagnosis of unstable angina pectoris and developing myocardial infarction.[58–60] Recent studies of patients with unstable angina point to T cell activation as an initiating or modulatory event in the inflammatory process.[61,62]

The research into mechanisms of myocardial infarction has been hampered by the lack of suitable animal models. Most studies on the pathogenesis of infarction have been performed on the hearts of dogs after coronary ligature. Obviously, the events following coronary ligature may be quite different from those occurring during plaque activation and thrombosis.

We observed that apoE-KO mice that had been on atherogenic diets for more than 8–9 months showed cardiac scars reminiscent of healed infarcts. This suggested to us that hypercholesterolemic mice may develop coronary atherosclerosis and myocardial infarction. An angiographic and histologic analysis showed coronary stenosis and occluding plaques in apoE$^{-/-}$ × LDLR$^{-/-}$ mice that had been fed 0.15% cholesterol for more than 8 months.[63] Such mice were then exposed to a mental stress test while monitored for ECG changes by telemetric surveillance. In such mice, mental stress led to significant STU depressions concomitant with leakage of the intracellular myocardial protein, troponin T, to the systemic circulation.[63] Histological analysis showed loss of dehydrogenase activity.[63] These findings support the conclusion that the mice developed myocardial infarction when exposed to the stress test.

To further characterize the process leading from coronary atherosclerosis to myocardial infarction, we exposed anesthetized apoE$^{-/-}$ × LDLR$^{-/-}$ mice to hypoxia.[63] A few minutes of hypoxia (10% oxygen in the ventilator) led to STU segment elevations reminiscent of those occurring in myocardial infarction in man, troponin T leakage, and loss of dehydrogenase activity. All these changes could be prevented by pretreatment with an endothelin A receptor blocker. This indicates that hypoxia elicits myocardial infarction in hypercholesterolemic mice by causing endothelin-dependent vasoconstriction in the atherosclerotic coronary artery.[63] It will now be important to identify other mediators involved in the process leading from silent coronary atherosclerosis to acute myocardial infarction, and to determine whether interference with such mediators can be used to prevent or treat myocardial infarction.

CONCLUSIONS

A large number of experimental and clinical studies have established that the immune system plays an important pathogenetic role in atherosclerosis. Current data imply innate immunity as necessary for lesion formation and this has led investigators to conclude that atherosclerosis is an inflammatory disease. The role of adaptive immunity is more complex—it is present throughout disease development and general immune defects reduce the extent of disease in experimental models. However, specific defects may have entirely different effects and it is likely that certain effector mechanisms of adaptive immunity are proatherogenic while others may be atheroprotective.

Attempts to treat or prevent atherosclerosis by modulating immune activity have been successful in experimental models. Current interest focuses on specific antigens such as oxLDL, heat shock protein 60, and macromolecular components of *Chlamydia pneumoniae*. In addition, it is possible that modulation of immunologically nonspecific inflammatory reactions may be useful for treating atherosclerosis. Finally, inflammatory markers have already proven to be useful for the diagnosis of active plaques and acute coronary syndromes. All these data imply that the immune system plays an active role in atherosclerosis, which can therefore be viewed as an inflammatory vascular response to a metabolic disturbance.

REFERENCES

1. HANSSON, G.K. 1997. Cell-mediated immunity in atherosclerosis. Curr. Opin. Lipidol. **8:** 301–311.
2. ROSS, R. 1999. Atherosclerosis—an inflammatory disease. N. Engl. J. Med. **340:** 115–126.
3. BRESLOW, J.L. 1996. Mouse models of atherosclerosis. Science **272:** 685–688.
4. PIEDRAHITA, J.A., S.H. ZHANG, J.R. HAGAMAN, P.M. OLIVER & N. MAEDA. 1992. Generation of mice carrying a mutant apolipoprotein E gene inactivated by gene targeting in embryonic stem cells. Proc. Natl. Acad. Sci. USA **89:** 4471–4475.
5. PLUMP, A.S., J.D. SMITH, T. HAYEK *et al.* 1992. Severe hypercholesterolemia and atherosclerosis in apolipoprotein E-deficient mice created by homologous recombination in ES cells. Cell **71:** 343–353.
6. ISHIBASHI, S., J. HERZ, N. MAEDA, J.L. GOLDSTEIN & M.S. BROWN. 1994. The two-receptor model of lipoprotein clearance: Tests of the hypothesis in "knockout" mice lacking the low density lipoprotein receptor, apolipoprotein E, or both proteins. Proc. Natl. Acad. Sci. USA **91:** 4431–4435.
7. DANSKY, H.M., S.A. CHARLTON, M.M. HARPER & J.D. SMITH. 1997. T and B lymphocytes play a minor role in atherosclerotic plaque formation in the apolipoprotein E-deficient mouse. Proc. Natl. Acad. Sci. USA **94:** 4642–4646.
8. GUPTA, S., A.M. PABLO, X.C. JIANG, N. WANG, A.R. TALL & C. SCHINDLER. 1997. IFN-γ potentiates atherosclerosis in apoE knock-out mice. J. Clin. Invest. **99:** 2752–2561.
9. MOSMANN, T.R. & S. SAD. 1996. The expanding universe of T-cell subsets: Th1, Th2 and more. Immunol. Today **17(3):** 138–146.

10. ZHOU, X., G. PAULSSON, S. STEMME & G.K. HANSSON. 1998. Hypercholesterolemia is associated with a Th1/Th2 switch of the autoimmune response in atherosclerotic apo E-knockout mice. J. Clin. Invest. **101:** 1717–1725.
11. PAIGEN, B., A. MORROW, C. BRANDON, D. MITCHELL & P.A. HOLMES. 1985. Variation in susceptibility to atherosclerosis among inbred strains of mice. Atherosclerosis **57:** 65–73.
12. NICOLETTI, A., S. KAVERI, G. CALIGIURI, J. BARIÉTY & G.K. HANSSON. 1998. Immunoglobulin treatment reduces atherosclerosis in apo E knockout mice. J. Clin. Invest. **102:** 910–918.
13. KAZATCHKINE, N.M. & S.V. KAVERI. 1999. Immunomodulation of autoimmune disease with normal polyspecific immunoglobulin G (intravenous immunoglobulin). *In* The Decade of Autoimmunity. Y. Shoenfeld, Ed.: 409–419. Elsevier. Amsterdam.
14. MACH, F., U. SCHONBECK, G.K. SUKHOVA, T. BOURCIER, J.Y. BONNEFOY, J.S. POBER & P. LIBBY. 1997. Functional CD40 ligand is expressed on human vascular endothelial cells, smooth muscle cells, and macrophages—implications for CD40-CD40 ligand signaling in atherosclerosis. Proc. Natl. Acad. Sci. USA **94:** 1931–1936.
15. MACH, F., U. SCHONBECK, G. K. SUKHOVA, E. ATKINSON & P. LIBBY. 1997. Reduction of atherosclerosis in mice by inhibition of CD40 signalling. Nature **394:** 200–203.
16. STEINBERG, D. 1997. Low density lipoprotein oxidation and its pathobiological significance. J. Biol. Chem. **272:** 20963–20966.
17. WATSON, A.D., N. LEITINGER, M. NAVAB, K.F. FAULL, S. HÖRKKÖ, J.L. WITZTUM, W. PALINSKI, D. SCHWENKE, R.G. SALOMON, W. SHA, G. SUBBANAGOUNDER, A.M. FOGELMAN & J.A. BERLINER. 1997. Structural identification by mass spectrometry of oxidized phospholipids in minimally oxidized low density lipoprotein that induce monocyte/endothelial interactions and evidence for their presence in vivo. J. Biol. Chem. **272:** 3597–13607.
18. NAVAB, M., J.A. BERLINER, A.D. WATSON *et al.* 1996. The Yin and Yang of oxidation in the development of the fatty streak. A review based on the 1994 George Lyman Duff Memorial Lecture. Arterioscler. Thromb. Vasc. Biol. **16(7):** 831–842.
19. KUME, N., M.I. CYBULSKY & M.A. GIMBRONE. 1992. Lysophosphatidylcholine, a component of atherogenic lipoproteins, induces mononuclear leukocyte adhesion molecules in cultured human and rabbit arterial endothelial cells. J. Clin. Invest. **90:** 1138–1144.
20. MATTSSON-HULTÉN, L., H. LINDMARK, U. DICZFALUSY, I. BJÖRKHEM, M. OTTOSSON, Y. LIU, G. BONDJERS & O. WIKLUND. 1996. Oxysterols present in atherosclerotic tissue decrease the expression of lipoprotein lipase messenger RNA in human monocyte-derived macrophages. J. Clin. Invest. **97:** 461–468.
21. SEIFERT, P.S., F. HUGO, J.J. TRANUM, U. ZHRINGER, M. MUHLY & S. BHAKDI. 1990. Isolation and characterization of a complement-activating lipid extracted from human atherosclerotic lesions. J. Exp. Med. **172:** 547–557.
22. PALINSKI, W., S. YLÄ-HERTTUALA, M.E. ROSENFELD *et al.* 1990. Antisera and monoclonal antibodies specific for epitopes generated during oxidative modification of low density lipoprotein. Arterioscl. Thromb. **10:** 325–335.
23. HÖRKKÖ, S., E. MILLER, E. DUDL, P. REAVEN, L.K. CURTISS, N.J. ZVAIFLER, R. TERKELTAUB, S.S. PIERANGELI, D.W. BRANCH, W. PALINSKI & J.L. WITZTUM. 1996. Antiphospholipid antibodies are directed against epitopes of oxidized phospholipids. Recognition of cardiolipin by monoclonal antibodies to epitopes of oxidized low density lipoprotein. J. Clin. Invest. **98:** 815–825.
24. YLÄ-HERTTUALA, S., W. PALINSKI, M.E. ROSENFELD *et al.* 1989. Evidence for the presence of oxidatively modified low density lipoprotein in atherosclerotic lesions of rabbit and man. J. Clin. Invest. **84:** 1086–1095.
25. WITZTUM, J.L. & D. STEINBERG. 1991. Role of oxidized low density lipoprotein in atherogenesis. J. Clin. Invest. **88:** 1785–1792.
26. GRIFFITH, R.L., G.T. VIRELLA, H.C. STEVENSON & V.M. LOPES. 1988. Low density lipoprotein metabolism by human macrophages activated with low density lipoprotein immune complexes. A possible mechanism of foam cell formation. J. Exp. Med. **168:** 1041–1059.

27. HOLVOET, P., G. PEREZ, Z. ZHAO, E. BROUWERS, H. BEMAR & D. COLLEN. 1995. Malondialdehyde modified low density lipoprotein in patients with atherosclerotic disease. J. Clin. Invest. **95:** 2611–2619.
28. PALINSKI, W., S. HÖRKKÖ, E. MILLER *et al.* 1996. Cloning of monoclonal autoantibodies to epitopes of oxidized lipoproteins from apolipoprotein E-deficient mice. Demonstration of epitopes of oxidized low density lipoprotein in human plasma. J. Clin. Invest. **98**(3): 800–814.
29. STEMME, S., J. HOLM & G.K. HANSSON. 1992. T lymphocytes in human atherosclerotic plaques are memory cells expressing CD45RO and the integrin VLA-1. Arterioscl. Thromb. **12:** 206–211.
30. PAULSSON, G., X. ZHOU, E. TÖRNQUIST & G.K. HANSSON. 2000. Oligoclonal T cell expansions in atherosclerotic lesions of apoE-deficient mice. Arterioscler. Thromb. Vasc. Biol. **20:** 10–17.
31. FREIGANG, S., S. HÖRKKÖ, E. MILLER, J.L. WITZTUM & W. PALINSKI. 1998. Immunization of LDL receptor-deficient mice with homologous malondialdehyde-modified and native LDL reduces progression of atherosclerosis by mechanisms other than induction of high titers of antibodies to oxidative neoepitopes. Arterioscl. Thromb. Vasc. Biol. **18:** 1972–1982.
32. STEMME, S., L. RYMO & G.K. HANSSON. 1991. Polyclonal origin of T lymphocytes in human atherosclerotic plaques. Lab. Invest. **65**(654): 654–660.
33. SWANSON, S.J., A. ROSENZWEIG, J.G. SEIDMAN & P. LIBBY. 1994. Diversity of T-cell antigen receptor V—gene utilization in advanced human atheroma. Arterioscl. Thromb. **14:** 1210–1214.
34. NICOLETTI, A., G. CALIGIURI, I. TÖRNBERG, K. KODAMA, S. STEMME & G.K. HANSSON. 1999. The macrophage scavenger receptor type A directs modified proteins to antigen presentation. Eur. J. Immunol. **29:** 512–521.
35. SALONEN, J.T., S. YLÄ-HERTTUALA, R. YAMAMOTO *et al.* 1992. Autoantibody against oxidized LDL and progression of carotid atherosclerosis. Lancet **339:** 883–887.
36. BERGMARK, C., R. WU, U. DE FAIRE, A.K. LEFVERT & J. SWEDENBORG. 1995. Patients with early-onset peripheral vascular disease have increased levels of autoantibodies against oxidized LDL. Arterioscler. Thromb. Vasc. Biol. **15:** 441–445.
37. PALINSKI, W., E. MILLER & J.L. WITZTUM. 1995. Immunization of low density lipoprotein (LDL) receptor-deficient rabbits with homologous malondialdehyde-modified LDL reduces atherogenesis. Proc. Natl. Acad. Sci. USA **92:** 821–825.
38. AMELI, S., A. HULTGÅRDH-NILSSON, J. REGNSTRÖM *et al.* 1996. Effect of immunization with homologous LDL and oxidized LDL on early atherosclerosis in hypercholesterolemic rabbits. Arterioscl. Thromb. Vasc. Biol. **16:** 1074–1079.
39. GEORGE, J., A. AFEK, B. GILBURD, H. LEVKOVITZ, A. SHAISH, I. GOLDBERG, Y. KOPOLOVIC, G. WICK, Y. SHOENFELD & D. HARATS. 1998. Hyperimmunization of apo-E-deficient mice with homologous malondialdehyde low-density lipoprotein suppresses early atherogenesis. Atherosclerosis **138:** 147–152.
40. WICK, G., G. SCHETT, A. AMBERGER, R. KLEINDIENST & Q. XU. 1995. Is atherosclerosis an immunologically mediated disease? Immunol. Today **16:** 27–33.
41. MAYR, M., B. METZLER, S. KIECHL, J. WILLEIT, G. SCHETT, Q. XU & G. WICK. 1999. Endothelial cytotoxicity mediated by serum antibodies to heat shock proteins of *Escherichia coli* and *Chlamydia pneumoniae*: immune reactions to heat shock proteins as a possible link between infection and atherosclerosis. Circulation **99:** 1560–1566.
42. KUO, C.C., A.M. GOWN, E.P. BENDITT & J.T. GRAYSTON. 1993. Detection of *Chlamydia pneumoniae* in aortic lesions of atherosclerosis by immunocytochemical stain. Arterioscl. Thromb. **13:** 1501–1504.
43. MUHLESTEIN, J.B., J.L. ANDERSON, E.H. HAMMOND, L. ZHAO, S. TREHAN, E.P. SCHWOBE & J.F. CARLQUIST. 1998. Infection with *Chlamydia pneumoniae* accelerates the development of atherosclerosis and treatment with azithromycin prevents it in a rabbit model. Circulation **24:** 633–636.
44. MOAZED, T.C., L.A. CAMPBELL, M.E. ROSENFELD, J.T. GRAYSTON & C.C. KUO. *Chlamydia pneumoniae* infection accelerates the progression of atherosclerosis in apolipoprotein E-deficient mice. J. Infect. Dis. **180:** 238–241.

45. HU, H., G.N. PIERCE & G. ZHONG. 1999. The atherogenic effects of chlamydia are dependent on serum cholesterol and are specific to *Chlamydia pneumoniae*. J. Clin. Invest. **103**: 747–753.
46. VAN DER WAL, A.C., A.E. BECKER, C.M. VAN DER LOOS & P.K. DAS. 1994. Site of intimal rupture or erosion of thrombosed coronary atherosclerotic plaques is characterized by an inflammatory process irrespective of the dominant plaque morphology. Circulation **89**(1): 36–44.
47. DAVIES, M.J., N. WOOLF, P. ROWLES & P.D. RICHARDSON. 1994. Lipid and cellular constituents of unstable human aortic plaques. Basic Res. Cardiol. **1**: 33–40.
48. MORENO, P.R., E. FALK, I.F. PALACIOS, J.B. NEWELL, V. FUSTER & J.T. FALLON. 1994. Macrophage infiltration in acute coronary syndromes. Implications for plaque rupture. Circulation **90**(2): 775–778.
49. KAARTINEN, M., A. PENTTILÄ & P.T. KOVANEN. 1994. Accumulation of activated mast cells in the shoulder region of human coronary atheroma, the predilection site of atheromatous rupture. Circulation **90**: 1669–1678.
50. FALK, E., P. SHAH & V. FUSTER. 1995. Coronary plaque disruption. Circulation **92**: 657–671.
51. LIBBY, P. 1995. Molecular bases of the acute coronary syndromes. Circulation **91**: 2844–2850.
52. LIBBY, P., G.K. HANSSON & J.S. POBER. 199. Atherogenesis and inflammation. *In* Molecular Basis of Cardiovascular Disease. K.R. Chien, Ed.: 349–366. W.B. Saunders. Philadelphia.
53. DAVIES, M.J. & A. THOMAS. 1985. Plaque fissuring—the cause of acute myocardial infarction, sudden ischaemic death and crescendo angina. Br. Heart J. **53**: 363–373.
54. SCHEIBENBOGEN, C., H. MOSER, S. KRAUSE & R. ANDREESEN. 1992. Interferon-γ–induced expression of tissue factor activity during human monocyte to macrophage maturation. Haemostasis **22**: 173–178.
55. MARMUR, J.D., M. ROSSIKHINA, A. GUHA *et al.* 1993. Tissue factor is rapidly induced in arterial smooth muscle after balloon injury. J. Clin. Invest. **91**: 2253–2259.
56. CONWAY, E.M., R. BACH, R.D. ROSENBERG & W.H. KONIGSBERG. 1989. Tumor necrosis factor enhances expression of tissue factor MRNA in endothelial cells. Thromb. Res. **53**(3): 231–241.
57. DAVIES, M.J. 1996. Stability and instability: two faces of coronary atherosclerosis. Circulation **94**: 2013–2020.
58. LIUZZO, G., L.M. BIASUCCI, J.R. GALLIMORE *et al.* 1994. Prognostic value of C-reactive protein and plasma amyloid A protein in severe unstable angina. N. Engl. J. Med. **331**: 417–424.
59. LIUZZO, G., L.M. BIASUCCI, A.G. REBUZZI, R. GALLIMORE, G. CALIGIURI, G.A. LANZA, G. QUARANTA, C. MONACO, M.B. PEPYS & A. MASERI. 1996. Plasma protein acute-phase response in unstable angina is not induced by ischemic injury. Circulation **94**: 2373–2380.
60. MASERI, A. Inflammation, atherosclerosis, and ischemic events—exploring the hidden side of the moon. N. Engl. J. Med. **336**: 1014–1016.
61. NERI SERNERI, G.G., R. ABBATE, A.M. GORI *et al.* 1992. Transient intermittent lymphocyte activation is responsible for the instability of angina. Circulation **86**: 790–797.
62. CALIGIURI, G., F. SUMMARIA, G. LIUZZO & A. MASERI. 1996. Time course of T-lymphocyte activation and of C-reactive protein in unstable angina: relation to prognosis. Circulation **94**(Suppl, 1): I-571.
63. CALIGIURI, G., B. LÉVY, J. PERNOW, P. THORÉN & G.K. HANSSON. 1999. Myocardial infarction mediated by endothelin receptor signaling in hypercholesterolemic mice. Proc. Natl. Acad. Sci. USA **96**: 6920–6924.

Questions and Answers

P. LIBBY (*Brigham and Women's Hospital, Boston, MA, USA*): You are making rapid progress on so many fronts and it is hard to know where to start. I think it will be very informative to look at the brains of the elderly apoE mice that have been stressed in your experiment for two reasons: one is that you are not increasing the oxygen demand with this stress, because it is a mixed model of supply-and-demand change, and it is hard to get a handle around it physiologically for that reason. The second reason is that there may also be a contributing atheroembolic event from the very severe proximal disease that these animals get. Stroke is a very important problem and this model may provide useful new information.

HANSSON: It is a very good point. We see occasional strokes. It does not occur as reproducibly as myocardial infarction. I absolutely agree, it will be important to look into that.

G.M. RUBANYI (*Berlex Biosciences, Richmond, VA, USA*): Excellent model; we were all looking for something like that. Have you tried anticoagulants/antithrombotics? Would they prevent any of these events? An ETA receptor antagonist would be suggesting, but not proving a vasospastic component. And the follow-up is, have you looked at angiogenesis, whether or not you lose collaterals, and whether that is what causes the events?

HANSSON: We are doing the anticoagulant experiments right now. I agree it also would be important to look at angiogenesis. We have stored the tissue for it, but we have not had a chance to look into it yet.

J.H. CAMPBELL (*University of Queensland, Brisbane, Australia*): Your smooth muscle cells present oxidized LDL to T lymphocytes by the same mechanism as macrophages, i.e., taking them up through the scavenger receptor as you showed today. What is the relative importance of smooth muscle cells versus macrophages as antigen-presenting cells in the inflammatory response of atherosclerosis?

HANSSON: That question has been a controversy for 10 years now. It is clear that the smooth muscle cells cannot present antigens to naive T cells and start an immune response. They don't seem to be very good at presenting to memory cells or cells that have already been activated either. There is even a suggestion that they may produce an inhibitor of T cell activation. There may also be a lack of co-factors but it looks like, depending on the exact culture conditions, they may cause an inhibition or a slight stimulation as third-party cells. However, they don't seem to be good at presenting antigen. Whether they somehow influence macrophage–T cell interaction is still an open question, I believe.

M.A. GIMBRONE (*Brigham and Women's Hospital, Boston, MA, USA*): I enjoyed every part of your presentation. I just want to focus on the middle part of your talk and the use of the word "immunity," which usually has a connotation of memory and specificity. Are the phenomena that you are describing to us specific and do they imply a "memory" in the sense that immune mechanisms typically are called such?

HANSSON: I would say that there is indirect, but not direct, evidence for that. In several experimental models, protection against atherosclerosis is paralleled by increased titers of the oxidized LDL antibodies and cellular immune response to oxidized LDL. It can be accomplished by transferring cells that carry adaptive immunity; now we would like to substitute for these cells a specific antibody or some kind of more purified antigen-specific lymphocyte.

GIMBRONE: That is a very specific way to go. I am just concerned about the general context in which we often discuss this. Cytokines, which were originally described as short-range messages between cells of the immune system, clearly are neither specific to the immune system nor are they conferring messages or effects that are necessarily immunity per se. Many cells can make cytokines. Certain cells of the immune system are professional makers of cytokines. How much of this will turn out to be immunity in the classic sense, and how much of this will be cytokine milieu in a more cell-biological sense?

HANSSON: My guess is that cytokines as effectors of the immune response will turn out to be important in this situation. But it is unlikely that transfer of cytokines would confer protection in the experiments I mentioned.

G.S. GETZ (*University of Chicago, Chicago, IL, USA*): Did you notice any change in the lipids when you did splenectomy or adoptive transfer?

HANSSON: No significant effect on cholesterol levels in the mice

A.R. TALL (*Columbia University, New York, NY, USA*): Have you had a chance to look at whether there is a change in T cell population in the immnuoprotected mice? Do they get more Th1 T cells in their lesions?

HANSSON: We have not been able to stain Th1 cells in lesions yet. We are trying to look by RTPCR.

S. HORIUCHI (*Kumamoto University, Kumamoto, Japan*): Your immune response is dramatically decreased when the knock-out mice were MSR knock-out mice. We have observed that macrophages from MSR knock-out mice have decreased adhesiveness to the vessel wall or other cells. Could your decrease in the immune response be explained by this decreased adhesiveness to T lymphocytes?

HANSSON: I don't think so. All our data fit with a role for SR-A in the processing of antigen. I believe that other mechanisms like ICAM and CD4 hooking on to the T cell receptors, etc. would be sufficient to put the cells in close contact for a long enough time to cause activation.

S. HORIUCHI: Autoantibodies against the oxidized LDL have been reported. Maybe your experiments really show that. Can you make antibody specific to oxidized BSA when you use oxidized BSA instead of oxidized LDL?

HANSSON: We do not have any data regarding that possibility.

Inflammation and Atherosclerosis
Atherosclerotic Lesions in Takayasu Arteritis

FUJIO NUMANO,[a] YUKIO KISHI, AKIRA TANAKA, MIHO OHKAWARA, TSUNEKAZU KAKUTA, AND YASUSHI KOBAYASHI

Third Department of Internal Medicine, Tokyo Medical and Dental University, Tokyo, Japan

ABSTRACT: Takayasu arteritis is a chronic vasculitis, mainly involving the aorta and its main branches as well as the coronary and pulmonary arteries, causing stenosis and/or obstruction due to thrombus formation or dilatation due to aneurysmal formation and/or rupture of the involved arteries. These characteristic anomalies resulted from ischemia of retinal arteries due to the obstruction of cervical vessels. In Western countries this disease is also known as "pulseless disease," because the pulse is frequently absent due to the obstruction of subclavian or brachial arteries. The pathogenesis of this morbid condition is still unknown. Epidemiologically, it is found mostly in female patients and is more prevalent in Asian and Latin American countries. Affected areas consist of a mixture of both active, productive inflammatory lesions, and old fibrous lesions. Autoimmune processes stimulated by viral infection and other unknown causative factors may play an important role under these pathophysiological conditions because HLA analysis revealed a statistically significant high frequency of haplotype A24-B52-DR2 in these patients in Japan. Documentation of atherosclerotic complications in young female patients with Takayasu arteritis who are generally free from traditional atherosclerosis risk factors may be clinical evidence that inflammation is indeed an important risk factor in atherogenesis.

INTRODUCTION

Recent progress in vascular biology has made great contributions to the elucidation of atherogenesis and consequently to the development of new therapeutic approaches for atherosclerotic disorders.[1–3] It could be said that this new world began with the discoveries of thromboxane A_2 by Samuelsson and colleagues in 1974[4,5] and platelet-derived growth factor (PDGF) by Ross in 1975.[6,7] In fact, the discovery of thromboxane A_2 marks the beginning of the exploration of the relationship between platelets and vascular endothelium in thrombogenesis. Research on PDGF and the subsequent discovery of various cytokines in atherogenesis[8,9] led to the current focus on the role of inflammation in atherogenesis.[1,10–12] Observing an increased level of C-reactive protein and leukocytosis in patients with unstable angina pectoris, Maseri studied the relationship between inflammation and severity of atherosclerosis. Although he could not find a positive relationship, he stressed that the

---

[a]Address for correspondence: Fujio Numano, M.D., Professor of Internal Medicine, Tokyo Medical and Dental University, 1-5-45 Yushima, Bunkyo-ku, Tokyo 113-8519, Japan. Voice: 81-3-5803-5224; fax: 81-3-5684-2033.
numano.med3@med.tmd.ac.jp

inflammation had a great influence on atherosclerosis and/or angina attacks in these patients.[13] Through his brilliant achievement in the field of vascular biology, Ross also concluded that atherosclerosis is an inflammatory disease.[1]

INFLAMMATION AND ATHEROSCLEROSIS

The story of the role of inflammation in atherosclerosis began in the first years of the twentieth century. Virchow proposed an important role of inflammation in atherogenesis,[14,15] but, his theory was not supported by the subsequent experimental discovery by Anitichow that rabbits fed with egg yolk developed atherosclerotic lesions in their aortas.[16] Based on this report, the lipid theory became the leading concept of atherogenesis for a very long time.[17,18]

However, there have been many papers dealing with the relationship between inflammation and atherosclerosis in the history of atherosclerotic research. In 1915, Albutt reported the existence of inflammatory cells around the vasa vasorum beneath human atherosclerotic lesions. Schwartz also found a positive relationship between inflammatory changes in adventitia and the severity of atherosclerosis.[20] Fabricum suggested the important roles of virus infection in atherosclerosis and Minich succeeded in experimentally inducing atherosclerosis in rabbits infected by herpes virus.[21–23]

Observing edematous changes in arteries of rabbits treated by endotoxin, Shimamoto and colleagues proposed an important role for vascular injury caused by substances including inflammatory ones.[24,25] Numano and colleagues experimentally confirmed that thromboxane A_2 induces vascular damage in rabbits and that substances preventing such vascular injury, including anti–thromboxane A_2 substance, have a preventive effect against experimentally induced atherosclerosis.[26–28]

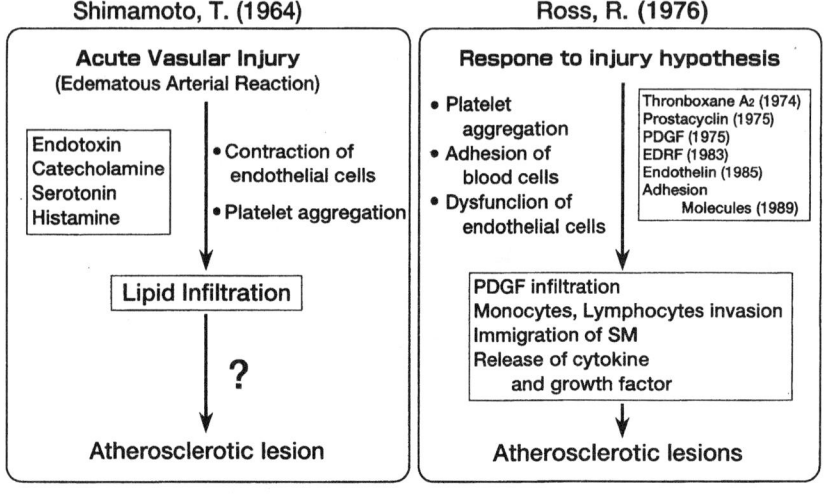

FIGURE 1. How atherosclerosis develops from vascular injury.

After discovering PDGF, as well as other growth factors and cytokines in macrophages and/or vascular smooth muscles, Ross proposed the important role of "response to vascular injury" in atherogenesis.[7] He has greatly contributed to the elucidation of how atherosclerosis can develop from vascular injury (FIG. 1).

TAKAYASU ARTERITIS

Takayasu arteritis is a chronic vasculitis, mainly involving the aorta and its main branches as well as the coronary and pulmonary arteries, causing stenosis and/or obstruction due to thrombus formation or dilatation due to aneurysmal formation and/or rupture of the involved arteries[29,30] (FIG. 2).

This disease has been called Takayasu arteritis in honor of Mikito Takayasu who was the first to report peculiar anastomosis of blood vessels in the optic fundi in a young female patient.[31] It was found shortly thereafter that these characteristic anomalies resulted from ischemia of retinal arteries due to the obstruction of cervical vessels. In Western countries this disease is also known as "pulseless disease," because the pulse is frequently absent due to the obstruction of subclavian or brachial arteries[33] (FIG. 3).

The pathogenesis of this morbid condition is still unknown. Epidemiologically, it is found mostly in female patients and is more prevalent in Asian and Latin American countries.[29,30]

Takayasu arteritis is characterized histologically as a "panarteritis," involving all layers of the arterial wall, including intimal fibrous thickening and/or typical atheromatous lesions, destruction of medial smooth muscles and elastic layers, cellular infiltration and collagenous fibrosis in the media and thickened adventitia with cellular infiltration around vasa vasorum[35] (FIG. 4). Pathological studies usually reveal intact areas between affected areas in arteries ("skipped lesion"). Affected areas consist of a mixture of both active, productive inflammatory lesions, and old fibrous lesions. However, more recent studies report disappearance of the skipped lesions and, in turn, development of atherosclerotic lesion.[34,35]

These inflammatory lesions originate in the vasa vasorum and are followed by cellular infiltration mainly composed of T cells invading the outer layer of the media and/or its neighboring adventitia[35] (FIGS. 5 and 6). At this stage, positive production of inflammatory cytokines and/or adhesion molecules around these areas is remarkable, suggesting a chemotactive activity of T cell and monocytes.[36]

Autoimmune processes stimulated by viral infection and other unknown causative factors may play an important role under these pathophysiological conditions because HLA analysis revealed a statistically significant high frequency of haplotype A24-B52-DR2 in these patients in Japan.[29,35,37,38] Destruction of medial smooth muscles and elastic fibers follows in the media and rapid progress of these changes occasionally result in aneurysmal formation and/or dissecting aneurysm.

Once the intima is invaded by inflammatory changes, such as cellular infiltration and/or migration of smooth muscle cells, edematous changes are encountered in the intima, which are naturally followed by infiltration of various substances like lipids and blood cells, including monocytes from the bloodstream (FIG. 7). In fact, as shown in FIGURE 8, we sometimes observe characteristic intimal change in typical smooth muscle cell proliferation with irregular fibrous changes. This characteristic histological feature is called "arteriocirrhosis."

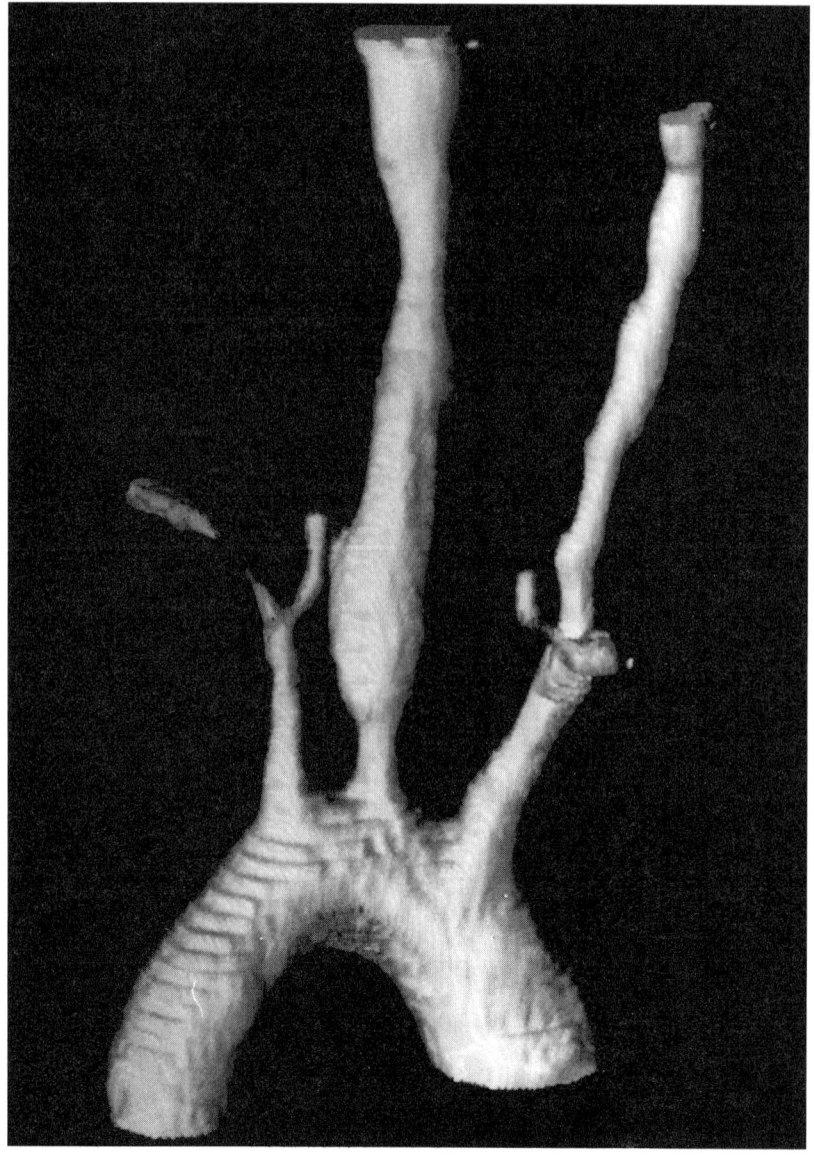

FIGURE 2. Three-dimensional computed tomograph of cervical arteries in a 24-year-old male with Takayasu arteritis.

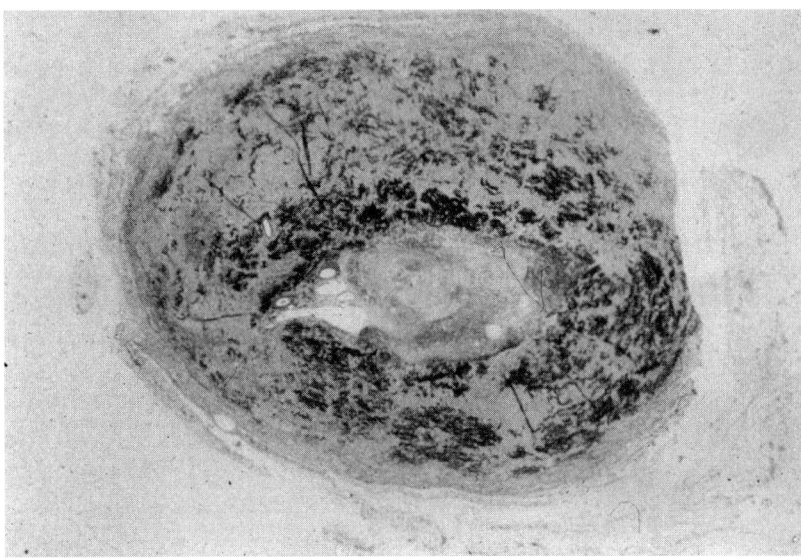

FIGURE 3. Obstruction by organized thrombus of an axillary artery in a 52-year-old female with Takayasu arteritis.

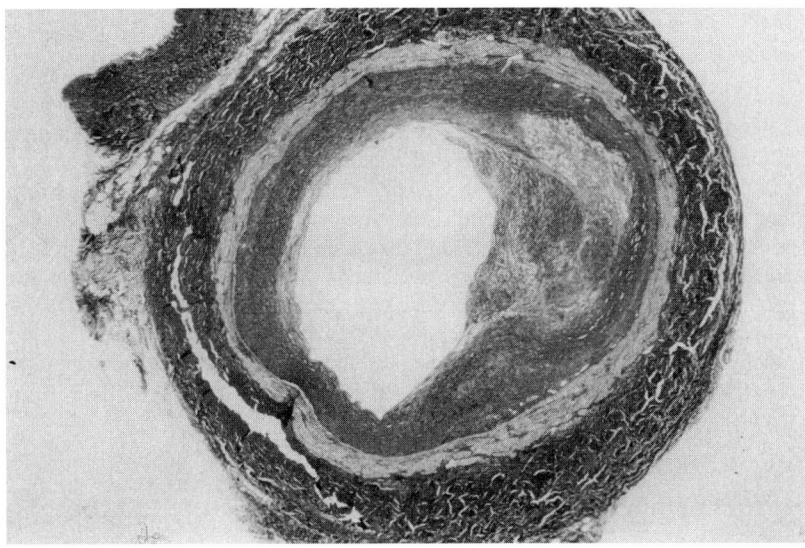

FIGURE 4. Subclavian artery of a 48-year-old female with Takayasu arteritis (Azan-Mallory staining, ×10). Note: Fibrous change in thickened intima with typical atherosclerotic lesions, destruction of medial layer, and thickened adventitia.

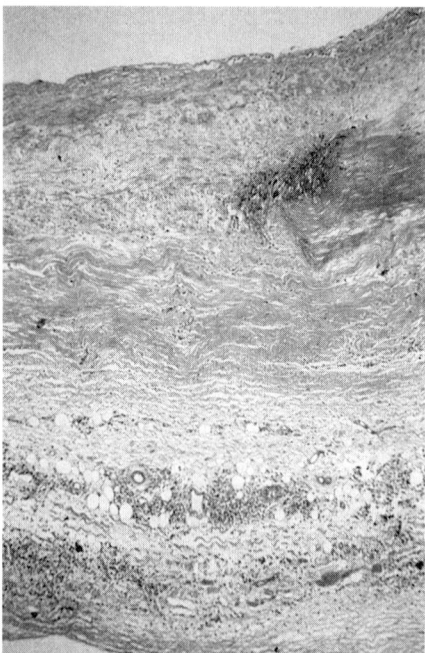

FIGURE 5. Aorta of a 48-year-old female with Takayasu arteritis (HE staining, ×5). Note: Cellular infiltration from adventitia through media and to intima.

At present, early diagnosis has become easier due to MRI, CT and other diagnostic modalities, and thereby facilitating treatment at an early stage. As a result, the prognosis for this morbid condition has improved remarkably and most patients can enjoy an added ten to twenty years of life, although they do not reach normal Japanese life expectancy. Thus, atherosclerotic disorders are now becoming more serious complications than ever among patients with Takayasu arteritis (FIG. 9). FIGURE 10 demonstrates typical atherosclerotic changes found in the thoracic aorta of a 52-year-old patient with Takayasu arteritis who died of rupture of the ascending aorta.

At this late stage, it is rather difficult to differentiate Takayasu arteritis and atherosclerotic lesions. The important aspects in differentiating both diseases are the destruction and fibrous changes in the medial layer, typical cellular infiltration and/or thickened adventitia in Takayasu arteritis (FIG. 4).

INFLAMMATION AS RISK FACTOR OF ATHEROSCLEROSIS

Takayasu arteritis is characterized by a high prevalence in young females. Ross and McKusick once called this disease "young female arteritis."[39] In Japan, 89% of patients are female and many of them were in their twenties.[40,41] Most of these patients are found to be nonsmokers with normolipidemia, free from diabetes mellitus,

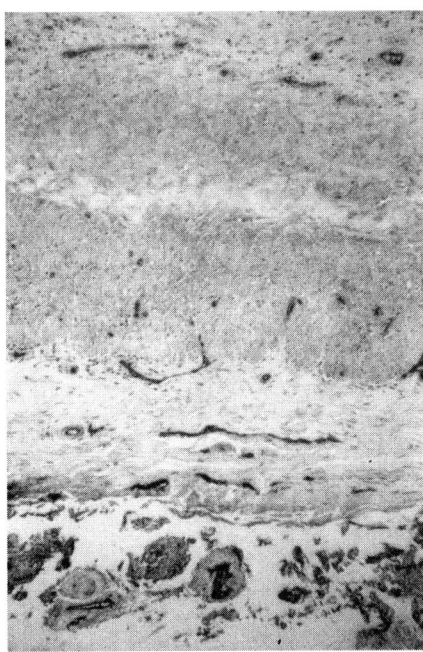

FIGURE 6. MCP-1 activity in vasa vasorum in the aorta of a 48-year-old female with Takayasu arteritis (Immunohistochemical staining, ×5).

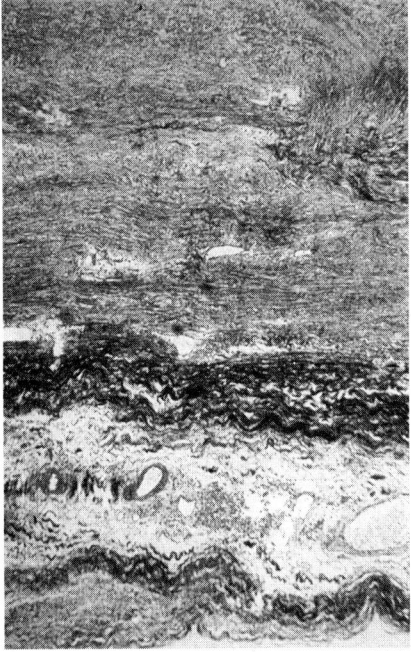

FIGURE 7. Aortic wall of a 42-year-old female (Azan-Mallory staining, ×7). Note: Cellular infiltration is remarkable around vasa vasorum in adventitia and in media.

72   ANNALS NEW YORK ACADEMY OF SCIENCES

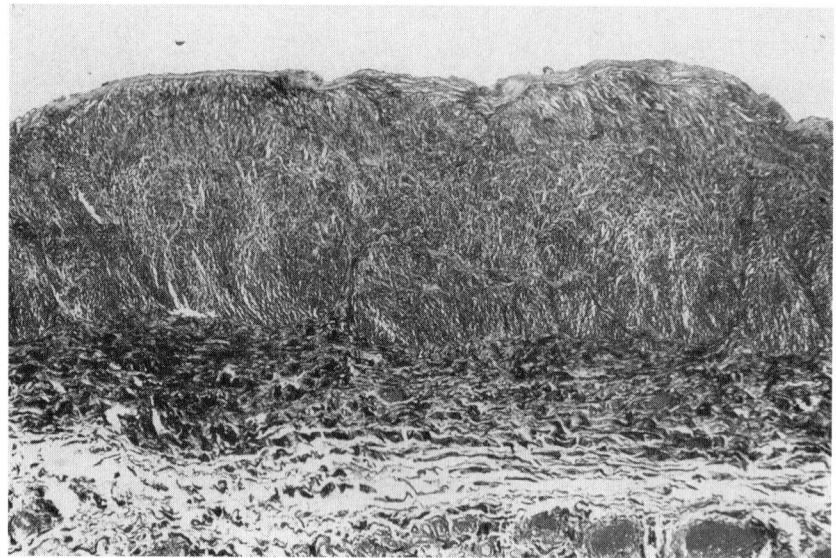

FIGURE 8. Subclavian artery of a 42-year-old female with Takayasu arteritis (Azan-Mallory staining, ×45). Note: Smooth muscle cell proliferation in intima with irregular fibrous networks, representative of "arteriocirrhosis." Complete destruction of medial layer, replaced by fibrosis, and thickened adventitia.

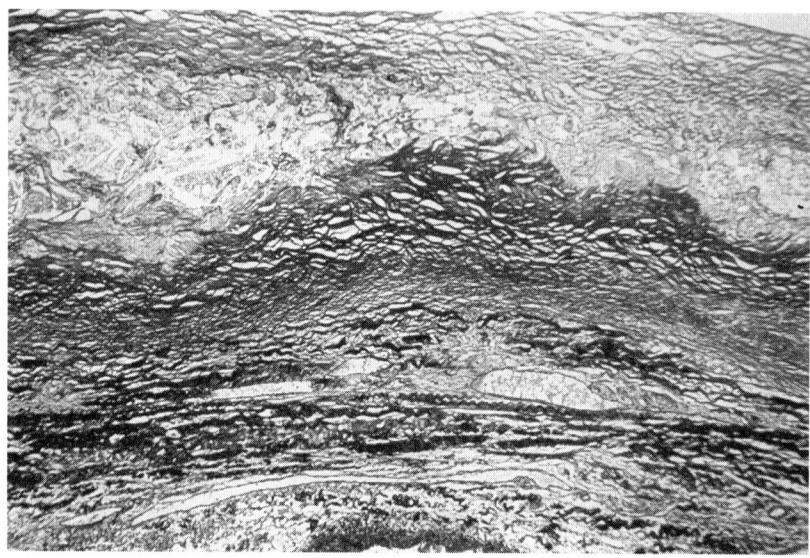

FIGURE 9. Arterial atherosclerotic lesion of a 42-year-old male with Takayasu arteritis (Azan-Mallory staining, ×45).

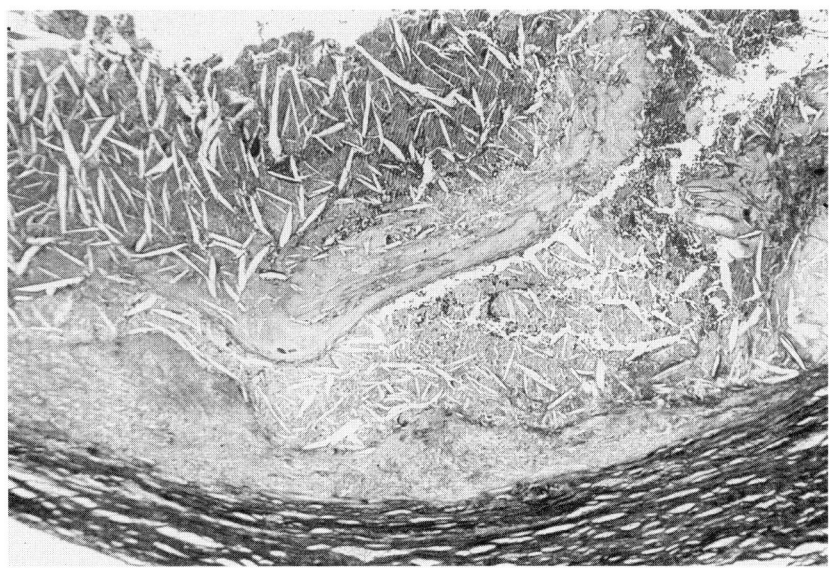

FIGURE 10. Dissected typical atheromatous lesions in the aortic wall of a 52-year-old female with Takayasu arteritis (Azan-Mallory staining, ×7).

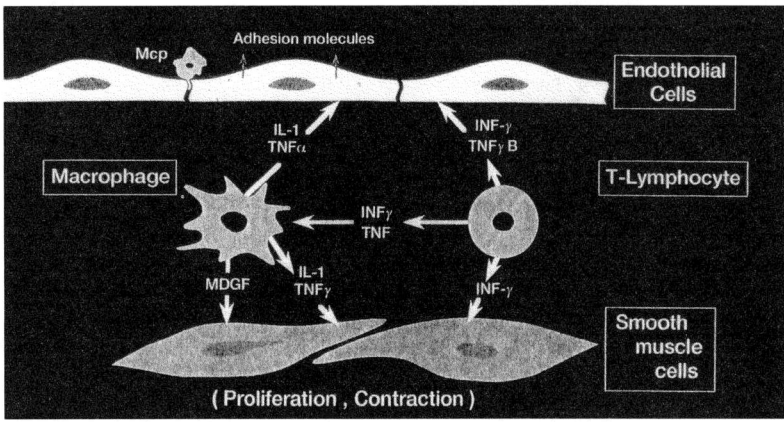

FIGURE 11. Inflammatory cells and cytokines in the pathogenesis of atherosclerosis.

and with normal blood pressure (unless renovascular hypertension due to renal arteritis is present). They also experience regular menstruation and occasionally present with hyperestrogenism.[42] Thus, there are usually no risk factors for atherosclerosis. Nevertheless atherosclerotic lesions were frequently found at autopsy in these patients, strongly suggesting that inflammation is an important risk factor in the causation and progression of atherosclerosis. Confirming T cells and leukocytes found by Stary in early lesions of infant aortas, suggested an important role for inflammation in the initiation and progression of atherosclerosis.[43,44] More recently, much progress in vascular biology clearly demonstrated significant roles of cytokines produced by endothelial cells, smooth muscle cells, macrophages, and even lymphocytes in the progression of atherosclerosis[1,2,8] (FIG. 11)—further stressing the importance of the process of inflammation in the arterial wall. Though many papers experimentally demonstrated the role of inflammation, it is very difficult to confirm this role clinically because of the many risk factors, such as hypertension, diabetes mellitus, and hyperlipidemia, simultaneously present. Documentation of atherosclerotic complications in young female patients with Takayasu arteritis who are generally free from such risk factors may be clinical evidence that inflammation is indeed an important risk factor in atherogenesis.

THE ADVENTITIA AND ATHEROSCLEROSIS

These processes may also focus on the role of the adventitia and/or vasa vasorum in atherosclerosis. As mentioned earlier, several papers dealt with a positive correlation between atherosclerotic lesions and adventitial inflammation. Prescott and colleagues showed that placing an endotoxin-soaked thread in the adventitia along the rat femoral artery was followed by leukocyte migration into the vessel wall from both the luminal and adventitial sides, and within a week by the appearance of smooth muscle cell–rich vascular lesions on the luminal surface adjacent to the thread.[45,46] She also observed that concurrent treatment with dexamethasone blocked formation of these lesions. Chignier demonstrated intimal lesions composed of cells morphologically identified as smooth muscle cells at the area in the aorta where the adventitia was surgically removed 30 days earlier.[47] The picture of "arteriocirrhosis" shown in FIGURE 8 may be a clinical demonstration analogous to Prescott's experimental observation.

In Takayasu arteritis, vasa vasorum plays an important role in initiation of the inflammatory process. Injury of endothelial cells in the vasa vasorum causes cellular infiltration out of vasa vasorum and leakage of various inflammatory cytokines. Wilcox observed arteritis, again stressing the role of adventitial inflammation in atherosclerotic disorders.[48,49] Wissler also strongly suggests the importance of combined immunological and lipid imbalance in atherogenesis.[11]

Takayasu arteritis is known for its linkage disequilibrium with HLA genes, which may initiate and accelerate this morbid condition. In addition, viral infection is also strongly suspected as an initial key maker of this disease.[37,38,50] Recently, Weck experimentally produced a gamma-herpes virus–induced vasculitis.[51] These results may be of help in the search for mechanisms by which viral infection or genetic factors could cause atherosclerosis.

REFERENCES

1. ROSS, R. 1999. Atherosclerosis: An inflammatory disease, N. Engl. J. Med. **340:** 115–126.
2. ROSS, R. 1993. The pathogenesis of atherosclerosis—a perspective for the 1990s. Nature **362:** 801–809.

3. BERLINER, J.A, M. NAVAB & A.M. FOGELMA. 1995. Atherosclerosis: Basic mechanisms. Circulation **91:** 2488–2496.
4. HAMBERG, M., J. SVENSSON & B. SAMUELSSON. 1974. Thromboxanes: A new group of biologically active compounds derived from prostaglandin endoperoxides. Proc. Natl. Acad. Sci. USA **72:** 2994–2998.
5. SAMUELSSON, B., M.M. TVASCHLERS, D.G. WALKER & A.M. SELIGMAN. 1976. New trends in prostaglandin research. In Advances in Prostaglandin and Thromboxane Research. B. Samuelsson & R. Paoletti, Eds.: 1–6. Raven Press. New York.
6. ROSS, R., J. GLOMSET, B. KARIYA & L. HARKER. 1974. A platelet-dependent serum factor that stimulates the proliferation of smooth muscle cells in vitro. Proc. Natl. Acad. Sci. USA **71:** 1207–1210.
7. ROSS, R. & J.A. GLOMSET. 1976. The pathogenesis of atherosclerosis. N. Engl. J. Med. **295:** 369–377, 420–425.
8. NUMANO, F. 1984. Cyclic nucleotides, prostaglandins and ischemic heart disease. Adv. Cycl. Nucl. Protein Phosph. Res. **17:** 661–670.
9. LIBBY, P. & R. ROSS. 1996. In Cytokines and Growth Regulatory Molecules in Atherosclerosis and Coronary Artery Disease. Vol. 1. V. Fuster, R. Ross & E.J. Topol, Eds.: 585–594. Lippincott-Raven. Philadelphia.
10. HANSSON, G.K. 1995. Immune and inflammatory mechanisms in pathogenesis of atherosclerosis. J. Atheroscl. Thromb. **1(1):** 6–9.
11. WISSLER, R.W. 1996. PDAY Group. Atheroarteritis: a combined immunological and lipid imbalance. Int. J. Card. **54(1):** 11–23.
12. BLACK, D. & C.F. REILLY. 1997. Inflammatory mechanisms in atherosclerosis. Inflamm. Res. **46:** 237–241.
13. MASER, A. 1997. Inflammation, atherosclerosis and ischemic events: exploring the hidden side of the moon. N. Engl. J. Med. **336:** 1014–1016.
14. VIRCHOW, R. 1852. Über parenchymatose entzundung. Virch. Arch. Path. Anat. **4:** 261–324.
15. BREDT, H. 1969. The morphology of arteriosclerosis. In Atherosclerosis. F.G. Schettler & G.S. Boyd, Eds.: 1–48. Elsevier. Amsterdam.
16. ANITSCKOW, N. & S. CHALALOW. 1913. Über experimentelle cholesterin steatose und ihre bedeutung fur die entstehung einiger pathologischer Prozesse. Path. Anat. **24:** 1–10.
17. NAPOLI, C., F. D'ARMINTO & F.P. MANCINI. 1997. Fatty streak formation occurs in human fetal aortas and is greatly enhanced by maternal hypercholesterolemia. J. Clin. Invest. **100:** 2680–2690.
18. STEINBERG, D. 1997. Low density lipoprotein oxidation and its pathobiological significance. J. Biol. Chem. **272:** 20963–20966.
19. ALBUTT, C. 1915. Diseases of the arteries including angina pectoris. p. 468. Macmillan Co. London.
20. SCHWARTZ, C.J. & J.R.A. MITCHELL. 1962. Cellular infiltration of the human adventitia associated with atheromatous plaques. Circulation **26:** 73–78.
21. FABRICAN, C.G., J. FABRICAN, M.M. LITENTA & C.R. MINICH. 1978. Virus induced atherosclerosis. J. Exp. Med. **148:** 335–340.
22. MINICH, C.R., J. FABRICAN, C.G. FABRICAN & M.M. LIRENTA. 1979. Atherosclerosis induced by infection with a herpes virus. Am. J. Pathol. **6:** 673–706.
23. KANER, R.J. & D.P. HAJJAR. 1996. In Viral Activation of Thrombo-atherosclerosis in Atherosclerosis and Coronary Artery Disease. V. Fuster, R. Ross & E. Topol, Eds.: 569–584. Raven Publishers. Philadelphia
24. SHIMAMOTO, T. 1963. The relationships of edematous reaction in arteries to atherosclerosis and thrombosis. J. Atherosclerosis **3:** 87–102.
25. SHIMAMOTO, T., M. KOBAYASHI & F. NUMANO. 1972. Infiltration of α-globulin, fibrinogen and β-lipoprotein into blood vessel wall by atherogenic stress visualized by immunofluorescence. Proc. Jap. Acad. **49:** 336–341.
26. NUMANO, F. M. YAJIMA, K. NISHIYAMA, K. SHIMOKADO, F. NUMANO, K. SASAGAWA & R. MORIWAKI. 1982. Effect of thromboxane A_2 injection on the rabbits coronary artery. Exp. Mol. Pathol. **37:** 118–132.
27. NUMANO, F. 1980. Chemotherapy of atherosclerosis. Jap. Circ. J. **44:** 55–68.

28. NUMANO, F., H. MAEZAWA, T. SHIMAMOTO & K. ADACHI. 1976. Changes of cyclic-AMP and cyclic-AMP phosphodiesterase in the progression and regression of experimental atherosclerosis. Ann. N.Y. Acad. Sci. **275:** 311–320.
29. NUMANO, F. 1999. Takayasu arteritis—beyond pulselessness. Int. Med. **38:** 226–232.
30. NUMANO, F. & Y. KOBAYASHI. 1996. Takayasu arteritis. Clinical characteristics and the role of genetic factors in its pathogenesis. Vasc. Med. **1:** 227–2633.
31. NUMANO, F. & T. KAKUTA. Takayasu arteritis: five doctors in the history of Takayasu arteritis. Int. J. Card. **54** (1): 1–10.
32. SHIMIZU, K. & K. SANO. 1951. Pulseless disease. J. Neuropathol. Clin. Neurol. **1:** 137–147.
33. OHTA, K. 1940. Eirn seltener, Fall von beiderseitigem Carotis-Subclavia verschluss—Ein Beitrag zur pathologie der Anastomosis peripapillaris des Auges mit fehlendem Radial puls. Trans. Soc. Pathol. Jpn. **30:** 680–690.
34. HOTTCHI, M. 1992. Pathological study on Takayasu arteritis. Heart Vessels Suppl **7:** 11–17.
35. NUMANO, F. 2000. Takayasu arteritis. *In* Inflammatory Diseases of Blood Vessels. G.S. Hoffman & C. Weyand, Eds. Cleveland. In press.
36. NOGUCHI, S., F. NUMANO, M.B. GRAVANIS & J.N. WILCOX. 1998. Increased levels of soluble forms of adhesion molecules in Takayasu arteritis. Int. J. Cardiol. Suppl **1:** 23–33.
37. NUMANO, F., I. ISOHISA, H. MAEZAWA & T. JUJI. 1979. HLA antigens in Takayasu's disease. Amer. Heart J. **98:** 153–159.
38. KIMURA, A., H. KITAMURA, Y. DATE & F. NUMANO. 1996. Comparative analysis of HLA genes in Takayasu arteritis. Int. J. Cardiol. **54** (Suppl 1): 61–69.
39. ROSS, R.S. & V.A. MCKUSICK. 1953. Aortic arch syndrome diminished or absent pulses in arteries arising from arch of aorta. Arch. Int. Med. **92:** 701–710.
40. KOIDE, K. 1992. Takayasu arteritis in Japan. Heart Vessels Suppl 7: 48–54.
41. NAGASAWA, T. 1996. Current status of large and small vessel vasculitis in Japan. Int. J. Cardiol. **54** (Suppl 1): 91–98.
42. NUMANO, F. & T. SHIMAMOTO. 1971. Hypersecretion of estrogen in Takayasu's disease. Amer. Heart J. **81:** 591–596.
43. STARY, H.C. 1996. The histological classification of atherosclerotic lesions in human coronary arteries. *In* Atherosclerosis and Coronary Artery Disease. V. Fuster, R. Ross & E.J. Topol, Eds. 1: 463–474. Lippincott-Raven. Philadelphia.
44. JONASSON, L., J. HOLM, O. SKALLI, G. BONDJERS & G.K. HANSSON. 1986. Regional accumulation of T cells, macrophages and smooth muscle cells in the human atherosclerotic plaque. Arteriosclerosis **6:** 131–138.
45. PRESCOTT, M.F., C.K. MCBRIDE & M. COURT. 1989. Development of intimal lesions after leucocyte migration into the vascular wall. Am. J. Pathol. **135:** 835–846.
46. PRESCOTT, M.F., C.K. MCBRIDE, C.M. VENTURINI & S.C. GERHARDT. 1989. Leucocyte stimulation of intimal lesion formation is inhibited by treatment with diclofenac sodium and dexamethasone. J. Cardiovasc. Pharm. **14**(Suppl 6): 76–81.
47. CHIGNIER, E. & R. ELROY. 1986. Adventitial reaction of small artery provokes endothelial loss and intimal hyperplasia. Surg. Gynecol. Obstet. **163:** 327–334.
48. WILCOX, J.N. & N.A. SCOTT. 1996. Potential role of the adventitia in arteritis and atherosclerosis. Int. J. Cardiol. **54**(Suppl 1): 21–35.
49. WILCOX, J.N., N.A. NEIKEN, S.R. COUGHLIN, D. GORDON & T.J. SCHALL. 1992. Local expression of inflammatory cytokines in human atherosclerosis plaques. J. Ather. Thromb. **1**(Suppl 1): 10–13.
50. NUMANO, F. 1998. Takayasu arteritis, Buerger disease and inflammatory abdominal aortic aneurysms. Is there a common pathway in their pathogenesis? Int. J. Cardiol. **60**(Suppl 1): 5–10.
51. WECK, K.E., A.J. DALCANTO, J.D. GOULD, A.K. O'GUIN, K.A. ROTH, J.E. SAFFITY, S.H. SPECK, H.W. VIRGIN & J. MURINE. 1997. Herpes virus 68 causes severe large vessel arteritis in mice lacking interferon-responsiveness. Nature Med. **3:** 1346–1353.

Gene Therapy for Heart Transplantation-Associated Coronary Arteriosclerosis[a]

MITSUAKI ISOBE,[b,c] JUN-ICHI SUZUKI,[d] RYUICHI MORISHITA,[e] YASUFUMI KANEDA,[e] AND JUN AMANO[f]

[c]*Department of Cardiovascular Medicine, Tokyo Medical and Dental University, Tokyo, Japan*

[d]*First Department of Internal Medicine,* [f]*Second Department of Surgery, Shinshu University, Matsumoto, Japan*

[e]*Osaka University Medical School, Osaka, Japan*

ABSTRACT: Cardiac allograft arteriosclerosis, which limits the long-term survival of recipients, cannot be prevented by conventional therapies. The arteriopathy is characterized by diffuse intimal thickening made up of proliferative smooth muscle cells. To test the hypothesis that cell cycle–regulatory genes play crucial roles in the development of this arteriopathy *in vivo* gene therapy targeting cell division cycle (cdc) 2 kinase was attempted in murine cardiac allografts using hemagglutinating virus of Japan (HVJ)–liposome method. Antisense cdc 2 kinase oligodeoxynucleotide (ODN) was transfected into the allografts by intraluminal injection during the operation and the allografts were harvested at 4 weeks after transplantation. Coronary intimal thickening had developed in sense ODN-treated allografts and ICAM-1 and VCAM-1 were enhanced in these arteries. PDGF mRNA was also detected. Antisense cdc 2 kinase ODN inhibited intimal hyperplasia. These data indicate that antisense cdc 2 kinase modulates gene expression and inhibits smooth muscle cell proliferation of graft arteries.

INTRODUCTION

Heart transplantation is now widely accepted as a way of treating patients with end stage heart failure. However, graft coronary arteriopathy remains as a major limitation for extended survival following cardiac transplantation. At least 40% of transplanted hearts develop angiographically detectable graft coronary disease within 5 years of transplantation.[1,2] This same phenomenon is also present in renal, lung, and liver allografts and has been designated chronic rejection. This graft vasculopathy usually diffusely involves both epicardial and intramuscular arteries. This feature differentiates graft vasculopathy from usual coronary atherosclerosis and makes it difficult to treat patients by aortocoronary bypass grafting or percutaneous translu-

---

[a]This study was supported by Research Grant for Immunology, Allergy and Organ Transplant, Ministry of Health and Welfare, Ministry of Science, Culture, Sports and Education, and grants from Uehara Foundation.

[b]Address for correspondence: Mitsuaki Isobe, M.D., Department of Cardiovasclar Medicine, Tokyo Medical and Dental University, 1-5-45 Yushima, Bunkyo-ku, Tokyo 113-8519, Japan. Voice: 81-3-5803-5951; fax: 81-3-5803-0238.
isobemi.med3@med.tmd.ac.jp

minal coronary angioplasty. Retransplantation can be done successfully in some cases, where early diagnosis permits, but graft vasculopathy frequently recurs in a second graft.[3] Therapeutic efficacy of currently used immunosuppressive drugs to prevent or treat graft vasculopathy has not been proved. Many efforts have focused on the effects of platelet-stabilizing agents, calcium antagonists, HMG CoA reductase inhibitors, and angiotensin-converting enzyme inhibitors.[4] However, clinical utility of these agents has been uncertain to date.

What is less clear are the mechanisms responsible for producing these changes. This is generally thought to be the result of direct immunological injury to the coronary arteries. We have demonstrated that proliferation of vascular smooth muscle cells is an outstanding feature of graft vasculopathy in rat and non-human primate models.[5] Based on these observations we developed gene therapy approaches to prevent this arteriopathy by inhibiting vascular smooth muscle cell proliferation.[6,7] Transfection of antisense cyclin-dependent kinase (cdk) 2 kinase oligodeoxynucleotide (ODN) to a murine model of chronic rejection resulted in marked reduction of intimal thickening of the cardiac allograft coronary arteries. We hypothesized that enzyme cell cycle division (cdc) 2 kinase also plays an important role in the smooth muscle cell proliferation in this process because inhibition of arterial neointimal formation by antisense cdc 2 kinase ODN after balloon angioplasty in rat carotid injury model was reported.[8] Previously we have shown that cdc 2 kinase mRNA is enhanced in chronically rejected monkey heart allografts.[9] This investigation was aimed to explore the effects of antisense cdc 2 kinase on the prevention of this disease.

MATERIALS AND METHODS

Preparation of HVJ-Liposome

The liposome, hemagglutinating virus of Japan (HVJ), and ODN were prepared as described before[6] according to the methods of Morishita and colleagues.[10] The sequences of antisense and sense cdc 2 kinase ODN are: antisense 5'-GTC-TTC-CAT-AGT-TAC-TCA-3'; sense 5'-TGA-GTA-ACT-ATG-GAA-GAC-3'.[8] These ODN were provided by Greiner Japan Co. (Tokyo, Japan).

Heterotopic Cardiac Transplantation in Mice and in Vivo Gene Transfer

Adult male DBA/2 (H-2^d) and B10.D2 (H-2^d) mice (age 4–6 weeks) were obtained from the Japan Charles River (Tokyo). They were housed in plastic cages with free access to food and water. Donor hearts were heterotopically transplanted into recipient mice as described before.[11,12] DBA/2 mice were used as donors and B10.D2 as recipients. DBA/2 mice were used for isograft control study.

HVJ-liposome complex with antisense ($N = 4$) or sense ($N = 4$) ODN was transfected into the allografts. A group of recipient mice transplanted with cardiac allografts received no treatment. After the transfection, donor hearts were immediately transplanted into recipients. No immunosuppression was given to recipient mice. Graft survival was assessed by graft palpation. Cardiac allografts and isografts were excised at day 28. Donor hearts were divided and stored in 10% buffered formalin at room temperature in OCT compound and cryogenic tubes at −80°C.

Pathological Analysis

Cardiac allografts were sectioned transversely. Serial sections were stained with Elastica van Gieson (EvG) to highlight the internal elastic lamina (IEL). The percentage of the lumen occluded by intimal thickening was calculated by two independent observers. The sections were photographed, videodigitized, and processed using an image analysis system (NIH Image). The area encompassed by the lumen and IEL was traced carefully and the area of luminal stenosis in each cross section was calculated according to the formula: luminal occlusion = (IEL area − luminal area)/IEL area.[6]

For immunohistochemistry, serial sections were incubated with primary antibodies against ICAM-1 (YN1/1.7) or VCAM-1 (M/K-2) (ATCC, Rockville, MD). Antibody-biotin conjugate was detected with Vectastain ABC Kit (Vector, Burlingame, CA). Enzyme activity was detected with diaminobenzidine.[13] Scoring of the intensity of expression was: 0, no visible staining; 1, few cells with faint staining; 2, moderate staining; and 3, intense diffuse staining.

Expression of PDGF mRNA was evaluated by *in situ* RT-PCR in the murine heart treated with antisense or sense ODN as described.[14] Scoring was: 0, no visible staining; 1, few cells with faint staining; 2, moderate staining; and 3, intense diffuse staining.

Statistical Analysis

All data are expressed as mean ± SD. Findings for percentages of intimal area and expression scores were compared among the grafts using Scheffes ANOVA. Values of $p < 0.05$ were considered significant.

RESULTS

All cardiac allografts and isografts in mice kept beating when they were excised. Native hearts and isografts did not show intimal hyperplasia of coronary arteries. In contrast, allografts showed varying degrees of intimal thickening in their arteries. In

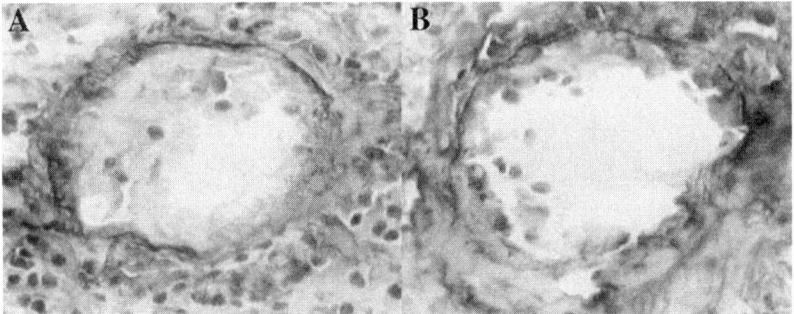

FIGURE 1. Representative pathological findings of graft coronary arteries 28 days after transplantation stained with Elastica van Gieson. (**A**) Severe intimal hyperplasia in a graft from a mouse transfected with sense ODN to cdc 2 kinase. (**B**) Suppression of intimal hyperplasia in a cardiac allograft transfected with antisense ODN to cdc 2 kinase.

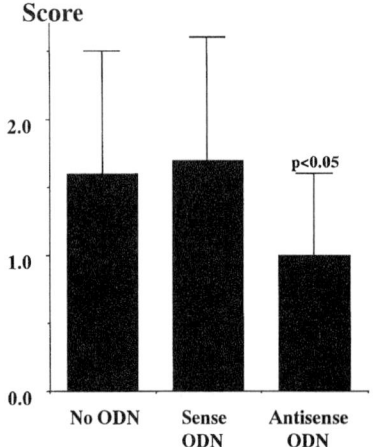

FIGURE 2. Comparison of intimal thickening score among mice treated with or without ODN. Mice treated with antisense cdc 2 kinase ODN show significant reduction of intimal thickening as compared with nontreated or sense ODN-transfected mice.

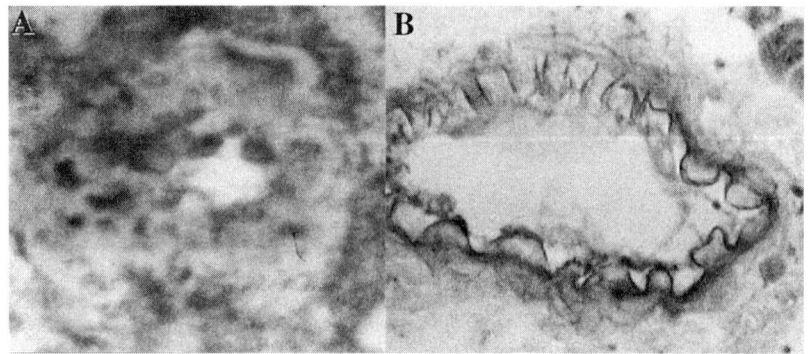

FIGURE 3. Representative cases of ICAM-1 expression in coronary arteries of cardiac allografts 28 days after transplantation. **(A)** An allografted heart from a mouse transfected with sense ODN. Dense staining of infiltrating cells and adjacent endothelial cells in the thickened intima is seen. **(B)** An allograft from a mouse transfected with antisense cdc 2 kinase ODN. Intimal thickening was suppressed and only a faint staining of ICAM-1 is noted.

the allograft without ODN transfection or with sense cdc 2 kinase ODN transfection, extensive thickening of intima was observed (FIG. 1). The thickening score of arteries treated with antisense cdc 2 kinase was significantly less than those treated with sense ODN ($p < 0.05$) (FIG. 2).

In isografts ($N = 2$) and normal hearts, expression of ICAM-1 and VCAM-1 was very weak. As shown in FIGURES 3 and 4, allografts treated with sense ODN showed marked expression of both adhesion molecules. In contrast, expression of these molecules was significantly suppressed in allografts treated with antisense ODN to cdc 2 kinase.

Expression of PDGF mRNA was observed in sense ODN–treated allografts, but that was suppressed in the allografts transfected with antisense ODN (FIG. 5).

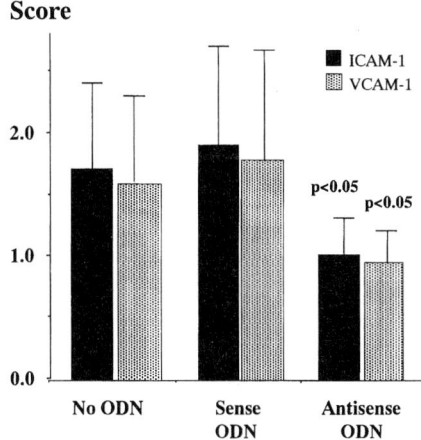

FIGURE 4. Comparisons of ICAM-1 and VCAM-1 expression among mice treated with or without ODN. Mice transfected with antisense cdc 2 kinase ODN show significant reduction in ICAM-1 and VCAM-1 expression as compared with nontreated or sense ODN-transfected mice.

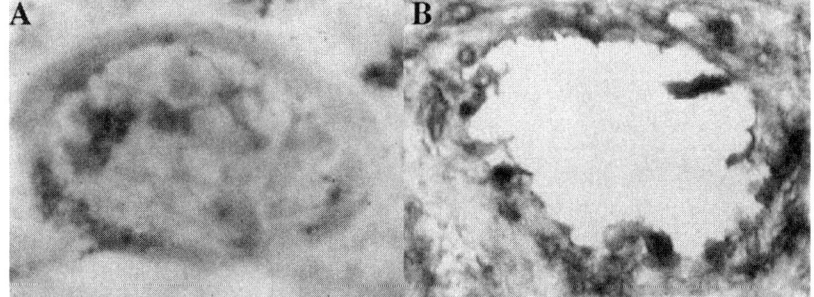

FIGURE 5. PDGF mRNA expression in coronary arteries of cardiac allografts. (**A**) An allograft from a mouse transfected with sense cdc 2 kinase ODN. Staining of infiltrating cells and adjacent endothelial cells in the thickened intima is found. (**B**) An allograft from a mouse transfected with antisense cdc 2 kinase ODN. Intimal thickening and expression of PDGF mRNA are suppressed.

DISCUSSION

One of the purposes of the present study was to demonstrate the involvement of cdc 2 kinase in the process of intimal thickening in graft coronary arteries. We showed that intraluminal administration of antisense ODN to cdc 2 kinase is effective in preventing the development of intimal hyperplasia after transplantation in a murine model.

Cdc 2 kinase, one of the cell cycle–regulatory genes, regulates the common pathway of cell cycle progression and plays an important role in cell transition through the G2/M phase.[8,10] Because proliferation of smooth muscle cells is an essential step in the intimal hyperplasia in chronic cardiac allograft rejection, induction of cdc 2 kinase in our model of monkey cardiac heart transplantation[9] supported the idea that this molecule could be a target of gene therapy for prevention of graft vasculopathy. Using *in situ* RT-PCR technique, in the previous study we showed cdc 2 kinase transcription in the media and in the thickened intima of coronary arteries in chronically rejected cardiac monkey allografts.

Previously we have shown the effects of antisense cdk 2 kinase transfection in preventing graft vasculopathy in the same model of murine cardiac allograft transplantation.[6] From our experience, the effect of antisense cdc 2 kinase ODNs is almost same as that of antisense cdk 2 kinase ODN. Based on these experimental data we are interested in the multipotential transcription factor E2F. E2F forms a complex with cyclin A and cdk2 kinase, both of which are critical to the process of cell growth and proliferation.[15,16] We assume that double-stranded DNA with high affinity for E2F acting as a decoy (E2F decoy) could inhibit cell cycle–regulatory gene expression and smooth muscle cell proliferation in our model of cardiac transplant–associated vasculopathy.[16] The experiment is currently underway.

In the present study we showed the suppression of adhesion molecules expression.[13] Transendothelial migration of inflammatory cells contributes to smooth muscle cell proliferation.[17] It has been shown that expression of VCAM-1 in the vascular endothelium increased in association with atherogenesis[18] and acute cellular cardiac rejection.[19] Similar findings are known in ICAM-1 expression. Therefore, expression of VCAM-1 and ICAM-1 could provide a molecular marker for early arteriosclerosis. ICAM-1 was strongly and diffusely expressed in the thickened intima of the allografts in recipients treated with sense cdc 2 kinase ODN, while ICAM-1 expression was almost nonexistent in the grafts from mice that received antisense ODN to cdc 2 kinase.

In this study we demonstrated the efficacy of antisense cdc 2 kinase ODN by HVJ-liposome method to prevent graft vasculopathy in a murine model. Since intraluminal delivery of ODN during the interval between donation and implantation is clinically feasible, graft arteriopathy after transplantation is potentially a good application of this gene therapy. However, there are many issues to be solved before the feasibility of clinical application of this technology is determined. The most appropriate target molecule, vectors, and routes of gene delivery, duration of effectiveness, and safety of the methods should be investigated. Clinical utility, safety, and long-term efficacy of this new technology to prevent graft coronary arteriosclerosis should be tested in larger animal models.

ACKNOWLEDGMENTS

We would like to thank Midori Oike and Rie Shiohara for their technical assistance.

REFERENCES

1. GAO, S.Z., J.S. SCHROEDER, E.L. ALDERMAN, S.A. HUNT, J.F. SILVERMAN, V. WIEDERHOLD & E.B. STINSON. 1987. Clinical and laboratory correlates of accelerated coronary artery disease in the cardiac transplant patient. Circulation **76:** V56–61.
2. GAO, S.Z., E.L. ALDERMAN, J.S. SCHROEDER, J.F. SILVERMAN & S.A. HUNT. 1988. Accelerated coronary vascular disease in the heart transplant patient: coronary arteriographic findings. J. Am. Coll. Cardiol. **12:** 334–340.

3. GAO, S.Z., J.S. SCHROEDER, S. HUNT & E.B. STINSON. 1988. Retransplantation for severe accelerated coronary artery disease in heart transplant recipients. Am. J. Cardiol. **62:** 876–881.
4. FURUKAWA, Y., A. MATSUMORI, T. HIROZANE & S. SASAYAMA. 1996. Angiotensin II receptor antagonist TCV-116 reduces graft coronary artery disease and preserves graft status in a murine model. A comparative study with captopril. Circulation **93:** 333–339.
5. SUZUKI, J., M. ISOBE, M. AIKAWA, M. KAWAUCHI, I. SHIOJIMA, N. KOBAYASHI, A. TOJO, K. KIMURA, T. NISHIKAWA, T. SAKAI, M. SEKIGUCHI, Y. YAZAKI & R. NAGAI. 1996. Nonmuscle and smooth muscle myosin heavy chain expression in rejected cardiac allografts—a study in rat and monkey models. Circulation **94:** 1118–1124.
6. SUZUKI, J., M. ISOBE, R. MORISHITA, M. AOKI, S. HORIE, Y. OKUBO, Y. KANEDA, Y. SAWA, H. MATSUDA, T. OGIHARA & M. SEKIGUCHI. 1997. Prevention of graft coronary arteriosclerosis by antisense cdk2 kinase oligonucleotide. Nature Med. **3:** 900–903.
7. SUZUKI, J., M. ISOBE, R. MORISHITA, M. AOKI, S. YAMAZAKI, Y. KANEDA, Y. SAWA, H. MATSUDA, T. OGIHARA, S. HORIE, Y. OKUBO & M. SEKIGUCHI. 1998. Antisense Cdk2 kinase oligodeoxynucleotide inhibits ICAM-1 expression in murine cardiac allograft arteriopathy. Transplant. Proc. **30:** 89–90.
8. MORISHITA, R., G.H. GIBBONS, K.E. ELLISON, M. NAKAJIMA, L. ZHANG, Y. KANEDA, T. OGIHARA & V.J. DZAU. 1993. Single intraluminal delivery of antisense cdc 2 kinase and proliferating-cell nuclear antigen oligonucleotides results in chronic inhibition of neointimal hyperplasia. Proc. Natl. Acad. Sci. USA **90:** 8474–8478.
9. SCHOENBECK, A., M. ISOBE, J. SUZUKI, M. KATO, N. KITAZAWA, J. AMANO, M. ENDOH, M. KAWAUCHI, S. TAKAMOTO & M. SEKIGUCHI. 1997. Expression of cell division cycle 2 kinase transcription in chronically rejected cardiac allografts of non-human primates. Heart Vessels **12:** 275–279.
10. MORISHITA, R., G.H. GIBBONS, K.E. ELLISON, M. NAKAJIMA, H. VON DER LEYEN, L. ZHANG, Y. KANEDA, T. OGIHARA & V.J. DZAU. 1994. Intimal hyperplasia after vascular injury is inhibited by antisense cdk 2 kinase oligonucleotides. J. Clin. Invest. **93:** 1458–1464.
11. ISOBE, M., E. HABER & B.A. KHAW. 1991. Early detection of rejection and assessment of cyclosporine therapy by indium-111 antimyosin imaging in mouse heart allografts. Circulation **84:** 1246–1255.
12. ISOBE, M., H. YAGITA, K. OKUMURA & A. IHARA. 1992. Specific acceptance of cardiac allograft after treatment with anti-ICAM-1 and anti-LFA-1. Science **255:** 1125–1127.
13. SUZUKI, J., M. ISOBE, S. YAMAZAKI, S. HORIE, Y. OKUBO & M. SEKIGUCHI. 1997. Inhibition of accelerated coronary atherosclerosis with short-term blockade of intercellular adhesion molecule-1 and lymphocyte function associated antigen-1 in a heterotopic murine model of heart transplantation. J. Heart Lung Transplant. **16:** 1141–1148.
14. SUZUKI, J., M. ISOBE, S. YAMAZAKI, S. HORIE, Y. OKUBO & M. SEKIGUCHI. 1998. Sensitive diagnosis of cardiac allograft rejection by detection of cytokine transcription in situ. Cardiovasc. Res. **40:** 307–313.
15. PAGANO, M., G. DRAETTA & D.P. JANSEN. 1992. Association of cdk2 kinase with the transcription factor E2F during S phase. Science **255:** 1144–1147.
16. MORISHITA, R., G.H. GIBBONS, M. HORIUCHI, K.E. ELLISON, M. NAKAMA, L. ZHANG, Y. KANEDA, T. OGIHARA & V.J. DZAU. 1995. A gene therapy strategy using a transcription factor decoy of the E2F binding site inhibits smooth muscle proliferation in vivo. Proc. Natl. Acad. Sci. USA **92:** 5855–5859.
17. OSBORN, L., C. HESSION, R. TIZARD, C. VASSALLO, S. LUHOWSKYJ, G. CHIROSSO & R. LOBB. 1989. Direct expression cloning of vascular cell adhesion molecule-1, a cytokine-induced endothelial protein that binds to lymphocytes. Cell **59:** 1203–1211.
18. CYBULSKY, M.I. & M.A. GIMBRONE JR. 1991. Endothelial expression of a mononuclear leukocyte adhesion molecule during atherogenesis. Science **251:** 788–791.
19. OROSZ, C.G., R.G. OHYE, R.P. PELLETIER, A.M. BUSKIRK, E. HAUNG, C. MORGAN, P.W. KINCADE & R.M. FERGUSON. 1993. Treatment with anti-vascular cell adhesion molecule 1 monoclonal antibody induces long-term murine cardiac allograft acceptance. Transplantation **56:** 453–460.

Role of Endothelin-1 in Atherosclerosis[a]

JIANGLIN FAN,[b] HIROYUKI UNOKI, SATOSHI IWASA, AND
TERUO WATANABE

Department of Pathology, Institute of Basic Medical Sciences, University of Tsukuba, Tsukuba, Ibaraki 305-8575, Japan

ABSTRACT: Increased evidence has shown that endothelin-1 (ET-1) derived from the arterial cells is involved in the development of atherosclerosis. ET-1 and ET receptors are upregulated in both human and experimental animal atherosclerotic lesions. Plasma ET-1 levels are significantly elevated in hypercholestolemic subjects and cholesterol-fed animals. We hypothesized that plasma lipoproteins such as LDL and HDL retained in the arterial wall can affect ET-1 production and secretion, thereby sustaining vascular functions. Using a two-chamber culture system, we have demonstrated that endothelial cells (ECs) show a polar secretion of ET-1; the majority of ET-1 are secreted toward the basal side of the vessels. Furthermore, we found that LDL enhances whereas HDL inhibits the ET-1 secretion from ECs in a polarized pattern. In order to demonstrate ET receptor distribution in the lesion, we recently studied both human and apoE-KO mice. Our study showed that there is an increased expression of ETB receptors in foamy macrophages in the lesions. More importantly, medial smooth muscle cells (SMCs) beneath the foam cell lesions exhibited a higher intensity of ETB receptor immunoreactivity than those located in foam cell–free areas. In such an area, ET-1 immunoreactivity is also increased. These results suggest that accumulation of foamy macrophages may modulate the shift of ET receptor subtypes from ETA to ETB in SMCs and an enhanced ET system mediated by ETB receptors may play a pivotal role in the progression of atherosclerosis. This notion has been further supported by a recent finding that administration of ET receptor antagonists resulted in a significant reduction of atherosclerosis in apoE-KO mice.

INTRODUCTION

Endothelin-1 (ET-1) is a 21-amino acid peptide with potent vasoactive properties. ET-1 was originally isolated from the supernatant of porcine aortic endothelial cells (ECs) and was found to exhibit vasocontrictive activity.[1] Since then, it has been found that ET-1 is produced by a number of organs and tissues and possesses diverse physiological and pathophysiological functions.[2–4] Three endothelins, known as ET-1, ET-2, and ET-3, have been found. They are encoded by separate genes and exert their functions by binding with two subtypes of endothelin receptors, denoted as the

---

[a]This work was supported by grants-in-aid for scientific research from the Ministry of Education, Science, and Culture of Japan, and Japan Society for the Promotion of Sciences (JSPS-RFTF96I00202).

[b]Address for correspondence: Dr. Jianglin Fan, Department of Pathology, Institute of Basic Medical Sciences, University of Tsukuba, Tsukuba, 305-8575, Japan. Voice: 81-298-53-3262; fax: 81-298-53-3262.

j-lfan@md.tsukuba.ac.jp

endothelin A (ETA) and endothelin B (ETB) receptors. Activation of ETA receptors on the surface of medial smooth muscle cells (SMCs) produces vascular contraction, whereas activation of ETB receptors on the endothelium induces relaxation of the medial SMCs through the release of prostacyclin and nitric oxide.[4]

There is increasing evidence showing that ET-1 released by ECs may be involved in the development of atherosclerosis. ET-1 has been observed in ECs, vascular SMCs, and macrophages in atherosclerotic lesions.[5–9] Although it remains unclear what roles ET-1 plays in the vascular wall, it has been demonstrated that ET-1 can induce expression of endothelial cell adhesion molecules,[10] serve as a chemotactic agent for monocytes, and induce monocyte chemoattractant protein-1 (MCP-1) production.[11,12] Moreover ET-1 is a mitogenic factor that stimulates the migration and proliferation of vascular SMCs,[13] thereby maintaining the atherosclerotic process. Furthermore, it has been found that selective blockade of the ETA receptor resulted in the reduction of fatty streak formation in cholesterol-diet fed hamsters[14] and apoE-KO mice.[15] Taken together, these findings suggest that ET-1 may provide a link between hypercholesterolemia and the development of atherosclerosis. Two unanswered questions regarding the local production of ET-1 are how is it regulated in the arterial wall and how is it modulated by oxidized low density lipoproteins (ox-LDLs)? Here we will review recent progress in determining the role of ET-1 in atherosclerosis, with emphasis on lipoprotein effects on the ET-1 production by ECs in a polarized manner.

EXPRESSION OF ET-1 AND ET RECEPTORS IN ATHEROSCLEROTIC LESIONS

Several studie have shown that ET-1 expression may be upregulated in atherosclerotic lesions, both in humans and experimental animals.[5–9] ET-1 distribution in atherosclerotic lesions is rather ubiquitous, including distribution in ECs, SMCs, and macrophages. A recent study in our laboratory showed that T lymphocytes also express ET-1 in atherosclerotic lesions.[16] In apoE-KO mice, the level of ET-1 mRNA in the aorta was threefold higher than that in control mice.[17] Since ET-1 exerts its functions via binding with ET receptors, the ET receptor distribution has also been investigated in both humans and ApoE-KO mice. It seems that macrophage-derived foam cells express predominantly ETB receptor rather than ETA receptor in the lesions.[16,17] In addition, there is a tendency for SMCs beneath the foam cell lesions to show increased expression of the ETB receptor compared to SMCs located far from the foam cell lesions, which mainly show ETA receptor expression.[16] Thus, this study suggested that foam cells may modulate the ET receptor subtype switch from ETA to ETB in vascular SMCs and that the more active ET system mediated by ETB receptors may play an active role in the progression of atherosclerosis.

HYPERCHOLESTEROLEMIA AND ET-1

Since ET-1 and its receptors are abundantly expressed in the atherosclerotic lesions, it is hypothesized that hypercholesterolemia may modulate ET-1 production during the development of atherosclerosis. To test this hypothesis, we used choles-

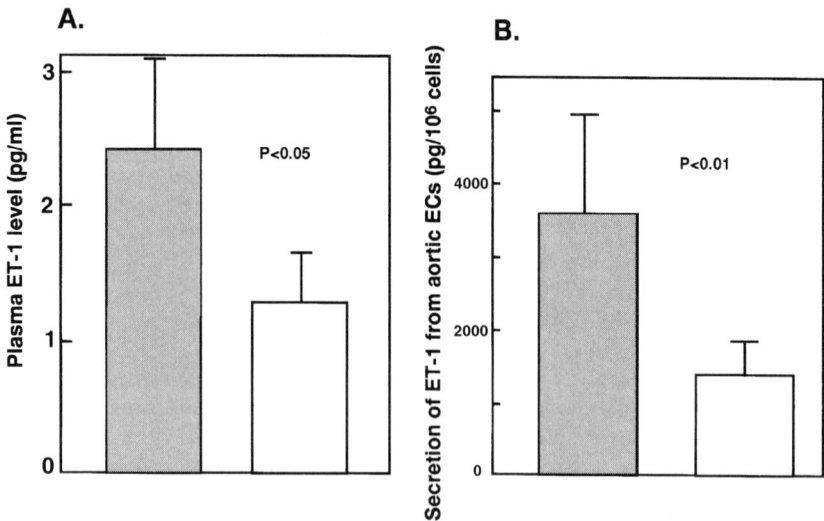

FIGURE 1. Hypercholesterolemia induces increased release of ET-1 in the plasma (**A**) of cholesterol-fed rabbits and in the conditioned medium of aortic endothelial cells (**B**) ($N = 15$). The rabbits were fed either a chow diet or cholesterol-rich (1%) diet for 12 weeks and the plasma ET-1 level was analyzed by ELISA. Aortic endothelial cells from either control or cholesterol-fed rabbits were isolated and cultured for 24 h in the presence of serum-free medium. The ET-1 level in the conditioned medium was quantitated by ELISA. (From Uyama et al.[18] Reproduced with permission.)

terol-fed rabbits as an atherosclerotic model and investigated the ET-1 production induced by hypercholesterolemia.[18] After 12 weeks of the cholesterol-rich diet, the plasma ET-1 concentration in hypercholesterolemic rabbits was increased by 1.8-fold compared to that in normal rabbits (FIG. 1A), suggesting that elevated cholesterol in the plasma can stimulate ET-1 production. Similar results were also reported in human hypercholesterolemic patients[19] and cholesterol-fed rats.[20] To determine whether the increased ET-1 levels were derived from ECs, we collected aortic ECs and cultured them for 24 hours. As shown in FIGURE 1B, there was an increase of about 2.7-fold in the level of ET-1 in the conditioned medium of hypercholesterolemic rabbit ECs compared with the conditioned medium of cells from normal rabbit aorta.[18] This result indicates that hypercholesterolemia can modulate the functions of ECs, including ET-1 production.

During the course of atherosclerotic progression, plasma atherogenic lipoproteins, such as LDLs, accumulate in the arterial intima and subsequent oxidative modification of LDLs may then occur.[21,22] Since oxidation of LDLs can take place within the vascular wall, it is conceivable that oxLDLs may influence EC-derived ET-1 production and secretion. We therefore investigated whether native LDL and oxidized LDL modulate ET-1 production from ECs. We hypothesized that atherogenic lipoproteins, especially oxLDLs formed within the arterial wall, may enhance ET-1 secretion towards the subintimal space, thereby stimulating SMC migration

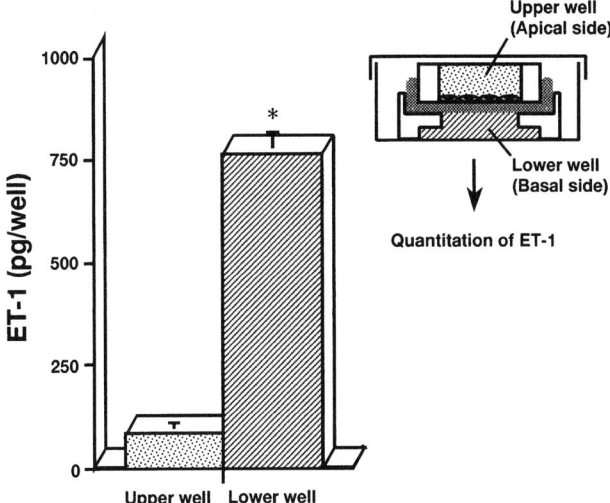

FIGURE 2. Polarized secretion of ET-1 by ECs cultured in the two-chamber culture model system. Amounts of ET-1 secretion in each upper and lower well after incubation with a serum-free medium for 24 h were assayed by specific ELISA. ET-1 secreted into the upper well was regarded as ET-1 secretion toward the apical side, and ET secreted into the lower well as ET-1 secretion toward the basal side, respectively. The inset shows a schematic representation of this experiment. Values are expressed as the mean ± SD of three independent experiments ($N = 6$). (From Unoki et al.[24] Reproduced with permission.)

and proliferation. To address this issue, we analyzed ET-1 production directed toward different sides of the ECs, namely the apical versus basal sides, by using a two-chamber culture system. This two-chamber culture system, which resembles an arterial intima, consists of an amnion membrane on which human umbilical vein endothelial cells (HUVECs) are cultured. The upper well and lower well, separated by cultured ECs, are referred to as the luminal and abluminal sides of the arterial intima, respectively.[23]

A critical advantage of using this two-chamber culture system is that ECs show well-developed junctional devices, which are normally not present in the ECs cultured on plastic dishes. The development of the intercellular junctional apparatus was confirmed by transmission electron microscopy and immunofluorescent staining with antibodies against tight-junction associated protein, ZO-1, and adherens-junction associated protein, α-catenin.[24] Selective expression of these proteins provides the basis for the polarized nature of ECs cultured on the amnion.

To investigate whether ET-1 is secreted from the EC monolayer in a polar fashion, we initially analyzed ET-1 secretion toward the upper well, designated as the apical side, and toward the lower well, designated as the basal side.[24] The media in the apical and basal sides were collected and analyzed by ELISA separately. We found that approximately 90% of the total amount of ET-1 was released towards the basal side (FIG. 2). This polarized secretion of ET-1 was also found when HUVECs were stimulated with IL-1β and INF-γ. When HUVECs were cultured in the presence of IL-

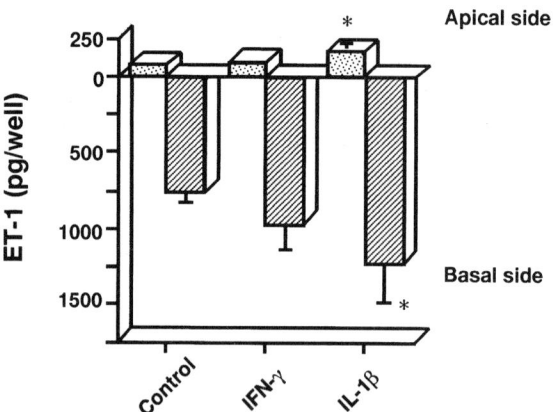

FIGURE 3. Effects of IL-1β and INF-γ on ET-1 secretion. IL-1β (10 ng/ml) and INF-γ (5 ng/ml) were loaded in the upper well and incubated with HUVECs for 4 hours. The amount of ET-1 in the medium in each well was measured by ELISA in triplicate. Values are expressed as the mean ± SD of three independent experiments ($N = 6$). *$p<0.05$ vs. the corresponding control.

1β (10 ng/ml) and INF-γ (5 ng/ml) for 4 hours, ET-1 secretion into the lower well was significantly increased compared to that from unstimulated HUVECs (FIG. 3). Since cytokines can be produced by a number of cell types in the atherosclerotic lesion,[25] ET-1 may be upregulated in paracrine or autocrine fashions to enhance the lesion development. The importance of this polarized secretion of EC-derived ET-1 is that ET-1 may modulate the medial SMC functions in physiological and pathophysiological states.

ET-1 SECRETION STIMULATED BY LDL AND HDL

To examine the effects of lipoproteins on ET-1 secretion, HUVECs were incubated with serum-free media containing either native LDLs (nLDLs) or oxLDLs (100 μg protein/ml) for 4 hours. When nLDLs or oxLDLs were loaded in the upper well, there was a 48% and a 61% increase of ET-1 release, respectively, from ECs in the upper well (FIG. 4). However, the amount of ET-1 in the opposite side (lower well) was significantly reduced (by 45% with nLDLs and 38% with oxLDLs). When nLDLs or oxLDLs were added to the lower well, there was a 23% and a 53% increase, respectively, of ET-1 production in the lower well, with a concomitant 26% decrease of ET-1 in the upper well. In addition, compared to the experiments in which nLDLs or oxLDLs were added in the upper well, there was an increase (13% for nLDLs and 20% for oxLDLs) in the total amount of ET-1 released (upper well + lower well) when nLDLs or oxLDLs were loaded in the lower well. Modulation of ET-1 production by these LDLs appeared to be correlated with the side where the LDLs were loaded, i.e., release of ET-1 was stimulated on that side. Thus, when either nLDLs or oxLDLs were loaded on the apical side, they stimulated ET-1 release

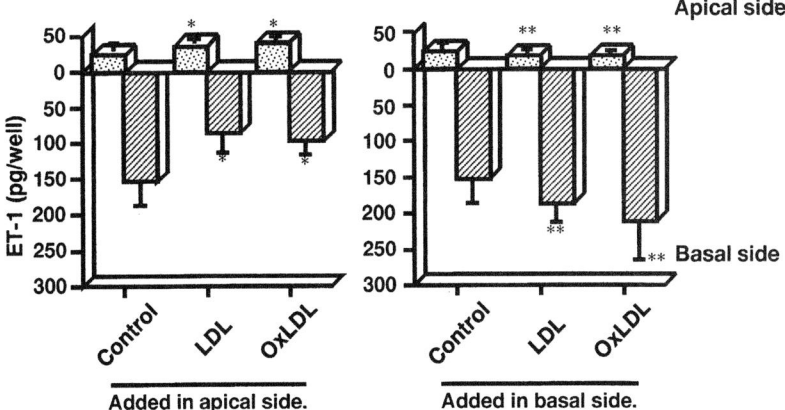

FIGURE 4. Effects of LDLs on ET-1 secretion. Lipoproteins were loaded in the upper well or in the lower well, and incubated with HUVECs for 4 hours. Native LDLs (100 μg/ml) and oxLDLs (100 μg/ml) were used in these experiments. The amount of ET-1 in the medium in each well was measured by ELISA in triplicate. Values are expressed as the mean ± SD of three independent experiments ($N = 6$). *$p < 0.05$ vs. the corresponding control. (From Unoki et al.[24] Reproduced with permission.)

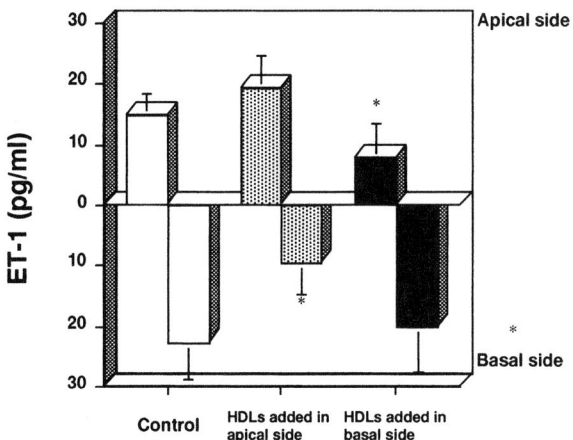

FIGURE 5. Effects of HDLs on ET-1 secretion. HDLs (50 μg/ml) were loaded in the upper well or in the lower well, and incubated with ECs for 4 hours. The ET-1 amount in each well was quantitated by ELISA. HDLs significantly reduced the ET-1 secretion toward the side of the well opposite to that on which the HDLs were loaded. Values are expressed as the mean ± SD of three independent experiments ($N = 6$). *$p < 0.05$ vs. the corresponding control. (From Unoki et al.[24] Reproduced with permission.)

towards the apical side with a simultaneous decrease of ET-1 in the lower well (basal side), and the converse was also true.

Since plasma HDL is considered to provide protection against atherosclerosis,[26] we also examined whether HDLs would influence ET-1 secretion in this system. When HDLs (50 µg/ml) were loaded on the apical side, there was a significant decrease (57%) of ET-1 secretion on the basal side, accompanied by a modest increase of ET-1 secretion on the apical side (FIG. 5). When HDLs were loaded on the basal side, there was a significant reduction (46%) of ET-1 secretion on the apical side, with only a slight decrease of ET-1 secretion on the basal side (FIG. 5). These results suggest that HDLs inhibit the secretion of ET-1 towards the side opposite of that where the HDLs are present. In conclusion, our current results provide evidence that nLDLs and oxLDLs may act as potential endogenous mediators of the increased release of ET-1 in hyperlipidemia and atherosclerosis, whereas HDLs may exert anti-atherogenic effects by inhibiting ET-1 release in a polar manner.

BLOCKADE OF THE ET RECEPTORS INHIBITS ATHEROSCLEROSIS

Since the ET system plays a potential role in the development of atherosclerosis, the effects of ET receptor antagonists on lesion development have been investigated recently. Kowala and colleagues showed that administration of selective ET_A receptor antagonist BMS-182874 (75~150 µmol/kg) to cholesterol-fed hamsters resulted in a significant reduction of fatty streak areas compared to controls.[14] More recently, Barton and colleagues showed that in apoE-KO mice fed a Western-type diet for 30 weeks, administration of ET_A receptor antagonist LU135252 (50 mg/kg/day) led to a 31% reduction of aortic atherosclerosis without changes in lipid profiles and systolic blood pressure.[15] Their study also showed that ET_A receptor antagonists may inhibit atherosclerosis by restoring NO-mediated endothelial functions. Because our studies showed that ET_B rather than ET_A receptors are predominantly expressed in macrophages and foam cells, we examined whether ET_B receptors may be involved in the lesion development. We used a non-selective dual $ET_{A/B}$ receptor antagonist, SB209670 (10 mg/kg/day), to treat apoE-KO mice fed a Western-type diet for 12 weeks. Our preliminary study showed that SB209670 treatment significantly reduced the total cholesterol in the plasma but did not affect the systolic and mean blood pressure. Compared to control mice, SB209670-treated mice had 58% reduced aortic lesions.[27] It seems that the anti-atherosclerosis effect of SB209670 in apoE-KO mice is not due to its cholesterol-lowering effect, since the lesion reduction was still present when compared with cholesterol-matched control mice. This work is still underway in our laboratory, but it is anticipated that ET receptor blockage may open an avenue for the treatment of atherosclerosis in the future.

SUMMARY

Recent studies have provided strong evidence that the ET system may be involved in the development of atherosclerosis. Hypercholesterolemia as a major risk factor for human atherosclerosis can lead to an increased level of ET-1 in the plasma. EC-derived ET-1 is secreted in a polar fashion. Thus, LDL, especially oxidized LDL, can enhance

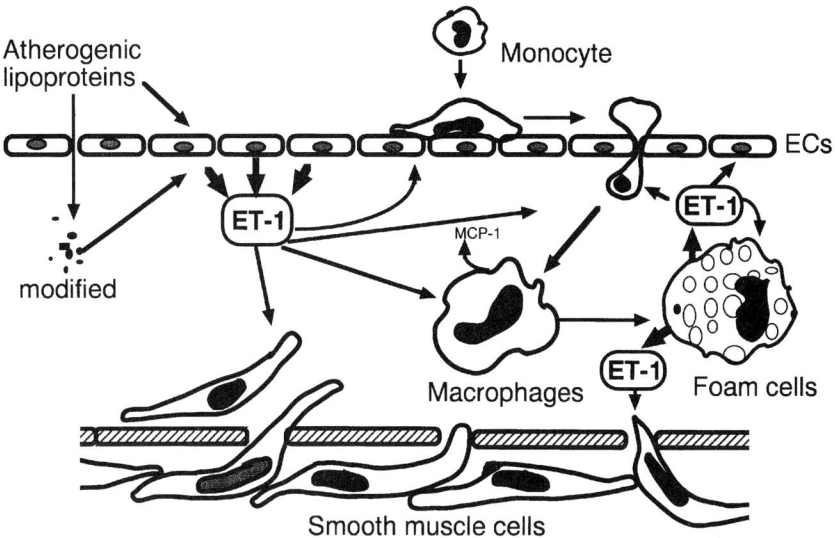

FIGURE 6. Postulated roles of ET-1 in atherosclerosis. Plasma atherogenic lipoproteins (LDL and β-VLDL) either in native form or in a modified form such as oxidized can stimulate endothelial cells to secrete a large amount of ET-1 in a polarized fashion towards the medial smooth muscle cells. Increased ET-1 in the intima may induce expression of endothelial cell adhesion molecules thereby resulting in monocyte adherence to endothelial cells. ET-1 also can directly attract monocyte migration or indirectly by inducing MCP-1 release from macrophage. Since ET-1 secretion from ECs is largely directed towards the media, the smooth muscle cell proliferation and migration may occur when there is a high concentration of ET-1 in the intimal space. Thus, increased ET-1 in the intima may facilitate the lesion development. With the advance of the lesions, macrophages take up lipids and are converted into foam cells. In such a circumstance, these foam cells can become the major source of ET-1 in the fatty streak. Through binding to ETB receptors on macrophages, ET-1 may act on macrophages themselves via autocrine or paracrine mechanism, which may lead to the development of the lesions.

ECs to produce large amounts of ET-1 towards the medial SMCs whereas HDL, as a protective lipoprotein, can inhibit the EC-derived ET-1 production. The increased ET-1 in the arterial wall may play multiple functional roles in the lesion development. For example, excess ET-1 may facilitate local monocyte migration, and through a local paracrine system, ET-1 may initiate SMC proliferation and migration (FIG. 6). With the advancement of the lesions, accumulated macrophages take up lipids, are transformed into foam cells, and constitute the major parts of the fatty streak. In return, these foam cells may become the major source of ET-1 to maintain the progression of the lesions (FIG. 6). In coronary arterial atherosclerosis, macrophage-derived ET-1 may contribute to hypervasoconstriction, which leads to abnormal coronary vasomotion in patients with unstable angina. This may also explain why vasospastic events occur preferentially at the site of atherosclerotic lesions.[9] The availability of different antagonists for ET receptors also provides an alternative way to study ET-1 functions in lesion development. Current studies indicate that these antagonists may be valuable in the treatment of atherosclerosis in the future.

ACKNOWLEDGMENTS

We thank Drs. H. Uyama and T. Kobayashi for their contributions to this study.

REFERENCES

1. YANAGISAWA, M., H. KURIHARA, S. KIMURA, Y. TOMOBE, M. KOBAYASHI, Y. MITSUI, Y. YAZAKI, K. GOTO & T. MASAKI. 1988. A novel potent vasoconstrictor peptide produced by vascular endothelial cells. Nature **332:** 411–415.
2. RUBANYI, G.M. & M.A. POLOKOFF. 1994. Endothelins: molecular biology, biochemistry, pharmacology, physiology, and pathophysiology. Pharmacol. Rev. **46:** 325–415.
3. TAMIRISA, P., W.H. FRISHMAN & A. KUMAR. 1995. Endothelin and endothelin antagonism: roles in cardiovascular health and disease. Am. Heart J. **130:** 601–610.
4. GOTO, K., H. HAMA & Y. KASUYA. 1996. Molecular pharmacology and pathophysiological significance of endothelin. Jpn. J. Pharmacol. **72:** 261–290.
5. LERMAN, A., B.S. EDWARDS, J.W. HALLETT, D.M. HEUBLEIN, S.M. SANDBERG & J.C. BURNETT, JR. 1991. Circulating and tissue endothelin immunoreactivity in advanced atherosclerosis. N. Engl. J. Med. **325:** 997–1001.
6. TOKUNAGA, O., J. FAN, T. WATANABE, M. KOBAYASHI, T. KUMAZAKI & Y. MITSUI. 1992. Endothelin. Immunohistologic localization in aorta and biosynthesis by cultured human aortic endothelial cells. Lab. Invest. **67:** 210–217.
7. LERMAN, A., M.W.I. WEBSTER, J.H. CHESEBRO, W.D. EDWARDS, C.M. WEI, V. FUSTER & J.C. BURNETT, JR. 1993. Circulating and tissue endothelin immunoreactivity in hypercholesterolemic pigs. Circulation **88:** 2923–2928.
8. WINKLES, J.A., G.F. ALBERTS, E. BROGI & P. LIBBY. 1993. Endothelin-1 and endothelin receptor mRNA expression in normal and atherosclerotic human arteries. Biochem. Biophys. Res. Commun. **191:** 1081–1088.
9. ZEIHER, A.M., C. IHLING, K. PISTORIUS, V. SCHACHINGER & H.E. SCHAEFER. 1994. Increased tissue endothelin immunoreactivity in atherosclerotic lesions associated with acute coronary syndromes. Lancet **344:** 1405–1406.
10. MCCARRON, R.M., L. WANG, D.B. STANIMIROVIC & M. SPATZ. 1993. Endothelin induction of adhesion molecule expression on human brain microvascular endothelial cells. Neurosci. Lett. **156:** 31–34.
11. ACHMAD, T.H. & G.S. RAO. 1992. Chemotaxis of human blood monocytes toward endothelin-1 and the influence of calcium channel blockers. Biochem. Biophys. Res. Commun. **189:** 994–1000.
12. HELSET, E., T. SILDNES & Z.S. KONOPSKI. 1994. Endothelin-1 stimulates monocytes in vitro to release chemotactic activity identified as interleukin-8 and monocyte chemotactic protein-1. Mediators Inflammation **3:** 155–160.
13. JANAKIDEVI, K., M.A. FISHER, P.J. DEL VECCHIO, C. TIRUPPATHI, J. FIGGE & A.B. MALIK. 1992. Endothelin-1 stimulates DNA synthesis and proliferation of pulmonary artery smooth muscle cells. Am. J. Physiol. **263**(Cell. Physiol. 32): C1295–C1301.
14. KOWALA, M.C., P.M. ROSE, P.D. STEIN, N. GOLLER, R. RECCE, S. BEYER, M. VALENTINE, D. BARTON & S.K. DURHAM. 1995. Selective blockade of the endothelin subtype A receptor decreases early atherosclerosis in hamsters fed cholesterol. Am. J. Pathol. **146:** 819–826.
15. BARTON, M., C.C. HAUDENSCHILD, L.V. DUSCIO, S. SHAW, K. MUNTER & T.F. LUSCHER. 1998. Endothelin ETA receptor blockade restores NO-mediated endothelial function and inhibits atherosclerosis in apolipoprotein E-deficient mice. Proc. Natl. Acad. Sci. USA **95:** 14367–14372.

16. IWASA, S., J. FAN, T. SHIMOKAMA, M. NAGATA & T. WATANABE. 1999. Increased immunoactivity of endothelin-1 and endothelin B receptor in human atherosclerotic lesions. A possible role in atherogenesis. Atherosclerosis **146:** 93–100.
17. KOBAYASHI, T. *et al.* 2000. Pathol. Int. (In press.)
18. UYAMA, H., S. HARAOKA, T. SHIMOKAMA, K. GOTO, K. DOHI & T. WATANABE. 1996. Diet-induced hypercholesterolemia increases endothelin-1 release by aortic endothelial cells. Pathobiology **64:** 238–332.
19. HAAK, H.T., W. MARZ, E. JUNGMANN, S. HAUSSER, R. SIEKMEIER, W. GROSS & K.H. USADEL. 1994. Elevated endothelin levels in patients with hypercholesterolemia. Clin. Invest. **72:** 580–584.
20. MIYAUCHI, T., Y. SUGISHIMA, M. MATSUDA, H. SAKAI, N. SUZUKI, T. MASAKI & K. GOTO. 1992. Increased plasma concentration of endothelin-1 in cholesterol-fed rats. Atherosclerosis **93:** 257–259.
21. STEINBERG, D., S. PARTHASARATHY, T.E. CAREW, J.C. KHOO & J.L. WITZTUM. 1989. Beyond cholesterol. Modifications of low-density lipoproteins that increase its atherogenicity. N. Engl. J. Med. **320:** 915–924.
22. WITZTUM, J.L. & D. STEINBERG. 1991. Role of oxidized low density lipoprotein in atherogenesis. J. Clin. Invest. **88:** 1785–1792.
23. YAMADA, T., J. FAN, T. SHIMOKAMA, O. TOKUNAGA & T. WATANABE. 1992. Induction of fatty streak-like lesions in vitro using a culture model system simulating arterial intima. Am. J. Pathol. **141:** 1435–1444.
24. UNOKI, H., J. FAN & T. WATANABE. 1999. Low density lipoproteins modulate endothelial cells to secrete endothelin-1 in a polarized pattern: a study using a culture model system simulating arterial intima. Cell Tissue Res. **295:** 89–99.
25. KISHIKAWA, H., T. SHIMOKAMA & T. WATANABE. 1993. Localization of T lymphocytes and macrophages expressing IL-1, IL-2 receptor, IL-6 and TNF in human aortic intima. Role of cell-mediated immunity in human atherogenesis. Virch. Arch. A Pathol. Anat. Histol. Pathol. **423:** 433–442.
26. KASHYAP, M.L. 1989. Basic considerations in the reversal of atherosclerosis: significance of high density lipoproteins in stimulating reverse cholesterol transport. Am. J. Cardiol. **63:** 56H–59H.
27. IWASA, S., J. FAN, T. MIYAUCHI & T. WATANABE. 1999. Circulation (Suppl I) **100:** I-474.

Questions and Answers

E. RAINES (*University of Washington, Seattle, WA, USA*): Do you know anything about the characteristics of the lesions in the animals treated with your antagonist?

FAN: No, we do not. We have just started to evaluate the lesions.

G.K. HANSSON (*Karolinska Hospital, Stockholm, Sweden*): Concerning the human lesions, there seems to be some ETA receptor–expressing cells, as well. Have you been able to characterize these any further?

FAN: The ETA receptors are mainly expressed by the smooth muscle cells. We have one paper about to be published that shows that there is a shift from A to B receptor expression within these smooth muscle cells. Especially when you look at the lesions below the fatty streak, the smooth muscle cells predominantly show the B receptor expression. If you look at the smooth muscle cells far from the lesions, they mainly show the A receptors. We don't know why the A shifted to the B, but it seems to be interesting.

HANSSON: Could it be a possible explanation why one often sees dilatation in the artery at sites of lesions? In the normal media, the size of the artery is increased while the lumen is substantially reduced. Maybe the cells are switched from a contractile to a more relaxing response. Also, do you think it is possible to use ETB blockade to treat atherosclerosis? Wouldn't you worry about vasoconstriction and eliciting ischemia?

FAN: Unfortunately, we don't have the ETB-selective antagonist, so we cannot answer this question right now.

P. GANZ (*Brigham and Women's Hospital, Boston, MA, USA*): The immunohistochemistry has actually suggested a large amount of immunoreactive ET-1 in certain kinds of human lesions, especially the unstable plaques. But I was wondering what your thoughts are about the functional importance of this endothelin-1 in human coronary arteries. There is one paper published, where they used bosantin, the mixed ETA/ETB antagonist and they were not able to demonstrate major changes when they blocked the endothelin system in the human coronary artery. With this mixed agent the changes were rather modest. We have used an ETA-specific antagonist, BQ123, and again the changes that we have seen in a small number of patients to date has been rather modest as well, which raises the question of how important really is ET-1 in the regulation of vascular tone in the human coronary artery. Do you have any data that are not published or are you aware of any data?

FAN: No, we don't have any human data regarding coronary artery. There are two reports, one from the United States and another from Switzerland. Both used the A receptor antagonist and both showed a reduction of lesion development. Compared to our result, the lesion reduction was smaller. They had only 30% and our results show a 60% reduction of the lesions.

H. YAMAMOTO (*Kanazawa University, Kanazawa, Japan*): I have a question about the polarity you demonstrated in the co-culture system. You administered cytokines from the basal side. Were the concentrations of those similar to those occurring *in vivo* in various physiological or pathological conditions?

FAN: We don't know what concentration is optimal. Regarding the *in vivo* concentration, we refer to several papers. We started with an optimal concentration to stimulate the endothelial cells. As for IL-1, we used 10 ng, for interferon-γ we used 5 ng. It is maximal concentration in the experiments reported by others.

YAMAMOTO: The second questions concerns the physiologic significance of ET-1 system in the development of atherosclerosis. Several years ago, Dr. Kurihara at Tokyo University developed a mouse deficient in ET-1. Has your diet-induction of atherosclerosis been studied in that model?

FAN: Unfortunately, both ET-1 and ET receptor knockout homozygous mice suffer from embryonically lethal phenotypes.

F.W. LUSCINSKAS (*Brigham and Women's Hospital, Boston, MA, USA*): Your system is interesting for the polarized secretion of endothelial cells. We are using HUVEC in a culture system. Ordinarily their permeability in various people's laboratories is much less than epithelial cells: thus demonstrating polarized secretion is interesting. Can you distinguish whether it is a polarized secretion, or, in view of the small size of endothelin, could it be selective transport?

FAN: We do not have data on that point.

Oxidized-LDL and Atherosclerosis

Role of LOX-1

TORU KITA,[a] NORIAKI KUME, MASAYUKI YOKODE, KENJI ISHII,
HIDENORI ARAI, HISANORI HORIUCHI, HIDEAKI MORIWAKI,
MANABU MINAMI, HIROHARU KATAOKA, AND YOSHIO WAKATSUKI

Graduate School of Medicine, Kyoto University, Department of Geriatric Medicine, Kyoto, Japan 606-8507

ABSTRACT: The accumulation of substantial numbers of monocyte/macrophages and activated T lymphocytes in focal areas of the arterial intima appears to be a hallmark of atherosclerosis. Our report demonstrated that lysophosphatidylcholine (lyso-PC), a polar phospholipid component that is increased in atherosclerotic lipoproteins, such as oxidized LDL and remnant lipoproteins in diabetic and Type 3 hyperlipidemia, can upregulate adhesion molecules for monocytes and T lymphocytes, and growth factors, such as heparin-binding epidermal growth factor-like growth factor and PDGF A and B chains. Recently, we identified the novel receptor for oxidized LDL, named LOX-1. We summarize the importance of the interaction between oxidized LDL and its receptor, LOX-1, in terms of early stage atherogenesis.

A large variety of different risk factors, such as smoking, shear stress, hypertension, hypercholesterolemia, diabetes mellitus, obesity, and aging, lead to endothelial activation and/or dysfunction, which can elicit a series of cellular interactions that culminate in the lesions of atherosclerosis. There is a great deal of research on how hypercholesterolemia, especially hyperLDL-cholesterolemia and remnant lipoproteinemia, leads to the activation of endothelial cells and the formation atherosclerotic lesions.[1–3] Although hypertension is an established risk factor for the development of atherosclerosis, the underlying molecular mechanisms have not been elucidated. There are several lines of experimental, epidemiological, and even clinical evidence that indicate that hyperlipidemia, especially hyperLDL-cholesterolemia and remnant lipoproteinemia, plays an essential role for the formation of atherosclerosis. Strong clinical evidence is shown in the patients with familial hypercholesterolemia and Type 3 hyperlipidemia. Hypertension also plays an important role in the pathogenesis of atherosclerotic plaque formation. It has been suggested that hypertensive patients with high renin profiles, who are likely to be associated with increased plasma angiotensin II (Ang II) levels, have a higher risk for myocardial infarction than those with low renin profiles.[4,5] In several experimental studies with hyperlipidemic animal models, it has been suggested that an interaction of the renin-angiotensin system and hyperLDL-cholesterolemia could play an

---

[a]Address for correspondence: Toru Kita, M.D., Graduate School of Medicine, Kyoto University, Department of Geriatric Medicine, 54 Kawahara-cho, Shogoin, Sakyo-ku, Kyoto, 606-8507, Japan.

tkita@kuhp.kyoto-u.ac.jp

important role in atherogenesis. In addition, it has been shown that angiotensin-converting enzyme (ACE) inhibitors reduce atherosclerotic formation in several experimental animal models, such as Watanabe heritable-hyperlipidemic (WHHL) rabbits and cholesterol-fed mice and monkeys.[6–9]

OXIDIZED LDL AND ITS RECEPTOR (LOX-1)

The earliest events in atherosclerosis have suggested that monocyte recruitment into lesions might involve the activation and/or dysfunction of vascular endothelial cells, in other words, endothelial adhesiveness for circulating monocytes and T-lymphocytes in the subendothelial spaces. This endothelial activation and/or dysfunction has been implicated in the pathogenesis of atherosclerosis, characterized by intimal thickening and lipid deposition in the arterial wall, i.e., "fatty steak."[2] This earliest type of lesion is a pure inflammatory lesion, consisting only of monocyte-derived macrophages and T lymphocytes.[10] Goldstein and Brown suggested that once LDL molecules are chemically modified, such as acetyl-LDL, they are taken up by macrophages and become foam cells using an *in vitro* system. Oxidative modification appeared to be a biologically plausible modification of LDL *in vivo*. The importance of Ox-LDL in atherosclerosis was first established through the use of the antioxidant probucol in studies of a genetic hyperlipidemic rabbit (WHHL rabbit).[3,11] Furthermore, accumulating evidence suggests that Ox-LDL is a key component in the formation of atherosclerosis[3,11,12]: Ox-LDL is a chemoattractant for monocytes[13] and is cytotoxic for endothelial cells in culture.[14] Also, Ox-LDL has a mitogenic activity for macrophages and smooth muscle cells.[15] Ox-LDL is recognized by the scavenger receptors on the surface of macrophage membrane and macrophage becomes foam cells. Incorporation of Ox-LDL into macrophages is mediated by at least six membrane proteins (such as the class A scavenger receptor and the class B scavenger receptor, such as CD36, SRBI, etc.[16,17]). Horiuchi and colleagues demonstrated that endocytosed lysophosphatidylcholine (lyso-PC), through class A scavenger receptor, plays an essential role in Ox-LDL–induced macrophage proliferations.[18] Nagy and colleagues showed that Ox-LDL activates CD36-mediated Ox-LDL uptake through a PPARγ-dependent transcriptional signaling pathway. They identified two major oxidized lipid components of Ox-LDL — 9HODE (9-hydroxyoctadecadienoic acid) and 13HODE (13-hydroxyoctade cadienoic acid)— as endogenous activators and ligands of PPARγ.[19,20]

With regard to the biological effect on endothelial cells, Ox-LDL and its lipid constituents (such as lyso-PC) impair endothelial production of nitric oxide (NO)[21] and induce the endothelial expression of leukocyte adhesion molecules and smooth muscle growth factors, which may be involved in atherosclerosis.[22–24] It has been suggested that vascular endothelial cells in culture and *in vivo* internalize and degrade Ox-LDL through a receptor-mediated pathway that does not involve the macrophage scavenger receptors thus far reported.[25] Sawamura and colleagues first identified LOX-1 as a critical molecule that is responsible for Ox-LDL uptake by endothelial cells.[26,27] The expression of endothelial LOX-1 is induced by TNF-α and shear stress.[28,29] Moreover, in animal models, such as WHHL rabbit and spontaneous hypertensive rat (SHR), LOX-1 is expressed in the endothelial cells.[30–33] As we have had no evidence of foam cell formation of endothelial cells either *in vitro* or *in vivo*, Ox-LDL uptake by LOX-1 in vascular endothelium may not result in massive lipid accumulation. Nevertheless it is highly likely that Ox-LDL taken up via LOX-1 in vascular endothelium may cause endothelial activation and/or dysfunction, since a variety of biological effects of Ox-LDL and its lipid constituents on endothelial cells have been reported. Physiological levels of laminar fluid flow shear stress transcriptionally induced LOX-1 expression in BAECs by a mechanism dependent on intracellular Ca^{2+} mobilization as shown by Murase and colleagues.[29] Endothelial expression of LOX-1 may also be dynamically modulated *in vivo* in response to dynamic changes in blood flow.[29] An *in vivo* study by Nagase and colleagues suggested this possibility.[31] Although pathophysiological consequences of Ox-LDL uptake by vascular endothelial cells through LOX-1 remain to be fully clarified, modulated expression of this novel Ox-LDL receptor by inflammatory stimuli and fluid mechanical stimuli may play an important role in the selective localization of atherosclerotic lesions in the vascular tissues.

We already know that macrophages incorporate Ox-LDL through a scavenger receptor, such as class A and CD36, and are converted into foam cells. Recently, it has been demonstrated that LOX-1 is expressed in human and murine macrophages.[34–36] Expression of LOX-1 is induced by TNF-α in macrophages,[36] and it is of interest how LOX-1 could be regulated by TNF-α in macrophages. The functional role of LOX-1 in macrophages is to be further determined.

HYPERTENSION AND ATHEROSCLEROSIS

Endothelial cells have been known to play numerous physiological roles in maintenance of vascular tonus. Among the molecules involved in these events, prostacyclin (PGI_2), endothelin (ET), Ang II, and NO have attracted increasing attention by many researchers. Vasomotor tone of the artery appears to be controlled by the constant action of NO.[2] Inhibition of formation of NO or PGI_2 would permit opposing forces of vasodilation, i.e., the action of vasoconstrictors such as ET, Ang II, or thromboxane A_2. Vasoconstriction has been indicated to be important in maintenance of vascular lumen according to the change in mechanical stress and progression of the lesions of atherosclerosis. There are several lines of evidence that LDL from hypertensive patients is more susceptible to oxidation than LDL from normotensive controls. In addition, hypertensive patients with elevated plasma Ang II levels show a fivefold increased incidence of myocardial infarction compared with normal or decreased levels of Ang II.[5,37] Treatment of patients with left ventricular dysfunction using angiotensin-converting enzyme (ACE) inhibitors reduces the incidence of recurrent myocardial infarction and its mortality.[38] In addition to the role as vasoactive substance, Ang II directly induces oxidative stress in the vasculature. It generates superoxide anions by activating NADH/NADPH oxidase in cultured rat aortic smooth muscle cells and in the aortas of rats that were made hypertensive by infusion of Ang II.[39,40] Capers and colleagues showed a marked inflammatory response, characterized by the infiltration of monocytes/macrophages in the aortas made hypertensive by infusion of Ang II.[41] Chen and colleagues demonstrated that Ang II directly stimulates MCP-1 gene expression in the vasculature via the AT-1 receptor.[42] Keidar and colleagues demonstrated that Ang II stimulates macrophage-mediated oxidation of LDL. They also showed that Ang II enhanced the uptake and oxidation of monocytes and macrophages. Li and colleagues showed for the first time, the presence of AT-1 receptor in HCAECs and that Ang II increases uptake of Ox-LDL by HCAECs in a concentration-dependent manner.[43] This increased uptake is due to the upregulation of LOX-1 caused by Ang II.

Ang II caused a concentration-dependent increase in Ox-LDL uptake by HCAECs and enhanced Ox-LDL–mediated cell injury.This study may explain the previous report that LOX-1 expression was found to be upregulated in SHR in which Ang II expression is increased.[32] We still do not know whether endothelial cells are injured via LOX-1 in SHR or other animal models. However, a recent study by Rueckschloss and colleagues[44] demonstrated that LOX-1 is downregulated in arteries of patients undergoing therapy with ACE inhibitors. In the near future we should be able to answer the following questions: By what molecular mechanisms does Ang II upregulate LOX-1? How does incorporated Ox-LDL by LOX-1 injure endothelial cells? Furthermore, we still do not know the physiological and even pathophysiological actions of LOX-1 molecules *in vivo*. We continue to study how LOX-1 is regulated both *in vitro* and *in vivo* and how LOX-1 recognizes Ox-LDL.[45]

REFERENCES

1. BROWN, M.S. & J.L. GOLDSTEIN. 1986. A receptor-mediated pathway for cholesterol homeostasis. Science **232:** 34–47.
2. RUSSELL, R. 1993. The pathogenesis of atherosclerosis: A perspective for the 1990s. Nature **362:** 801–809.
3. STEINBERG, D. 1997. Low density lipoprotein oxidation and its pathobiological significance. J. Biol. Chem. **272:** 20963–20968.
4. KEIDAR, S., M. KAPLAN, C. SHAPIRA, J.G. BROOK & M. AVIRAM. 1994. Low density lipoprotein isolated from patients with essential hypertension exhibits increased propensity for oxidation and enhanced uptake by macrophages: A possible role for angiotensin II. Atherosclerosis **107:** 71–84.
5. ALDERMAN, M.H., S. MADHAVAN, W.L. OOI, H. COHEN, J.E. SEALEY & J.H. LARAGH. 1991. Association of the renin-sodium profile with the risk of myocardial infarction in patients with hypertension. N. Engl. J. Med. **324:** 1098–1104.
6. CHOBANIAN, A.V., C.C. HAUDENSCHILD, C. NICKERSON & S. HOPE. 1992. Trandolapril inhibits atherosclerosis in the Watanabe heritable hyperlipidemic rabbit. Hypertension **20:** 473–477.
7. FURUKAWA, Y, A. MATSUMORI, T. HIROZANE & S. SASAYAMA. 1996. Angiotensin II receptor antagonist TVC-116 reduces graft coronary artery disease and preserves graft status in a murine model: a comparative study with captopril. Circulation **93:** 333–339.
8. DZAU, V.J., G.H. GIBBONS, H.P. COOKE & N. OMOIGUL. 1993. Vascular biology and medicine in the 1990s: scope, concepts, potentials, and perspectives. Circulation **87:** 705–719.
9. ALBERG, G. & P. FERRER. 1990. Effects of captopril on atherosclerosis in cynomolgus monkeys. J. Cardiovasc. Pharmacol. **15(5):** S65–S72.
10. ROSS, R. 1999. Atherosclerosis—an inflammatory disease. N. Engl. J. Med. **340(2):** 115–126.
11. KITA, T., Y. NAGANO, M. YOKODE, K. ISHII, N. KUME, A. OOSIMA *et al.* 1987. Probucol prevents the progression of atherosclerosis in Watanabe heritable hyperlipidemic rabbit, an animal model for familial hypercholesterolemia. Proc. Natl. Acad. Sci. USA **84:** 5928–5931.
12. YLA-HERTTUALA, S. W. PALINSKI, M.E. ROSENFELD, S. PARTHASARATHY, T.E. CAREW, S. BUTLER *et al.* 1989. Evidence for the presence of oxidatively modified low density lipoprotein in atherosclerotic lesions of rabbit and man. J. Clin. Invest. **84:** 1086–1095.

13. QUINN, M.T., S. PARTHASARATHY, L.G. FONG & D. STEINBERG. 1987. Oxidatively modified low density lipoproteins: a potential role in recruitment and retention of monocyte/macrophages during atherogenesis. Proc. Natl. Acad. Sci. USA **84:** 2995–2998.
14. HESSLER, J.R., D.W. MOREL, L.J. LEWIS & G.M. CHISOLM. 1983. Lipoprotein oxidation and lipoprotein-induced cytotoxicity. Arteriosclerosis **3:** 215–222.
15. YUI, S., T. SASAKI, A. MIYAZAKI, S. HORIUCHI & M. YAMAZAKI. 1993. Induction of murine macrophage growth by modified LDLs. Arterioscler. Thromb. **13:** 331–337.
16. KRIEGER, M. 1997. The other side of scavenger receptors: pattern recognition for host defense. Curr. Opinion Lipidol. **8:** 275–280.
17. YLA-HERTTUALA, S. 1998. Is oxidized low-density lipoprotein present *in vivo*? Curr. Opin. Lipidol. **9:** 337–344.
18. SAKAI, M., M. SHINCHIRI, H. HAKAMATA & S. HORIUCHI. 1998. Endocytosed lysophosphatidylcholine, through the scavenger receptor, plays an essential role in oxidized low-density lipoprotein-induced macrophage proliferation. Trends Cardiovasc. Med. **8:** 119–124.
19. NAGY, L., P. TONTONOZ, J.G.A. ALVAREZ, H. CHEN & R.M. EVANS. 1998. Oxidized LDL regulates macrophage gene expression through ligand activation of PPARγ. Cell **93:** 229–240.
20. TONTONOZ, P., L. NAGY, J.G.A. ALVAREZ, V.A. THOMAZY & R.M. EVANS. 1998. PPARγ promotes monocyte/macrophage differentiation and uptake of oxidized LDL. Cell **93:** 241–252.
21. KUGIYAMA, K., S.A. KEMS, J.D. MORRISETT, R. ROBERTS & P.D. HENRY. 1990. Impairment of endothelium-dependent arterial relaxation isolecithin in modified low-density lipoproteins. Nature **344:** 160–162.
22. KUME, N., M.I. CYBULSKY, JR. & M.A. GIMBRONE. 1992. Lysophosphatidyl-choline, a component of atherogenic lipoproteins, induces mononuclear leukocyte adhesion molecules in cultured human and rabbit arterial endothelial cells. J. Clin. Invest. **90:** 1138–1144.
23. KUME, N. & M.A. GIMBRONE, JR. 1994. Lysophosphatidylcholine transcriptionally induces growth factor gene expression in cultured human endothelial cells. J. Clin. Invest. **93:** 907–911.
24. OCHI, H., N. KUME, E. NISHI, H. MORIWAKI, M. MASUDA, K. FUJIKAWA & T. KITA. 1998. Tyrosine phosphorylation of platelet endothelial cell adhesion molecule-1 induced by lysophosphatidyl-choline in cultured endothelial cells. Biochem. Biophys. Res. Commun. **243:** 862–868.
25. KUME, N., H. ARAI, C. KAWAI & T. KITA. 1991. Receptors for modified low-density lipoproteins on human endothelial cells: different recognition for acetylated low-density lipoprotein and oxidized low-density lipoprotein. Biochim. Biophys. Acta **1091:** 63–67.
26. SAWAMURA, T., N. KUME, T. AOYAMA, H. MORIWAK, H. HOSHIKAWA, Y. ARIBA, T. TANAKA, S. MIWA, Y. KATSURA, T. KITA & T. MASAKI. 1997. An endothelial receptor for oxidized low-density lipoprotein. Nature **386:** 73–77.
27. AOYAMA, T., T. SAWAMURA, Y. FURUTANI, R. MATSUOKA, M. YOSHIDA, H. FUJIWARA & T. MASAKI. 1999. Structure and chromosomal assignment of the human lectin-like oxidized low-density lipoprotein receptor-I (Lox-1) gene. Biochem. J. **339:** 177–184.
28. KUME, N., T. MURASE, H. MORIWAKI, T. AOYAMA, T. SAWAMURA, T. MASAKI & T. KITA. 1998. Inducible expression of lectin-like oxidized LDL receptor-1 in vascular endothelial cells. Circ. Res. **83:** 322–327.
29. MURASE, T., N. KUME, R. KORENAGA, J. ANDO, T. SAWAMURA, T. MASAKI & T. KITA. 1998. Fluid shear stress transcriptionally induces lectin-like oxidized low density lipoprotein receptor- 1 in vascular endothelial cells. Circ. Res. **83:** 328–333.
30. KATAOKA, H., N. KUME, S. MIYAMOTO, M. MINAMI, H. MORIWAKI, T. MURASE, T. SAWANMURA, T. MASAKI, N. HASHIMOTO & T. KITA. 1999. Expression of lectin like oxidized LDL receptor-I human atherosclerosis lesions. Circulation **99:** 3110–3117.
31. NAGASE, M., S. HIROSE, T. SAWAMURA, T. MASAKI & T. FUJITA. 1997. Enhanced expression of endothelial oxidized low-density lipoprotein receptor (Lox-1) in hypertensive rats. Biochem. Biophys. Res. Commun. **237:** 496–498.
32. NAGASE, M., S. HIROSE & T. FUJITA. 1998. Unique repetitive sequence and unex-

pected regulation of expression of rat endothelial receptor for oxidized low-density lipoprotein. Biochem. J. **330:** 1417–1422.
33. NAGASE, M., J. ABE, K. TAKAHASHI, J. ANDO, S. HIROSE & T. FUJITA. 1998. Genomic organization and regulation of expression of the lectin-like oxidized low-density lipoprotein receptor (Lox-1) gene. J. Biol. Chem. **278:** 33702–33707.
34. MORIWAKI, H., N. KUME, T. SAWAMURA, T. AOYAMA, H. HOSHIIKAWA, H. OCHI, H. NISHI, E. MASAKI & T. KITA. 1998. Ligand specificity of Lox- 1, a novel endothelial receptor for oxidized low density lipoprotein. Arterioscler. Thromb. Vasc. Biol. **18:** 1541–1547.
35. YOSHIDA, H., N. KONDRATENKO, S. GREEN, D. STEINBERG & O. QUEHENBERGER. 1998. Identification of the lectin-like receptor for oxidized low-density lipoprotein in human macrophages and its potential role as a scavenger receptor. Biochem. J. **334:** 9–13
36. MORIWAKI, H., N. KUME, H. KATAOKA, T. MURASE, T. SAWAMURA, T. MASAKI & T. KITA. 1998. Expression of lectin-like oxidized low density lipoprotein receptor-1 in human and murine macrophages-upregulated expression by TNF-α. FEBS Lett. **440:** 29–32.
37. CAMBIEN, F., O. POIRER, L. LECERF, A. EVENS, J.P. CAMBOU, G. ARVOILER, G. LUC, J.M. BARD, L. BARA & S. RICHARD. 1992. Deletion polymorphism in the gene for angiotensin-converting enzyme is a potent risk factor for myocardial infarction. Nature **359:** 641–644.
38. PITT, B. 1994. Angiotensin-converting enzyme inhibitors in patients with coronary atherosclerosis. Am. Heart J. **128:** 1328–1332.
39. GRIENDLING, K.K., C.A. MINIERI, J.D. OLLERENSHAW & R.W. ALEXANDER. 1994. Angiotensin II stimulates NADH and NADPH oxidase activity in cultured vascular smooth muscle cells. Circ. Res. **74:** 1141–1148.
40. RAJAGOPALAN, S., S. KURZ, T. MUNZEL, M. TARPEY, B.A. GREEMAN, K.K. GRIENDLING & D.G. HARRISON. 1996. Angiotensin II mediated hypertension in the rat increases vascular superoxide production via membrane NADH/NADPH oxidase activation: contribution to alterations of vasomotor tone. J. Clin. Invest. **97:** 1916–1923.
41. CAPERS, Q.I., R.W. ALEXANDER, P. LOU, H. DE LEON, J.N. WILCOX, N. ISHIZAKA, A.B. HOWARD & V.V.R. TAYLOR. 1997. Monocyte chemoattractant protein-1 expression in aortic tissues of hypertensive rats. Hypertension **30:** 1397–1402.
42. CHEN, X.-L., P.E. TUMMALA, M.T OLBRYCH, R.W. ALEXANDER & R.M. MEDFORD. 1998. Angiotensin II induces monocyte chemoattractant protein-1 gene expression in rat vascular smooth muscle cells. Circ. Res. **83:** 952–959.
43. LI, D.Y., Y.C. ZHANG, N.H. PHILLIPS, T. SAWAMURA & J.L. MEHTA. 1999. Upregulation of endothelial receptor for oxidized low-density lipoprotein (LOX-l) in cultured human coronary artery endothelial cells by angiotensin II type 1 receptor activation. Circ. Res. **84:** 1043–1049.
44. RUECKSCHLOSS, U., H. MORAWLETZ, H. HACH, K. HAKIM, H.R. ZERKOWSKI & J. HOLTZ. 1997. The endothelial receptor for oxidized low-density lipoprotein is downregulated in arteries of patients under therapy with angiotensin converting enzyme inhibitors. Circulation **96**(Suppl I): 1–21 (Abstract 115).
45. KITA, T. 1999. Lox-1, a possible clue to the missing link between hypertension and atherogenesis. Circ. Res. **84:** 1113–1115.

Questions and Answers

R. WISSLER (*University of Chicago, Chicago, IL, USA*): Should we assume that if there is no oxidized LDL, there will be no lesions, no atherosclerosis?

KITA: I don't think so. For instance, atherosclerotic lipoproteins, such as B-VLDL, its remnant, or glycated LDL, are also important for the formation of atherosclerosis. Therefore, oxidized LDL is one of the key molecules, but not the only one.

A.R. TALL (*Columbia University, New York, NY, USA*): I would like to pursue two different lines that came through your talk. One is related to the uptake of oxidized

LDL by the endothelium. What are the consequences of that, because the endothelial cell is not thought to become a foam cell, and yet as you showed lysophosphatidylcholine can induce the expression of abnormal molecules in endothelium. The lysophosphatidylcholine is of course quite water soluble, so it probably does not need a receptor to get inside the cell. What is the molecular mechanism that might connect endothelial expression of LOX-1 with endothelial dysfunction?

KITA: So far, we don't have any data that explains the endothelial dysfunction except for Dr. Lee's study. But we have confirmed that LOX-1 expression by endothelial cells cannot transform them into foam cells. Once oxidized LDL is taken up by macrophages, lysophosphatidylcholine is released, and that might modulate endothelial function.

G. HANSSON (*Karolinska Hospital, Stockholm, Sweden*): I'd like to ask about the T cell activation data. You showed that if you give lysophosphatidylcholine to the T cells, they started secreting gamma-HBGF. Our understanding of this activation is that it requires crosslinking of receptors on the cell surface, the antigen bound to the MHC molecule of the antigen-presenting cell being recognized by the T cell receptors together with some adhesion molecules. These data would suggest that there is an entirely different mechanism of T cell activation that is independent of antigen-receptor complexes. If that is correct, it could have tremendous implications in immunology. Alternatively, the lysophosphatidylcholine could be a co-activator or a co-stimulant and I wonder whether you have looked into this possibility.

KITA: You are right, actually I did not present precisely our data. They required IL-2 first, so we think lysophsphatidylcholine might be a co-activator of the T cells.

HANSSON: Do you know if all T cells are activated or only a fraction of them, which would be entirely compatible with an antigen or a superantigen being involved?

KITA: Yes, so far, we saw no monoclonality of T cells in atherosclerotic lesions. Whether or not it required a certain antigen we still don't know. According to Dr. Yamamoto's data from Tohoku University, they cloned all immunoglobulin messenger RNAs and they found that there is monoclonality of them.

S. HORIUCHI (*Kumamoto University, Kumamoto, Japan*): The question I have is related to the Alan Tall's question, whether LOX-1 is a binding type receptor or an endocytotic type receptor. In the atherosclerotic lesion with LOX-1 expression can you observe the endothelial cell localized to some other smooth muscle cell and macrophage in the intima, but something to do with foam cells is much more activated?

KITA: We still don't know, but there are at least four phosphorylation sites, so we have to make sure whether or not it is a receptor-mediated type or endocytotic. We don't know.

M. GIMBRONE (*Brigham and Women's Hospital, Boston, MA, USA*): Two very quick questions interrelated with endothelium and LOX-1. Is it truly at the surface of the endothelial cell? You showed histochemistry in cross-section so I can't tell. Is it at the cell surface? If so, is it shed? Can it be detected in serum as a marker? The second question: Your data, which we will see in the poster session, indicate that TNF can activate endothelium to upregulate LOX-1 at message and protein levels. If that is true, then LOX-1 becomes an endothelial activation antigen, cytokine-inducible. Is it present in inflammatory lesions not related to atherosclerosis?

KITA: We are not certain. We are now asking whether LOX-1 is expressed in patients with various forms of inflammatory vasculitis.

GIMBRONE: Have you actually looked in serum from people with atherosclerosis for shed receptor?

KITA: Dr. Kataoka is making the antibody. He may answer this at his poster session.

H. TANAKA (*Tokyo Medical Dental University, Tokyo, Japan*): Does LOX-1 bind only oxidized LDL? Does it also bind other lipoproteins? How about remnant lipoprotein particles?

KITA: LOX-1 cannot bind to LDL or remnant particles. It can bind to apoptotic cells that recognize the phosphatidyl cell molecules, but only the oxidized LDL as lipoprotein. LOX-1 does not bind acetyl-LDL.

Receptors and Lipid Transfer Proteins in HDL Metabolism

DAVID L. SILVER,[a] XIAN-CHENG JIANG, TAKESHI ARAI, CAN BRUCE, AND ALAN R. TALL

Division of Molecular Medicine, Department of Medicine, Columbia University, New York, New York 10032, USA

ABSTRACT: It is believed that HDL exerts its anti-atherogenic effects through the process of delivering cholesterol from peripheral tissues back to the liver for removal from the body (i.e., reverse cholesterol transport). The metabolic life cycle of HDL lipid and apolipoproteins during reverse cholesterol transport involves both its modification in plasma by lipid transfer proteins and the clearance from plasma of HDL lipid and protein mediated by hepatic cell surface proteins. We review recent work from our laboratory that focuses on specific metabolic steps in reverse cholesterol transport and the results of altering these steps on plasma HDL levels and atherosclerosis. Recently, SR-BI was shown to be an authentic HDL receptor mediating the selective uptake of HDL lipids into cells without degradation of HDL proteins. We discuss the evidence for additional receptor activity mediating HDL protein catabolism in the liver from studies in obese (*ob/ob*) mice, which have markedly increased HDL due to a defect in hepatic catabolism of apoA-I and apoA-II. In addition, we review recent findings that phospholipid transfer protein deficiency in mice results in markedly reduced HDL levels. Lastly, we highlight our findings that overexpression of SR-BI in LDL receptor–deficient mice results in decreased atherosclerosis.

In general, HDL levels are inversely related to atherosclerosis susceptibility in humans and mice.[1,2] The protective properties of HDL may be due to its role in reverse cholesterol transport and to its anti-oxidant and anti-inflammatory effects in the arterial wall. Low HDL is often accompanied by hypertriglyceridemia, obesity, and insulin resistance. Obese subjects characteristically have accelerated catabolism of HDL apolipoproteins.[3] A common belief is that low HDL cholesterol reflects increased core lipid exchange between HDL and triglyceride-rich lipoproteins, leading to modifications of HDL composition and size that result in increased catabolism of HDL particles.[4] HDL from hypertriglyceridemic subjects with low HDL is smaller and more susceptible to renal filtration and degradation.[5] Overall, there is evidence in humans and mice that variations in plasma HDL levels may be due to alterations in HDL apoprotein synthesis or catabolism.[3,6,7] HDL catabolism can be thought of as occurring in two compartments, the plasma and tissues. Within these two compartments there are numerous proteins that influence reverse cholesterol transport. For example, lipid transfer proteins (e.g., cholesteryl ester transfer protein, hepatic

---

[a]Address for correspondence: David L. Silver, Ph.D., Division of Molecular Medicine, Department of Medicine, Columbia University, Room 8-401, 630 W. 168 Street, New York, NY 10032. Voice: 212-305-4899; fax: 212-305-5052.
dls51@columbia.edu

lipase, and phospholipid transfer protein) in the plasma compartment can alter HDL levels, with either anti-atherogenic or pro-atherogenic consequences.[8] Hepatic HDL receptors can also have profound effects on plasma HDL levels.[9,10]

Here we review recent work from our laboratory that focuses on the mechanisms of HDL catabolism by the liver in terms of holo-HDL particle uptake and selective lipid uptake. We discuss the recent surprising finding that phospholipid transfer protein (PLTP) plays a major role in determining plasma HDL levels. Since alterations in the catabolism of HDL in either plasma or in tissues will likely have effects on reverse cholesterol transport, we end by examining the consequences of genetically altering reverse cholesterol transport on atherosclerosis.

HOLO-HDL PARTICLE UPTAKE BY THE LIVER: LESSONS FROM OBESE MICE

Recently, an authentic HDL receptor, scavenger receptor B-I (SR-BI), was shown to bind HDL in a specific fashion and to mediate the uptake of HDL cholesteryl esters in cells and tissues without degradation of HDL protein (i.e., selective uptake).[11] For example, mice deficient in SR-BI have substantially increased plasma HDL cholesteryl ester, but do not have defects in catabolism of HDL apoprotein,[12,13] indicating that this receptor is unlikely to mediate hepatic uptake of HDL protein. Extensive efforts have been made by many laboratories towards the identification of cellular HDL binding proteins, resulting in the identification of a number of HDL binding proteins.[9] Although these proteins do indeed bind to HDL apoproteins with various affinities, none so far has been shown to mediate the uptake and degradation of HDL apoproteins by the liver. Thus, it remains unclear how the hepatic catabolism of HDL apoproteins is mediated or regulated. The limited data on HDL apoprotein and cholesterol uptake indicate that the process involved in HDL apoprotein and cholesterol uptake are dissimilar to LDL. For example, LDL apoprotein and cholesterol are taken up and traffic together through the endosomal system, whereas HDL apoprotein and cholesterol may have different routes of entry into the cell with unknown fates within the cell.[10,14]

Intriguingly, two monogenic mouse obesity models, *ob/ob* and *db/db*, have been shown to have greatly increased plasma HDL cholesterol levels. Our interest in examining HDL catabolism in *ob/ob* mice has led to some insights into the processes of hepatic HDL catabolism. The high HDL levels in *ob/ob* mice contrast with obese humans with low HDL and other mouse models of obesity and diabetes, such as lethal yellow, tubby, and the brown adipose-ablated transgenic mouse UCP-DTA, all of which have normal HDL levels.[15,16] *Ob/ob* mice were found to have a nonsense mutation in the leptin gene,[17] and *db/db* mice were shown to have a splicing defect in the gene encoding the leptin receptor,[18] resulting in defective leptin production and signaling, respectively. Since *ob/ob* and *db/db* represent specific mutations in leptin and its receptor, these findings suggested to us that leptin might play a role in the regulation of HDL apoprotein metabolism. As an initial step in investigating this hypothesis, we have characterized HDL apoprotein metabolism in *ob/ob* and *db/db* mice and determined if leptin deficiency is responsible for the high HDL levels.

The primary defect leading to high plasma HDL levels in *ob/ob* mice could be due to either increased production of HDL or decreased catabolism. In *in vivo* HDL protein turnover studies using HDL radiolabeled on the protein moieties, we have recently shown that HDL catabolism by *ob/ob* livers is dramatically delayed.[19] In addition, this defect in HDL apoprotein catabolism was not accompanied by increases in expression of apoA-I or apoA-II, the major apolipoproteins of HDL.[19] In fact, we found that apoA-I mRNA levels were markedly reduced relative to wild-type levels.[19] Thus, the increased plasma levels in *ob/ob* mice are explained by decreased hepatic catabolism of HDL apoproteins. Moreover, we found that low dose levels of leptin administered to *ob/ob* mice significantly reduced plasma HDL levels and increased apoA-I mRNA levels to normal.[19] Importantly, *ob/ob* mice do not have reduced hepatic SR-BI levels relative to wild-type mice,[19] indicating that an as-yet-unidentified molecule(s) may mediate HDL protein uptake by the liver.

The *in vivo* HDL turnover studies are limited since they cannot reveal the mechanism at the cellular level by which HDL catabolism is defective in *ob/ob* mice, nor do they reveal how leptin regulates this process. Therefore, to explore HDL catabolism in wild-type and *ob/ob* mice at the cellular level, we have developed a primary mouse hepatocyte system. This system, compared to some previous reports with liver cell lines,[20–22] yields consistently high levels of specific HDL binding and uptake in wild-type hepatocytes. In order to achieve these levels of activity, extensive precautions were required during the isolation of primary hepatocytes. For example, if protease inhibitors were left out during the isolation procedure, only low levels of HDL protein cell association were observed.

Our present work has focused on utilizing primary hepatocytes to understand the process of holo-HDL particle uptake in wild-type and *ob/ob* mice. Interestingly, preliminary results indicate that the majority of HDL apoproteins that enter hepatocytes are not degraded by the lysosome, but rather are re-secreted by the cell (D.L. Silver and A.R. Tall, unpublished results) in what has been previously termed "retroendocytosis."[22–24] Moreover, the major defect in HDL catabolism by the *ob/ob* hepatocyte appears to be in the process of HDL binding and uptake that results in marked decreases in re-secretion or recycling of HDL particles and selective lipid uptake, with only a moderate reduction in HDL apoprotein degradation (D.L. Silver and A.R. Tall, unpublished results). Thus, given that *ob/ob* mice have high plasma levels of HDL and preliminary evidence indicates that this defect leads to reduced holo-HDL particle recycling and selective uptake, HDL recycling may play an important role in regulating plasma HDL cholesterol levels. Further comparisons of HDL catabolism and trafficking at the cellular level in both *ob/ob* and wild-type hepatocytes may aid in uncovering the molecular players involved in HDL catabolism by the liver.

TARGETED DISRUPTION OF PLTP REVEALS A MAJOR ROLE IN HDL METABOLISM

Targeted mutation of the mouse phospholipid transfer protein (PLTP) gene has revealed an essential role of PLTP in plasma lipoprotein metabolism. The ability of plasma to stimulate transfer of all of the major plasma phospholipids (PC, SM, PI, PE) and free cholesterol from vesicles into HDL was almost abolished in PLTP KO mice, indicating a unique contribution of the PLTP gene to these activities in the mouse. *In vitro* assays of PLTP activity always show significant background, reflecting spontaneous phospholipid transfer in the absence of plasma.[25] Thus, it was surprising that the rapid *in vivo* transfer of VLDL phospholipid into HDL was abolished in PLTP KO mice, indicating that there is little spontaneous transfer of VLDL phospholipids into HDL. Although it has long been suspected that the transfer of phospholipids and cholesterol from triglyceride-rich lipoproteins plays a role in the maintenance of HDL levels,[26] the magnitude of this contribution has never been quantified. The most dramatic aspect of the phenotype of homozygous PLTP KO mice was a marked 60–70% reduction in HDL levels, with major reductions in HDL PL, free cholesterol, cholesteryl ester (CE), and apoA-I. Thus, in the mouse the transfer of phospholipids and free cholesterol from triglyceride-rich lipoprotein into HDL is uniquely mediated by PLTP and plays a major role in the determination of levels of all of the principal components of HDL.

The reduced HDL levels in PLTP KO mice may reflect both decreased transfer of surface components from triglyceride-rich lipoprotein into HDL as well as altered stability of HDL particles. It is likely that PLTP has binding sites for phospholipid[27] and mediates phospholipid transfer by a carrier mechanism. PLTP may also have the capacity to bind and transfer free cholesterol.[28] Thus, it is likely that a block in the transfer of phospholipid and free cholesterol leads to depletion of these components in HDL. ApoA-I is secreted in association with triglyceride-rich lipoproteins, and the transfer of apoA-I from triglyceride-rich lipoproteins into HDL may depend on the transfer of phospholipids and free cholesterol. In addition to direct effects of decreased transfer, it is likely that the stability of HDL particles is altered in PLTP KO mice. The lipidation of protein-rich nascent HDL particles, dependent on PLTP activity, may lead to stabilization of these particles. Consistent with this suggestion, preliminary studies indicate hypercatabolism of HDL PC and apoA-I in PLTP KO mice (Jiang and Tall, unpublished observation).

Interestingly, the heterozygote KO mouse, while having a dose-related depletion of plasma phospholipid transfer activity, did not display significant changes in plasma lipoprotein levels. This suggests that normal plasma PLTP activity is more than sufficient to provide components for HDL. The transgenic overexpression of PLTP, thus, only produced a high HDL phenotype when crossed with apoA-I transgenic mice, where the excessive production of HDL protein may have outstripped the ability of PLTP to stimulate lipidation of nascent HDL.[28] In mice with massive overexpression (20–40-fold of PLTP by adenovirus injection),[29,30] it is possible that low HDL reflects destabilization of HDL particles owing to very high levels of surface active PLTP. Several lines of evidence have shown a role for PLTP in stimulating the formation of preβ-HDL particles.[28,29,31] The presence of much lower preβ-HDL in PLTP KO mice (17% of that of wild type) is consistent with a role of this activity in preβ-HDL formation. However, as opposed to overexpression experiments, the loss of PLTP activity in PLTP KO mice did not result in disproportionate changes in preβ-HDL, suggesting a role for other factors in determining the ratio of preβ/α-HDL.

On both chow and high fat diets, the most dramatic feature of the PLTP KO mouse phenotype was the reduced HDL levels. However, on the high fat diet, this was associated with an accumulation of lipids in the VLDL and LDL fraction. This occurred without elevation of plasma apoB or triglyceride levels, and presumably reflects the accumulation of phospholipid and free cholesterol-rich surface components of triglyceride-rich lipoprotein (TRL). Vesicular lipoproteins were identified by negative stain electron microscopy in the LDL region. These may appear on the high fat diet because of increased flux of TRL, leading to enhanced accumulation of surface components. Unexpectedly, there was also some accumulation of CE especially in VLDL. We carried out preliminary turnover studies with VLDL carrying radiolabeled CE to test the possibility that *in vivo* PLTP might play a role in transferring VLDL CE into HDL, however, there was no significant transfer in either wild type or PLTP KO mice (Jiang and Tall, unpublished observation). One possible explanation is that LCAT (lecithyl cholesterol acyl transferase) activity is diverted from HDL into VLDL in PLTP KO mice on the high fat diet. Another is that PLTP KO mice have a subtle defect in clearance of VLDL remnants.

The phenotype of the PLTP KO mouse, i.e., low HDL and high levels of non-HDL cholesterol, is usually associated with increased propensity to atherosclerosis. However, the increased LDL on the atherogenic diet predominantly reflects the presence of vesicular lipoproteins, which may have anti-atherogenic properties.[31] Preliminary analysis indicates that the vesicular lipoproteins are enriched in apoA-IV (Jiang, Qin and Tall, unpublished observation), and thus may resemble the particles accumulating in apoE KO/hepatic lipase KO mice, which appear to have anti-atherogenic properties.[32] The impact of the PLTP KO on atherogenesis will be tested by crossing with induced mutant strains with increased atherosclerosis susceptibility.

OVEREXPRESSION OF SR-BI RESULTS IN REDUCED ATHEROSCLEROSIS

In order to evaluate the relationship between lipoprotein metabolism and atherosclerosis, we studied the consequence of the overexpression of scavenger receptor type B class I (SR-BI) in mice. Overexpression of SR-BI results in decreased HDL cholesterol, increased selective uptake of HDL-CE in the liver, and an increase in biliary cholesterol content, suggesting an enhancement of reverse cholesterol transport.[33,34] The enhancement of reverse cholesterol transport by SR-BI may be related both to increased selective uptake of CE (cholesteryl ester) in the liver, as well as increased flux of free cholesterol between HDL and cell membrane.[35]

Recent SR-BI overexpression results in a marked decrease in atherosclerosis in LDL receptor-deficient (LDLR0) mice fed the high fat/cholesterol/bile salt diet, and no change in atherosclerosis in LDLR0 mice fed the high fat/cholesterol diet.[36] These diet/genotype combinations were chosen because they induce moderate elevations in total plasma cholesterol levels (i.e., 200–400 mg/dl) and a lipoprotein profile not dissimilar to human profiles. The atherosclerosis results were highly correlated with effects of SR-BI overexpression on levels of VLDL plus LDL cholesterol.[36] Although SR-BI overexpression dramatically lowered HDL levels irrespective of diet and LDL receptor genotype, this did not appear to be a major determinant of atherosclerosis. Because VLDL+LDL cholesterol was decreased on the low fat chow diet in both LDLR1 and LDLR0 mice expressing the SR-BI transgene, these studies suggest that the therapeutic overexpression of hepatic SR-BI could be anti-atherogenic.

A major effect of SR-BI overexpression was the lowering of LDL cholesterol and apoB levels, including both apoB100 and apoB48. This was seen in LDLR2 (wild type) and LDLR1 (heterozygote) mice on chow and high fat/cholesterol/bile salt diets and in LDLR0 mice on chow diet.[36] However, effects on VLDL cholesterol and apoB were more variable. VLDL cholesterol was slightly increased on the chow diet, markedly increased on the high fat/cholesterol diet, and decreased on the high fat/cholesterol/bile salt diet.[36] The mechanisms underlying these complex effects are uncertain. Although SR-BI has been shown to bind native LDL,[37] it is tempting to suggest that the LDL-lowering effects of SR-BI overexpression are related to increased removal from the circulation of either LDL itself or its precursors, i.e., VLDL remnants. Selective uptake from these particles could also be involved in the reduction in VLDL and LDL cholesterol. In contrast, the increase in VLDL cholesterol, apoB, and triglycerides that occurred on the high fat/cholesterol diet may have reflected increased VLDL secretion, perhaps due to increased hepatic uptake of fatty acids by SR-BI; this effect may be exaggerated by the high fat content of the diet. The failure to observe this response on the high fat/cholesterol/bile salt diet is likely related to the bile salt component.

The finding that the outcome of atherosclerosis studies in SR-BI transgenic mice is predominantly influenced by effects on VLDL and LDL cholesterol levels, although unexpected, is consistent with earlier mouse atherosclerosis studies. Thus, Young and co-workers[38] found a high correlation between extent of atherosclerosis and plasma total or non-HDL cholesterol levels in mice with different induced mutations of apoB. In contrast to these findings, reduction of HDL levels by apoA-I knock-out or cholesteryl ester transfer protein overexpression, while modifying the extent of lesions in some models, does not have a profound impact on atherosclerosis.[39,40] Perhaps the lack of predominance of HDL effects in SR-BI transgenic mice is related to opposing actions, i.e., the fractional clearance of HDL cholesterol by the liver is increased while HDL levels and pool size are decreased.[9] It is possible that moderate overexpression would result in a different spectrum of lipoprotein changes, and this merits further investigation.

The present results showing decreased atherosclerosis suggest that hepatic overexpression of SR-BI or its human homolog could have therapeutic benefits. The lowering of the atherogenic lipoprotein fraction, i.e., VLDL+LDL cholesterol and apoB levels was seen in both LDLR1 and LDLR0 mice on chow diets. Thus, this therapy could work independent of LDL receptor activity and could be synergistic with statins. In the context of a low fat diet, hepatic SR-BI overexpression could potentially provide a method for lowering LDL cholesterol in patients with familial hypercholesterolemia.

FUTURE PERSPECTIVES

The identification of SR-BI and the understanding of its functions are just beginning to shed light on the process of reverse cholesterol transport. However, work from our laboratory on obese mice and from others indicate that SR-BI may not be the sole hepatic HDL receptor. The next major challenge will be to identify the holo-HDL particle receptor (Receptor X, FIG. 1). We speculate that this receptor not only mediates HDL protein uptake, but may also contribute to cholesterol uptake. This idea is supported by our observations of HDL particle recycling, which could lead to the selective removal of HDL cholesterol inside the cell rather than on the plasma membrane. Experimentally increasing reverse cholesterol transport by increasing

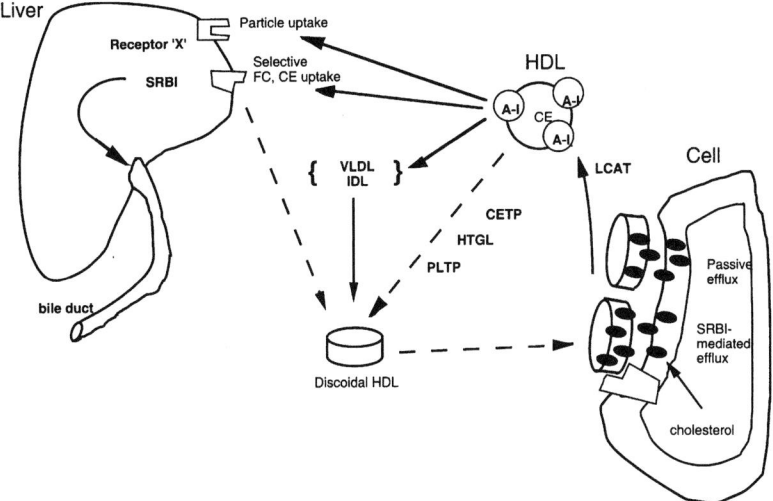

FIGURE 1. Reverse cholesterol transport. The primary recipient of tissue-cholesterol may be a phospholipid-rich, discoidal HDL particle, or free apoA-I. As cholesterol is esterified by LCAT, the discoidal HDL matures into a spherical form. Spherical HDL may then be further modified by both CETP and PLTP, resulting in increased discoidal HDL particles. HDL cholesteryl esters are then selectively taken up by the liver via SR-BI. An unidentified HDL particle receptor (Receptor X) is likely involved in the uptake and degradation of holo-HDL particles. Cholesterol movement (*solid lines*); the regeneration of nascent, phospholipid-rich discoidal HDL (*dashed lines*). CE, cholesteryl esters; CETP, cholesteryl ester transfer protein; FC, free cholesterol; HTGL, hepatic triglyceride lipase; IDL, intermediate-density lipoproteins; LCAT, lecithyl cholesterol acyl transferase; PLTP, phospholipid transfer protein; SR-BI, scavenger receptor BI; VLDL, very-low-density lipoprotein.

hepatic SR-BI activity in mice has been shown to have anti-atherogenic consequences. Reverse cholesterol transport may also be altered by manipulating PLTP activity in the plasma compartment. The information learned from analyzing PLTP-deficient mice has revealed that the inhibition of PLTP activity results in the production of discoidal apoA-IV–rich particles (FIG. 1). These particles may be good acceptors for cholesterol from extrahepatic tissues. Taken together, the data suggest that by increasing reverse cholesterol transport while increasing the plasma HDL pool size (e.g., by inhibition of Receptor X) might be the preferred therapeutic strategy.

REFERENCES

1. BRESLOW, J. 1994. Curr. Opin. Lipidol. **5:** 175–184.
2. MILLER, N. 1980. *In* Atherosclerosis: 500–503. Springer Publishing Co. New York.
3. FIDGE, N. P. NESTEL, T. ISHIKAWA, M. REARDON & T. BILLINGTON. 1980. Turnover of apoproteins A-I and A-II of high density lipoprotein and the relationship to other lipoproteins in normal and hyperlipidemic individuals. Metabolism **29:** 643–653.
4. TALL, A.R. & J.L. BRESLOW. 1996. *In* Atherosclerosis and Coronary Artery Disease: 105–128. Lippincott-Raven. Philadelphia.

5. HOROWITZ, B.S. et al. 1993. Increased plasma and renal clearance of an exchangeable pool of apolipoprotein A-I in subject with low levels of high density lipoprotein cholesterol. J. Clin. Invest. **91:** 1743–1752.
6. BRINTON, E.A., S. EISENBERG & J.L. BRESLOW. 19994. Human HDL cholesterol levels are determined by apoA-I fractional catabolic rate, which correlates inversely with estimates of HDL particle size. Effects of gender, hepatic and lipoprotein lipases, triglyceride and insulin level, and body fat distribution. Arterioscler. Thromb. **14:** 707–720.
7. MEHRABIAN, M. et al. 1993. Influence of the apoA-II gene locus on HDL levels and fatty streak development in mice. [Erratum published in Arterioscler. Thromb. 1993. 13: 466] Arterioscler. Thromb. **13:** 1–10.
8. TALL, A.R. 1998. An overview of reverse cholesterol transport. Eur. Heart J. **19**(Suppl A): A31–A35.
9. FIDGE, A.H. 1999. High density lipoprotein receptors, binding proteins, and ligands. J. Lipid Res. **40:** 187–201.
10. RIGOTTI, A. et al. 1997. Scavenger receptor BI—a cell surface receptor for high density lipoprotein. Curr. Opin. Lipidol. **8:** 181–188.
11. ACTON, S. et al. 1996. Identification of scavenger receptor SR-BI as a high density lipoprotein receptor [see Comments]. Science **271:** 518–520.
12. VARBAN, M.L. et al. 1998. Targeted mutation reveals a central role for SR-BI in hepatic selective uptake of high density lipoprotein cholesterol [see Comments]. Proc. Natl. Acad. Sci. USA **95:** 4619–4624.
13. RIGOTTI, A. et al. 1997. A targeted mutation in the murine gene encoding the high density lipoprotein (HDL) receptor scavenger receptor class B type I reveals its key role in HDL metabolism. Proc. Natl. Acad. Sci. USA **94:** 12610–12615.
14. BROWN, M.S, J. HERZ & J.L. GOLDSTEIN. 1997. LDL-receptor structure. Calcium cages, acid baths and recycling receptors [news; comment]. Nature **388:** 629–630.
15. NISHINA, P.M., S. LOWE, J. WANG & B. PAIGEN. 1994. Characterization of plasma lipids in genetically obese mice: the mutants obese, diabetes, fat, tubby, and lethal yellow. Metabolism **43:** 549–553.
16. HAMANN, A., J.S. FLIER & B.B. LOWELL. 1998. Obesity after genetic ablation of brown adipose tissue. Z. Ernahrungswiss. **37:** 1–7.
17. ZHANG, Y. et al. 1994. Positional cloning of the mouse obese gene and its human homologue. [Erratum published in Nature. 1995. 374: 479] [See Comments]. Nature **372:** 425–432.
18. LEE, G.H. et al. 1996. Abnormal splicing of the leptin receptor in diabetic mice. Nature **379:** 632–635.
19. SILVER, D.L., X.C. JIANG & A.R. TALL. 1999. Increased high density lipoprotein (HDL), defective hepatic catabolism of ApoA-I and ApoA-II, and decreased ApoA-I mRNA in *ob/ob* mice. Possible role of leptin in stimulation of HDL turnover. J. Biol. Chem. **274:** 4140–4146.
20. GUEUNDOUZI, K., X. COLLET, B. PERRET, H. CHAP & R. BARBARAS. 1998. Remnant high density lipoprotein2 particles produced by hepatic lipase display high-affinity binding and increased endocytosis into a human hepatoma cell line (HEPG2). Biochemistry **37:** 14974–14980.
21. TAMAI, T., W. PATSCH, D. LOCK & G. SCHONFELD. 1983. Receptors for homologous plasma lipoproteins on a rat hepatoma cell line. J. Lipid Res. **24:** 1568–1577.
22. KAMBOURIS, A.M., P.D. ROACH, G.D. CALVERT & P.J. NESTEL. 1990. Retroendocytosis of high density lipoproteins by the human hepatoma cell line, HepG2. Arteriosclerosis **10:** 582–590.
23. DELAMATRE, J.G., T.G. SARPHIE, R.C. ARCHIBOLD & C.A. HORNICK. 1990. Metabolism of apoE-free high density lipoproteins in rat hepatoma cells: evidence for a retroendocytic pathway. J. Lipid Res. **31:** 191–202.
24. TAKATA, K., S. HORIUCHI, A.T. RAHIM & Y. MORINO. 1988. Receptor-mediated internalization of high density lipoprotein by rat sinusoidal liver cells: identification of a nonlysosomal endocytic pathway by fluorescence-labeled ligand. J. Lipid Res. **29:** 1117–1126.

25. TALL, A.R. & P.H. GREEN. 1981. Incorporation of phosphatidylcholine into spherical and discoidal lipoproteins during incubation of egg phosphatidylcholine vesicles with isolated high density lipoproteins or with plasma. J. Biol. Chem. **256:** 2035–2044.
26. MJOS, O.D., O. FAERGEMAN, R.L. HAMILTON & R.J. HAVEL. 1975. Characterization of remnants produced during the metabolism of triglyceride-rich lipoproteins of blood plasma and intestinal lymph in the rat. J. Clin. Invest. **56:** 603–615.
27. BEAMER, L.J., S.F. CARROLL & D. EISENBERG. 1997. Crystal structure of human BPI and two bound phospholipids at 2.4 angstrom resolution. Science **276:** 1861–1864.
28. JIANG, X. *et al.* 1996. Increased prebeta-high density lipoprotein, apolipoprotein AI, and phospholipid in mice expressing the human phospholipid in mice expressing the human phospholipid transfer protein and human apolipoprotein AI transgenes. J. Clin. Invest. **98:** 2373–2380.
29. EHNHOLM, S. *et al.* 1998. Adenovirus mediated overexpression of human phospholipid transfer protein alters plasma HDL levels in mice. J. Lipid Res. **39:** 1248–1253.
30. LUSA, S., M. JAUHIAINEN, J. METSO, P. SOMERHARJU & C. EHNHOLM. 1996. The mechanism of human plasma phospholipid transfer protein-induced enlargement of high-density lipoprotein particles: evidence for particle fusion. Biochem. J. **313:** 275–282.
31. WILLIAMS, K.J., A.R. TALL, C. BISGAIER & R. BROCIA. 1987. Phospholipid liposomes acquire apolipoprotein E in atherogenic plasma and block cholesterol loading of cultured macrophages. J. Clin. Invest. **79:** 1466–1472.
32. BERGERON, N. *et al.* 1998. Lamellar lipoproteins uniquely contribute to hyperlipidemia in mice doubly deficient in apolipoprotein E and hepatic lipase. Proc. Natl. Acad. Sci. USA **95:** 15647–15652.
33. KOZARSKY, K.F. *et al.* 1997. Overexpression of the HDL receptor SR-BI alters plasma HDL and bile cholesterol levels. Nature **387:** 414–417.
34. WANG, N., T. ARAI, Y. JI, F. RINNINGER & A.R. TALL. 1998. Liver-specific overexpression of scavenger receptor BI decreases levels of very low density lipoprotein ApoB, low density ApoB, and high density lipoprotein in transgenic mice. J. Biol. Chem. **273:** 32920–32926.
35. JI, Y. *et al.* 1997. Scavenger receptor BI promotes high density lipoprotein-mediated cellular cholesterol efflux. J. Biol. Chem. **272:** 20982–20985.
36. ARAI, T., N. WANG, M. BEZOUEVSKI, C. WELCH & A.R. TALL. 1999. Decreased atherosclerosis in heterozygous low density lipoprotein receptor-deficient mice expressing the scavenger receptor BI transgene. J. Biol. Chem. **274:** 2366–2371.
37. ACTON, S.L., P.E. SCHERER, H.F. LODISH & M. KRIEGER. 1994. Expression cloning of SR-BI a CD36-related class B scavenger receptor. J. Biol. Chem. **269:** 21003–21009.
38. VENIANT, M.M. *et al.* 1997. Susceptibility to atherosclerosis in mice expressing exclusively apolipoprotein B48 and apolipoprotein B100. J. Clin. Invest. **100:** 180–188.
39. MAROTTI, K.R. *et al.* 1993. Severe atherosclerosis in transgenic mice expressing simian cholesteryl ester transfer protein. Nature **364:** 73–75.
40. LI, H., R.L. REDDICK & N. MAEDA. 1993. Lack of apoA-I is not associated with increased susceptibility to atherosclerosis in mice. Arterioscler. Thromb. **13:** 1814–1821.

Questions and Answers

R. WISSLER (*University of Chicago, Chicago, IL, USA*) Do you think for regulation of our HDL levels we should be regulating our receptors, or our synthesis, or both?

TALL: The bulk of the evidence now is indicating that synthesis would be the way to go. There are two examples; the first was a defect in cholesterol acyltransferase protein where HDL levels are increased, but overall these individuals have an excess of coronary heart disease. That is not necessarily the final word on this topic and it is more complicated than that, but I think the main lesson in physiology is the increase in HDL, thereby disrupting the clearance in that way. The second example is that the SR-BI knock-out mice, the attenuated mice, even though the lesson is not clear-cut, because there also are effects on apo-B lipoprotein in these mice. The increase in HDL that occurs in the male mice does not appear to provide any protection against atherosclerosis. So, I think in contrast, A-1 overexpression in the transgenic model is very protective.

S. HORIUCHI (*Kumamoto University, Kumamoto, Japan*): Are your data really convincingly showing that the SR-BI can function as a so-called C-selective uptake receptor? As you know very well, the HDL receptors usually have two different functions: one is C-selective uptake and the other is, as you just showed, the cholesterol efflux. In this sense, do your data also indicate that SR-BI may function as an efflux receptor and that HDL-dependent cholesterol uptake is really proportional to SR-BI expression by these cells?

TALL: Yes.

HORIUCHI: It appears that there is some difference in the mechanism between the C-selective uptake and cholesterol efflux from the peripheral cell to the HDL particle. Please comment.

TALL: The SR-BI enhances the flux of cholesterol and precholesterol in either direction across the cell membrane, and so the net movement depends really on the composition of HDL in the medium. In the case of cholesteryl ester, it enhances cellular uptake, but if you load the cell with cholesteryl ester it does not enhance efflux of cholesteryl ester. So, there is something different there, and I think that relates to compartmentalization in the cell. The cholesteryl ester inside the cell is compartmentalized away from the plasma membrane and the pool in the plasma membrane is very small, so it is not in equilibrium with what is in the medium. The equilibrium, which is enhanced by SR-BI, is not affected for cholesteryl ester. On a molecular level, I suspect there are common mechanisms. There are data showing that the CD36 will bind HDL, and yet it does not mediate selective uptake, nor does it mediate precholesterol efflux itself. So, HDL binding is not sufficient for either process.

G. GETZ (*University of Chicago, Chicago, IL, USA*): It has usually been assumed that apoprotein A-I mediates the interaction between SR-BI and HDL. Your last set of data on apo-E knock-out mice raises some questions about this. Would you like to comment on the ligand for SR-BI?

TALL: Yes, there are multiple ligands, apoA-I, as you said, and then, in a study from Krieger's laboratory a variety of HDL lipoproteins A2, apo-Cs can all promote binding of ligands to SR-BI. So, it is a rather promiscuous receptor; it also recognizes apo B lipoproteins. So, people then talk about pattern recognition receptors, but they don't really know what is going on. SR-BI recognizes many things, so I would suspect the effect of apo E knock-out is not simply absence of a specific ligand. There are so many potential ligands that I don't think the effect is related to the absence of the ligand. In this cartoon we had apo E tethering a lipoprotein to the cell surface; you know liver cells have apo E on their surface which helps capture the lipoprotein. So that capture process may be essential in the selective uptake. Alternatively, it is possible that the extreme hypocholesterolemia that these animals exhibit changes the plasma membrane composition in a way that it is no longer possible for selective uptake to occur. Either of those mechanisms are possible. We are trying to look into that now.

Scavenger Receptor Classes A and B

Their Roles in Atherogenesis and the Metabolism of Modified LDL and HDL

THEO J.C. VAN BERKEL,[a] MIRANDA VAN ECK, NICOLE HERIJGERS, KEES FLUITER, AND S. NION

Division of Biopharmaceutics, Leiden/Amsterdam Center for Drug Research, University of Leiden, 2300 RA Leiden, The Netherlands

ABSTRACT: Scavenger-receptor class A has been held responsible for the clearance of modified LDL from the blood circulation. However, in mice deficient in scavenger-receptor class A, the decay *in vivo* of acetylated LDL ($t_{1/2} < 2$ min), as well as tissue distribution and liver uptake (at 5 min 77.4 ± 4.6% of the injected dose) are not significantly different from control mice. The degradation capacity of acetylated LDL with liver endothelial cells, Kupffer cells, and peritoneal macrophages from knock-out mice was 58%, 63%, and 17% of the control, respectively, indicating that scavenger-receptor class A is relatively more important for the degradation of acetylated LDL and foam cell formation in peritoneal macrophages as compared to the liver cell types. This might explain the 60% reduction in atherosclerotic lesion area in scavenger-receptor–deficient apoE knock-out mice as compared to control apoE knock-out mice. Scavenger-receptor BI can facilitate selective uptake of cholesterol esters from HDL. A high cholesterol diet for two weeks induced an 80% downregulation of scavenger-receptor BI in the liver parenchymal cells while expression in liver macrophages is increased fourfold. The *in vivo* kinetics for the selective uptake of (oxidized) cholesterol esters from HDL correlate with the changes in scavenger-receptor BI expression. It is suggested that scavenger-receptor BI is subject to different regulatory mechanisms in parenchymal liver cells and macrophages related to a difference in function in these cell types.

INTRODUCTION

Macrophage-derived foam cells are an important feature of early atherosclerotic lesions.[1] Native LDL[1] does not provoke foam cell formation because effective accumulation of cholesterol esters is prevented by downregulation of the native LDL receptor.[2] Various modifications of LDL, including acetylation,[3] acetoacetylation,[4] malondialdehyde treatment,[5] and oxidation[6] lead to scavenger receptor–mediated uptake by macrophages, coupled to lipid accumulation with characteristics similar to that observed in atherosclerotic plaque.[7]

Some years ago it was established that when acetylated LDL (AcLDL) is injected *in vivo*, it is rapidly cleared from the blood by the liver.[8] The AcLDL receptor was partially purified from total liver with an estimated molecular mass of 220–250 kD.[9] Kodama and colleagues[10] purified a protein with a molecular mass of 220 kD from bovine lung membranes. This protein was subsequently cloned and it appeared that

[a]Corresponding author.

two scavenger receptor isoforms, called type I and type II, are generated by alternative splicing of a message encoded by a single gene.[11,12] Expression of both types of scavenger receptors has been detected in macrophages *in vitro*[11,13] and *in vivo*.[14,15] The major sites of expression *in vivo* are tissue macrophages, although liver endothelial cells are also immunostained with the monoclonal antibody 2F8.[16] The recent identification of additional scavenger receptors such as Marco,[17] macrosialin,[18,19] CD 36,[20] and scavenger receptor B1,[21] has introduced questions about their relative role and specificity in modified LDL recognition and uptake in the body.

The rapid clearance of AcLDL by the liver is accomplished mainly by liver endothelial cells,[22] while OxLDL is concentrated in Kupffer cells.[23] In an extension of studies with mouse peritoneal macrophages we assumed that AcLDL uptake is exerted by scavenger receptors class A types I and II, while a specific binding protein for OxLDL in Kupffer cells is observed,[23,24] and recently identified as macrosialin.[19] The generation of mice deficient in scavenger receptor class A types I and II[25] makes it possible to test whether these receptors indeed are mainly responsible for the clearance and metabolism of AcLDL. In addition the potential importance of other modified LDL receptors might become clear in such a model.

Acton and colleagues[26] recently provided the first piece of evidence that scavenger receptor class BI (SR-BI), a member of the CD 36 family,[21] binds HDL and can also mediate the selective uptake of HDL-cholesterol (HDL-CE). SR-BI was found to bind a broad spectrum of ligands, including both modified lipoproteins, native lipoproteins, and anionic phospholipids.[27] We recently showed that the selective uptake of HDL-CE by isolated rat liver parenchymal cells can be inhibited completely by ligands specific for SR-BI,[28] indicating that the expression of SR-BI can be solely responsible for the selective HDL-CE uptake in this cell type.

In vivo, SR-BI is expressed in the steroidogenic organs and liver of rodents,[26,29,30] which all display selective uptake of HDL-CE. In the steroidogenic tissues SR-BI expression is coordinately regulated with the steroidogenesis by adrenocorticotropic hormone (ACTH), human chorionic gonadotropin (hCG), and estrogen.[29,31] Furthermore, SR-BI expression in adrenals is upregulated in apoA-I knock-out mice, hepatic lipase knock-out mice, and LCAT knockout mice.[30,32] Unlike the steroidogenic tissues, SR-BI expression in the liver is downregulated by estrogen treatment of rats.[29] We showed recently that the downregulation of SR-BI expression in the liver is limited to the parenchymal cells and is correlated with a decrease in the selective HDL-CE uptake.[33] Surprisingly, SR-BI expression and the selective HDL-CE uptake is upregulated in Kupffer cells after ethinyl estradiol (EE)–treatment or a high cholesterol diet, pointing to a different regulatory response in tissue macrophages (Kupffer cells) as compared to parenchymal cells.[33] Our present goal was to analyze whether SR-BI may mediate the increased hepatic uptake of (oxidized) cholesterol esters *in vitro* and *in vivo*.

MATERIALS AND METHODS

Transgenic Mice

Mice deficient in type I and type II class A scavenger receptors were generated by disrupting exon 4 of the gene, which is essential for the formation of functional trimeric receptors.[25] 3-1 ES cells were transfected by electroporation and ES cells containing the disrupted allele were injected into C57Bl/6J blastocytes. Embryos were transferred into the uterus of ICR recipients. To obtain heterozygous mutants, chimeras were mated with ICR females. Brother-sister mating of heterozygotes were used to generate homozygous mutants (−/−) and controls (+/+), which were thus littermates. Mice heterozygous and homozygous for the mutation were normal in appearance, growth, and fertility. Deficiency was transmitted in a Mendelian fashion, as identified by southern blot analysis of tail DNA. Immunostaining of liver sections from wild-type animals, using monoclonal antibody 2F8,[16] detected class A scavenger receptors in liver endothelial cells and Kupffer cells, while in homozygous receptor-deficient mice no immunoreactive protein was detected.[25] 2F8 can bind to both type I and type II class A scavenger receptors, indicating the homozygous receptor-deficient mice are deficient in both type I and II receptor protein.

Serum Clearance in Vivo and Liver Association

In the scavenger receptor class A studies, 6–7-week-old mice were anesthetized by intraperitoneal injection of 2.1 mg of Nembutal®. The abdomens were opened and radiolabeled compounds were injected into the inferior vena cava at the level of the renal veins. The body temperature of the mice was maintained at 36.5–37°C by an infrared heating lamp. At the indicated times, 50 µl of blood was taken from the inferior vena cava at least 0.5 cm distal to the injection point. The samples were centrifuged for 2 min at $20,000 \times g$, and the radioactivity in the supernatants was counted. Liver lobules were tied off and excised at the indicated times. After weighing the lobule and counting its radioactivity, the total liver uptake was calculated using the assumption that 4.80% of the total body weight is contributed by the liver. The amount of liver that was tied off was 2–3% at each time point, so that at the longest circulation time still less than 15% of the total liver was removed. The percentage liver value is corrected for the amount of sample present in the entrapped blood based upon ^{3}H-labeled albumin measurements. When indicated, polyinosinic acid was injected as a bolus 1 min before the radiolabeled compound.

Cell Isolation Procedures

Mice or rats were anesthetized and injected with the radiolabeled compounds in a similar way as for the determination of the total liver uptake. At 10 min after injection the heart aorta was cannulated, and a liver perfusion was started with Hank's buffer, pH 7.4, plus HEPES (1.6 g/l) at 37°C. After a 10-min perfusion (flow rate, 14 ml/min), a lobule was tied off for determination of the total liver uptake. To separate the various cell types, the liver was subsequently subjected to perfusion with inclusion of 0.025% (w/vol) collagenase.

Endothelial cells and Kupffer cells were purified by centrifugal elutriation. Purity of the cells was assessed by phase-contrast microscopy. The purity of the endothelial cell preparation was higher than 90%, while Kupffer cell preparations contained 70–90% Kupffer cells, the rest being endothelial cells. The microscopical purity determinations were controlled by assessing the uptake of latex (size 0.8 µm) by Kupffer cells, while endothelial cells are negative. Calculation of the contribution of the different cell types to total liver uptake was performed as described.[8] A quantitative recovery of the radioactivity associated with total liver in the subsequently isolated cells was obtained by using the tyramine cellobiose–labeled AcLDL. This was checked for each individual cell-type isolation by comparing the calculated (from the relative contribution of the various cell types) and determined total liver association. Peritoneal macrophages (unstimulated) were collected from each genotype animal by lavage of the peritoneum with 10 ml PBS/1 mM EDTA. Cells were centrifuged for 10 min at 750g and subsequently purified on Nycodenz.

RESULTS

Serum Decay and Liver Association of AcLDL

The disappearance of AcLDL (5 µg) from the blood circulation in control mice proceeds at a rapid rate and 2 min after injection already more that 90% is removed (FIG. 1). The liver is mainly responsible for this rapid removal and at 5 min after injection 79.1 ± 4.6% (±S.D. N = 7) of the injected dose is liver-associated. Subsequently the radioactivity with the liver declines.

Surprisingly we observe no apparent difference in the clearance rate of AcLDL when injected into scavenger receptor class A type I, II knock-out (KO) mice. Also the initial kinetics of liver uptake are similar to control mice at 5 min after injection, 77.4 ± 6.3% (±S.D. N = 5) while there is also no significant difference in the decline in liver-associated radioactivity.

It might be assumed that at a low dose of AcLDL (5 µg), the capacity of the uptake system cannot be assessed, thus we injected also a higher dose (200 µg, FIG. 1). It appears that indeed the initial clearance is retarded, but again no significant difference in clearance and liver uptake between control and scavenger receptor KO mice was observed, indicating that scavenger receptors distinct from class A types I and II can mediate efficient clearance of AcLDL from the blood circulation. Initial data on the clearance of AcLDL in KO mice and wild-type mice have already been reported.[25]

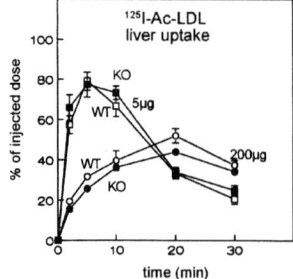 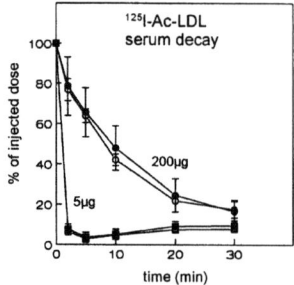

FIGURE 1. Liver uptake and serum decay of AcLDL at two doses in wild-type (WT) and KO mice (KO). ^{125}I-AcLDL (5 or 200 µg of apolipoprotein) was injected into anesthetized WT and KO mice, and the liver association and serum decay was determined. Bars represent S.E. for 5–7 animals for 5 µg and 3 animals for 200 µg. The liver value is corrected for serum radioactivity based upon ^{3}H-labeled albumin. *Open symbols* represent WT and *closed symbols* KO mice.

TABLE 1. *In vivo* distribution of ^{125}I-tyramine cellobiose labeled AcLDL in control and KO mice

	%ID/mg cell protein		Relative contribution (%)	
	Control mice	KO mice	Control mice	KO mice
Parenchymal cells	0.01 ± 0.00	0.02 ± 0.00	2.8 ± 1.8	5.7 ± 0.2
Endothelial cells	7.24 ± 0.11	6.05 ± 0.39 ($p < 0.05$)	74.4 ± 1.2	71.8 ± 1.1
Kupffer cells	2.93 ± 0.07	2.53 ± 0.34	22.9 ± 0.6	22.6 ± 1.3

Note: At 10 min after injection of ^{125}I-tyramine cellobiose-AcLDL (40 µg), parenchymal, endothelial and Kupffer cells were isolated. The amount of radioactivity as percentage of the injected dose (%ID) per mg cell protein was determined as well as the relative contribution of the different liver cell types to the total uptake by liver based upon the amount of protein each cell type contributes to total liver protein.[23]

Cellular Distribution of AcLDL in Liver

We have shown previously in rats that AcLDL is mainly taken up by endothelial cells. In agreement with these data we find now, also for control mice, that the highest specific uptake (per mg cell protein) is found to be associated with endothelial cells (TABLE 1). For the KO mice, essentially similar cellular uptake values were obtained, although the value for endothelial cells was 17% lower ($p = 0.04$). When the amount of protein contributed by each cell type to total liver was taken into account, it can be calculated which percentage the various liver cell types are responsible for the total liver uptake (TABLE 1). The mice endothelial cells indeed appear to be the main site for uptake of AcLDL. In principle, the relative contribution of the various cell types to the uptake of AcLDL appears to be similar for the KO mice as compared to the control mice.

Cell Association and Degradation of AcLDL by Isolated Cells

It was recently established that the degradation of AcLDL in thioglycolate-elicited peritoneal macrophages is reduced to less than one-third in knock-out mice as compared to control mice.[25] FIGURE 2(A) shows that the cell association of AcLDL with peritoneal macrophages of KO mice and wild-type mice is comparable while the degradation, in agreement with the earlier data, for the KO mice is 17% as compared to cells from wild-type mice. Similar experiments were performed with endothelial cells and Kupffer cells isolated from mouse liver (FIG. 2, B and C). The cell association and degradation of AcLDL by endothelial cells follows saturation kinetics, whereas for the cells isolated from KO mice the maximal cell association reaches a value 50% of the control cells. For AcLDL degradation with endothelial cells from the KO mice, the maximal value of degradation is 58% of that found with the wild-type endothelial cells.

For isolated Kupffer cells it also appears that the cell-association and degradation of AcLDL are lower for the cells from the scavenger receptor class A type I/II KO mice. The maximal cell association with the cells from KO mice reaches 53% of the control while for the degradation 63% is observed. It thus appears that for the isolated cells a significant proportion of the uptake and degradation is exerted by scavenger receptor class A types I/II. In agreement with data obtained with rat liver cells,[22]

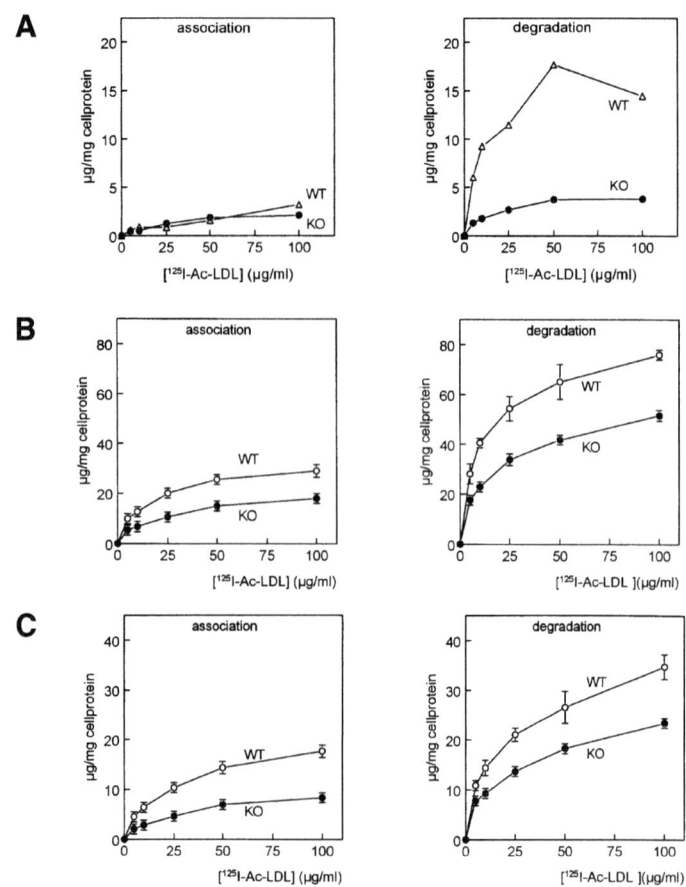

FIGURE 2. Cell-association and degradation of AcLDL by isolated peritoneal macrophages (**A**), endothelial (**B**), or Kupffer cells (**C**) from wild type (WT) and KO mice (KO) as function of the AcLDL concentration. The amount of ^{125}I-AcLDL was varied and the cell association or degradation is expressed as micrograms of apolipoprotein/mg cell protein. Incubation time was 2 h at 37°C and the values represent the mean ± S.E. (N = 3) for endothelial and Kupffer cells while peritoneal macrophages were isolated from 30 WT or 30 KO mice. *Open symbols* represent WT and *closed symbols* KO mice.

the metabolism of AcLDL by endothelial liver cells from control mice is more active (per mg cell protein) than that observed with Kupffer cells.

Inhibition of Selective Uptake of HDL-CEOH by Rat Liver Parenchymal Cells by Substrates of SR-BI

We showed earlier that the selective uptake of HDL-CE by parenchymal cells could almost be completely inhibited by OxLDL and liposomes containing phosphatidyl serine, e.g., known substrates for SR-BI.[28] As with native cholesterol esters,

TABLE 2. Capacities of cell association and degradation of AcLDL by Kupffer cells and endothelial liver cells from wild-type and scavenger receptor class A types I/II KO mice

	Kupffer cells Apparent V_{max} (µg/mg cell protein)		Endothelial cells Apparent V_{max} (µg/mg cell protein)	
	Cell association	Degradation	Cell association	Degradation
Wild-type mice	15.1 ± 2.2	21.4 ± 1.1	28.3 ± 4.2	65.0 ± 1.3
KO mice	8.0 ± 2.5	13.5 ± 1.7	14.1 ± 3.1	37.8 ± 2.7
Relative percentage of KO mice vs. wild-type mice	53.0%	63.0%	49.8%	58.2%

Note: Substrate curves ($N = 3$) were analyzed according to a single-site binding model using non-linear regression (Graph-PAD, ISIS Software).

the increased selective uptake of HDL-CEOH by the liver is mediated by the parenchymal cells *in vivo*. To answer the question of whether SR-BI is mediating this increased selective uptake of HDL-CEOH, the inhibitory effects of known SR-BI substrates on HDL-CEOH uptake by isolated parenchymal cells was compared with the inhibitory effects on the selective uptake of HDL-CE and HDL particle association as measured by iodinated HDL. Freshly isolated rat liver parenchymal cells were incubated for three hours at 37°C with HDL, either iodinated or labeled with [^{3}H]CE or [^{3}H]CEOH. At this time point the apparent association as calculated according to Pitmann of [^{3}H]CE labeled HDL (202 ± 14 ng HDL/mg cell protein) exceeds [^{125}I]-HDL (36 ± 3 ng HDL/mg cell protein) association 5.6 times, while the association of [^{3}H]CEOH-HDL (966 ± 150 ng HDL/mg cell protein) apparently exceeds [^{125}I]-HDL association 27 times. The ability of (modified) lipoproteins to compete for [^{125}I]-HDL and selective HDL-CE and HDL-CEOH uptake was tested by co-incubation with either 100 µg/ml LDL, AcLDL, OxLDL, and either neutral liposomes or liposomes containing phosphatidylserine (FIG. 3). Addition of either 100 µg/ml LDL or modified LDL did only marginally (<10%) decrease the cell association of [^{125}I]-HDL. [^{3}H]CE-HDL and [^{3}H]CEOH-HDL association was also not significantly affected by addition of LDL. However, addition of AcLDL led to a 35% and 30% inhibition, respectively, while OxLDL decreased [^{3}H]CE-HDL and [^{3}H]CEOH-HDL uptake for 75 ± 2.4% and 75 ± 5.4%, respectively. Liposomes consisting of phosphatidylcholine, cholesterol, and the anionic phospholipid phosphatidylserine inhibited both HDL-CE and HDL-CEOH uptake almost 50% (FIG. 3) while [^{125}I]-HDL association was increased. Neutral liposomes, consisting only of phosphatidylcholine and cholesterol, did not influence HDL-CE and HDL-CEOH uptake. The effective inhibition of the selective uptake of oxidized cholesterol esters, similarly as for native cholesterol esters from HDL, did not correlate with a similar inhibition of the HDL particle association.[28] Apparently the total amount of HDL binding sites in liver exceeds the amount of SR-BI–mediated binding sites, albeit these latter are efficiently coupled to selective uptake. This is in agreement with the limited amount of poly I–insensitive binding sites for OxLDL on parenchymal cells, as compared the total amount of HDL binding sites (less than 10%).

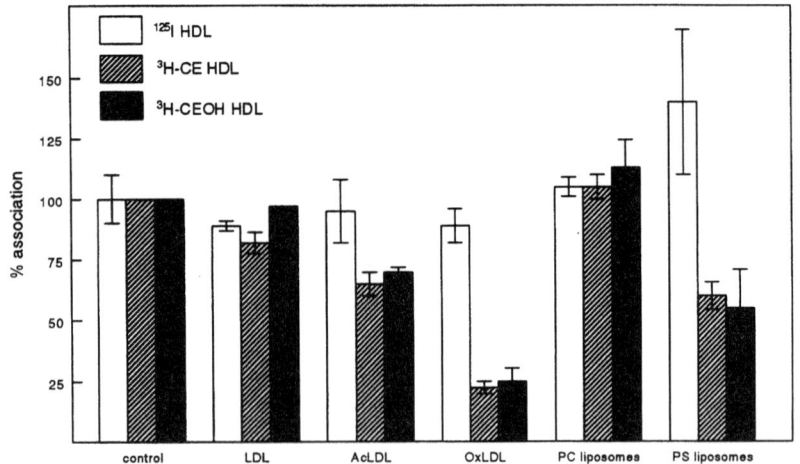

FIGURE 3. Effect of native and modified lipoproteins and neutral and phosphatidyl serine liposomes on the parenchymal cell association of HDL labeled with [^{125}I], [^{3}H]-CE, or [^{3}H]-CEOH. Rat liver parenchymal cells were incubated for 3 h at 37°C with 10 µg/ml labeled HDL in the absence or presence of 100 µg/ml unlabeled competitors in DMEM with 2% BSA. The 100% value for association of [^{3}H]-CE– or [^{3}H]-CEOH–labeled HDL was 202±14 ng and 966±150 ng HDL/mg cell protein, respectively. For [^{125}I]-HDL, association was 36±3 ng HDL/mg cell protein. The association is expressed as the percentage of the radioactivity obtained in the absence of competitor. The results are given as means ± S.E.M. ($N = 3$).

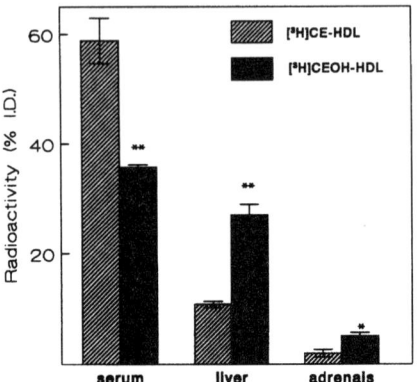

FIGURE 4. Tissue distribution of [^{3}H]-CEOH HDL and [^{3}H]-CE HDL at 30 minutes after injection in the rat. 300–400 µg (500,000 dpm) of [^{3}H]-CEOH HDL or [^{3}H]-CE HDL was injected into the vena cava inferior of anesthetized rats. Thirty minutes after injection the amount of radioactivity was determined after combustion in a Hewlett-Packard sample oxidizer 306 and counting for radioactivity. The total recovery of label was 94% and 86% of the injected dose for [^{3}H]-CEOH and [^{3}H]-CE HDL, respectively. Values are means ± S.E.M. of four experiments. **Extremely significant difference, $p < 0.005$. *Significant difference, $p < 0.05$ (unpaired Student's t test).

TABLE 3. SR-BI expression levels on parenchymal and Kupffer cell membranes

	Control	EE	High cholesterol diet
		\multicolumn{2}{c}{Percentage of control}	
PC	100 ± 4.5	15.2 ± 4.1**	25.0 ± 6.0**
KC	100 ± 5.0	388 ± 55.0**	310 ± 75.0*

Note: Cell membranes from parenchymal and Kupffer cells were isolated from control rats, rats treated with ethinyl estradiol (EE) (5 mg/kg) for 5 days, or from rats that had been fed a high-cholesterol diet for two weeks. Solubilized membrane proteins were subjected to SDS-PAGE and blotted onto nitrocellulose membranes. SR-BI was visualized by immunolabeling followed by enhanced chemiluminescence detection and quantitated.[21] Values are means ± S.E.M. of three experiments.
**Very significant difference, $p < 0.005$.
*Significant difference, $p = 0.05$ (unpaired Student's t-test).

Uptake of HDL-CEOH by the Liver and Adrenals in Vivo

The main uptake site of [^{3}H]-CEOH labeled HDL *in vivo* is the liver.[2] The liver uptake of [^{3}H]CEOH HDL 30 min after injection is 27.0 ± 1.9 percent of injection dose (ID%) (FIG. 4) and is 2.3-fold higher than the liver uptake of native HDL-CE ($N = 4$). When the adrenal uptake of [^{3}H]CEOH HDL is compared to the uptake of [^{3}H]CE HDL, a similar 2.6-fold difference in uptake is seen. Adrenal uptake at 30 min after injection was 2.0 ± 0.7 ID% and 5.1 ± 0.6% for [^{3}H]CE HDL and [^{3}H]CEOH HDL, respectively ($N = 4$). No other organs have a preferential uptake of HDL-CEOH as compared to native HDL-CE.

Intrahepatic Cellular Uptake in Vivo of HDL-CEOH: Effect of 17α-Ethinyl Estradiol Treatment or a High Cholesterol Diet on SR-BI Expression and HDL-CEOH Uptake

Treatment of rats with 17α-ethinyl estradiol (EE) for 5 consecutive days or a high cholesterol diet for two weeks lowers expression of SR-BI in the liver parenchymal cells, while the expression of SR-BI in the Kupffer cells was increased as previously reported (TABLE 3).[32] Furthermore it was found that the induced changes in hepatic SR-BI expression were well correlated to changes in the selective uptake of HDL-CEOH.[33] In order to test whether the changes in SR-BI expression induced by either EE treatment or a high cholesterol diet also affected the increased selective uptake of HDL CEOH, the liver uptake of [^{3}H]CEOH labeled HDL was determined, as well as the association of iodinated HDL in order to analyze total particle association. To identify the changes in the cellular uptake sites for [^{3}H]CEOH HDL, parenchymal cells and liver tissue macrophages (Kupffer cells) were isolated (FIG. 5). Treatment of rats with EE for 5 days resulted in a significant 50% decrease in [^{3}H]CEOH-HDL uptake by the liver, while uptake of ^{125}I-labeled HDL did not change significantly (data not shown). Thus the selective uptake of HDL-CEOH was greatly inhibited by treatment of rats with EE, in accordance with the supposed role of SR-BI as the mediator of selective HDL-CEOH uptake. This decrease in selective uptake of HDL-CEOH by the liver can be explained by a 64% decrease in [^{3}H]CEOH-HDL uptake

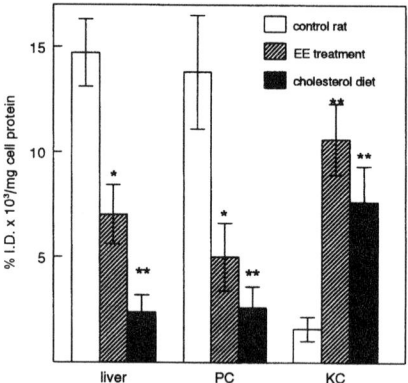

FIGURE 5. *In vivo* distribution of [^{3}H]-CEOH HDL between parenchymal and Kupffer cells, at 10 min after injection in ethinyl estradiol–treated rats, rats fed with a high cholesterol diet, or control rats. Control rats (*open bars*), or rats treated with EE (5 mg/kg) for 5 days (*hatched bars*), or rats put on a high cholesterol diet for two weeks (*solid bars*). At 10 min after injection of [^{3}H]-CEOH HDL, the liver was perfused and parenchymal cells (PC) and Kupffer cells (KC) were isolated at 4°C. Values expressed as the percentage of the injected dose × 10^3/mg of cell protein, are means ± S.E.M. of five experiments. **Very significant difference, $p < 0.01$. *Significant difference, $p < 0.05$ (unpaired Student's t test).

by the parenchymal cells after EE treatment. In contrast, the Kupffer cells showed a significant 6.6-fold increase ($p < 0.05$) in uptake of [^{3}H]CEOH-HDL.

Rats were also fed a high cholesterol diet for two weeks. This diet increased the plasma cholesterol levels 20-fold as compared to the control animals as previously described,[33] while total cholesterol concentration in the liver increased more than tenfold. The total cellular cholesterol concentration in parenchymal cells increased from the control value of 11 ± 0.9 ng/mg cell protein up to 136 ± 18 ng/mg cell protein ($N = 3$, ±S.E.M.), while the cholesterol content in the Kupffer cells increased from 6.8 ± 0.2 ng/mg cell protein in the control animals to 155 ± 66 ng/mg cell protein after the two-week diet ($N = 3$, ±S.E.M.). This diet resulted in a very significant ($p < 0.01$) 80% decrease in selective uptake of [^{3}H]CEOH-HDL by the liver (FIG. 5). The two-week high cholesterol diet inhibited only the parenchymal cell uptake of [^{3}H]CEOH-HDL (81%), while Kupffer cell uptake of [^{3}H]CEOH-HDL was increased almost fivefold. The decrease in HDL-CEOH uptake by the parenchymal cells and increase in HDL-CEOH uptake by the Kupffer cells after either EE treatment or high cholesterol diet is similar to that found with native HDL-CE and correlates with the induced changes in hepatic SR-BI expression.[33]

DISCUSSION

Scavenger receptors are implicated in the pathological deposition of cholesterol esters during atherogenesis. The cloning and characterization[11,12] of scavenger receptor class A types I/II have now led to the creation of receptor-deficient mice.[25] Besides by southern analysis, receptor deficiency has also been shown by the absence of immunostaining by the anti-murine scavenger receptor class A types I/II monoclonal antibody (2F8) of liver sinusoidal cells in the KO mice.[25] More than a decade ago we showed that upon injection of AcLDL in rats, these particles were rapidly removed by the blood circulation and that liver endothelial cells were the main site of uptake.[22] We assumed that the scavenger receptor class A types I/II were responsible for this uptake because the *in vitro* interaction of AcLDL with liver endothelial cells and Kupffer cells possessed characteristics similar to those described for this type of scavenger receptor. It is therefore surprising to observe that upon injection of AcLDL into KO mice a rapid clearance and liver uptake is observed. Moreover, the murine liver endothelial cell appears to be the major liver site for AcLDL uptake both in control and receptor-deficient mice. We do not consider the 17% inhibition in uptake of AcLDL by endothelial cells in the KO mice a very significant reflection of receptor deficiency (although the p value was <0.05). Also, the injection of a higher dose of AcLDL (200 µg) did not lead to a significant effect on the decay or liver uptake, although the kinetics clearly point to a partial saturation of the uptake system. From these data, we have to conclude that alternative uptake systems for AcLDL must be present in the liver endothelial cells and Kupffer cells that can compensate for the absence of scavenger receptor class A types I/II and thus this receptor concentration is not rate limiting *in vivo*. Furthermore the degradation of AcLDL was not hampered *in vivo* in the KO mice.

Studies *in vitro* with isolated mouse endothelial cells, Kupffer cells, and peritoneal macrophages were performed to assess whether the capacity of the individual cell types to interact with AcLDL is hampered by the absence of scavenger receptor class A types I/II. For peritoneal macrophages it is clear, as also briefly reported recently,[25] that the degradation of AcLDL is especially affected (in KO cells the maximal degradation is 17% of the cells from control mice), Lougheed and colleagues[39] also recently reported an 80% reduction of AcLDL degradation in macrophages from scavenger receptor class A types I/II KO mice. For the isolated endothelial cells and Kupffer cells, we observe that the maximal degradation of AcLDL in the cells from KO mice reaches a value of 58% and 63% of the cells from wild-type mice, respectively. These data indicate that the scavenger receptor class A types I/II are of quantitative importance for the degradation of AcLDL by these cell types. The surprising observation that a 40–50% reduction in cell-association and degradation of AcLDL by KO mice liver endothelial and Kupffer cells *in vitro* is not reflected in a concomitant delay in clearance *in vivo* might be caused by the extremely rapid recycling of the alternative scavenger receptors. It might also be possible that *in vivo* initial binding to proteoglycans may mask the receptor deficiency. Apparently an excess capacity is present *in vivo* for the turnover of modified lipoproteins and other potential ligands for scavenger receptors. It must be concluded that alternative still-unidentified receptors are present that can take over the function of scavenger receptor class A types I/II. Whether these receptors are related to recently described scavenger receptors such as Marco,[17] macrosialin,[18,19] CD36,[20] and scavenger receptor BI (SR-BI)[21] is unknown and awaits characterization.

The liver and steroidogenic tissues are mainly responsible for the clearance of native HDL cholesteryl esters from the blood circulation. SR-BI is now held responsible for mediating the selective uptake of native HDL-CE by these organs.[26,29,30] The presence of hydroxyl groups in oxidized cholesterol esters yields a better solubility in water, enabling the cholesteryl hydroxides to transfer more efficiently through an aqueous phase between HDL and cellular membranes. This might explain the increased cellular uptake of HDL-CEOH. However, based upon our previous *in vivo* experiments, it was concluded that this increased solubility did not lead to an increased uptake by all cell types, but just the parenchymal cells within the liver. In addition, the adrenals, which are known to have a high expression of SR-BI, show a similar increased uptake of HDL-CEOH as compared to native HDL-CE. Apparently, a cell-specific process is mediating uptake of oxidized cholesterol esters *in vivo*, as for the uptake of native cholesterol esters. We now suggest that indeed the increased selective uptake of oxidized cholesterol esters as compared to native cholesterol esters is mediated by SR-BI. We obtained five points of evidence for this involvement. (1) The increased selective uptake of HDL-CEOH by isolated parenchymal cells can be blocked by OxLDL, AcLDL, and phosphatidylserine liposomes to a similar extent as native cholesterol ester uptake. (2) The effect of OxLDL is not influenced by the simultaneous presence of poly I, indicating a poly I–insensitive site for OxLDL interaction. (3) *In vivo* the increased uptake of oxidized as compared to native cholesterol esters in untreated rats is only exerted by the parenchymal cells of the liver and by the adrenals, the cellular sites where SR-BI is expressed. (4) Within the liver the uptake of oxidized cholesterol esters is similarly regulated by estradiol treatment or a high cholesterol diet of rats as for native cholesterol esters, whereby the *in vivo* uptake by parenchymal cells is decreased while the uptake by Kupffer cells is increased. These latter changes parallel the expression of SR-BI as analyzed on western blots. (5) The SR-BI transfected CHO cells show a very efficient selective uptake of oxidized cholesterol esters, exceeding particle association 20 times at 30 min of incubation while oxidized cholesterol ester uptake at this time point is 3.4 times higher than for native cholesterol esters. It thus appears that SR-BI is a major determinant for the selective uptake of oxidized cholesterol esters, leaving only a low percentage contribution for other receptors.

CONCLUSION

The mechanism for the more effective cellular uptake of oxidized cholesterol esters as compared to native cholesterol esters from HDL by SR-BI is presently unclear. The higher solubility of oxidized cholesterol esters as compared to native cholesterol esters might either facilitate the interaction of CEOH from HDL with the active site of SR-BI, or facilitate its further transport into the cell. Whatever its mechanism it might be concluded that the association of enzymatic activities with HDL together with the efficient clearance route of HDL-associated oxidized cholesterol esters, as exerted by SR-BI on liver parenchymal cells, may work synergistically to detoxify lipid hydroperoxides and thereby protect LDL from oxidation *in vivo*. This scavenging function of SR-BI for oxidized lipids is in line with the expected function of a member of the scavenger receptor family.

REFERENCES

1. STEINBERG, D. 1988. Atheroscler. Rev. **18:** 1–23.
2. BROWN, M.S., S.K. BASU, J.R. FALCK, Y.K. HO & J.L. GOLDSTEIN. 1980. J. Supramol. Struct. **13:** 67–81.

3. GOLDSTEIN, J.L., Y.K. HO, S.K. BASU & M.S. BROWN. 1979. Proc. Natl. Acad. Sci. USA **76:** 333–337.
4. MAHLEY, R.W., T.L. INNERARITY, K.H. WEISGRABER & S.Y. OH. 1979. J. Clin. Invest. **64:** 743–750.
5. FOGELMAN, A.M., I. SCHECHTER, J. SEAGER, M. HOKOM, J.S. CHILD & P.A. EDWARDS. 1980. Proc. Natl. Acad. Sci. USA **77:** 2214–2218.
6. PARTHASARATHY, S., U.P. STEINBRECHER, J. BARNETT, J.L. WITZTUM & D. STEINBERG. 1985. Proc. Natl. Acad. Sci. USA **82:** 3000–3004
7. BROWN, M.S. & J.L. GOLDSTEIN. 1983. Annu. Rev. Biochem. **52:** 223–261.
8. VAN BERKEL, TH.J.C., J.F. NAGELKERKE, L. HARKES & J.K. KRUIJT. 1982. Biochem. J. **208:** 493–503.
9. DRESEL, H.A., E. FRIEDRICH, D.P. VIA, H. SINN, R. ZIEGLER & G. SCHETTLER. 1987. EMBO J. **6:** 319–326.
10. KODAMA, T., P. REDDY, C. KISHIMOTO & M. KRIEGER. 1988. Proc. Natl. Acad. Sci. USA **85:** 9238–9242.
11. KODAMA, T., M. FREEMAN, L. ROHRER, J. ZABRECKY, P. MATASUDAIRA & M. KRIEGER. 1990. Nature (London) **343:** 531–535.
12. ROHRER, L., M. FREEMAN, T. KODAMA, M. PENMAN & M. KRIEGER. 1990. Nature **343:** 570–572.
13. ASHKENAS, J., M. PENMAN, E. VASILE, M. FREEMAN & M. KRIEGER. 1993. J. Lipid Res. **34:** 983–1000.
14. YLÄ-HERTTUALA, S., M.E. ROSENFELD, S. PARTHASARATHY, E. SIGAL, T. SÄRKIOJA, J.L. WITZTUM & D. STEINBERG. 1991. J. Clin. Invest. **87:** 1146–1152.
15. NAITO, M., T. KODAMA, A. MATSUMOTO, T. DOI & K. TAKAHASHI. 1991. Am. J. Pathol. **139:** 1411–1423.
16. HUGHES, D.A., I.P. FRASER & S. GORDON. 1995. Eur. J. Immunol. **25:** 466–473.
17. ELOMAA, O., M. KANGAS, C. SAHLBERG, J. TUUKKANEN, R. SORMUNEN, A. LIAKKA, I. THESLEFF, G. KRAAL & K. TRYGGVASON. 1995. Cell **80:** 603–609.
18. RAMPRASAD, M.P., W. FISCHER, J.L. WITZTUM, G.R. SAMBRANO, O. QUEHENBERGER & D. STEINBERG. 1995. Proc. Natl. Acad. Sci. USA **92:** 9580–9584.
19. VAN VELZEN, A.G., R.P. DA SILVA, S. GORDON & TH.J.C. VAN BERKEL. 1997. Biochem. J. **322:** 411–415.
20. ENDEMANN, G., L.W. STANTON, K.S. MADDEN, C.M. BRYANT, R.T. WHITE & A.A. PROTTER. 1993. J. Biol. Chem. **268:** 11811–11816.
21. ACTON, S.L., P.E. SCHERER, H.F. LODISH & M. KRIEGER. 1994. J. Biol. Chem. **269:** 21003–21009.
22. NAGELKERKE, J.F., K.P. BARTO & TH.J.C. VAN BERKEL. 1983. J. Biol. Chem. **258:** 12221–12227.
23. VAN BERKEL, TH.J.C., Y.B. DE RIJKE & J.K. KRUIJT. 1991. J. Biol. Chem. **266:** 2282–2289.
24. DE RIJKE, Y.B. & TH.J.C. VAN BERKEL 1994. J. Biol. Chem. **269:** 824–827.
25. SUZUKI, H., Y. KURIHARE, M. TAKEYA, N. KAMADA, M. KATAOKA, K. JISHAGE, O. UEDA, H. SAKAGUCHI, T. HIGASHI, T. SUZUKI, Y. TAKASHIMA, Y. KAWABE, O. CYNSHI, Y. WADA, M. HONDA, H. KURIHARA, H. ABURATANI, T. DOI, A. MATSUMOTO, S. AZUMA, T. NODA, Y. TOYODA, H. ITAKURA, Y. YAZAKI, S. HORIUCHI, K. TAKAHASHI, J.K. KRUIJT, TH.J.C. VAN BERKEL, U.P. STEINBRECHER, S. ISHIBASHI, N. MAEDA, S. GORDON & T. KODAMA. 1997. Nature **386:** 292–296.
26. ACTON, S., A. RIGOTTI, K.T. LANDSCHULZ, S. XU, H.H. HOBBS & M. KRIEGER. 1996. Science **271:** 518–520.
27. RIGOTTI, A., S. ACTON & M. KRIEGER.1995. J. Biol. Chem. **270:** 16221–16224.
28. FLUITER, K. & TH.J.C. VAN BERKEL. 1997. Biochem. J. **326:** 515–519.
29. LANDSCHULZ, K.T., R.K. PATHAK, A. RIGOTTI, M. KRIEGER & H.H. HOBBS. 1996. J. Clin. Invest. **98:** 984–995.
30. WANG, N., W. WENG, J.L. BRESLOW & A.R. TALL. 1996. J. Biol. Chem. **271:** 21001–21004.
31. RIGOTTI, A. 1996. J. Biol. Chem. **271:** 33545–33549.
32. NG, D.S., O.L. FRANCONE, T.M. FORTE, J. ZHANG, M. HAGHPASSAND & E.M. RUBIN. 1997. J. Biol. Chem. **272:** 15777–15781.

33. FLUITER, K., D.R. VAN DER WESTHUYZEN & TH.J.C. VAN BERKEL. 1998. J. Biol. Chem. **273:** 8434–8438.

Questions and Answers

A.R. TALL (*Columbia University, New York, NY, USA*): Your demonstration that SRBI actually mediates the reverse transport of oxidized lipid is, I think, very important. You have shown this for cholesterol esters. Oxidized phospholipids in plasma and peroxidase may play some role in clearing. But I suspect that the capacity of the system you have described is so much larger that it will turn out to be much more important than the peroxidase, for example. Have you looked at oxidized phospholipid uptake?

VAN BERKEL: No, we did not look specifically at the phospholipids, but when you look at the speed of the uptake of the oxidized cholesteryl esters, I can only agree that this must be the major route of removal, because when you analyze the data in the rats you can see that within 10 minutes, 50–60% is removed. I anticipate that the oxidized phospholipids also are a substrate for SRBI uptake.

S. HORIUCHI (*Kumamoto University, Kumamoto, Japan*): The plasma clearance of radiolabeled acetyl- LDL in the wild-type mice and the MSRA knock-out mice is comparable, but in isolated liver cells, such as hepatocytes and Kupffer cells, your data showed some 40% decrease. How do you explain that kind of inconsistency?

VAN BERKEL: I think it is very difficult to look at the capacity of these receptor systems *in vivo*, because receptor expression on the membrane has to be rate limiting. Apparently *in vivo* this receptor expression is not rate limiting under these conditions, although we tried to saturate the system by having an increased concentration of acetylated LDL. A second explanation may be that when we isolate the cells we may remove additional receptor systems that are important *in vivo*.

HORIUCHI: In our experience, the MSRA knock-out mice endothelial cells or Kupffer cells have remarkably reduced adhesiveness to the tissue culture well. That may have something to do with the difference between *in vitro* and *in vivo*.

VAN BERKEL: Not in our experiments We noticed this difference in adhesion and therefore isolated the cells and incubated them directly in suspension. We have data at the moment that the adhesion of the endothelial and Kupffer cells is lower and also that the amount of Kupffer cells in the scavenger receptor A knock-out animals is lower than in control animals. I agree that adhesion is an additional property of scavenger receptor class A.

HORIUCHI: Oxidized LDL is effectively taken up by these Kupffer cells or endothelial cells. After the intravenous injection of modified LDL, can you find some foam cell formation by Kupffer cells or endothelial cells, similar to macrophages? Is there a difference between these cell types?

VAN BERKEL: You can induce a rapid, massive uptake *in vivo* of oxidized LDL by the cells, and you can confer a foam cell–like appearance. You can also study *in vivo* the transfer of the cholesteryl esters from these cells. So, we have done experiments in which we labeled cholesteryl esters in oxidized LDL; they are taken up by the cells and then we follow a rapid uptake in 10 minutes, and then the release. We also can analyze the kinetics of the release to HDL, and then analyze subsequent uptake by parenchymal cells and secretion into the bile.

H. HAKAMATA (*University of California, San Francisco, CA, USA*): What is the source of your beta-VLDL?

VAN BERKEL: Beta-VLDL is obtained from rats fed a high cholesterol diet for two weeks. It is apoA-rich. We also isolated beta-VLDL from mice. There is no difference between the rat and mouse beta-VLDL.

CD36 in Atherosclerosis

The Role of a Class B Macrophage Scavenger Receptor

ANDREW C. NICHOLSON, MARIA FEBBRAIO, JIHONG HAN,
ROY L. SILVERSTEIN, AND DAVID P. HAJJAR[a]

Center of Vascular Biology, Cornell University Medical College, 1300 York Avenue, New York, New York, USA

ABSTRACT: CD36, an 88 kD transmembrane glycoprotein, is an important receptor for oxidized lipoproteins. Unlike the LDL receptor, expression of CD36 is upregulated by this pro-atherogenic particle, and binding and uptake perpetuates a cycle of lipid accumulation and receptor expression. This effect is, in part, mediated by the transcription factor, peroxisome proliferator activated receptor-γ (PPARγ), and its ligands. We have found that specific inhibitors of protein kinase C (PKC) reduce basal mRNA expression of CD36 and block induction of CD36 mRNA and protein by oxidized LDL (OxLDL) and a PPARγ ligand. In addition, PKC inhibitors block both PPARγ mRNA and protein expression. These results suggest that activation of CD36 gene expression by OxLDL involves activation and translocation of PKC with subsequent PPARγ activation. More recently, we have generated a mouse null for CD36, and crossed it with the atherogenic Apo E null strain. Evaluation of lesion development in these animals will allow us to assess the *in vivo* contribution of CD36 to the pathogenesis of atherosclerosis.

CD36 is a type B scavenger receptor, a family of receptors that includes SR-BI, an HDL receptor.[1] CD36 is expressed by monocyte/macrophages,[2] platelets,[3] microvascular endothelial cells,[4] and adipose tissue.[5] Like the type A scavenger receptors,[6] CD36 recognizes a broad variety of ligands including OxLDL,[7,8] anionic phospholipids,[9] apoptotic cells,[10] thrombospondin (TSP),[11] collagen,[12] and *Plasmodium falciparum*–infected erythrocytes.[13] Unlike the class A receptors, which recognize the oxidized apoprotein portion of the lipoprotein particle,[14] CD36 binds to the lipid moiety of OxLDL.[8] Binding of OxLDL to CD36-transfected cells is inhibited by anionic phospholipid vesicles.[9] CD36 may also bind HDL,[15] however SR-BI mediates uptake of HDL CE with much greater efficiency than CD36.[16]

We have shown that half or more of the binding of OxLDL by human monocyte-derived macrophages is inhibited by anti-CD36 antibodies.[8] CD36-transfected cells bind OxLDL in a saturable manner. Binding, internalization, and degradation of OxLDL was increased fourfold in CD36-transfected cells relative to cells transfected with vector alone.[8] LDL and acetylated LDL (AcLDL) bind equally to control and CD36-transfected cells.[8]

---

[a]Address for correspondence: David. P. Hajjar, Ph.D., Weill Medical College of Cornell University, Department of Pathology, A–626, 1300 York Avenue, New York, NY 10021. Voice: 212-746-6470; fax: 212-746-8789.
dphajjar@mail.med.cornell.edu

Expression of CD36 in monocyte/macrophages is dependent both on the differentiation state as well as exposure to soluble mediators[17,18] We studied the effect of lipoproteins, native LDL, and modified LDL (AcLDL and OxLDL) on the expression of CD36 in J774 cells, a murine macrophage cell line.[19] Exposure to lipoproteins resulted in a marked induction of CD36 mRNA expression (four- to eightfold). Maximum induction was observed 2 h after treatment with AcLDL and at 4 h with LDL and OxLDL. Expression of CD36 mRNA persisted for 24 h with each treatment group. Induction of CD36 mRNA expression was paralleled by an increase in CD36 protein as determined by Western blot, with the greatest induction by OxLDL (fourfold). In the presence of actinomycin D, treatment of macrophages with LDL, AcLDL, or OxLDL did not affect CD36 mRNA stability, implying that CD36 mRNA was transcriptionally regulated by lipoproteins.[19] Incubation of macrophages with cholesterol acceptor proteins (BSA or HDL) reduced expression of CD36 mRNA in a dose-dependent manner.[19] The effects of lipoproteins on CD36 expression were mimicked by alterations in macrophage cellular cholesterol content.[20] Depletion of cellular cholesterol by treatment with β-cyclodextrins significantly decreased the expression of both CD36 mRNA and ^{125}I-OxLDL binding. In contrast, macrophages that are cholesterol-loaded with cyclodextrin:cholesterol complexes increased both CD36 mRNA expression and ^{125}I-OxLDL binding.[20] Results of these experiments demonstrate that unlike the LDL receptor, which is downregulated by cellular cholesterol, expression of CD36 is enhanced by cholesterol and downregulated by cholesterol efflux. These results further imply that macrophage expression of CD36 and foam cell formation in atherosclerotic lesions may be perpetuated by a cycle in which lipids continue to drive expression of a lipoprotein receptor in a self-regulatory manner.

The effect of OxLDL on CD36 is due, in part, to its ability to activate the transcription factor, PPARγ (peroxisome proliferator activated receptor-γ).[21,22] Other PPARγ ligands (15-deoxy$\Delta^{12,14}$ prostaglandin J2, 15d-PGJ2) and the thiazolidinedione class of antidiabetic drugs also increase CD36 expression.[21,22]

We evaluated signaling pathways involved in the induction of CD36 mRNA. Treatment of RAW264.7 cells (a murine macrophage cell line) with protein kinase C (PKC) activators (diacylglycerol and ingenol) upregulated CD36 mRNA expression. Specific inhibitors of PKC reduced CD36 expression in a time-dependent manner. In contrast, protein kinase A (PKA) and cyclic AMP agonists had no effect on CD36 mRNA expression. PKC inhibitors reduced basal expression of CD36 and blocked induction of CD36 mRNA by 15d-PGJ2 and OxLDL. In addition, PKC inhibitors decreased both PPARγ mRNA and protein expression. Treatment of human monocytes with OxLDL, but not 15d-PGJ2, resulted in increased expression of PKC-α as well as its translocation from the cytosol to the plasma membrane. Finally, PKC inhibitors blocked induction of CD36 protein surface expression by OxLDL and 15d-PGJ2 in human monocytes, as determined by flow cytometry. These results demonstrate that activation of CD36 gene expression by OxLDL involves initial activation and translocation of PKC with subsequent PPARγ activation.

Generation of null and transgenic mice, in which specific genes are targeted, has led to an important leap forward in our ability to understand the pathogenesis of atherosclerosis. Before the invention of these techniques, mice were all but resistant to atherosclerosis and therefore not useful. Mouse models are valuable because mice can be studied in large numbers, the genetics of many strains are well documented, inbred strains provide virtual clones in which to do experiments, environmental factors can be altered, and crossbreeding and now, genetic techniques, allow manipulation of genetic factors. To date, there are several important murine models, including Apo E and LDL receptor nulls, which have been created specifically to mimic human atherosclerosis. We hypothesized that targeting a receptor for OxLDL on the macrophage may alter the course of disease by delaying or preventing foam cell and fatty streak formation and perhaps by preventing alteration of the vessel wall due to macrophage actions. To test this hypothesis, we created a mouse null in CD36.

Our research indicates that there is a substantial reduction in the binding and internalization of OxLDL by macrophages from these animals. To test whether this is now protective against atherosclerosis, and thus a potential target for therapeutic intervention, we have backcrossed the CD36 null mouse to the Apo E null, to provide the high cholesterol, atherosclerotic environment. Studies are currently underway to assess the role of CD36 in the pathogenesis of this disease and the relationship of diet and other factors. Already, we have established that CD36 null mice have altered lipoprotein metabolism: there is an increase in plasma cholesterol, triacylglycerol, and non-esterified fatty acids. The increased cholesterol is in the form of HDL, and the increase in triacylglycerol is in the form of vLDL. We believe the alterations we observe in lipid metabolism are due to the role of CD36 as a long chain fatty acid transporter, and that this mouse establishes a physiological role for these controversial proteins. Further study is necessary, however, to unequivocally establish this to be the case. The results of these studies will give us greater understanding of the mechanism of diseases like atherosclerosis and diabetes, and allow identification of risk factors and potential therapeutic drugs. Animal models such as ours are essential to the study of complex human diseases in which these parameters can only be assessed in the intact animal.

REFERENCES

1. ACTON, S., R. ATTILIO, K. LANDSCHULTZ, S. XU, H. HOBBS & M. KRIEGER. 1996. Identification of scavenger receptor SR-B1 as a high density lipoprotein receptor. Science **271**: 518.
2. TALLE, M., P. RAO, E. WESTBERG, N. ALLEGAR, M. MAKOWSKI, R. MITTLER & G. GOLDSTEIN. 1983. Patterns of antigenic expression on human monocytes as defined by monoclonal antibodies. Cell. Immunol. **78**: 83.
3. LI, Y.S., Y.J. SHYY, J.G. WRIGHT, A.J. VALENTE, J.F. CORNHILL & P.E. KOLATTUKUDY. 1993. The expression of monocyte chemotactic protein (MCP-1) in human vascular endothelium in vitro and in vivo. Mol. Cell Biochem. **126**: 61.
4. GREENWALT, D., R. LIPSKY, C. OCKENHOUSE, H. IKEDA, N. TANDON & G. JAMIESON. 1992. Membrane glycoprotein CD36: A review if its roles in adherence, signal transduction, and transfusion medicine. Blood **80**: 1105.
5. ABUMRAD, N., M.R. EL-MAGHRABI, E. AMRI, E. LOPEZ & P. GRIMALDI. 1993. Cloning of a rat adipocyte membrane protein implicated in binding or transport of long-chain fatty acids that is induced during preadipocyte differentiation. J. Biol. Chem. **268**: 17665.
6. KRIEGER, M., S. ACTON, J. ASHKENAS, A. PEARSON, M. PENMAN & D. RESNICK. 1993. Molecular flypaper, host defense, and atherosclerosis. J. Biol. Chem. **268**: 4569.
7. ENDEMANN, G., L. STANTON, K. MADDEN, K. BRYANT, R.T. WHITE & A. PROTTER. 1993. CD36 is a receptor for oxidized low density lipoprotein. J. Biol. Chem. **268**: 11811.
8. NICHOLSON, A., S.F.A. PEARCE & R. SILVERSTEIN. 1995. Oxidized LDL binds to CD36 on human monocyte-derived macrophages and transfected cell lines. Evidence implicating the lipid moiety of the lipoprotein as the binding site. Arterioscl. Thromb. **15**: 269.
9. RIGOTTI, A., S. ACTON & M. KRIEGER. 1995. The class B scavenger receptors SR-B1 and CD36 are receptors for anionic phospholipids. J. Biol. Chem. **270**: 16221.

10. REN, Y., R. SILVERSTEIN, J. ALLEN & J. SAVILL. 1995. CD36 gene transfer confers capacity for phagocytosis of cells undergoing apoptosis. J. Exp. Med. **181:** 1857.
11. ASCH, A., J. BARNWELL, R. SILVERSTEIN & R. NACHMAN. 1987. Isolation of the thrombospondin membrane receptor. J. Clin. Invest. **79:** 1054.
12. TANDON, N., U. KRALISZ & G. JAMIESON. 1989. Identification of GPIV (CD36) as a primary receptor for platelet-collagen adhesion. J. Biol. Chem. **264:** 7576.
13. BARNWELL, J., C. OCKENHOUSE & D. KNOWLES. 1985. Monoclonal antibody OKM5 inhibits the in vitro binding of *Plasmodium falciparum* infected erythrocytes to monocytes, endothelial, and C32 melanoma cells. J. Immunol. **135:** 3494.
14. PARTHASARATHY, S., L. FONG, D. OTERO & D. STEINBERG. 1987. Recognition of solubilized apoproteins from delipidated, oxidized low density lipoprotein (LDL) by the acetyl-LDL receptor. Proc. Natl. Acad. Sci. USA **84:** 537.
15. CALVO, D., D. GOMEZ-CORONADO, Y. SUAREZ, M. LASUNCION & M.A. VEGA. 1998. Human CD36 is a high affinity receptor for the native lipoproteins HDL, LDL, and VLDL. J. Lipid Res. **39:** 777.
16. CONNELLY, M.A., S. KLEIN, S. AZHAR, N. ABUMRAD & D L. WILLIAMS. 1999. Comparison of class B scavenger receptors, CD36 and scavenger receptor BI (SR-BI), shows that both receptors mediate high density lipoprotein-cholesteryl ester selective uptake but SR-BI exhibits a unique enhancement of cholesteryl ester uptake. J. Biol. Chem. **274:** 41.
17. HUH, H.-Y., S.F.A. PEARCE, L. YESNER & R.L. SILVERSTEIN. 1996. Regulated expression of CD36 during monocyte-to-macrophage differentiation: Potential role of CD36 in foam cell formation. Blood **87:** 2020.
18. YESNER, L., H. HUH, S.F.A. PEARCE & R. SILVERSTEIN. 1996. Regulation of monocyte CD36 and thrombospondin-1 expression by soluble mediators. Arterioscl. Thromb. **16:** 1019.
19. HAN, J., D.P. HAJJAR, M. FEBBRAIO & A.C. NICHOLSON. 1997. Native and modified low density lipoproteins increase the functional expression of the macrophage class B scavenger receptor, CD36. J. Biol. Chem. **272:** 21654.
20. HAN, J., D.P. HAJJAR, J.M. TAURAS & A.C. NICHOLSON. 1999. Cellular cholesterol regulates expression of the macrophage type B scavenger receptor, CD36. J. Lipid Res. **40:** 830–838
21. TONTONOZ, P., L. NAGY, J. ALVAREZ, V. THOMAZY & R. EVANS. 1998. PPARγ promotes monocyte/macrophage differentiation and uptake of oxidized LDL. Cell **93:** 241.
22. NAGY, L., P. TONTONOZ, J. ALVAREZ, H. CHEN & R. EVANS. 1998. Oxidized LDL regulates macrophage gene expression through ligand activation of PPARγ. Cell **93:** 229.

Questions and Answers

P. LIBBY (*Brigham and Women's Hospital, Boston, MA, USA*): Could you give us a better idea about the type of substrate you tried in your macrophage uptake experiments? What is oxidized LDL? How did you make it? How oxidized was it? Have you looked at minimally modified LDL and acetylated LDL?

FEBBRAIO: We utilized copper oxidized LDL for 10 h at 37°C, so this is minimally modified, using the procedure first described by Endemann.

LIBBY: Just for comparison, can you tell us what the T-BARS values were?

FEBBRAIO: I do not have that data with me.

LIBBY: I am not a lipoprotein person, so I am allowed to be totally naive and ask what is the fatty acid sensor in the liver? We do have an idea what the cholesterol sensor is. What is the fatty acid sensor? Has anyone thought about PPAR as the sensor?

FEBBRAIO: We are thinking that way, but we don't have any data.

T.J.C. VAN BERKEL (*University of Leiden, Leiden, the Netherlands*): I am interested in your oxidized LDL data with the macrophages, because you showed a diminishment of binding and cell association. But, we know that the CD36 is not really rapidly internalizing oxidized LDL. What are the data on the degradation of oxidized LDL? That is especially relevant for foam cell biology, because the rate of degradation will be an important factor in foam cell formation.

FEBBRAIO: I agree that it is very important to know the degradation data, and our laboratory is pursuing this question.

A.R. TALL (*Columbia University, New York, NY, USA*): The HDL increase of 40% is surprising. In the studies done comparing CD36 with SRBI, there is a small effect on selective uptake of HDL cholesteryl ester uptake in the CD36 overexpressing cells. It is in the range of 10–20% of that mediated by SRBI. So, when you consider the SRBI null mouse actually has a twofold increase in HDL cholesterol, and you have got 40%. So you have got about a fifth of what the true SRB1 null is. It is not inconceivable that residual activity of CD36 that has been shown has been deemphasized, because that is the way people wanted to deal with the information, but maybe that peripheral expression of CD36 in adipose muscle and heart actually is mediating enough selective uptake, so when you knock it out you get a 40% increase in HDL cholesterol.

FEBBRAIO: In our hands, we do not observe significant CD36-dependent HDL uptake. It is clear that CD36 binds HDL, but in our experiments, there is no appreciable CD36-dependent uptake of ^{125}I-HDL. These results are similar to those reported by Krieger.

TALL: Not really. If you look at the data that William's laboratory presented at AHA, it is not different to the Krieger lab data. If you actually look at the numbers, there is a small residual effect. Anyway, I would not eliminate that as an explanation. The second question I have is, the fact that you have lower glucose and insulin levels is actually really interesting and your explanation is quite plausible, but directly contradicts the recent paper in *Nature Genetics* by James Scott's group, which claims that in the hypertensive insulin-resistant rat a fairly major part of the insulin resistance is due to a null mutation in CD36. So, I wonder what your thoughts were about that discrepancy.

FEBBRAIO: Actually, I spoke to him, because we were very surprised. You are right, his conclusion is that insulin dysregulation in the rat was due to CD36 and I felt almost bad to say that our mice are not in the same situation. It turns out that there is a duplication in the wild-type rats of the CD36 gene, and then he has a deletion in the SHR rats, and part of that deletion has not been mapped. It could be that there is another gene in there. I would hope that it is not, I would hope that CD36 plays a role in this, or it could be a big difference between rats and mice, like there are lipid differences.

TALL: How did you control for the genetic background modifiers? Did you have littermate controls?

FEBBRAIO: Everything is done with littermate controls. These are four times crossed to C57Bl-6. I think both of us are wishing to work together to see the difference. There are strain differences between mice. In fact, I was recently doing a search and C57Bl-6 mice, 6J, which is what we are on, can be considered to be relatively diabetes resistant. So another possibility is that we need to backcross to a different strain of mouse. It could be also diet. Right now we had them on a normal chow diet and we have put them on a high cholesterol diet for the atherogenic studies. There are supposedly diabetes-inducing diets that we need to try next. But I agree with you, it is a little bit difficult. The other thing he told me is that the rat is less of a pure background than the mice that we are dealing with, because apparently in the genetics of the SHR there are different strains even within the SHR.

T. KITA (*Kyoto University, Kyoto, Japan*): Among cardiomyopathy patients, some patients have no CD36 molecules. Did you check whether your CD36 knockout mice have cardiomegaly or have you looked at the size of the myocyte?

FEBBRAIO: We actually did look into this. We have some preliminary data that the hearts of the null animals are larger. We have done echocardiography in unanesthetized mice and observed dilation of the left ventricle in the null animals. We are currently continuing the study, and, as you saw, the BMIPP data are very suggestive that there has been a change in metabolism. This is also what Dr. Tanaka has thought to be the mechanism in his cardiomyopathy patients.

KITA: How about skeletal muscle?

FEBBRAIO: The size of the skeletal muscle? We have not looked at that.

H. BISCHOFF (*Bayer AG, Germany*): It was very interesting to hear that the relationship may be to carbohydrate metabolism. What was the insulin in the fasting state in these animals?

FEBBRAIO: I remember it was in the normal range in the fasting state. But the kit we used had a very narrow range at the part of the curve that was considered normal. So, to get the exact number we need to do more and better samples.

BISCHOFF: How many animals did you use per group?

FEBBRAIO: We were using five at a time and we have done it three times. We also segregated male from female and that did not seem to make a difference. We also looked at old versus young animals and obtained similar results. Next we would like to see the difference on a high fat diet versus the normal chow.

BISCHOFF: I was somewhat surprised that you made the relationship between the fasting glucose and the insulin response to glucose load. These are usually two different things because the fasting blood glucose is controlled by the liver and glucose production and glucagon/insulin ratio and not by the insulin response to glucose load. What was the glucose response to the glucose load?

FEBBRAIO: You are asking if I measured both insulin and glucose at the same time? We first measured glucose by giving a glucose load; that was one curve. And in a subsequent experiment we measured insulin levels.

Animal Models for Hyperinsulinemia and Insulin Resistance

HIDEKI ABE[a] AND NOBUHIRO YAMADA[b,c]

[a]*Hepatobiliarypancreatic Division, Department of Surgery, Graduate School of Medicine, University of Tokyo, Tokyo, Japan*

[b]*Institute of Clinical Medicine, University of Tsukuba, Ibaragi, Japan*

ABSTRACT: The direct effect of endogenous insulin on the atherosclerotic process has not been well understood. To clarify this question, we performed pancreas transplantation in Wistar Shionogi (WS) rats. Hyperinsulinemia was not related to coronary risk factors such as dyslipidemia and hypertension in transplanted rats. After 9 months of transplantation, the cholesterol ester contents of the aortas of transplanted WS rats were significantly higher than in the control rats. The effects of insulin resistance on coronary risk factors were examined in mice deficient in insulin substrate-1–deficient (IRS-1) mice, a nonobese animal model of insulin resistance. Blood pressure and plasma triglyceride levels were significantly higher in IRS-1–deficient mice than in normal mice. Impaired endothelium-dependent vascular relaxation was also observed in IRS-1–deficient mice. Furthermore, lipoprotein lipase activity was lower than in normal mice, suggesting impaired lipolysis was involved in the increased plasma triglyceride levels under insulin-resistant conditions.

INTRODUCTION

Various risk factors for atherosclerosis have been identified from epidemiological studies.[1–3] In particular, hyperinsulinemia is considered to be an important risk factor for coronary artery disease.[4–8] The insulin-resistant state, which is usually related to hyperinsulinemia, is often associated with a clustering of coronary risk factors such as hypertension, glucose intolerance, obesity, hypertriglyceridemia, and low plasma high density lipoprotein (HDL)-cholesterol levels. These lead to an increased risk of cardiovascular disease, presumably due to promotion of atherosclerosis,[6,7] but the mechanism associated with these coronary risk factors in subjects with hyperinsulinemia or insulin resistance is not clearly understood.

The present study determines whether endogenous insulin or insulin resistance itself accelerates the progression of atherosclerosis by minimizing the effects of insulin resistance on atherogenesis. The present study also examines whether the clustering syndrome of coronary risk factors is under the influence of insulin resistance in non-obese insulin receptor substrate-1–deficient (IRS-1) mice.[8] The pheno-

---

[c]Address for correspondence: Nobuhiro Yamada, M.D., Ph.D., Institute of Clinical Medicine, University of Tsukuba, 1-1-1 Tennoudai, Tsukuba-shi, Ibaragi 305-8575, Japan. Voice: 81-0298-53-3051; fax: 81-0298-53-3051.

ymdnbhr@igaku.md.tsukuba.ac.jp

type of IRS-1 knockout mice resembles that of non insulin-dependent diabetes mellitus at the prediabetes stage with insulin resistance.

MATERIALS AND METHODS

Animals and Animal Treatment

Male, 8–10-week-old Wistar Shionogi (WS) rats weighing 250–300 g were used for pancreas transplantation. Recipient rats received syngeneic whole pancreas isolated from donor rats of similar age, sex, and weight. All the rats were fed normal laboratory chow *ad libitum*. Sham operation was performed in control rats.

Subsequently, female mice homozygous for targeted disruption of the IRS-1 gene and female wild-type mice that were offspring of heterozygous mice were examined. The genotype of the mice was confirmed by the polymerase chain reaction method. All the mice were fed normal laboratory chow *ad libitum*.

Studies of Hyperinsulinemia Model

Blood samples were obtained from a tail vein under ether anesthesia and the concentrations of plasma glucose and insulin were determined, under *ad libitum* feeding in the morning 2, 4, 6, and 8 months after transplantation. Nine months after transplantation, body weight was determined, and blood pressure was measured at a tail artery using an automatic machine. The concentrations of plasma glucose, insulin, plasma cholesterol, HDL-cholesterol, and triglyceride were also determined.

The entire aorta from the aortic valve to the iliac bifurcation, except for the site of the anastomosis, was removed and carefully cleaned of loose adventitial tissue. The portions of ascending aorta adjacent to the heart and descending aorta distal to the left subclavian artery were used for microscopic examinations. We measured the thickness of the intima and the media at three randomly selected sites per section of aorta, and measured the cholesteryl ester content of the whole aorta.[9] Total lipid extracts were prepared by homogenizing three times in chloroform/methanol (2:1).

Studies of Insulin Resistance Model

Blood pressure was measured at a tail artery in a restrained condition using an automatic machine, and in an unrestrained condition using a perfluorocarbon cannula inserted into the femoral artery.

Nine homozygous and 11 wild-type mice (20–25 weeks old) were decapitated, and a section of the thoracic aorta between the aortic arch and diaphragm was removed and placed in oxygenated, modified Krebs-Henseleit solution. The aorta was cleaned of loosely adhering fat and connective tissue and cut into rings (3 mm long). The relaxation response to acetylcholine (ACh) and sodium nitroprusside (SNP) was expressed as a percentage of the decreased tension in contractile force induced by $3 \times 10^{-8} - 1 \times 10^{-7}$ M U46619, a derivative of thromboxane A_2. For the relaxation studies, the aortic rings were precontracted with $3 \times 10^{-8} - 1 \times 10^{-7}$ M U46619. When the U46619-induced contraction reached a plateau, ACh ($10^{-9} - 10^{-5}$ M) and SNP ($10^{-9} - 10^{-5}$ M) were added cumulatively. Each aortic ring was exposed to only one relaxant agent.

The blood of 2–3, 4–5, 6–12-month-old homozygous ($N = 17$) and wild-type mice ($N = 21$) was collected following a 6-h fast. Blood was collected from the retroorbital plexus using heparin-coated capillaries. High performance liquid chromatography (HPLC) was applied to show elution peaks of the two major lipoprotein classes, apoB-containing lipoproteins and HDL.

After the 6-h fast, post-heparin plasma of 6–12-month-old homozygous ($N = 12$) and wild-type ($N = 16$) mice was taken 3 min after a bolus injection of heparin (100 units/kg) into the external jugular vein. Lipoprotein lipase (LPL) activity was assayed by the method described by Nilsson-Ehle and Schotz.[10] LPL activity in adipose tissue derived from utero-ovarian region was assayed as described.[11]

Statistical Analysis

Data were analyzed by the Mann-Whitney U test and expressed as mean ± SD. A value of $p < 0.05$ was considered to be statistically significant.

RESULTS

Studies of Hyperinsulinemia Model

The plasma insulin concentrations of WS transplanted rats ($N = 6$) were significantly higher in each determination than those of WS control rats ($N = 6$). The plasma insulin concentrations of WS transplanted rats were 139% (transplant/control: 82 ± 33/59 ± 20 pmol/1) to 179% (transplant/control: 102 ± 43/57 ± 19 pmol/1) those of WS control rats, whereas the plasma glucose concentrations of WS transplanted rats were not significantly different from those of WS control rats.

Nine months after transplantation, the body weights in WS transplanted rats were significantly greater than those in WS control rats. There were no differences in blood pressure levels between WS control and WS transplanted rats. Plasma total cholesterol and triglyceride levels were significantly greater in WS control rats than in WS transplanted rats.

Microscopical examination of the aorta demonstrated no apparent increase in intimal thickness in both groups of WS rats. To evaluate atherogenic changes in aorta before histological changes have developed, we measured cholesterol contents in aortas. The cholesterol ester content of the aorta was significantly greater in transplanted WS rats than in control WS rats. The cholesterol ester in transplanted ($N = 10$) and control WS rats ($N = 13$) was 3.8 ± 2.1 and 1.9 ± 1.0 mg/g dry tissue, respectively ($p < 0.01$). Plasma insulin levels were positively correlated with cholesterol ester contents in the aorta, and those corrected values by plasma cholesterol levels have highly significant correlation with plasma insulin levels.[12]

Studies of Insulin Resistance Model

In the restrained condition, systolic arterial blood pressure was significantly higher in homozygous mice than in wild-type mice (147 ± 11 mm Hg versus l23 ± 24 mm Hg, $p < 0.01$). In the unrestrained condition, systolic, diastolic, and mean arterial blood pressure were all significantly higher in homozygous mice than in wild-type mice. The systolic/diastolic pressure was 132 ± 14/89 ± 16 mm Hg in homozygous mouse and 119 ± 15/79 ± 12 mm Hg in wild-type mouse. The mean blood pressure was 110 ± 12 mm Hg in homozygous mice and 99 ± 10 mm Hg in wild-type mice, $p < 0.01$. Pulse pressure and pulse rate did not differ significantly between homozygous and wild-type mice.

ACh caused concentration-dependent relaxation in aortic strips. This relaxation was significantly reduced in aortic strips from homozygous mice compared to wild-type mice. In contrast, relaxation caused by SNP (10^{-9}–10^{-5} M), which is an endothelium-independent agent and activates soluble guanylate cyclase, did not differ significantly between homozygous and wild-type mice.

Plasma triglyceride level following 6-h fast in homozygous mice was significantly higher than wild-type mice at each measurement. This difference was 1.6-fold at 2–3 months old (homozygous/wild-type: 51.2 ± 23.8/33.1 ± 19.8 mg/dl) and 1.7-fold at 4–5 months old (homozygous/wild-type: 47.9 ± 19.3/28.4 ± 8.0 mg/dl). Plasma cholesterol and free fatty acid levels did not differ significantly between the two groups. HPLC analysis of the lipoprotein profiles revealed no significant difference in plasma HDL-cholesterol.

LPL activity in the post-heparin plasma after the 6-h fast was significantly lower in homozygous mice than in wild-type mice, whereas hepatic triglyceride lipase activity did not differ significantly between the two groups. LPL activity in adipose tissue was also significantly lower in homozygous mice than in wild-type mice.[13]

DISCUSSION

Hyperinsulinemia plays a role in the development of atherosclerosis through the pathophysiologic process related to insulin resistance, hyperlipidemia, glucose intolerance, and hypertension; however, the effects of insulin itself on atherogenesis are not clear. Animal models relevant to human hyperinsulinemia and insulin resistance, such as the db/db mouse, ob/ob mouse,[14] and OLETF rat[15] are not suitable for studying the effects of insulin on atherogenesis, because hyperinsulinemia is a result of insulin resistance in those animal models.

Pancreas transplantation is a useful model with which to evaluate effects of endogenous insulin on the artery by minimizing the insulin resistance and the adverse effects of exogenous insulin injection. Although plasma insulin levels in transplanted rats were approximately twice as high as those in control rats, we found that plasma glucose levels in recipient rats were maintained at normal physiologic levels. Plasma glucose levels may be adjusted to normal by relatively high plasma glucagon levels in the transplanted rats. In the present study, although hyperinsulinemia was not related to coronary risk factors, such as dyslipidemia and hypertension, in transplanted rats after 9 months of transplantation, the cholesterol ester content of the aorta was significantly greater in transplanted rats than in control rats. Plasma insulin concentrations were well correlated to cholesterol ester contents in the aorta. Increased and regulated insulin secretion may affect cellular functions of the arterial wall and atherosclerotic processes.

Insulin resistance is often associated with atherosclerotic disease in subjects with obesity, impaired glucose tolerance, and hyperinsulinemia, and several researchers have recently suggested that insulin resistance contributes to the pathogenesis of atherosclerosis. The effects of insulin resistance on coronary risk factors were examined in IRS-1–deficient mice, a non-obese animal model of insulin resistance. Blood pressure and plasma triglyceride levels were significantly higher in IRS-1–deficient mice than in normal mice. Impaired endothelium-dependent vascular relaxation was also observed in IRS-1–deficient mice. Furthermore, lipoprotein lipase activity was lower than in normal mice, suggesting impaired lipolysis to be involved in increased plasma triglyceride levels under insulin-resistant conditions. Thus, insulin resistance plays an important role in the clustering of coronary risk factors, which may accelerate the progression of atherosclerosis in subjects with insulin resistance.

We estimated blood pressure in a non-obese animal model of insulin resistance under two different conditions, restrained and unrestrained conditions. Blood pressure under both conditions was significantly higher in IRS-1–deficient mice than in control mice. Thus, hypertension appears to occur as a result of pathophysiological abnormalities caused by IRS-1 deficiency rather than increased sympathetic activity during the experiment. Furthermore, secondary hyperinsulinemia may have been responsible for the hypertension in the present animal model. However, in our hyperinsulinemia model with transplanted pancreas, hyperinsulinemia did not affect blood pressure, despite a twofold increase in plasma insulin following pancreas transplantation. Similar plasma insulin levels were observed in the IRS-1–deficient mice and therefore do not likely influence blood pressure. Thus, insulin resistance rather than hyperinsulinemia appears to be the primary cause of hypertension in IRS-1–deficient mice. A recent study reported that mice lacking the gene for endothelial nitric oxide synthase are hypertensive,[16] suggesting that a resulting impairment in endothelium-dependent vascular relaxation is involved in the pathophysiology of hypertension. Endothelium-dependent relaxation of the aorta was reduced in IRS-1–deficient mice, whereas endothelium-independent relaxation did not differ between IRS-1–deficient and control mice.

In conclusion, endogenous hyperinsulinemia influences the process of atherosclerosis by enhancing accumulation of cholesterol ester in the arterial wall without causing hyperlipidemia, hypertension, and glucose intolerance. Insulin resistance plays an essential role both in the clustering of coronary risk factors such as hypertension and hypertriglyceridemia and in the reduced endothelium-dependent vascular relaxation. Endothelium dysfunctions, such as impaired endothelium-dependent vascular relaxation, have been considered to be closely related to the pathogenesis of atherosclerosis.

REFERENCES

1. ZAVARONI, I. *et al.* 1987. Evidence that multiple risk factors for coronary artery disease exist in individuals with abnormal glucose tolerance. Am. J. Med. **83:** 609–612.
2. KANNEL W.B. *et al.* 1971. Systolic versus diastolic blood pressure and risk of coronary artery disease: the Framingham study. Am. J. Cardiol. **27:** 335–346.
3. FULLER, J.H. *et al.* 1980. Coronary-heart-disease risk and impaired glucose tolerance: the Whitehall study. Lancet **1**(8183): 1373–1376.
4. CONSENSUS CONFERENCE. 1985. Lowering blood cholesterol to prevent heart disease. J. Am. Med. Assoc. **253:** 2080–2086.
5. FERRANNINI, E. *et al.* 1987. Insulin resistance in essential hypertension. N. Engl. J. Med. **317:** 350–357.
6. KAPLAN, N.M. 1989. The deadly quartet. Arch. Intern. Med. **149:** 1514–1520.
7. REAVEN, G.M. 1988. Banting lecture. Role of insulin resistance in human disease. Diabetes **37:** 1595–1607.

8. TAMEMOTO, H. *et al.* 1994. Insulin resistance and growth retardation in mice lacking insulin receptor substrates Nature **372:** 182–186.
9. YAMADA, N. *et al.* 1992. Apolipoprotein E prevents the progression of atherosclerosis in WHHL rabbits. J. Clin. Invest. **89:** 706–711.
10. NILSSON-EHLE, P. & M.C. SCHOTZ. 1976. A stable, radioactive substrate emulsion for assay of lipoprotein lipase. J. Lipid Res. **17:** 536–541.
11. SHIMADA, M. *et al.* 1993. Overexpression of human lipoprotein lipase in transgenic mice. J. Biol. Chem. **268:** 17924–17929.
12. ABE, H. *et al.* 1998. Hypertension, hypertriglyceridemia, and impaired endothelium-dependent vascular relaxation in mice lacking receptor substrates. J. Clin. Invest. **101:** 1784–1788.
13. ABE, H. *et al.* 1996. Hyperinsulinemia accelerates accumulation of cholesterol ester in aorta of rats with transplanted pancreas. Diabetologia **39:** 1276–1283.
14. HUNT, C.E. *et al.* 1976. Animal models of diabetes and obesity, including the PBB/Ld mouse. Fed. Proc. **35:** 1206–1217.
15. KAWANO, K. *et al.* 1992. Spontaneous long-term hyperglycemic rat with diabetic complications, Otsuka Long-Evans Tokushima Fatty (OLETF) Strain. Diabetes **41:** 1422–1428.
16. HUANG, P.L. *et al.* 1995. Hypertension in mice lacking the gene for endothelial nitric oxide synthase. Nature **377:** 239–242.

Lipid Lowering Reduces Proteolytic and Prothrombotic Potential in Rabbit Atheroma[a]

MASANORI AIKAWA[b] AND PETER LIBBY

Cardiovascular Division, Department of Medicine, Brigham and Women's Hospital, Harvard Medical School, Boston, Massachusetts 02115, USA

ABSTRACT: Thrombus formation at sites of atheromatous plaque disruption cause most acute coronary events such as myocardial infarction and unstable angina. Lesional macrophages and smooth muscle cells produce matrix metalloproteinases (MMPs) and tissue factor (TF), the molecules likely contribute to plaque rupture and thrombus formation. Recent clinical studies have suggested that lipid lowering can reduce the incidence of acute coronary events. We have recently determined the effects of long-term dietary lipid lowering on atheroma of high-cholesterol-fed rabbits. Lipid lowering diminished macrophage accumulation, reduced expression and activity of MMPs, and increased interstitial collagen accumulation in rabbit atheroma. Expression and activity of TF in atheroma also substantially decreased during lipid lowering. Dietary lipid lowering also promoted accumulation of mature smooth muscle cells expressing less MMPs and TF in the plaque's fibrous cap. These results suggest potential mechanisms by which lipid lowering reduces acute coronary events in patients by decreasing proteolytic and prothrombotic activity within the atheroma.

INTRODUCTION

Rupture of atherosclerotic plaque participates in the pathogenesis of thrombus formation and consequent acute coronary syndromes, including unstable angina, acute myocardial infarction, or cardiac sudden death.[1–3] Rupture-prone lesions usually contain prominent accumulation of inflammatory cells, such as macrophages, underlying a thin and collagen-poor fibrous cap.[4,5] Macrophage-rich areas are frequently found in coronary plaques of patients with acute coronary syndromes.[6] Macrophages within atheroma overexpress a number of inflammatory mediators, various matrix-degrading enzymes, and tissue factor (TF, a strong activator of blood coagulation).[7–9] Extracellular matrix including collagens confer strength on the plaque's fibrous cap. Enzymes including matrix metalloproteinases (MMPs) expressed in atheroma may weaken the plaque's protective fibrous cap and may promote plaque disruption.[3] Lesional macrophages also overexpress TF, a strong activator of blood coagulation.[10] TF may accelerate thrombus formation at sites of rupture. The pro-

---

[a]The studies referred to here were supported by grants from the National Heart, Lung, and Blood Institute to Peter Libby (HL-34634, PO1 HL48743) and a Research Fellowship Award from the Japan Heart Foundation to Masanori Aikawa.

[b]Address for correspondence: Masanori Aikawa, M.D., Ph.D., Cardiovascular Division, Brigham and Women's Hospital, Harvard Medical School, 221 Longwood Avenue, LMRC 309, Boston, MA 02115. Voice: 617-732-7093; fax: 617-732-6961.

maikawa@bics.bwh.harvard.edu

teolytic and the prothrombotic potential produced by lesional macrophages may prove decisive in determining the onset of acute coronary events.

INCREASED PROTEOLYTIC AND PROTHROMBOTIC ACTIVITY IN ATHEROMA MAY TRIGGER PLAQUE DISRUPTION AND THROMBUS FORMATION

Accumulating evidence has suggested an important role for members of the MMP family in the pathogenesis of plaque disruption. Lesional macrophages, smooth muscle cells (SMCs), and endothelial cells produce various MMPs.[8,9] Henney and colleagues provided evidence for MMP-3 (stromelysin-1) expression in human atheroma.[11] Galis and colleagues demonstrated the protein expression of MMPs, including MMP-1 (collagenase-1), MMP-2 (gelatinase-A), MMP-3, and MMP-9 (gelatinase-B), in human atherosclerotic lesions.[12,13] Nikkari and colleagues and Brown and colleagues also reported MMP-1 and MMP-9 expression in human atheroma.[14,15] Human atheroma also contain MMP-7 (matrilysin) and MMP-12 (macrophage elastase).[16,17] Sukhova and colleagues recently showed that MMP-13 (collagenase-3) in human atheroma colocalizes with degraded collagen detected by a specific antibody to the collagenase cleavage site of collagen.[18] Shah and colleagues demonstrated that conditioned media of cultured macrophages can digest collagen obtained from the human fibrous cap.[19] These results support the concept that MMPs produced by macrophages play an important role in onset of acute coronary events.

TF likely plays an important role in pathogenesis of thrombus formation at sites of atheromatous plaque disruption resulting in acute coronary events.[10] Wilcox and colleagues and Drake and colleagues reported expression of this membrane-bound glycoprotein in human atheroma and adventitial fibroblast-like cells.[20,21] Thiruvikraman and colleagues detected TF *in situ* using digoxigenin-labeled coagulation factors VIIa and X, co-factors of TF, in human atherosclerotic plaques and in experimental arteriosclerosis.[22] Hatakeyama and colleagues reported a similar pattern of TF expression in human aorta.[23] Marmur and colleagues detected TF activity in human coronary atheroma.[24] Recent studies have suggested increased expression and activity of TF in atherectomy specimens obtained from patients with acute coronary syndromes.[25–28] These findings support the important role of TF in determining the thrombogenicity of atheroma, and hence their propensity to provoke acute vascular complications.

LIPID LOWERING AS A POTENTIAL THERAPY FOR PLAQUE STABILIZATION

Recent clinical trials have repeatedly shown that lipid lowering with HMG-CoA reductase inhibitors achieves a 30–40% reduction rate in the incidence of acute coronary events.[29–32] These benefits do not appear to accrue so much from improvement in luminal caliber, but from functional changes in the atheroma itself that are commonly termed "stabilization."[33,34] However, the precise molecular and cellular mechanisms that underlie lesion stabilization leading to this striking clinical benefit remain speculative. One potential mechanism might be reduced expression of proteins, including MMPs and TF, that may trigger plaque disruption and thrombus formation.

Several studies in animals with atherosclerosis demonstrated that lipid lowering decreased inflammatory cells (including macrophages) and increased connective tissue in atheroma.[35–39] Combined with clinical evidence, these findings suggest that lipid lowering can improve inflammation and may decrease plaque instability and thrombogenicity.

Dietary Lipid Lowering Reduces Proteolytic Activity and Increases Collagen Accumulation

To test the hypothesis that lipid lowering ameliorates features associated with plaque stability, we determined effects of dietary lipid lowering on atheroma of hypercholesterolemic rabbits.[40] Using balloon injury and an atherogenic diet (0.3% cholesterol and 4.7% coconut oil) for a period of 4 months, we produced experimental atheroma in 30 rabbits (FIG. 1). At that time 15 rabbits were sacrificed (Baseline

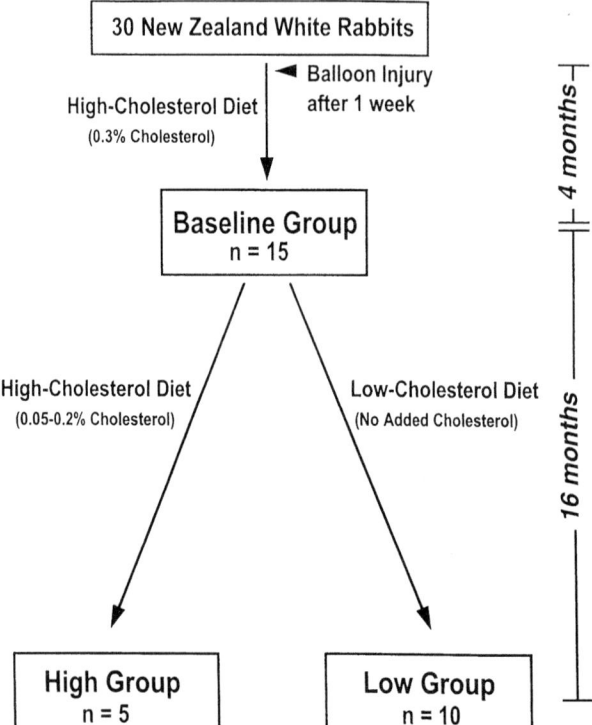

FIGURE 1. Experimental protocol. Thirty New Zealand White male rabbits were fed igh-cholesterol diet for 4 months to create the atheroma. The balloon injury by Fogarty emolectomy catheter of the thoracic aortas was performed 1 week after initiation of the therogenic diet. Fifteen rabbits sacrificed at 4 months comprised the "Baseline" group. ive animals continued the atherogenic diet ("High" group), and the remaining animals conumed a chow diet with no added cholesterol and fat for 16 months ("Low" group). (From ikawa et al.[41] Reproduced with permission.)

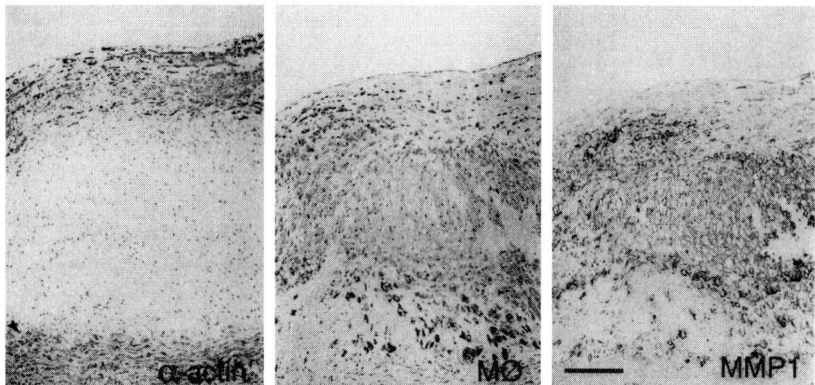

FIGURE 2. The rabbit aortic lesions after 4 months of high-cholesterol diet contain numerous macrophages expressing MMP-1 (collagenase-1). RAM11-positive macrophages accumulate in the intima beneath a thin smooth muscle layer detected by anti–α-actin antibody. MMP-1 is predominantly expressed by macrophages. The *arrowhead* indicates the internal elastic lamina. Scale bar: 200 μm. Original magnification: ×100. (From Aikawa *et al.*[40] Reproduced with permission.)

group). The remaining animals were divided into two groups: five animals continued on a cholesterol-enriched diet (0.05–0.2%) for 16 more months (High group), and 10 animals consumed a purified chow diet with no added cholesterol or fat for 16 months (Low group).

Rabbit aortic atheroma after 4 months of atherogenic diet contained prominent macrophage accumulation underlying a thin smooth-muscle layer resembling the fibrous cap of human atheroma (FIG. 2). Lesional macrophages in the baseline lesions expressed high levels of MMP-1 (collagenase-1) detected by immunohistochemistry using anti–rabbit MMP-1 monoclonal antibody. Aortic rings from these rabbits elaborated proteolytic activity ascribable to MMP-2, MMP-3, and MMP-9 (detected by SDS-PAGE substrate zymography for gelatin, casein, and elastin). After 16 months of dietary lipid lowering, however, the number of macrophages in atheroma decreased substantially and expression of MMP-1 was almost undetectable, while MMP-1 expression persisted in the atheroma of High-group animals (FIG. 3). Proteolytic activity by MMPs also decreased by lipid lowering. Interestingly, picrosirius red polarization (a histochemical indicator of the major arterial interstitial collagens types I and III) revealed a marked increase in collagen accumulation in the intima of the Low-group animals after lipid lowering (FIG. 4). These results suggest that lipid lowering yields a reduction in macrophages producing proteolytic activity, and in turn permits collagen accumulation, a key determinant of plaque stability.

Lipid Lowering Reduces Expression and Activity of TF

We also demonstrated that along with reduced macrophage number, long-term dietary lipid lowering reduces mRNA, protein expression, and biological activity of TF, another potential contributor to acute coronary events.[41] Before lipid lowering, the atherosclerotic rabbit aortas express high levels of TF mRNA detected by RT-

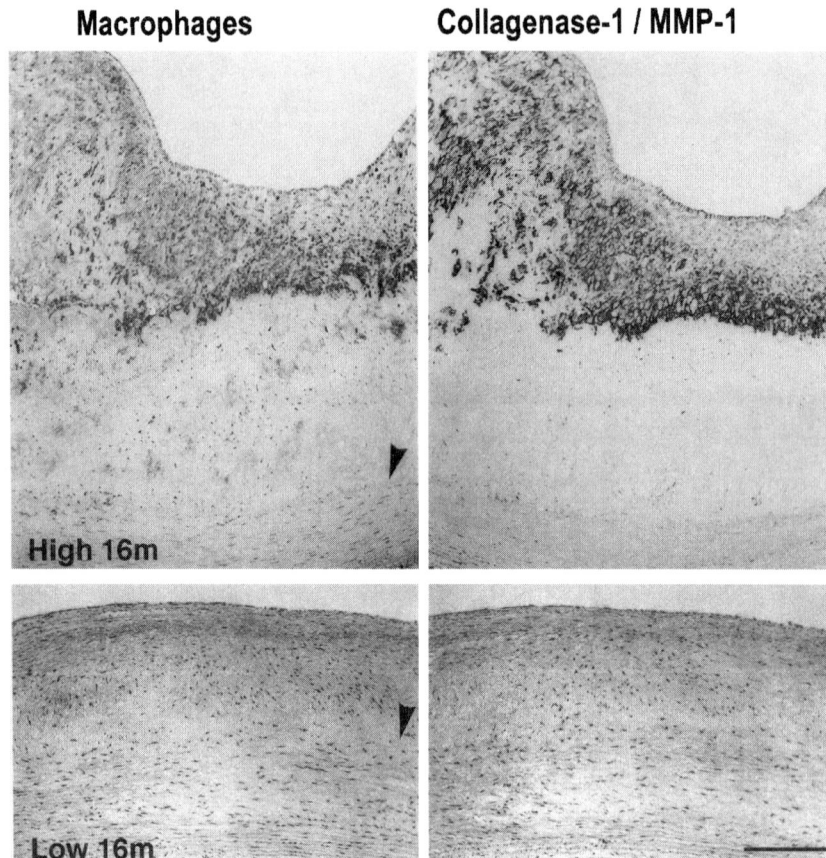

FIGURE 3. Reduced expression of MMP-1 associated with decrease in number of lesional macrophages. (*Top*) Macrophages within the lesion of the High group animal after an additional 16 months of the atherogenic diet continue to express MMP-1 strongly. (*Bottom*) 16 months after cessation of the high-cholesterol diet, MMP-1 and macrophages are almost undetectable. *Arrowheads* indicate the internal elastic lamina. Scale bar: 200 μm. Original magnification: ×100. (Modified from Aikawa *et al.*[40])

PCR. Immunohistochemistry using an anti–rabbit TF antibody revealed overexpression of TF protein by macrophages in rabbit atheroma of the Baseline and High groups; some intimal SMCs and endothelial cells also expressed this procoagulant. We furthermore demonstrated presence of functionally active TF protein by using an *in situ* binding assay for its co-factors, factors VIIa and X.[22] Digoxigenin-labeled factors VIIa and X bound specifically in rabbit atheroma and colocalized well with immunoreactive TF in atheroma of the Baseline-group animals (FIG. 5, top panels). The atherosclerotic rabbit aortas also contained enzymatically active TF, detected by using a chromogenic assay that measured generation of factor Xa.

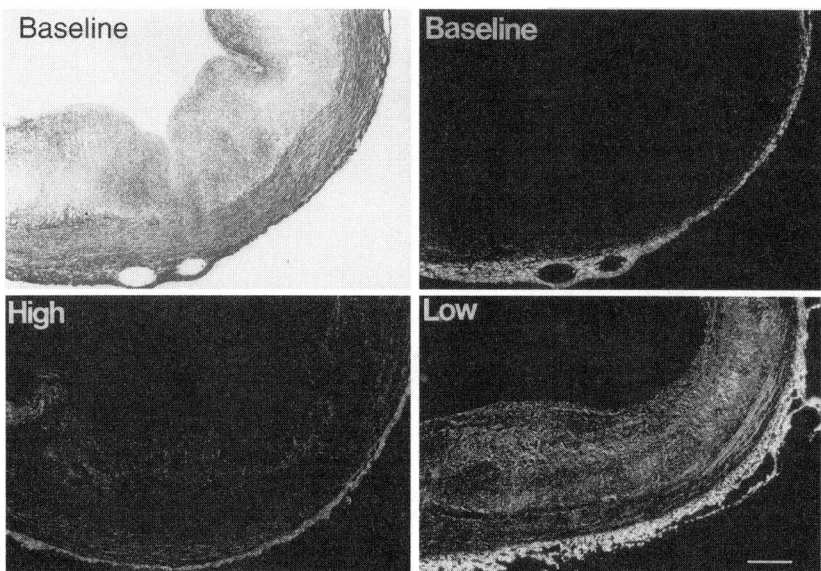

FIGURE 4. Interstitial collagen content in the aortic intima detected by the picrosirius red polarization method. (*Top left*) Picrosirius red staining without polarized light on the rabbit aorta after 4 months of the atherogenic diet (baseline) shows the thickened intima of the aorta. (*Top right*) The serial aortic section from the baseline lesion shows positive picrosirius red staining under polarized light in the media and adventitia only. (*Bottom left*) The aortic lesion of the High group animal that continued the atherogenic diet for 16 months shows some increase in interstitial collagen content with time. (*Bottom right*) The aorta of the Low-group animal after 16 months of dietary lipid lowering contains abundant interstitial collagen within the intima. Scale bar: 400 μm. Original magnification: ×40. (From Aikawa et al.[40] Reproduced with permission.)

After 16 months of lipid lowering by diet, TF mRNA and protein expression decreased in association with reduced macrophage number. *In situ* binding of TF to factors VIIa and X, as well as factor Xa generating activity also decreased in atheroma of the Low-group animals (FIG. 5, bottom panels). These results suggest a potential mechanism by which lipid lowering reduces acute coronary events in patients at risk by decreasing procoagulant activity within the atheroma.

Lipid Lowering Promotes Accumulation of More Mature SMCs in the Fibrous Cap

Intimal SMCs differ from medial SMCs with respect to gene expression, function, and morphology.[42] Smooth muscle–specific myosin heavy chain isoforms (SM1 and SM2) are useful markers for smooth muscle differentiation/maturation, applicable to determining the phenotype of intimal SMCs *in situ*.[43,44] SMCs in the fibrous cap of the human coronary artery show an immature phenotype as determined by decreased expression of SM1 and SM2, while medial SMCs express both

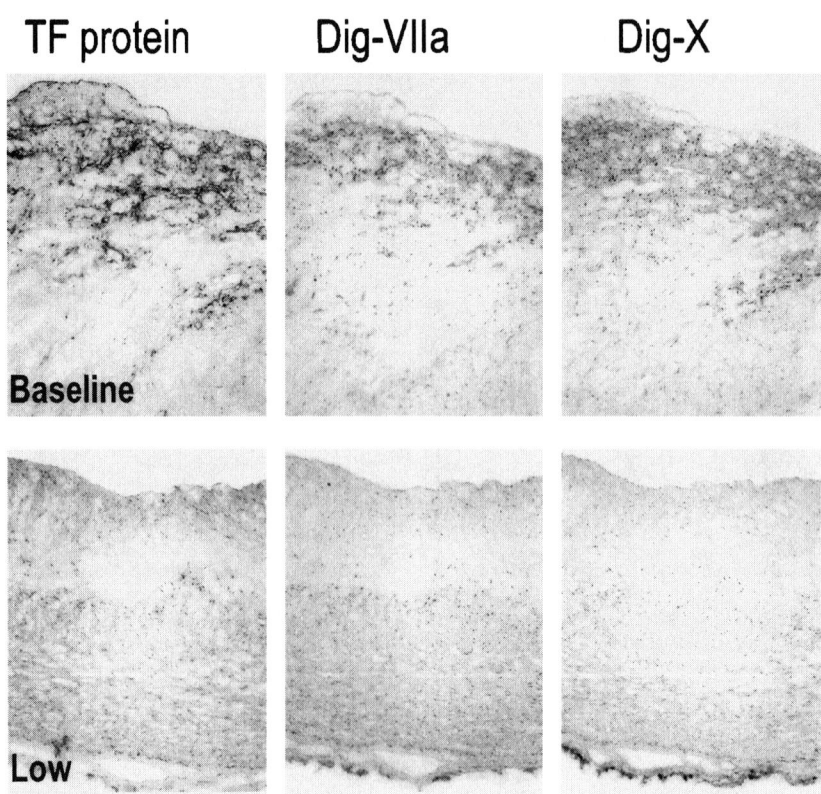

FIGURE 5. *In situ* binding of TF to the coagulation factors VIIa and X. Functionally active TF that can bind factors VIIa and X was detected by use of *in situ* binding assay using digoxigenin-labeled factors VIIa and X (DigVIIa and DigX). (*Top*) Intense staining for DigVIIa and DigX colocalized with protein expression of TF on rabbit atheroma after 4 months of high-cholesterol feeding (baseline). (*Bottom*) Staining of DigVIIa and DigX decreased in the aortic intima of Low group animal after 16 months of lipid lowering whereas the adventitia displayed positive staining. TF was also almost undetectable in the intima. Scale bar: 200 μm. Original magnification: ×100. (Modified from Aikawa *et al.*[41])

myosins.[43] Intimal SMCs overexpress MMPs including MMP-1, MMP-3, and MMP-9, and TF.[12,20] In the fibrous cap of rabbit atheroma from the Baseline group, SMCs exhibited immature phenotype indicated by reduced expression of SM1 and SM2 (FIG. 6, top panels). However, after 16 months of dietary lipid lowering, intimal SMCs expressed both SM1 and SM2 consistent with a more mature phenotype of medial SMCs (FIG. 6, bottom panels).[45] Electron microscopy also determined accumulation of mature SMCs with features typical of the "contractile" phenotype.[45] Kockx and colleagues reported a similar accumulation of "contractile"-type SMCs in rabbit atheroma after dietary lipid lowering determined by electron microscopy.[46]

Immature SMCs in rabbit atheroma expressed MMP-3 and MMP-9. However, more mature SMCs after dietary lipid lowering expressed lower levels of MMP-3

Baseline

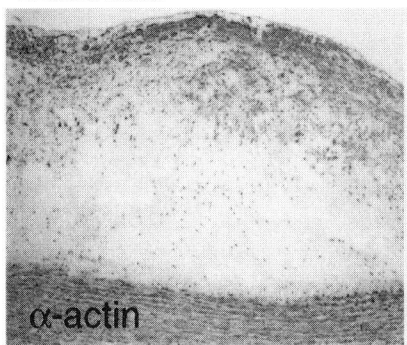 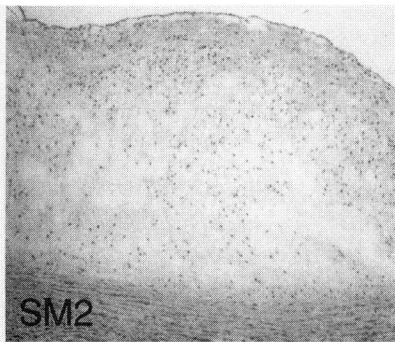

After Lipid Lowering

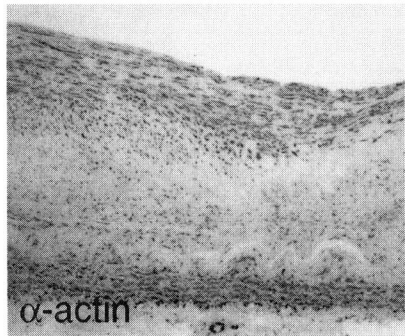 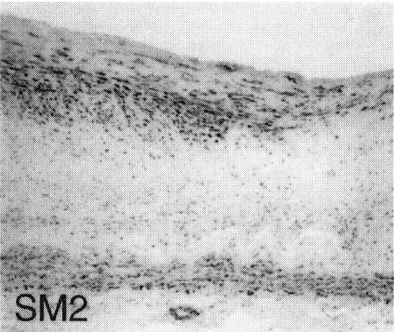

FIGURE 6. Phenotype of intimal SMCs in plaque's fibrous cap of rabbit atheroma determined by expression of α-smooth muscle actin and a myosin heavy chain isoform (SM2) specific to mature smooth muscle. SM2-positive SMCs were less numerous than α-actin–positive cells, whereas medial SMCs stained positive for both α-actin and SM2. After 16 months of lipid lowering, many intimal SMCs stained positively for both α-actin and SM2, indicating that intimal SMCs exhibit a mature phenotype similar to medial SMCs. The *arrowhead* indicates the internal elastic lamina. Scale bar: 200 μm. Original magnification: ×100. (Modified from Aikawa *et al.*[44])

and MMP-9.[45] Intimal SMCs also express TF. However, after 16 months of lipid lowering, TF expression by intimal SMCs substantially decreased.[41] These findings regarding accumulation of more mature SMCs provide additional insights into the mechanisms of lipid lowering's effects on the biology of atheroma.

Platelet-derived growth factor B-chain (PDGF-B) can suppress SMC differentiation/maturation.[47] We found that SMC maturation occurred in association with decreased PDGF-B expressed by lesional macrophages,[45] suggesting that diminished macrophage number plays yet another important role in plaque stabilization by promoting accumulation of more normal SMCs expressing fewer MMPs and less TF.

UNANSWERED QUESTIONS AND FUTURE DIRECTIONS

This article has discussed effects of dietary lipid lowering on lesional macrophages and SMCs in rabbit atheroma. Reduced number of macrophages producing proteolytic and prothrombotic activity may play a critical role in stabilization of atheroma during lipid lowering. Accumulation of mature SMCs, expressing fewer MMPs and less TF, in the fibrous cap also likely contribute to plaque stabilization by lipid lowering. However, the molecular and cellular mechanisms by which lipid lowering reduces macrophage number and promotes maturation of SMCs are not known.

Atherosclerotic arteries produce excess reactive oxygen species (ROS) such as superoxide anion (O_2^-), which promote oxidative modification of LDL.[48] Oxidized LDL (oxLDL) can alter functions of vascular wall cells including endothelial cells. Oxidized LDL and its derivatives increase endothelial expression of molecules, such as vascular cell adhesion molecule 1 (VCAM-1), that contribute to monocyte recruitment.[49,50] One possible result of decreased macrophage accumulation might be reduced oxidative stress and endothelial activation due to lipid lowering.

Macrophages in atheroma can proliferate.[51–53] Macrophage proliferation may play an important role not only in progression of atherosclerosis but also in pathogenesis of unstable plaque formation. Reduced accumulation of macrophages during lipid lowering might result from reduced proliferation.[53] Sakai and colleagues demonstrated that HMG-CoA reductase inhibitors suppress macrophage proliferation *in vitro*.[54] However, *in vivo* evidence regarding this issue remains scant and molecular mechanisms of macrophage proliferation have not yet been shown.

Lipid lowering by HMG-CoA reductase inhibitors reduces acute coronary events in patients.[29–32] This article has discussed how lipid lowering by diet alone in hypercholesterolemic rabbits can ameliorate criteria associated with plaque instability and thrombogenicity. However, some evidence has suggested that clinical benefits of HMG-CoA reductase inhibitors may result from direct effects on lesional cells independent of reductions in LDL.[31,32,55] Accumulating *in vitro* data suggest that HMG-CoA reductase inhibitors inhibit proliferation of SMCs and macrophages, modulate immune function, and suppress prothrombotic potential. Nevertheless, it should still be noted that many such experiments have used rather high doses of HMG-CoA reductase inhibitors. Thus, further *in vivo* experiments should address whether HMG-CoA reductase inhibitors have similar effects *in vivo* at doses relevant to clinical practice. However, even if the so-called pleiotropic effects of HMG-CoA reductase inhibitors turn out not to be important at clinically employed doses, the dietary studies in rabbits described here establish beyond a doubt that lipid lowering per se can ameliorate features of plaque associated with instability and clinical events.

ACKNOWLEDGMENTS

We acknowledge our colleagues and collaborators Elena Rabkin, Sami J. Voglic, Seigo Sugiyama, Yoshikatsu Okada, Ryozo Nagai, Frederick J. Schoen, Mark B. Taubman, John T. Fallon, and Christopher C. Hill, who contributed to the experiments described. We also thank Karen E. Williams for her editorial expertise.

REFERENCES

1. FUSTER, V., L. BADIMON, J.J. BADIMON & J.H. CHESEBRO. 1992. The pathogenesis of coronary artery disease and the acute coronary syndromes (1). N. Engl. J. Med. **326:** 242–250.
2. FUSTER, V., L. BADIMON, J.J. BADIMON & J.H. CHESEBRO. 1992. The pathogenesis of coronary artery disease and the acute coronary syndromes (2). N. Engl. J. Med. **326:** 310–318.
3. LIBBY, P. 1995. Molecular bases of the acute coronary syndromes. Circulation **91:** 2844–2850.
4. DAVIES, M.J., P.D. RICHARDSON, N. WOOLF, D.R. KATZ & J. MANN. 1993. Risk of thrombosis in human atherosclerotic plaques: role of extracellular lipid, macrophage, and smooth muscle cell content. Br. Heart J. **69:** 377–381.
5. VAN DER WAL, A.C., A.E. BECKER, C.M. VAN DER LOOS & P.K. DAS. 1994. Site of intimal rupture or erosion of thrombosed coronary atherosclerotic plaques is characterized by an inflammatory process irrespective of the dominant plaque morphology. Circulation **89:** 36–44.
6. MORENO, P.R., E. FALK, I.F. PALACIOS, J.B. NEWELL, V. FUSTER & J.T. FALLON. 1994. Macrophage infiltration in acute coronary syndromes. Implications for plaque rupture. Circulation **90:** 775–778.
7. LIBBY, P., Y.J. GENG, M. AIKAWA, U. SCHOENBECK, F. MACH, S.K. CLINTON, G.K. SUKHOVA & R.T. LEE. 1996. Macrophages and atherosclerotic plaque stability. Curr. Opin. Lipidol. **7:** 330–335.
8. DOLLERY, C.M., J.R. MCEWAN & A.M. HENNEY. 1995. Matrix metalloproteinases and cardiovascular disease. Circ. Res. **77:** 863–868.
9. CELENTANO, D.C. & W.H. FRISHMAN. 1997. Matrix metalloproteinases and coronary artery disease: a novel therapeutic target. J. Clin. Pharmacol. **37:** 991–1000.
10. TAUBMAN, M.B., J.T. FALLON, A.D. SCHECTER, P. GIESEN, M. MENDLOWITZ, B.S. FYFE, J.D. MARMUR & Y. NEMERSON. 1997. Tissue factor in the pathogenesis of atherosclerosis. Thromb. Haemost. **78:** 200–204.
11. HENNEY, A.M., P.R. WAKELEY, M.J. DAVIES, K. FOSTER, R. HEMBRY, G. MURPHY & S. HUMPHRIES. 1991. Localization of stromelysin gene expression in atherosclerotic plaques by in situ hybridization. Proc. Natl. Acad. Sci. USA **88:** 8154–8158.
12. GALIS, Z.S., G.K. SUKHOVA, M.W. LARK & P. LIBBY. 1994. Increased expression of matrix metalloproteinases and matrix degrading activity in vulnerable regions of human atherosclerotic plaques. J. Clin. Invest. **94:** 2493–2503.
13. GALIS, Z.S., G.K. SUKHOVA, R. KRANZHOFER, S. CLARK & P. LIBBY. 1995. Macrophage foam cells from experimental atheroma constitutively produce matrix-degrading proteinases. Proc. Natl. Acad. Sci. USA **92:** 402–406.
14. NIKKARI, S.T., K.D. O'BRIEN, M. FERGUSON, T. HATSUKAMI, H.G. WELGUS, C.E. ALPERS & A.W. CLOWES. 1995. Interstitial collagenase (MMP-1) expression in human carotid atherosclerosis. Circulation **92:** 1393–1398.
15. BROWN, D.L., M.S. HIBBS, M. KEARNEY, C. LOUSHIN & J.M. ISNER. 1995. Identification of 92-kD gelatinase in human coronary atherosclerotic lesions. Association of active enzyme synthesis with unstable angina. Circulation **91:** 2125–2131.
16. HALPERT, I., U.I. SIRES, J.D. ROBY, S. POTTER-PERIGO, T.N. WIGHT, S.D. SHAPIRO, H.G. WELGUS, S.A. WICKLINE & W.C. PARKS. 1996. Matrilysin is expressed by lipid-laden macrophages at sites of potential rupture in atherosclerotic lesions and localizes to areas of versican deposition, a proteoglycan substrate for the enzyme. Proc. Natl. Acad. Sci. USA **93:** 9748–9753.
17. MATSUMOTO, S., T. KOBAYASHI, M. KATOH, S. SAITO, Y. IKEDA, M. KOBORI, Y. MASUHO & T. WATANABE. 1998. Expression and localization of matrix metalloproteinase-12 in the aorta of cholesterol-fed rabbits: relationship to lesion development. Am. J. Pathol. **153:** 109–119.
18. SUKHOVA, G., U. SCHOENBECK, E. RABKIN, F. SCHOEN, A. POOLE, R. BILLINGHURST & P. LIBBY. 1999. Evidence of increased collagenolysis by interstitial collagenases-1 and -3 in vulnerable human atheromatous plaques. Circulation **99:** 2503–2509.

19. SHAH, P.K., E. FALK, J.J. BADIMON, A. FERNANDEZ-ORTIZ, A. MAILHAC, G. VILLAREAL-LEVY, J. T. FALLON, J. REGNSTROM & V. FUSTER. 1995. Human monocyte-derived macrophages induce collagen breakdown in fibrous caps of atherosclerotic plaques. Potential role of matrix-degrading metalloproteinases and implications for plaque rupture. Circulation **92:** 1565–1569.
20. WILCOX, J.N., K.M. SMITH, S.M. SCHWARTZ & D. GORDON. 1989. Localization of tissue factor in the normal vessel wall and in the atherosclerotic plaque. Proc. Natl. Acad. Sci. USA **86:** 2839–2843.
21. DRAKE, T.A., J.H. MORRISSEY & T.S. EDGINGTON. 1989. Selective cellular expression of tissue factor in human tissues. Implications for disorders of hemostasis and thrombosis. Am. J. Pathol. **134:** 1087–1097.
22. THIRUVIKRAMAN, S.V., A. GUHA, J. ROBOZ, M.B. TAUBMAN, Y. NEMERSON & J.T. FALLON. 1996. In situ localization of tissue factor in human atherosclerotic plaques by binding of digoxigenin-labeled factors VIIa and X. Lab. Invest. **75:** 451–461.
23. HATAKEYAMA, K., Y. ASADA, K. MARUTSUKA, Y. SATO, Y. KAMIKUBO & A. SUMIYOSHI. 1997. Localization and activity of tissue factor in human aortic atherosclerotic lesions. Atherosclerosis **133:** 213–219.
24. MARMUR, J.D., S.V. THIRUVIKRAMAN, B.S. FYFE, A. GUHA, S.K. SHARMA, J.A. AMBROSE, J.T. FALLON, Y. NEMERSON & M.B. TAUBMAN. 1996. Identification of active tissue factor in human coronary atheroma. Circulation **94:** 1226–1232.
25. ANNEX, B.H., S.M. DENNING, K.M. CHANNON, M.H. SKETCH, JR., R.S. STACK, J.H. MORRISSEY & K.G. PETERS. 1995. Differential expression of tissue factor protein in directional atherectomy specimens from patients with stable and unstable coronary syndromes. Circulation **91:** 619–622.
26. MORENO, P.R., V.H. BERNARDI, J. LOPEZ-CUELLAR, A.M. MURCIA, I.F. PALACIOS, H.K. GOLD, R. MEHRAN, S.K. SHARMA, Y. NEMERSON, V. FUSTER & J.T. FALLON. 1996. Macrophages, smooth muscle cells, and tissue factor in unstable angina. Implications for cell-mediated thrombogenicity in acute coronary syndromes. Circulation **94:** 3090–3097.
27. ARDISSINO, D., P.A. MERLINI, R. ARIENS, R. COPPOLA, E. BRAMUCCI & P.M. MANNUCCI. 1997. Tissue-factor antigen and activity in human coronary atherosclerotic plaques. Lancet **349:** 769–771.
28. KAIKITA, K., H. OGAWA, H. YASUE, M. TAKEYA, K. TAKAHASHI, T. SAITO, K. HAYASAKI, K. HORIUCHI, A. TAKIZAWA, Y. KAMIKUBO & S. NAKAMURA. 1997. Tissue factor expression on macrophages in coronary plaques in patients with unstable angina. Arterioscler. Thromb. Vasc. Biol. **17:** 2232–2237.
29. SCANDINAVIAN SIMVASTATIN SURVIVAL STUDY GROUP. 1994. Randomised trial of cholesterol lowering in 4444 patients with coronary heart disease: the Scandinavian Simvastatin Survival Study (4S). Lancet **344:** 1383–1389.
30. SHEPHERD, J., S.M. COBBE, I. FORD, C.G. ISLES, A.R. LORIMER, P.W. MACFARLANE, J.H. MCKILLOP & C.J. PACKARD. 1995. Prevention of coronary heart disease with pravastatin in men with hypercholesterolemia. West of Scotland Coronary Prevention Study Group. N. Engl. J. Med. **333:** 1301–1307.
31. SACKS, F.M., M.A. PFEFFER, L.A. MOYE, J.L. ROULEAU, J.D. RUTHERFORD, T.G. COLE, L. BROWN, J.W. WARNICA, J.M. ARNOLD, C.C. WUN, B.R. DAVIS & E. BRAUNWALD. 1996. The effect of pravastatin on coronary events after myocardial infarction in patients with average cholesterol levels. Cholesterol and Recurrent Events Trial investigators. N. Engl. J. Med. **335:** 1001–1009.
32. DOWNS, J.R., M. CLEARFIELD, S. WEIS, E. WHITNEY, D.R. SHAPIRO, P.A. BEERE, A. LANGENDORFER, E.A. STEIN, W. KRUYER & A.M. GOTTO, JR. 1998. Primary prevention of acute coronary events with lovastatin in men and women with average cholesterol levels: results of AFCAPS/TexCAPS. Air Force/Texas Coronary Atherosclerosis Prevention Study. J. Am. Med. Assoc. **279:** 1615–1622.
33. BROWN, B.G., X.Q. ZHAO, D.E. SACCO & J.J. ALBERS. 1993. Lipid lowering and plaque regression. New insights into prevention of plaque disruption and clinical events in coronary disease. Circulation **87:** 1781–1791.
34. LIBBY, P. & M. AIKAWA. 1998. New insights into plaque stabilisation by lipid lowering. Drugs **56:** 9–13.

35. ARMSTRONG, M.L. & M.B. MEGAN. 1972. Lipid depletion in atheromatous coronary arteries in rhesus monkeys after regression diets. Circ. Res. **30:** 675–680.
36. ARMSTRONG, M.L. & M.B. MEGAN. 1975. Arterial fibrous proteins in cynomolgus monkeys after atherogenic and regression diets. Circ. Res. **36:** 256–261.
37. SMALL, D.M., M.G. BOND, D. WAUGH, M. PRACK & J.K. SAWYER. 1984. Physicochemical and histological changes in the arterial wall of nonhuman primates during progression and regression of atherosclerosis. J. Clin. Invest. **73:** 1590–1605.
38. KAPLAN, J.R., S.B. MANUCK, M.R. ADAMS, J.K. WILLIAMS, T.C. REGISTER & T.B. CLARKSON. 1993. Plaque changes and arterial enlargement in atherosclerotic monkeys after manipulation of diet and social environment. Arterioscler. Thromb. **13:** 254–263.
39. SHIOMI, M., T. ITO, T. TSUKADA, T. YATA, Y. WATANABE, Y. TSUJITA, M. FUKAMI, J. FUKUSHIGE, T. HOSOKAWA & A. TAMURA. 1995. Reduction of serum cholesterol levels alters lesional composition of atherosclerotic plaques. Effect of pravastatin sodium on atherosclerosis in mature WHHL rabbits. Arterioscler. Thromb. Vasc. Biol. **15:** 1938–1944.
40. AIKAWA, M., E. RABKIN, Y. OKADA, S.J. VOGLIC, S.K. CLINTON, C.E. BRINCKERHOFF, G.K. SUKHOVA & P. LIBBY. 1998. Lipid lowering by diet reduces matrix metalloproteinase activity and increases collagen content of rabbit atheroma: a potential mechanism of lesion stabilization. Circulation **97:** 2433–2444.
41. AIKAWA, M., S.J. VOGLIC, S. SUGIYAMA, E. RABKIN, M.B. TAUBMAN, J.T. FALLON & P. LIBBY. 1999. Dietary lipid lowering reduces tissue factor expression in rabbit atheroma. Circulation. In press.
42. SCHWARTZ, S.M., D. DEBLOIS & E.R. O'BRIEN. 1995. The intima. Soil for atherosclerosis and restenosis. Circ. Res. **77:** 445–65.
43. AIKAWA, M., P.N. SIVAM, M. KURO-O, K. KIMURA, K. NAKAHARA, S. TAKEWAKI, M. UEDA, H. YAMAGUCHI, Y. YAZAKI, M. PERIASAMY & R. NAGAI. 1993. Human smooth muscle myosin heavy chain isoforms as molecular markers for vascular development and atherosclerosis. Circ. Res. **73:** 1000–1012.
44. AIKAWA, M., Y. SAKOMURA, M. UEDA, K. KIMURA, I. MANABE, S. ISHIWATA, N. KOMIYAMA, H. YAMAGUCHI, Y. YAZAKI & R. NAGAI. 1997. Redifferentiation of smooth muscle cells after coronary angioplasty determined via myosin heavy chain expression. Circulation **96:** 82–90.
45. AIKAWA, M., E. RABKIN, S.J. VOGLIC, H. SHING, R. NAGAI, F.J. SCHOEN & P. LIBBY. 1998. Lipid lowering promotes accumulation of mature smooth muscle cells expressing smooth muscle myosin heavy chain isoforms in rabbit atheroma. Circ. Res. **83:** 1015–1026.
46. KOCKX, M.M., G.R. DE MEYER, N. BUYSSENS, M.W. KNAAPEN, H. BULT & A.G. HERMAN. 1998. Cell composition, replication, and apoptosis in atherosclerotic plaques after 6 months of cholesterol withdrawal. Circ. Res. **83:** 378–387.
47. HOLYCROSS, B.J., R.S. BLANK, M.M. THOMPSON, M.J. PEACH & G.K. OWENS. 1992. Platelet-derived growth factor-BB-induced suppression of smooth muscle cell differentiation. Circ. Res. **71:** 1525–1532.
48. WITZTUM, J.L. 1994. The oxidation hypothesis of atherosclerosis. Lancet **344:** 793–795.
49. KUME, N., M.I. CYBULSKY & M.A. GIMBRONE, JR. 1992. Lysophosphatidylcholine, a component of atherogenic lipoproteins, induces mononuclear leukocyte adhesion molecules in cultured human and rabbit arterial endothelial cells. J. Clin. Invest. **90:** 1138–1144.
50. KHAN, B.V., S.S. PARTHASARATHY, R.W. ALEXANDER & R.M. MEDFORD. 1995. Modified low density lipoprotein and its constituents augment cytokine- activated vascular cell adhesion molecule-1 gene expression in human vascular endothelial cells. J. Clin. Invest. **95:** 1262–1270.
51. ROSENFELD, M.E. & R. ROSS. 1990. Macrophage and smooth muscle cell proliferation in atherosclerotic lesions of WHHL and comparably hypercholesterolemic fat-fed rabbits. Arteriosclerosis **10:** 680–687.
52. REKHTER, M.D. & D. GORDON. 1995. Active proliferation of different cell types, including lymphocytes, in human atherosclerotic plaques. Am. J. Pathol. **147:** 668–677.
53. RAINES, E.W., M.E. ROSENFELD & R. ROSS. 1996. The role of macrophages. *In* Atherosclerosis and Coronary Artery Disease. V. Fuster & E.J. Topol, Eds.: 539–555. Lippincott-Raven Publishers. Philadelphia.

54. SAKAI, M., S. KOBORI, T. MATSUMURA, T. BIWA, Y. SATO, T. TAKEMURA, H. HAKAMATA, S. HORIUCHI & M. SHICHIRI. 1997. HMG-CoA reductase inhibitors suppress macrophage growth induced by oxidized low density lipoprotein. Atherosclerosis **133:** 51–59.
55. RIDKER, P.M., N. RIFAI, M.A. PFEFFER, F.M. SACKS, L.A. MOYE, S. GOLDMAN, G.C. FLAKER & E. BRAUNWALD. 1998. Inflammation, pravastatin, and the risk of coronary events after myocardial infarction in patients with average cholesterol levels. Cholesterol and Recurrent Events (CARE) Investigators. Circulation **98:** 839–844.

Mechanisms of Vascular Atrophy and Fibrous Cap Disruption

ALEXANDER W. CLOWES[a] AND SCOTT A. BERCELI

Division of Vascular Surgery, University of Washington, Seattle, Washington 98195, USA

ABSTRACT: The process of plaque destabilization and rupture remains an area of intense investigation. While reductions in lumen cross-sectional area induced by early, non-occlusive lesions are compensated by remodeling and expansion of the artery, further plaque enlargement leads to an uncompensated reduction in lumen area and an increase in surface shearing forces. We hypothesize that these local increases in wall shear stress lead to a reduction in smooth muscle cell proliferation and increase in cell death. Using a primate prosthetic graft model, we have observed that alterations in nitric oxide and platelet-derived growth factor metabolism are important regulators of intimal growth and regression. We suggest that these factors may also be influential in the process of fibrous cap atrophy and plaque rupture.

While early atherosclerotic plaques are of limited clinical significance, it is their development into complicated Type IV and V lesions that is associated with the onset of clinical symptoms. Disruption of these plaques has now been established as the initiating event leading to the sudden onset of thromboembolic complications.[1] Localized endothelial denudation with superficial thrombosis does occur over advanced atherosclerotic plaques, but the microscopic platelet thrombi are often self-limited and resolve promptly without clinical symptoms.[2,3] Instead, it is the deep intimal injuries with fracture of the plaque cap and exposure of the underlying necrotic core, that most commonly lead to acute arterial occlusion. Pathologic examination of these specimens has identified an unstable plaque phenotype, characterized by a large pool of extracellular lipid and a macrophage-rich, smooth muscle cell–poor fibrous cap.[4]

Fracture of the plaque is governed by the interplay between local circumferential wall stress and the tensile strength of the overlying fibrous cap.[3] The fibrous cap is a dynamic structure. Its composition and configuration are influenced by the local biologic and biomechanical environment.[5,6] As such, it is this balance between smooth muscle cell proliferation and matrix synthesis on one hand and smooth muscle cell death and matrix degradation on the other that dictates plaque stability. Much insight has been gained in understanding this process through examination of pathologic specimens. The fibrous caps of advanced lesions exhibit a predominance of macrophages, few smooth muscle cells, and a high percentage of cells undergoing apoptosis.[7] The colocalization of cells demonstrating substantial DNA fragmenta-

---

[a]Address for correspondence: Alexander W. Clowes, Division of Vascular Surgery, University of Washington, BB 442 HSB-Box 356410, Seattle, WA 98195-6410.
clowes@u.washington.edu

tion with sites of plaque rupture further supports these concepts.[8] While the events surrounding fibrous cap rupture have been well described, the underlying remodeling process that leads to plaque instability is only beginning to be understood. Foremost is the influence of biomechanical forces on this remodeling process.[6]

Arterial remodeling in response to alterations in the hemodynamic environment has been proposed as one of the primary regulators of vessel geometry and the atherosclerotic process.[9] With the initial development of a fatty streak and the progression to a complicated lesion, the resulting reduction in lumen cross-sectional area is compensated by vessel enlargement.[10,11] The remodeling process continues in an effort to maintain a physiologic level of wall shear stress. However, as plaque enlargement exceeds the ability of the artery to dilate, the resulting reduction in lumen area results in an increase in surface shear forces. In addition, the altered topography created by the advanced atheromatous plaque creates local perturbations in the flow field. It is these disturbances in the flow field, and the corresponding changes in local wall shearing forces, which we propose have a significant role in thinning of the fibrous cap and the development of the unstable plaque phenotype.

SHEAR STRESS AND INTIMAL HYPERPLASIA

Since the initial observations of Zarins and Glagov[12] demonstrating the influence of shear stress on lesion localization, many investigators have examined the mechanisms underlying these effects. In our laboratory we have used a primate prosthetic graft model, with or without placement of a distal fistula, to investigate the influence of shear on intimal hyperplasia. Like the calcified diseased artery, the graft is rigid and lacks the ability to dilate in response to increased blood flow and shear stress. Bilateral aorto-iliac PTFE grafts are implanted simultaneously with the placement of bilateral femoral arteriovenous fistula (AVF) (FIG. 1). Following a 2-month peri-

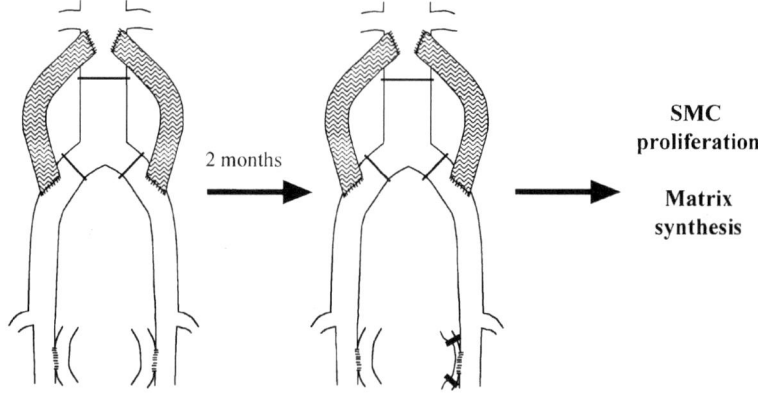

FIGURE 1. Prosthetic graft "flow switch" experimental design.

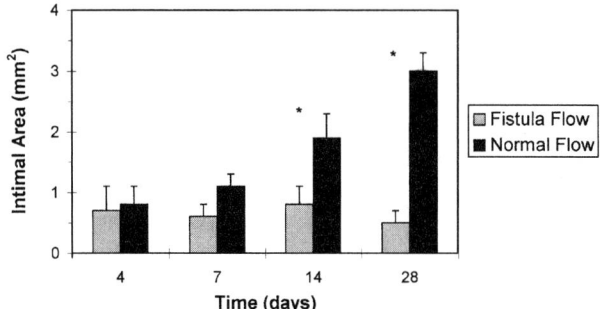

FIGURE 2. Intimal area time course progression after flow switch for fistula-flow and normal-flow grafts. All values are mean ± SEM for each group ($N = 5$). *$p < 0.05$ for fistula compared to normal flow grafts at 14 and 28 days. (Adapted from Geary *et al.*[13])

od, during which the grafts develop an endothelialized intima, one of the fistulae is ligated. In response to fistula ligation and reduction in blood flow, neointimal smooth muscle cells begin to proliferate; a maximum is reached at 4 days and returns to baseline by 14 days. A corresponding increase in intimal areas is also observed at both 14 and 28 days (FIG. 2).[13]

To determine if the intimal thickening process is reversible, we have employed a "reverse flow switch" model (FIG. 3). Bilateral aorto-iliac bypass grafts are implanted without the presence of distal fistulae. The intima develops under normal flow conditions for two months, and at the end of this period a distal fistula is placed in one leg. Grafts are harvested after an additional two-month period. One graft has

Reverse Flow Switch

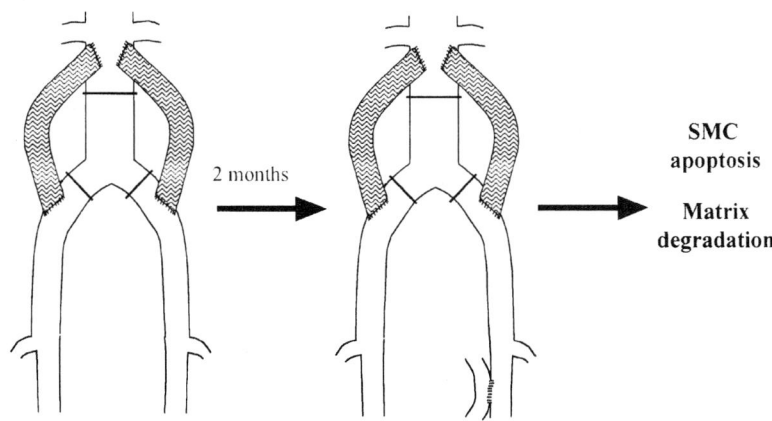

FIGURE 3. Prosthetic graft "reverse flow switch" experimental design.

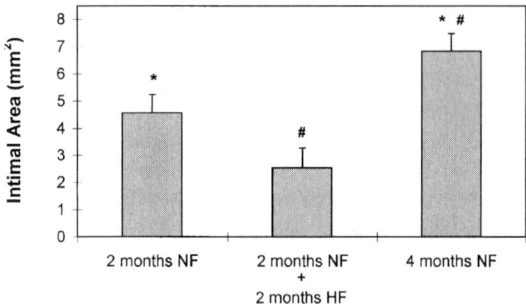

FIGURE 4. Intimal areas of "reverse flow switch" grafts subjected to two months of normal flow (NF), two months of normal flow followed by two months of high flow (HF), or four months of normal flow. All values are mean ± SEM for each group ($N = 8$). $*p < 0.05$ for two months NF versus four months NF. $^{\#}p < 0.05$ for two months NF + two months HF versus four months NF. (Adapted from Mattsson et al.[14])

been exposed to normal flow for four months and the second graft exposed to normal flow for two months followed by high flow for two months. Intimal area and smooth muscle cell proliferation decrease in response to the increase in wall shear stress (FIG. 4). The atrophy of the intima is due to loss of matrix and cells and is apparent by seven days after the switch from normal to high flow (Davies, Kenagy, Fischer, Berceli, and Clowes, unpublished results). Northern blot analysis of the graft intimas demonstrates a fourfold increase in endothelial cell nitric oxide synthase (ecNOS) expression in the specimens exposed to high flow. Immunohistochemistry demonstrates that the increase in expression is confined to the endothelium.[14]

MECHANISM OF FIBROUS CAP ATROPHY

While the process and underlying mechanisms of fibrous cap atrophy and plaque rupture are clearly multifactorial, we believe local alterations in wall shear stress to be one determinant of plaque instability (FIG. 5). Initial reductions in lumen cross-sectional area created by the developing plaque are compensated by vessel enlargement and normalization of shear. However, further increases in plaque volume, uncompensated by vessel dilation, lead to local regions of elevated shear stress along the protruding plaque. This locally perceived increase in shear promotes an increase in dilating factors (e.g., nitric oxide) and a decrease in growth promoting or survival factors (e.g., platelet-derived growth factor). In combination, these effects act to decrease smooth muscle cell proliferation, reduce smooth muscle cell migration, and increase smooth muscle cell apoptotic death. In addition, matrix is lost on account of decreased synthesis and increased degradation.[15,16] This process of fibrous cap atrophy is modeled by the response of the baboon graft neointima subjected to an increase in shear stress.

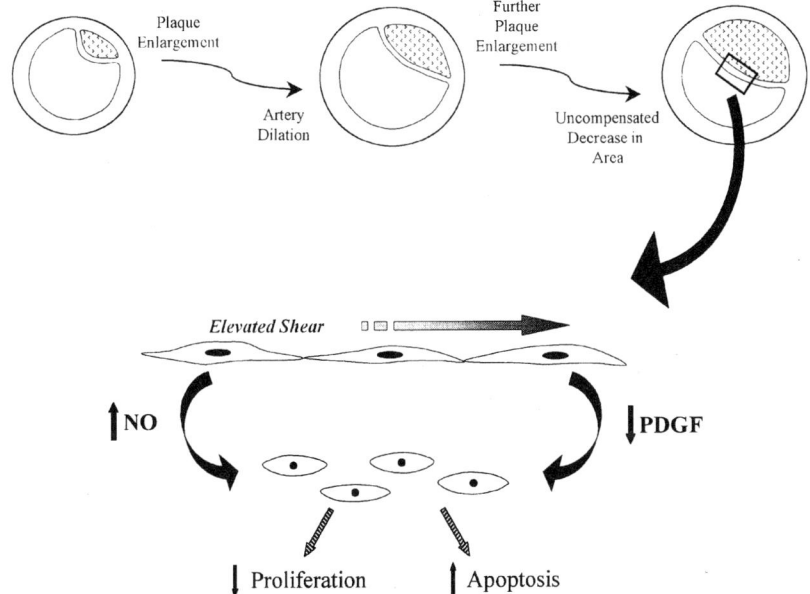

FIGURE 5. Initial enlargement of the atherosclerotic plaque is compensated by an increase in cross-sectional area and normalization of shear. However, further plaque enlargement leads to reduced lumen area and an increase shear forces. This promotes an increase in NO and reduction in PDGF synthesis by the endothelium. These changes reduce smooth muscle cell proliferation and increase apoptosis, thereby promoting fibrous cap atrophy.

NITRIC OXIDE

Through experiments on the flow-dependent regulation of arterial diameter, the role of endothelial-derived nitric oxide (NO) in maintaining vascular tone has been elucidated. While the influence of wall shear stress on NO synthesis both *in vitro* and *in vivo* has been well described,[17–19] the mechanism of mechanotransduction by the endothelial cell remains an area of intense research.[20,21] Activation of shear-regulated ion channels and deformation of the cytoskeleton have been suggested as possible mediators of the imposed strains.[22] Recent data support these hypotheses, demonstrating both an early calcium-dependent and a late calcium-independent activation of NOS. This early response acts through phospholipase C, leading to the influx of calcium, activation of NOS, and substantial but short-lived release of NO. The late response involves activation of a small GTP-binding protein, stimulation of calcium-independent C and mitogen-activated protein kinases, and reduced but prolonged release of NO.[23]

Recent investigations have suggested NO as an important regulatory molecule in the pathophysiology of arterial disease. NO inhibits smooth muscle cell proliferation and can increase apoptotic cell death.[24] Both cGMP-dependent and cGMP-independent pathways have been identified as regulators of smooth muscle proliferation and apoptosis,[25–28] however the detailed mechanisms remain to be fully described. The biologic response of smooth muscle and endothelial cells to NO differ, where NO enhances endothelial proliferation and reduces endothelial apoptosis.[29,30] The intracellular signaling pathways that account for these differences remain to be further explored.

Experimental evidence supports a role for NO in the response to injury and vascular remodeling process *in vivo*. Studies performed in our laboratory demonstrate an increase in injury-induced intimal thickening in animals treated with an NO inhibitor. (Fischer and Clowes, 1999, unpublished) The local application of an NO donor or the NO precursor L-arginine reduces neointimal area in vein grafts or balloon-dilated arteries, respectively.[31,32] The inhibition of neointima formation, which occurs in response to elevated flow, is also mediated by NO, since NOS blockade prevents the normal remodeling process and adaptation to increased wall shear.[33]

While most studies have investigated the role of NO in intimal growth and its effect on smooth muscle cell proliferation, recent investigation has focused on the influence of NO on the process of intimal regression and cell death. Local application of L-arginine to atherosclerotic lesions results in an increase in apoptotic cell death, via a cGMP-independent mechanism.[34] This increase in cell death was almost exclusively localized to the intimal macrophages and not to the smooth muscle cells. The process of NO-induced smooth muscle cell apoptosis established in cell culture has yet to be demonstrated *in vivo*.

PLATELET-DERIVED GROWTH FACTOR

The flow-dependent regulation of PDGF-A and -B chain expression by endothelial cells in culture has been well characterized.[35,36] This response appears linked to the temporal gradient of the shear, with abrupt changes in flow being the most potent stimulus for increased gene expression.[37] Recent investigations have identified a GC-rich shear-stress response element in the promoter regions of both A and B chain genome. Binding of egr-1 and NFκB to these promoter sites is linked to the shear-induced transcription of these growth factors.[38,39] This flow-regulated PDGF synthesis appears dependent on the local production of endothelial-derived NO.[37] Both egr-1 and NFκB expression has been demonstrated to be inversely related to NO concentrations, with endogenous NO synthesis or exogenous NO donors downregulating both transcription factors and inhibiting the shear-induced expression of PDGF.

The mitogenic and migratory effects of the various PDGF isoforms have been extensively investigated by our group.[40] *In vitro*, the PDGF-BB isoform stimulates both smooth muscle cell proliferation and migration, whereas PDGF-AA stimulates only proliferation and inhibits migration. Of recent interest is the influence of PDGF on the process of cell death. Smooth muscle cells harvested from normal and atherosclerotic arterial segments and examined in cell culture both demonstrate an increase in apoptosis in response to withdrawal of PDGF-AA and -BB. The plaque-derived cells exhibit greater sensitivity to the growth factors.[41]

Exposure of normal arteries to increased flow induces a downregulation of both endothelial PDGF-A and -B chain expression.[42] We have investigated the flow-dependent regulation of PDGF using our flow-switch prosthetic graft model (FIG. 1). Northern blots prepared from four-day animals demonstrate a 2.9-fold increase in

PDGF-A chain mRNA expression in response to the reduction in flow. *In situ* hybridization confirms this finding, demonstrating an increase in PDGF-A expression in the intima of reduced-flow grafts. While occurring across the entire intima, this increase in PDGF-A was most prominent in the intact endothelial layer. PDGF-α and -β receptors, also examined by Northern blot analysis, are also increased (2.1- and 1.7-fold, respectively), but these differences did not reach statistical significance. Interestingly, PDGF-B chain expression is present in only very small quantities in both high and reduced flow grafts.[43]

The physiologic impact of these changes was investigated in our laboratory using chimeric antibodies against both the PDGF-α and -β receptors. Using our flow-switch model, we have found a significant reduction in the ratio of high-flow to normal-flow intimal areas in animals treated with antibodies to PDGF-β receptors. (Davies and Clowes, 1999, unpublished material) Interestingly, this effect seems predominantly mediated through reductions in the intimal area of normal flow grafts, where PDGF expression is most notable.

CONCLUSION

The process of plaque destabilization and rupture remains an area of intense investigation. While reductions in lumen cross-sectional area induced by early, nonocclusive lesions are compensated by remodeling and expansion of the artery, further plaque enlargement leads to an uncompensated reduction in lumen area and an increase in surface shearing forces. We hypothesize that these local increases in wall shear stress lead to a reduction in smooth muscle cell proliferation and an increase in cell death. While shear-induced lesion remodeling is an area of intense investigation, we have observed alterations in NO and PDGF metabolism to be important regulators of intimal growth and regression in our experimental prosthetic graft model. We suggest that these factors may also be influential in the process of fibrous cap atrophy and plaque rupture.

REFERENCES

1. DAVIES, M.J. & A.C. THOMAS. 1985. Plaque fissuring—the cause of acute myocardial infarction, sudden ischaemic death, and crescendo angina. Br. Heart J. **53:** 363–373.
2. DAVIES, M.J. 1994. Pathology of arterial thrombosis. Br. Med. Bull. **50:** 789–802.
3. DAVIES, M.J. 1996. Stability and instability: two faces of coronary atherosclerosis. The Paul Dudley White Lecture 1995. Circulation **94:** 2013–2020.
4. DAVIES, M.J., P.D. RICHARDSON, N. WOOLF, D.R. KATZ & J. MANN. 1993. Risk of thrombosis in human atherosclerotic plaques: role of extracellular lipid, macrophage, and smooth muscle cell content. Br. Heart J. **69:** 377–381.
5. LEE, R.T. & P. LIBBY. 1997. The unstable atheroma. Arterioscler. Thromb. Vasc. Biol. **17:** 1859–1867.
6. LIBBY, P., Y.J. GENG, G.K. SUKHOVA, D.I. SIMON & R.T. LEE. 1997. Molecular determinants of atherosclerotic plaque vulnerability. Ann. N.Y. Acad. Sci. **811:** 134–142; discussion 142–145.
7. KOCKX, M.M., G.R. DE MEYER, J. MUHRING, W. JACOB, H. BULT & A.G. HERMAN. 1998. Apoptosis and related proteins in different stages of human atherosclerotic plaques. Circulation **97:** 2307–2315.

8. CRISBY, M., B. KALLIN, J. THYBERG, B. ZHIVOTOVSKY, S. ORRENIUS, V. KOSTULAS & J. NILSSON. 1997. Cell death in human atherosclerotic plaques involves both oncosis and apoptosis. Atherosclerosis **130:** 17–27.
9. GLAGOV, S. 1994. Intimal hyperplasia, vascular modeling, and the restenosis problem. Circulation **89:** 2888–2891.
10. GLAGOV, S., E. WEISENBERG, C.K. ZARINS, R. STANKUNAVICIUS & G.J. KOLETTIS. 1987. Compensatory enlargement of human atherosclerotic coronary arteries. N. Engl. J. Med. **316:** 1371–1375.
11. ZARINS, C.K., M.A. ZATINA, D.P. GIDDENS, D.N. KU & S. GLAGOV. 1987. Shear stress regulation of artery lumen diameter in experimental atherogenesis. J. Vasc. Surg. **5:** 413–420.
12. ZARINS, C.K., D.P. GIDDENS, B.K. BHARADVAJ, V.S. SOTTIURAI, R.F. MABON & S. GLAGOV. 1983. Carotid bifurcation atherosclerosis. Quantitative correlation of plaque localization with flow velocity profiles and wall shear stress. Circ. Res. **53:** 502–514.
13. GEARY, R.L., T.R. KOHLER, S. VERGEL, T.R. KIRKMAN & A.W. CLOWES. 1994. Time course of flow-induced smooth muscle cell proliferation and intimal thickening in endothelialized baboon vascular grafts. Circ. Res. **74:** 14–23.
14. MATTSSON, E.J., T.R. KOHLER, S.M. VERGEL & A.W. CLOWES. 1997. Increased blood flow induces regression of intimal hyperplasia. Arterioscler. Thromb. Vasc. Biol. **17:** 2245–2249.
15. ARROYO, L.H. & R.T. LEE. 1999. Mechanisms of plaque rupture: mechanical and biologic interactions. Cardiovasc. Res. **41:** 369–375.
16. NEWBY, A.C. & A.B. ZALTSMAN. 1999. Fibrous cap formation or destruction—the critical importance of vascular smooth muscle cell proliferation, migration and matrix formation. Cardiovasc. Res. **41:** 345–360.
17. PAPADAKI, M., R.G. TILTON, S.G. ESKIN & L.V. MCINTIRE. 1998. Nitric oxide production by cultured human aortic smooth muscle cells: stimulation by fluid flow. Am. J. Physiol. **274:** H616–626.
18. KNUDSEN, H.L. & J.A. FRANGOS. 1997. Role of cytoskeleton in shear stress-induced endothelial nitric oxide production. Am. J. Physiol. **273:** H347–355.
19. HYRE, C.E., J.L. UNTHANK & M.C. DALSING. 1998. Direct *in vivo* measurement of flow-dependent nitric oxide production in mesenteric resistance arteries. J. Vasc. Surg. **27:** 726–732.
20. CHIEN, S., S. LI & Y.J. SHYY. 1998. Effects of mechanical forces on signal transduction and gene expression in endothelial cells. Hypertension **31:** 162–169.
21. ISHIDA, T., M. TAKAHASHI, M.A. CORSON & B.C. BERK. 1997. Fluid shear stress-mediated signal transduction: how do endothelial cells transduce mechanical force into biological responses? Ann. N.Y. Acad. Sci. **811:** 12–23; discussion 23–24.
22. LEHOUX, S. & A. TEDGUI. 1998. Signal transduction of mechanical stresses in the vascular wall. Hypertension **32:** 338–345.
23. TAKAHASHI, M., T. ISHIDA, O. TRAUB, M.A. CORSON & B.C. BERK. 1997. Mechanotransduction in endothelial cells: temporal signaling events in response to shear stress. J. Vasc. Res. **34:** 212–219.
24. BENNETT, M.R. 1999. Apoptosis of vascular smooth muscle cells in vascular remodelling and atherosclerotic plaque rupture. Cardiovasc. Res. **41:** 361–368.
25. POLLMAN, M.J., T. YAMADA, M. HORIUCHI & G.H. GIBBONS. 1996. Vasoactive substances regulate vascular smooth muscle cell apoptosis. Countervailing influences of nitric oxide and angiotensin II. Circ. Res. **79:** 748–756.
26. SARKAR, R., D. GORDON, J.C. STANLEY & R.C. WEBB. 1997. Dual cell cycle-specific mechanisms mediate the antimitogenic effects of nitric oxide in vascular smooth muscle cells. J. Hypertens. **15:** 275–283.
27. NISHIO, E., K. FUKUSHIMA, M. SHIOZAKI & Y. WATANABE. 1996. Nitric oxide donor SNAP induces apoptosis in smooth muscle cells through cGMP-independent mechanism. Biochem. Biophys. Res. Commun. **221:** 163–168.
28. NISHIO, E. & Y. WATANABE. 1997. Nitric oxide donor-induced apoptosis in smooth muscle cells is modulated by protein kinase C and protein kinase A. Eur. J. Pharmacol. **339:** 245–251.

29. TZENG, E., Y.M. KIM, B.R. PITT, A. LIZONOVA, I. KOVESDI & T.R. BILLIAR. 1997. Adenoviral transfer of the inducible nitric oxide synthase gene blocks endothelial cell apoptosis. Surgery **122:** 255–263.
30. KIM, Y.M., C.A. BOMBECK & T.R. BILLIAR. 1999. Nitric oxide as a bifunctional regulator of apoptosis. Circ. Res. **84:** 253–256.
31. FULTON, G.J., M.G. DAVIES, L. BARBER, J.L. GRAY, E. SVENDSEN & P.O. HAGEN. 1998. Local effects of nitric oxide supplementation and suppression in the development of intimal hyperplasia in experimental vein grafts. Eur. J. Vasc. Endovasc. Surg. **15:** 279–289.
32. BOSMANS, J.M., C.J. VRINTS, M.M. KOCKX, H. BULT, K.M. CROMHEEKE & A.G. HERMAN. 1999. Continuous perivascular L-arginine delivery increases total vessel area and reduces neointimal thickening after experimental balloon dilatation. Arterioscler. Thromb. Vasc. Biol. **19:** 767–776.
33. ELLENBY, M.I., C.B. ERNST, O.A. CARRETERO & A.G. SCICLI. 1996. Role of nitric oxide in the effect of blood flow on neointima formation. J. Vasc. Surg. **23:** 314–322.
34. WANG, B.Y., H.K. HO, P.S. LIN, S.P. SCHWARZACHER, M.J. POLLMAN, G.H. GIBBONS, P.S. TSAO & J.P. COOKE. 1999. Regression of atherosclerosis: role of nitric oxide and apoptosis. Circulation **99:** 1236–1241.
35. MITSUMATA, M., R.S. FISHEL, R.M. NEREM, R.W. ALEXANDER & B.C. BERK. 1993. Fluid shear stress stimulates platelet-derived growth factor expression in endothelial cells. Am. J. Physiol. **265:** H3–8.
36. HSIEH, H.J., N.Q. LI & J.A. FRANGOS. 1991. Shear stress increases endothelial platelet-derived growth factor mRNA levels. Am. J. Physiol. **260:** H642–H646.
37. BAO, X., C. LU & J.A. FRANGOS. 1999. Temporal gradient in shear but not steady shear stress induces PDGF-A and MCP-1 expression in endothelial cells: Role of NO, NFkappaB, and egr-1. Arterioscler. Thromb. Vasc. Biol. **19:** 996–1003.
38. KHACHIGIAN, L.M., K.R. ANDERSON, N.J. HALNON, M.A. GIMBRONE, JR., N. RESNICK & T. COLLINS. 1997. Egr-1 is activated in endothelial cells exposed to fluid shear stress and interacts with a novel shear-stress-response element in the PDGF A-chain promoter. Arterioscler. Thromb. Vasc. Biol. **17:** 2280–2286.
39. KHACHIGIAN, L.M., N. RESNICK, M.A. GIMBRONE, JR. & T. COLLINS. 1995. Nuclear factor-kappa B interacts functionally with the platelet-derived growth factor B-chain shear-stress response element in vascular endothelial cells exposed to fluid shear stress. J. Clin. Invest. **96:** 1169–1175.
40. KOYAMA, N., C.E. HART & A.W. CLOWES. 1994. Different functions of the platelet-derived growth factor-alpha and -beta receptors for the migration and proliferation of cultured baboon smooth muscle cells. Circ. Res. **75:** 682–691.
41. BENNETT, M.R., G.I. EVAN & S.M. SCHWARTZ. 1995. Apoptosis of human vascular smooth muscle cells derived from normal vessels and coronary atherosclerotic plaques. J. Clin. Invest. **95:** 2266–2274.
42. MONDY, J.S., V. LINDNER, J.K. MIYASHIRO, B.C. BERK, R.H. DEAN & R.L. GEARY. 1997. Platelet-derived growth factor ligand and receptor expression in response to altered blood flow *in vivo*. Circ. Res. **81:** 320–327.
43. KRAISS, L.W., R.L. GEARY, E.J. MATTSSON, S. VERGEL, Y.P. AU & A.W. CLOWES. 1996. Acute reductions in blood flow and shear stress induce platelet-derived growth factor-A expression in baboon prosthetic grafts. Circ. Res. **79:** 45–53.

Questions and Answers

G.M. RUBANYI (*Berlex Bioscience, Richmond, VA, USA*): Do you see evidence of inflammation under high-flow conditions; macrophage accumulation, for example?

CLOWES: We see occasional macrophages in the graft itself, but we don't see them penetrating into the intima.

RUBANYI: So, where does the urokinase-type plasminogen activator (UPA) come from?

CLOWES: UPA can be expressed either by the endothelium or the smooth muscle cells, or both. In injury situations, UPA typically is expressed by the smooth muscle cells.

RUBANYI: As far as apoptosis and nitric oxide are concerned, overwhelming evidence suggests that eNOS-produced NO is anti-apoptotic, if anything. But, how about redox enzymes? Have you looked at antioxidants, or the usual enzymes, e.g., SOD, catalase, and so on?

CLOWES: We have not, but we have gotten into the array game, too, and are busy looking into bar codes.

RUBANYI: Yes, because NO induces apoptosis if superoxide and peroxynitrate is produced. There is a lot of NO in the atherosclerotic plaque; there is no dilation, because concomitantly there is a lot of superoxide produced, and all the "bad things" happen rather than vasodilation.

CLOWES: I think that is a terrific suggestion.

P. GANZ (*Brigham and Women's Hospital, Boston, MA, USA*): I would like to make one comment to support your data. A member of our division, Scott Kinley, has looked at the predictors of restenosis after coronary angioplasty and, surprisingly, found that the Reynolds number, a predictor of unsteady shear stress, was a very good predictor of failure of restenosis under high-flow conditions. Maybe your grafts and the angioplasty situation are somewhat analogous.

M.A. GIMBRONE (*Brigham and Women's Hospital, Boston, MA, USA*): In your graft model, it is microvascular endothelium that is growing in, becoming the luminal lining. In the case of the carotid, even if it is a sick endothelium, it is large vessel endothelium, I am wondering, if those endothelial cells are at the same setpoint in terms of the repertory of genes they are expressing at the time of flow shift.

CLOWES: We will be able to look at that because we are going to look at the adjacent iliac artery that should have large vessel endothelium on it.

GIMBRONE: You have an excellent model to get at the age-old issue of what is the primary molder of endothelial phenotype. We all assume that the endothelium is not necessarily the same in the microvasculature of different organs, in large vessels versus small vessels, etc. But this is a beautiful model in which that switch is perhaps occurring.

Y. SATO (*Tohoku University, Sendai, Japan*): In your model you showed the increased activity of UPA and MMP-2, but in terms of the activation of MMP-2, have you ever checked whether membrane-type MMPs are activated in your system?

CLOWES: We haven't yet, but that is high on our list of things to do.

Roles of the AGE-RAGE System in Vascular Injury in Diabetes[a]

YASUHIKO YAMAMOTO,[b,c] SHO-ICHI YAMAGISHI,[c] HIDETO YONEKURA,[c]
TOSHIO DOI,[d] HIROKO TSUJI,[d] ICHIRO KATO,[e] SHIN TAKASAWA,[e]
HIROSHI OKAMOTO,[e] JOYNAL ABEDIN,[c] NOBUSHIGE TANAKA,[c]
SHIGERU SAKURAI,[c] HIDEYUKI MIGITA,[c] HIROYUKI UNOKI,[c] HUA WANG,[c]
TAKAHIRO ZENDA,[c] PING-SHENG WU,[c] YASUNORI SEGAWA,[f]
TOMOMI HIGASHIDE,[f] KAZUO KAWASAKI,[f] AND HIROSHI YAMAMOTO[b,c]

[c]*Department of Biochemistry, Kanazawa University School of Medicine,
13-1 Takara-machi, Kanazawa 920-8640, Japan*

[d]*Division of Artificial Kidney, Kyoto University Hospital, Shogoin Kawahara-cho,
Sakyo-ku, Kyoto 606-8507, Japan*

[e]*Department of Biochemistry, Tohoku University School of Medicine, 2-1 Seiryo-machi,
Aoba-ku, Sendai 980-8575, Japan*

[f]*Department of Ophthalmology, Kanazawa University School of Medicine,
13-1 Takara-machi, Kanazawa 920-8640, Japan*

> ABSTRACT: This study concerns whether advanced glycation endproducts (AGE) are related to microvascular derangement in diabetes, exemplified by pericyte loss and angiogenesis in retinopathy and by mesangial expansion in nephropathy. AGE caused a decrease in viable pericytes cultivated from bovine retina. On the other hand, AGE stimulated the growth and tube formation of human microvascular endothelial cells (EC), this being mediated by autocrine vascular endothelial growth factor. In AGE-exposed rat mesangial cells, type IV collagen synthesis was induced. Those AGE actions were dependent on a cell surface receptor for AGE (RAGE), because they were abolished by RAGE antisense or ribozyme. The AGE-RAGE system may thus participate in the development of diabetic microangiopathy. This proposition was supported by experiments with animal models; several indices characteristic of retinopathy were correlated with circulating AGE levels in OLETF rats. The predisposition to nephropathy was augmented in RAGE transgenic mice when they became diabetic.

INTRODUCTION

During prolonged diabetic exposure, small blood vessels are impaired as are larger vessels. This gives rise to so-called diabetic microangiopathy, exemplified by retinopathy and nephropathy, derangement in the eyes and the kidney, respectively. These vascular complications account for various disabilities and the short life ex-

---

[a]This work was supported by "Research for the Future" Program of the Japan Society for the Promotion of Science (97L00805).

[b]Address for correspondence: Hiroshi Yamamoto, M.D., Ph.D., Department of Biochemistry, Kanazawa University School of Medicine, 13-1 Takara-machi, Kanazawa 920-8640, Japan.

pectancy in diabetic patients. One of the histopathologic hallmarks of diabetic retinopathy is the loss of pericytes, which normally line the endothelium and regulate not only the growth but also the function of neighboring endothelial cells.[1] Focal angiogenesis is the other hallmark of retinopathy (clinically known as microaneurysms) wherein endothelial cells locally proliferate. Nephropathy is characterized by an expansion of the mesangial area due to accumulation of extracellular matrix, which can then result in diabetic glomerulosclerosis.

ADVANCED GLYCATION ENDPRODUCTS

We have noticed that a common factor causative of these microvascular changes is advanced glycation endproducts (AGE). Reducing sugars like glucose can react non-enzymatically at their carbonyl ends with the amino groups of proteins to form reversible Schiff bases and then Amadori compounds. Hemoglobin A_{1C}, a widely used index for monitoring blood glucose control, is an example of an Amadori compound. These early glycation products undergo further chemical reactions to become irreversibly cross-linked derivatives termed AGE. This reaction was first described by Maillard[2] in 1912, and is now known to proceed within our bodies during aging and to proceed at an extremely accelerated rate in diabetes.[3]

FIGURE 1 summarizes our hypothesis[4,5] that has been drawn mainly from experiments with microvascular endothelial cells, retinal pericytes, and renal mesangial cells in culture. AGE formed under hyperglycemic conditions could act on pericytes through

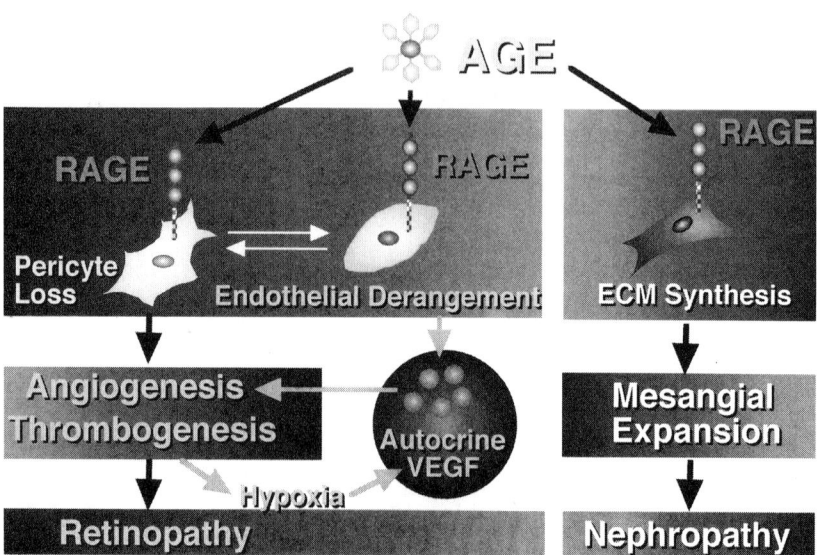

FIGURE 1. Possible roles of the AGE-RAGE system in the development of diabetic microangiopathy.[4,5]

interactions with the cell surface receptor for AGE (RAGE), to cause pericyte loss, which would in turn relieve the restriction of endothelial cell (EC) growth on one hand and reduce the ability of EC to produce prostacyclin on the other, thereby leading to angiogenesis and thrombogenesis. AGE-RAGE system would also take an active part in mesangial expansion through an induction of extracellular matrix synthesis by mesangial cells, the pericyte equivalent in renal glomeruli. On the other hand, AGE could directly act on EC through RAGE to cause angiogenesis and thrombogenesis. These events would lead to the development and exacerbation of diabetic microangiopathies.

AGE EFFECTS ON PERICYTES

We prepared AGE–bovine serum albumin (BSA) by incubating BSA with high concentrations of glucose and the administering it to cultured bovine retinal pericytes. When exposed to AGE-BSA, the growth curve of pericytes was shifted downward in a dose-dependent manner.[6] AGE also exhibited an acute toxicity to pericytes when assayed by the release of radioactivity from [^{3}H]2-deoxyglucose–labeled cells.

RECEPTOR FOR AGE

A variety of cells are known to express RAGE. It was initially isolated from bovine lung by the Stern and colleagues[7] at Columbia University in 1992. RAGE gene is expressed in pericytes as in EC.[6]

We conducted a confocal laser microscopic analysis in which pericytes were double-stained for AGE and for RAGE (FIG. 2). The antibody employed for AGE stain was labeled with Texas red, which on excitation yielded red fluorescence. RAGE immune complex was visualized with FITC, which looked green. When cells underwent tomography at 0.25-μm resolution, both red and green signals were marked in the cytoplasm. When one image was imposed on the other, the two fluorescent patterns mostly overlapped. This indicates that after the recognition by RAGE, AGE ligands could be internalized together with their receptors.

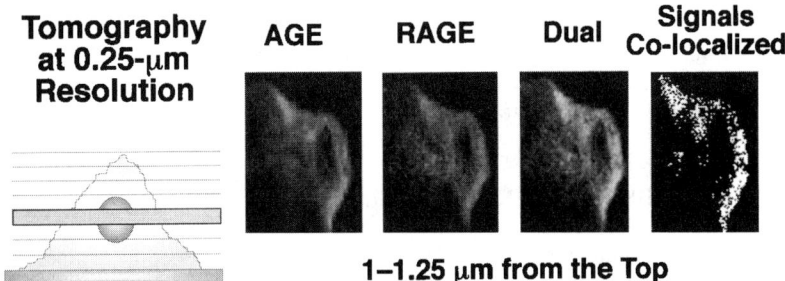

FIGURE 2. Confocal laser microscopic analysis of pericytes exposed to AGE.

RAGE ANTISENSE

Next, we employed an antisense strategy to ascertain the functional role of RAGE. A septadecamer oligodeoxyribonucleotide complement of the 5' region of RAGE mRNA was synthesized by phosphorothioate chemistry.[6,8] In the presence of the antisense, AGE-induced decrease in pericyte number was found to be protected against, while sense control effected no change.[6] This suggests that AGE action on pericytes is mediated by ligand-receptor interactions.

AGE EFFECTS ON ENDOTHELIAL CELLS

Contrasting with the case of pericytes, AGE supershifted the growth curve upward in a dose-dependent manner.[5,9] AGE also induced endothelial cell synthesis of DNA, and this was abolished not only by anti–AGE-BSA antibodies but also by antibodies against glycated RNase, suggesting that structures common to these AGE preparations are responsible for the growth promotion.[5] Control non-glycated BSA showed no stimulation. The results thus indicate that AGE are potentially angiogenic.

AGE were also found to inhibit prostacyclin-producing ability of EC.[9,10] The dosage giving the maximal inhibition was the same that most stimulated EC growth. Further, AGE increased the levels of mRNA coding for plasminogen activator inhibitor-1 (PAI-1) and of its protein product, and as well biologically assessed anti-fibrinolytic activity.[10] Accordingly, AGE are thrombogenic in two meanings. One is to decrease anti-thrombogenic activity, and the other to stabilize preformed fibrin clots.

Further, the AGE stimulation of EC DNA synthesis, the inhibition of prostacyclin synthesis, and the increase in immunoreactive PAI-1 were all abolished by RAGE antisense.[9,10] This is a confirmation by Western blotting that the antisense efficiently blocked translation of RAGE message.[10] The results thus indicate that the AGE actions on EC are also RAGE-mediated.

AGE-DRIVEN ANGIOGENESIS IS VEGF-MEDIATED

We have evidence that AGE-driven angiogenesis is mediated by autocrine VEGF[11] generated in EC themselves. First, AGE increased the level of mRNA coding for $VEGF_{121}$ and $VEGF_{165}$, the secretory forms of this growth factor, as well as their *de novo* synthesis in EC.[5] Second, a monoclonal anti-VEGF antibody could effectively neutralize the AGE-induced DNA synthesis in EC.[5] The antibody itself had no effect, indicating that this is not due to non-specific, toxic effects. Third, AGE doubled the total length of the endothelial tubes formed on Matri-gel, and the antibody against VEGF fully neutralized this induction.[5]

ROLE OF AGE-RAGE IN MESANGIAL EXPANSION

Doi and colleagues[12] at Kyoto University Hospital developed a hammerhead-type ribozyme against RAGE mRNA. The construct has catalytic RNA complement of RAGE message in the anti-codon region of transfer RNA. Flanking this segment are two *cis*-acting ribozymes to liberate the *trans*-acting one. This would ensure the secondary RNA structure essential for catalytic activity and efficient proximation of the RAGE ribozyme to the target in the cytoplasm. As a control, the same vector was used except for carrying anti-HIV ribozyme in place of the RAGE ribozyme. These expression vectors were introduced into rat mesangial cells. RAGE ribozyme–transfected cells expressed the ribozyme RNA and little RAGE mRNA. Those cells were also lightly stained for RAGE proteins. This indicates that the ribozyme works well, cleaving its expected target in cells where it is expressed.

When exposed to AGE, mesangial cell levels of mRNA coding for type-IV collagen increase. However, this was prevented in cells that carried the RAGE ribozyme. The results suggest that the AGE induction of collagen gene expression in mesangial cells is dependent on RAGE.

IN VIVO EVALUATION OF THE ROLES OF AGE-RAGE SYSTEM

OLETF Rats

Otsuka Long Evans Tokushima Fatty (OLETF) rats have been known as a good animal model for non-insulin-dependent diabetes mellitus. They are obese and hyperglycemic, and develop states that resemble human diabetic complications. Until recently, it has been thought that OLETF rats could not have retinopathy. However, the group at the Department of Ophthalmology, Kanazawa University,[13] demonstrated that this animal model does show a sign of diabetic retinopathy: that is, a delay in oscillatory potentials in the electroretinogram (ERG). This change in ERG has been established by this ophthalmology team as the earliest ocular sign detected in human diabetic patients.

When the light-evoked potentials were recorded in the eyes of OLETF rats, the peaks of oscillatory potentials were consistently delayed, compared with those in the control, non-diabetic rats, which have the identical genetic background. As OLETF rats aged, the level of circulating AGE increased gradually, and the latency of the oscillatory peak was correlated with that increase.[13] AGE level was also correlated with retinal contents of VEGF message.[13]

RAGE Transgenic Mice

In addition, transgenic mouse lines are now established that overexpress RAGE gene.[14] The transgene carries human RAGE genomic DNA linked to murine *flk-1* promoter (FIG. 3). This promoter is known to work strongly and specifically in vascular cells. Southern blot showed the presence of the RAGE transgene in the genome of each transgenic line. RT-PCR analysis with primers and a probe specific to human RAGE showed active transcription of the transgene. On Western blot, about a twofold increase in RAGE proteins was detected in tissues of the RAGE transgenic mice.

To stably induce diabetes in these transgenic lines, we employed a genetic approach. That is, RAGE transgenic mice were cross-bred with another transgenic line carrying human cDNA for inducible nitric oxide synthase (iNOS) under the control of insulin promoter. This line has been established in 1998 by Okamoto and colleagues at Tohoku University and develops insulin-dependent diabetes mellitus (ID-

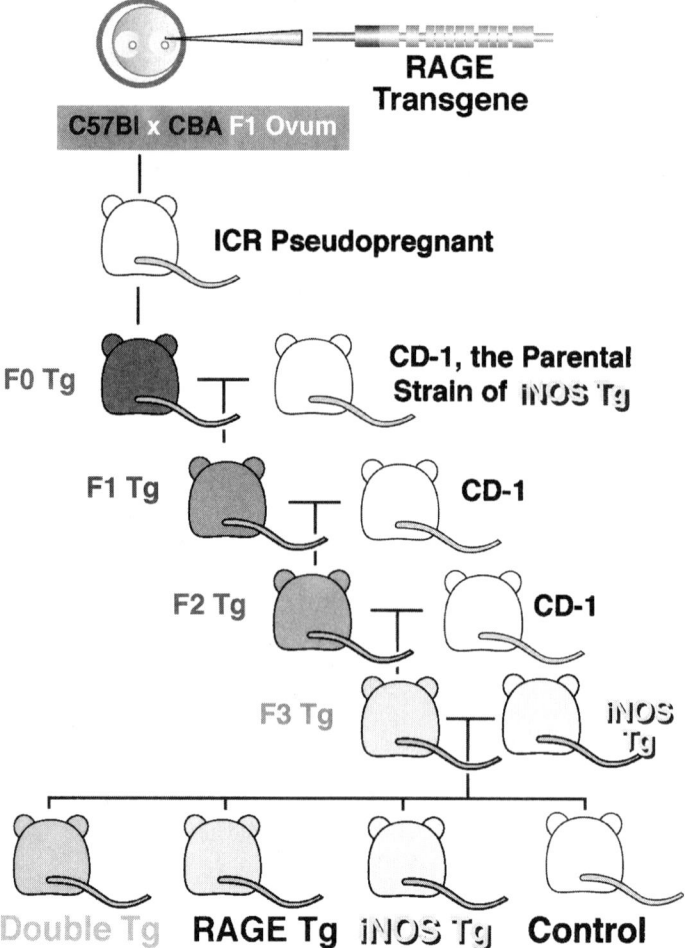

FIGURE 3. Cross-breeding of RAGE transgenic mice with genetically IDDM-prone iNOS transgenic mice.

DM) early after birth due to selective destruction of pancreatic β cells.[15] Because different parental strains were employed to produce the two transgenic animals, descendants from RAGE transgenic mice were successively mated with iNOS transgenic mice to unify the genetic background without influencing the susceptibility to IDDM[14] (FIG. 3). The resultant four groups of littermates, namely RAGE transgenic, iNOS transgenic, the double transgenic, and the non-transgenic, were used for analyses at F4.

As expected, RAGE transgenic and RAGE-iNOS double transgenic animals exhibited hyperglycemia, a high percent of hemoglobin A_{1C}, and elevated plasma AGE. One of the most striking findings was extraordinarily heavy kidneys in double transgenic mice. Histopathologic examinations of the kidneys revealed glomerulosclerotic changes with deposition of PAS-positive materials in the mesangial area in animals carrying the iNOS transgene alone and in those carrying the two transgenes. And, higher degrees of glomerular enlargement and glomerulosclerosis were noted more in the double transgenic than in the IDDM model animal without the RAGE transgene. Quantitative morphometry of more than 50 visual fields revealed the largest glomerular volume and the highest sclerosis index in RAGE-iNOS double transgenic mice. Albuminuria was also most prominent in the double transgenic. Further, the mesangial areas of the double transgenic animals were more heavily stained for type I collagen than those of the animals carrying the iNOS transgene alone.

Thus, it was concluded that renal vascular changes were augmented in RAGE transgenic animals when they became diabetic. And, because the AGE levels were almost invariant between the double transgenic and iNOS transgenic, the expression of RAGE gene would seem to be rate-limiting in the exacerbation of diabetic nephropathy. Whether the predisposition to retinopathy is augmented by RAGE overexpression remains to be determined.

CONCLUSION

Experiments with pericytes, EC, and mesangial cells in culture led to changes characteristic of diabetic microangiopathies that are at least in part accounted for by the AGE-RAGE system. The data obtained with animal models would seem to support this concept.

ACKNOWLEDGMENTS

We thank Shin-ichi Matsudaira, Reiko Kitamura, Tomoko Yachi, and Yuya Shichinohe for assistance; Fumiyoshi Ishidate for confocal laser microscopic analysis, and Hidenori Maeda and Kanako Kuwajima for illustrations.

REFERENCES

1. YAMAGISHI, S., K. KOBAYASHI & H. YAMAMOTO. 1993. Vascular pericytes not only regulate growth, but also preserve prostacyclin-producing ability and protect against lipid peroxide-induced injury of co-cultured endothelial cells. Biochem. Biophys. Res. Commun. **190:** 418–425.
2. MAILLARD L.C. 1912. Action des acides amines sur les sucres; formation des melanoidines par voie methodique. CR Acad. Sci. **154:** 66–68.
3. BROWNLEE, M., A. CERAMI & H. VLASSARA. 1988. Advanced glycosylation end products in tissue and the biochemical basis of diabetic complications. N. Engl. J. Med. **318:** 1315–1321.
4. YAMAGISHI, S., H. YONEKURA, Y. YAMAMOTO, H. FUJIMORI & H. YAMAMOTO. 1998. AGE and endothelial cells. J. Atheroscler. Thromb. **4:** 141–143.
5. YAMAGISHI, S., H. YONEKURA, Y. YAMAMOTO, K. KATSUNO, F. SATO, I. MITA, H. OOKA, N. SATOZAWA, T. KAWAKAMI, M. NOMURA & H. YAMAMOTO. 1997. Advanced glycation endproducts-driven angiogenesis in vitro: Induction of the growth and tube formation of human microvascular endothelial cells through autocrine vascular endothelial growth factor. J. Biol. Chem. **272:** 8723–8730.

6. YAMAGISHI, S., C.-C. HSU, M. TANIGUCHI, S. HARADA, K. OHSAWA, K. KOBAYASHI & H. YAMAMOTO. 1995. Receptor-mediated toxicity to pericytes of advanced glycosylation end products: A possible mechanism of pericyte loss in diabetic microangiopathy. Biochem. Biophys. Res. Commun. **213:** 681–687.
7. NEEPER, M., A.M. SCHMIDT, J. BRETT, S.D. YAN, F. WANG, Y-C.E. PNA, K. ELLISTON, D. STERN & A. SHAW. 1992. Cloning and expression of a cell surface receptor for advanced glycosylation end products of proteins. J. Biol. Chem. **267:** 14998–15004.
8. YAMAMOTO, Y., S. YAMAGISHI, C.-C. HSU & H. YAMAMOTO. 1996. Advanced glycation endproducts-receptor interactions stimulate the growth of human pancreatic cancer cells through the induction of platelet-derived growth factor-B. Biochem. Biophys. Res. Commun. **222:** 700–703.
9. YAMAGISHI, S., Y. YAMAMOTO, S. HARADA, C.-C. HSU, C.-C. & H. YAMAMOTO. 1996. Advanced glycosylation end products stimulate the growth but inhibit the prostacyclin-producing ability of endothelial cells through interactions with their receptors. FEBS Lett. **384:** 103–106.
10. YAMAGISHI, S., H. FUJIMORI, H. YONEKURA, Y. YAMAMOTO & H. YAMAMOTO. 1998. Advanced glycation endproducts inhibit prostacyclin production and induce plasminogen activator inhibitor-1 in human microvascular endothelial cells. Diabetologia **41:** 1435–1441.
11. NOMURA, M., S. YAMAGISHI, S. HARADA, Y. HAYASHI, T. YAMASHIMA, J. YAMASHITA & H. YAMAMOTO. 1995. Possible participation of autocrine and paracrine vascular endothelial growth factors in hypoxia-induced proliferation of endothelial cells and pericytes. J. Biol. Chem. **270:** 28316–28324.
12. TSUJI, H., N. IEHARA, T. MASEGI, M. IMURA, J. OHKAWA, H. ARAI, K. ISHII, T. KITA & T. DOI. 1998. Ribozyme targetting of receptor for advanced glycation end products in mesangial cells. Biochem. Biophys. Res. Commun. **245:** 583–588.
13. SEGAWA, Y., Y. SHIRAO, S. YAMAGISHI, T. HIGASHIDA, M. KOBAYASHI, K. KATSUNO, A. IYOBE, H. HARADA, F. SATO, H. MIYATA, H. ASAI, A. NISHIMURA, M. TAKAHIRA, T. SOUNO, Y. SEGAWA, K. MAEDA, K. SHIMA, A. MIZUNO, H. YAMAMOTO & K. KAWASAKI. 1998. Upregulation of retinal vascular endothelial growth factor mRNAs in spontaneously diabetic rats without ophthalmoscopic retinopathy. Ophthalmic Res. **30:** 333–339.
14. YAMAMOTO, Y. *et al.* In preparation.
15. TAKAMURA, T., I. KATO, N. KIMURA, T. NAKAZAWA, H. YONEKURA, S. TAKASAWA & H. OKAMOTO. 1998. Transgenic mice overexpressing type 2 nitric-oxide synthase in pancreatic β cells develop insulin-dependent diabetes without insulitis. **273:** 2493–2496.

Questions and Answers

H. HAKAMATA (*University of California, San Francisco, CA, USA*): AGE concentrations added to the medium of the endothelial cells and the pericytes were very different. How do you explain the *in vivo* situation?

YAMAMOTO: The dosage that caused maximum effect on endothelial cells was 50 µg/ml, on the other hand, the dosage that gave maximum effect on the pericytes was 2 mg/ml. Concerning the former, 50 µg/ml AGE is within the range reported in plasma of diabetic patients. So, in the case with endothelial cell dosage, that seems reasonable. The dosage that gave an effect in pericytes looks high, but it may be possible in tissues. Concerning the retinal environment in the diabetic state, a breakdown of the blood-retinal barrier has been reported.

HAKAMATA: What is the intracellular signal mediated by RAGE which may mediate cell death or cell growth? What is different?

YAMAMOTO: Nobody knows the second message after the receptor event. However, available evidence suggests that some oxidative stress in the cells may mediate the ligand-receptor interaction. However, obviously the consequence was quite different between endothelial cells and pericytes. Certainly the intracellular signaling event may differ in the two cell types. To resolve this important issue, the second message should be identified in each cell type.

A.R. TALL (*Columbia University, New York, NY, USA*): The transgenic overexpression of RAGE seems to result in expression in a number of tissues including the lung, depending on the vascularity, I guess. What is the level of expression of RAGE in comparison with the amount that would be present normally in endothelium in those tissues?

YAMAMOTO: The absolute value has not been determined. The most abundantly expressing tissue is the lung. When we calculated the relative ratio to recombinant RAGE protein, 1 µg of lung tissue contained several nanograms of RAGE protein. The endothelial cell level was about 25-fold lower than that.

TALL: The pathology that appears is primarily in the kidney. Is it possible that what you are looking at is actually substantial overexpression and you are getting soluble RAGE released into the bloodstream, which is then binding AGEs and forming some type of complex that is deposited in the kidney—rather than a cellular activation mechanism?

YAMAMOTO: It is possible. That has already been studied by Dr. Schmidt at your university. She administered soluble forms of RAGE and found that macroangiopathy of diabetic complication was prevented. But in my laboratory this approach has not been done.

TALL: Do you have soluble RAGE that has been released from the endothelium in circulation in your animals?

YAMAMOTO: We have never observed that vascular cells in culture released soluble RAGE proteins nor have we administered soluble RAGE proteins.

TALL: But *in vivo*, it might be interesting to see if this is happening.

YAMAMOTO: In collaboration with researchers at the Diabetic Center at Tokyo Women's Medical College, we surveyed more than 200 subjects, but none exhibited RAGE in plasma.

M.A. GIMBRONE (*Brigham and Women's Hospital, Boston, MA, USA*): In the natural setting, the advanced glycation endproducts would be occurring on multiple targets, some of which might be in the matrix or basement membrane on which the cells are adherent. You are providing, if I understand it correctly, the AGE-BSA stimulus as a soluble media addition. Have you ever tried to expose the endothelium or the pericytes to a surface that has AGE products absorbed onto it? Does that elicit different results than soluble RAGE?

YAMAMOTO: I did not, but other researchers did. Some similar results were obtained with soluble and fixed AGE, but among laboratories that employed either soluble or fixed AGE different results have been reported. Among those observations, what I think is very important, monocytes could adhere to fixed collagen matrix. This may be an additional aspect to the initiation of atherosclerosis. That observation was made by Professor Horiuchi.

S. HORIUCHI (*Kumamoto University, Kumamoto, Japan*): This RAGE receptor seems to be different from the endocytic receptor. You showed that ligand bound to

RAGE goes into the cytoplasm. This is something new. By what mechanism does ligand-bound RAGE go into the cell, particularly the cytoplasm?

YAMAMOTO: We have no clear answer at the moment, but confocal laser microscopic analysis data suggest that both receptor and ligand are internalized. It looks like an endocytosis mechanism.

HORIUCHI: In your elegant transgenic animal model, your RAGE transgenic mice and double transgenic mice had quite different kidney lesions. Doesn't that mean that transgenic mice have also expressed RAGE in that lesion? Is there any difference compared to the wild type?

YAMAMOTO: We have data. Using immunofluorescence histology, stronger fluorescence was marked in both endothelial cell pattern and mesangial pattern, but I did not show those data today.

HORIUCHI: Is the level of RAGE expression in your mice very high or not?

YAMAMOTO: That is not clear. The message level was very high beyond our expectation, but the level of protein product was only twofold higher than control. So some limiting factor may have worked in our experiments.

HORIUCHI: Because your transgene is human, you may be able to differentiate between the human RAGE and the endogenous mouse RAGE.

YAMAMOTO: The antibody employed for western blotting and for immunocytochemistry was raised against human recombinant RAGE, but it also recognizes mouse endogenous protein. The sizes of both human and murine proteins are invariant. We are now developing human-specific anti-RAGE antibodies.

Characterization of Atherosclerotic Plaques by Magnetic Resonance Imaging

ZAHI A. FAYAD [a–c] AND VALENTIN FUSTER [a]

[a]*The Zena and Michael A. Wiener Cardiovascular Institute*
[b]*Department of Radiology, Mount Sinai School of Medicine,
New York, New York 10029, USA*

ABSTRACT: The study of atherosclerotic disease during its natural history and after therapeutic intervention will enhance our understanding of the progression and regression of this disease and will aid in selecting the appropriate medical treatments or surgical interventions. Several invasive and noninvasive imaging techniques are available to assess atherosclerotic vessels. Most of these techniques are strong in identifying the morphological features of the disease, such as lumenal diameter and stenosis or wall thickness, and in some cases provide an assessment of the relative risk associated with the atherosclerosis. However, none of these techniques can fully characterize the composition of the atherosclerotic plaque in the vessel wall and, therefore, are incapable of identifying the vulnerable plaques. High-resolution, multi-contrast, magnetic resonance (MR) can non-invasively image vulnerable plaques, characterize plaques in terms of lipid and fibrous content, and identify the presence of thrombus or calcium. Application of MR imaging opens up whole new areas for diagnosis, prevention, and treatment (e.g., lipid-lowering drug regimens) of atherosclerosis.

ATHEROSCLEROTIC PLAQUES

Atherosclerosis, the leading cause of mortality and morbidity in Western societies, is a disease of the vessel wall that occurs in the carotid arteries, aorta, coronary arteries, and other peripheral arteries. Some of the consequences of this disease are thrombotic myocardial infarction, thromboembolic cerebral infarction, and aortic aneurysms.[1,2] The study of atherosclerotic disease during its progression and after therapeutic intervention will enhance our understanding of the natural history of this disease and will aid in selecting the appropriate medical treatments or surgical interventions.

According to the criteria of the American Heart Association Committee on Vascular Lesions, plaque progression can be subdivided into the five phases and different lesion types shown in FIGURE 1.[1,3–5] The "vulnerable" type IV and type Va lesions (phase 2) and the "complicated" type VI lesion (phase 4) are the most relevant to acute ischemic events. Type IV and type Va lesions, although not necessarily stenotic at angiography, may be prone to disruption because of their softness due to a high lipid content, thin fibrous cap, and macrophage-dependent chemical properties.[6] Type IV lesions consist of confluent cellular lesions with a great deal of extra-

---

[c]Address for correspondence: Zahi A. Fayad, Ph.D., Mount Sinai School of Medicine, Box 1234, New York, NY 10029. Voice: 212-241-6858; fax: 212-987-7462.
fayadz01@doc.mssm.edu

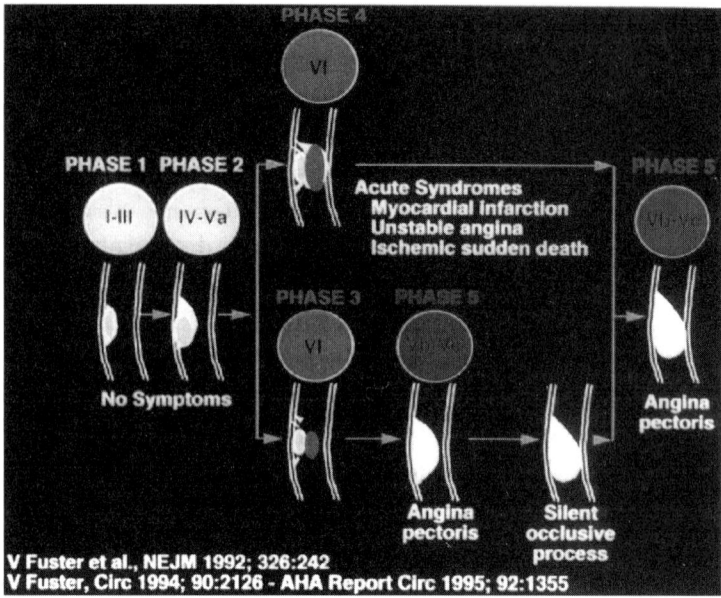

FIGURE 1. Phases and lesion morphology of progression of coronary atherosclerosis according to gross pathological and clinical findings. (Modified with permission from Fuster.[3])

cellular lipid intermixed with fibrous tissue covered by a fibrous cap, whereas type Va lesions possess a predominant extracellular lipid core also covered by a thin fibrous cap. Disruption of a type IV or type Va lesion leads to the formation of a thrombus or "complicated" type VI lesion. The lipid core is highly thrombogenic due to the tissue factor produced by macrophages.[7] The acute type VI lesion that results in an acute ischemic event, rather than being characterized by a small mural thrombus, consists of an occlusive thrombus.

MAGNETIC RESONANCE AS A TOOL FOR ATHEROSCLEROTIC PLAQUE CHARACTERIZATION

Several invasive (e.g., x-ray angiography,[8–10] intravascular ultrasound,[11,12] and angioscopy[13,14]) and noninvasive (surface B-mode ultrasound[15–17] and ultrafast computed tomography[18,19]) imaging techniques are available to assess atherosclerotic vessels. Most of these techniques are strong in identifying the morphological features of the disease such as lumenal diameter and stenosis or wall thickness. Some of the techniques provide an assessment of the relative risk associated with the atherosclerotic disease. However, none of these imaging methods can characterize the composition of an atherosclerotic plaque and, therefore, are incapable of identifying vulnerable plaques.

High-resolution magnetic resonance (MR) has emerged as the leading imaging modality for atherosclerotic plaque characterization. MR is a non-invasive, nondestructive imaging technique with excellent soft-tissue contrast that differentiates plaques components on the basis of biophysical and biochemical parameters (such as chemical composition and concentration, water content, physical state, molecular motion, or diffusion).

MAGNETIC RESONANCE STUDIES OF *EX VIVO* PLAQUES

Early work on applying MR techniques to the characterization of plaque focused on lipid assessment with nuclear magnetic resonance spectroscopy and chemical-shift imaging.[20–27] Unfortunately, the concentration of the lipid present in the plaque is very low in comparison with water and these techniques suffer from poor signal-to-noise.[21,24,28] Therefore, it has been difficult to extend these techniques to an *in vivo* setting. Current studies are focused on MR imaging of water protons.

Following an *ex vivo* MR imaging study of iliac artery specimens by Kaufman and colleagues,[29] Herfkens and colleagues[30] performed the first *in vivo* patient imaging study of aortic atherosclerosis. Only the anatomic or morphological features of the atherosclerotic lesions (such as wall thickening) and luminal narrowing were assessed.

MULTI-CONTRAST MAGNETIC RESONANCE PLAQUE IMAGING

With improvements of the MR techniques, high resolution and contrast imaging became possible and therefore allowed the study of the different plaque components using multi-contrast MR, generated by T1, T2, and proton-density weighting (PDW).[28,31–38]

Multiple studies have been previously performed to validate the MR assessment of different plaque components. In a recent study, we have analyzed 22 human carotid endarterectomy specimens with *ex vivo* MR and histopathological specimens.[39] Sixty-six cross-sections were matched between the multi-contrast MR images (partial T1-, T1-, heavily T1-, partial T2-, T2-, PDW-, and diffusion-weighted imaging) and histopathology. In each cross-section, the presence or absence of plaque components was prospectively identified on the MR images. The overall sensitivity and specificity for each component were very high. Calcification, fibrocellular tissue, lipid core, and thrombus were readily identified. Diffusion imaging, which probes

TABLE 1. Plaque characterization with magnetic resonance

	MR signal intensity		
	T1W	PDW	T2W
Ca^{2+}	– –	– –	– –
Lipid	+	+	–
Fibrocellular	+ +	+ +	+ +
Thrombus[a,b]	+ +	+	+/–

[a]Surface irregularities.
[b]Signal intensity less than fibrocellular.

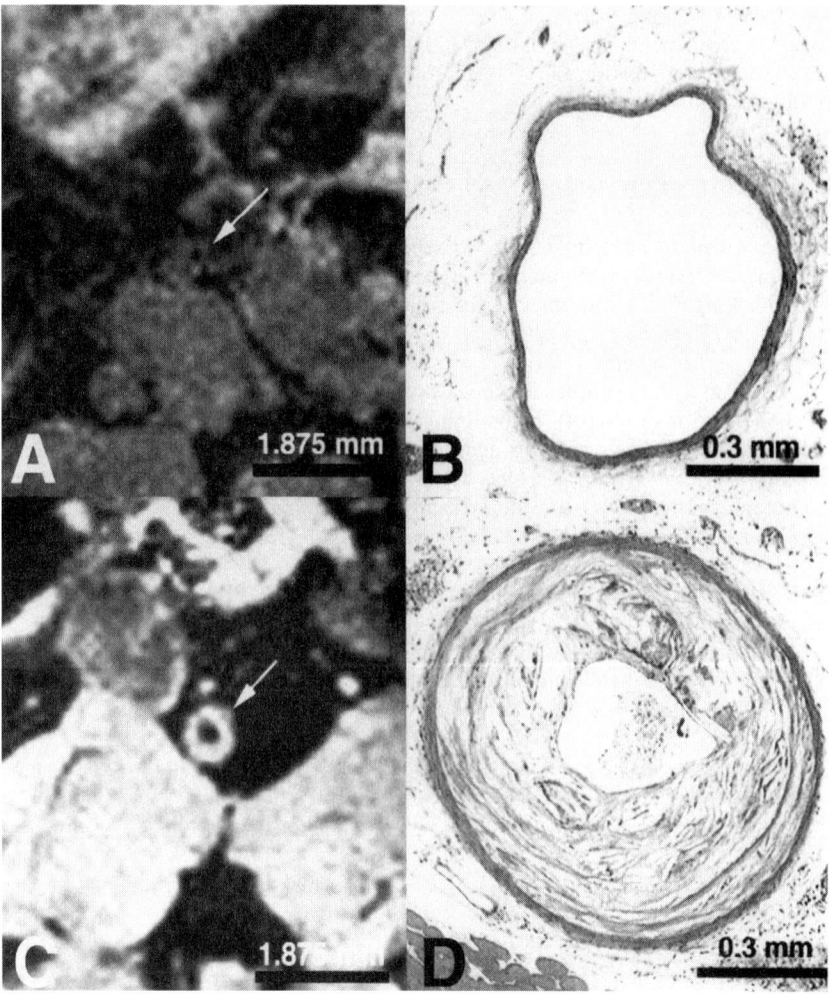

FIGURE 2. Magnetic resonance (MR) image (proton density-weighted) of the abdominal aorta (*arrow*) in a normal mouse and in an apolipoprotein E-knockout mouse (apoE-KO) showing differences between normal and atherosclerotic arteries. On all MR images the lumen is dark. The normal abdominal aorta wall thickness is approximately 50 μm and was not clearly visible at a spatial in-plane resolution of 97 μm. Wild-type mice were free of atherosclerotic lesions as shown on the MR images in **A** (magnified, see scale) and histopathology (**B**), as shown by the hematoxylin and eosin stain (original magnification ×40). A large atherosclerotic lesion (*arrow*) that encircles the abdominal aorta of a 12-month-old apoE-KO mouse is shown on the MR images in **C** (magnified). These findings correlated with histopathology as shown in **D** [hematoxylin and eosin stain (original magnification ×40)]. All the MR images have a pixel size of $97 \times 97 \times 500$ μm^3. The left kidney and spinal cord are used as anatomical landmarks to facilitate the comparison between MR images and histological sections. (Adapted from Fayad *et al.*[44])

the motion of the water molecules, was found to be useful for thrombus detection as also demonstrated by Toussaint and colleagues.[40]

Atherosclerotic plaque characterization by MR is based on the signal intensities (TABLE 1) and morphological appearance of the plaque on T1W, PDW, and T2W images as previously validated.[31,36,39] Lipid components are defined as hyperintense regions within the plaque on both T1W and PDW images, and hypointense on T2W images. Fibrocellular components are defined as hyperintense regions of the plaque on T1W, PDW, and T2W images. Calcium deposits are defined as hypointense regions within the plaque on T1W,[41,42] PDW, and T2W images.[36] Thrombotic plaques have marked irregularities on the luminal surface and are considered as hyperintense (less than most fibrocellular components) regions within the plaque on T1W, PDW, and T2W images. We note that perivascular fat, mainly composed of triglycerides, has a different appearance on MR than atherosclerotic plaque lipids. The plaque lipids consist primarily of unesterified cholesterol and cholesteryl esters.[28,43]

MAGNETIC RESONANCE STUDIES OF PLAQUES IN ANIMALS

Skinner and colleagues reported that *in vivo* MR plaque characterization is useful for studying the progression of experimental atherosclerosis in hypercholesterolemic rabbits and for imaging the plaque components (such as fibrous caps, necrotic cores, and intraplaque hemorrhage).[38] Since the pathogenesis of atherosclerosis is currently being investigated in genetically engineered small animals, we developed a noninvasive MR microscopy technique to study *in vivo* atherosclerotic lesions (without knowl-

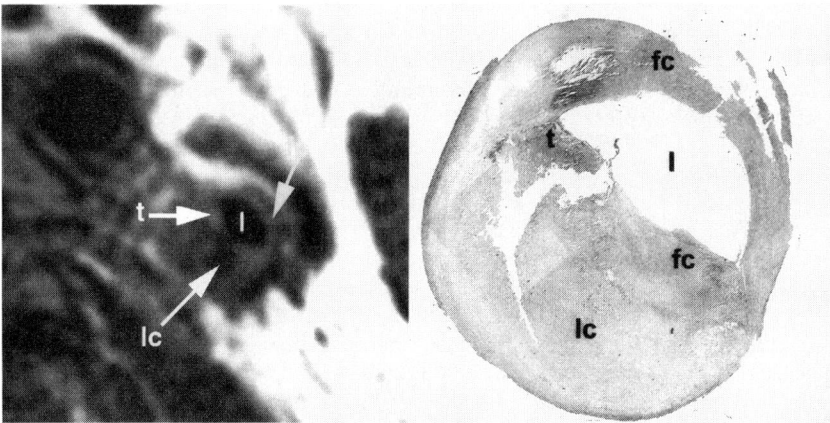

FIGURE 3. *In vivo* T2-weighted (T2W) of the left internal carotid artery. Plaque characterization was based on the information obtained from T1-, proton-density-, and T2-weighted MR images. The images were correlated with histopathology (combined mason & eosin stain). The lipid core (lc) is shown as dark on the T2W images. The fibrous cap (fc) is bright on the T2W images. Thrombus is detected as very bright signal intensity on the T2W images. (l) arterial lumen. The MR images are 3 mm thick, with an in-plane resolution of 450 μm.

edge of the lesion location or lesion type) in live apolipoprotein E knockout (apoE-KO) mice.[44] The spatial resolution was 0.0012–0.005 mm^3. The lumen and wall of the abdominal aorta and iliac arteries were identified on all images in apoE-KO ($N = 8$) and in wild-type mice ($N = 5$) on chow diet. Images obtained with MR were compared with corresponding cross-sectional histopathology ($N = 58$). MR accurately determined wall area in comparison to histopathology (slope = 1.0, r = 0.86). In addition, atherosclerotic lesions were characterized in terms of lesion shape and type. Lesion type was graded by MR according to morphological appearance/severity and by histopathology according to the American Heart Association classification (FIG. 2). There was excellent agreement between MR and histopathology in grading of lesion shape and type (slope = 0.97, r = 0.91 for lesion shape; slope = 0.64, r = 0.90 for lesion type). The combination of high-resolution MR microscopy and genetically engineered animals is a powerful tool to investigate serially and noninvasively the progression and regression of atherosclerotic lesions in an intact animal model and should greatly enhance basic studies of atherosclerotic disease.

MAGNETIC RESONANCE STUDIES OF HUMAN CAROTID ARTERY PLAQUES *IN VIVO*

A study performed in patients with advanced carotid atherosclerosis who were referred for endarterectomy, showed that MR allows the *in vivo* discrimination of lipid cores, fibrous caps, calcification, normal media, adventia, intraplaque hemorrhage, and acute thrombosis.[36] The relaxation constant T2 of various plaque components *in vivo* calculated before endarterectomy correlated closely with values obtained *in vitro* after surgery. An *in vivo* MR image before endarterectomy and histopathology after endarterectomy from a patient with a severe plaque in the left internal carotid artery is shown in FIGURE 3. Improvements in spatial resolution have been possible with the design of new phased-array coils[45] tailored for carotid imaging[46] and new imaging sequences, such as long echo train fast spin echo imaging with "velocity-selective" flow suppression (FIG. 4).[47,48]

IN VIVO HUMAN AORTIC PLAQUES MAGNETIC RESONANCE STUDIES

We have extended the *in vivo* MR atherosclerotic plaque characterization to the aorta.[47,49] The principal challenges associated with MR imaging of thoracic aorta are obtaining sufficient sensitivity for sub-millimeter imaging and exclusion of artifacts due to respiratory motion and blood flow. This study presents the use of a novel combination of fast MR imaging methods, which allow imaging of the thoracic aortic wall for the assessment of atherosclerotic plaque size, extent, and composition. Imaging was performed using a clinical MR system in 10 patients with aortic plaques identified by transesophageal echocardiography (TEE). Plaque composition and size were assessed from T1-, proton density-, and T2-weighted images. Matched MR and TEE cross-sectional aortic images were compared. MR examinations resulted in excellent, artifact-free images from all 10 patients. Comparison of MR and TEE images showed a strong correlation for plaque composition ($\chi^2 = 36.68$ and

$p = 0.0023$; $N = 25$) and mean maximum plaque thickness [(4.56 ± 0.21 mm measured by MR and 4.62 ± 0.31 mm by TEE) (r = 0.88, $N = 25$)]. A typical image of the descending thoracic aorta in a normal subject is shown in FIGURE 5. MR and TEE images from a patient with a lipid-rich (type Va) aortic plaque in the descending thoracic aorta is shown in FIGURE 6. Another patient with both a lipid-rich plaque (type Va) and a more stable fibrotic plaque (type Vc) is seen in FIGURE 7. Note the increased wall thickening of the descending thoracic aorta in the patients (FIGS. 6 and 7) compared to the normal subject (FIG. 5).

IN VIVO STUDIES OF HUMAN CORONARY ARTERY PLAQUES

The ultimate goal is the imaging of plaque *in vivo* in coronary arteries. Preliminary studies in a pig model of atherosclerosis showed that the difficulties of coronary wall imaging are due to the combination of cardiac and respiratory motion artifacts, the non-linear course of the coronary arteries, and the relatively small size as well as location of the coronary arteries.[50,51] For that purpose, we have developed a new method for high-resolution MR imaging of atherosclerotic plaque in the walls of human epicardial coronary arteries. A fast double inversion recovery fast spin echo sequence was developed on a 1.5T MR system.[52] The features of this sequence are short radiofrequency pulses, long echo train imaging, nonselective and selective inversion pulses that maximized the flow suppression due to outflow and minimized artifacts due to vessel motion, and flexible contrast capabilities (proton density- and T2-weighting). The achievable in-plane spatial resolution was 0.5–0.78 mm and the

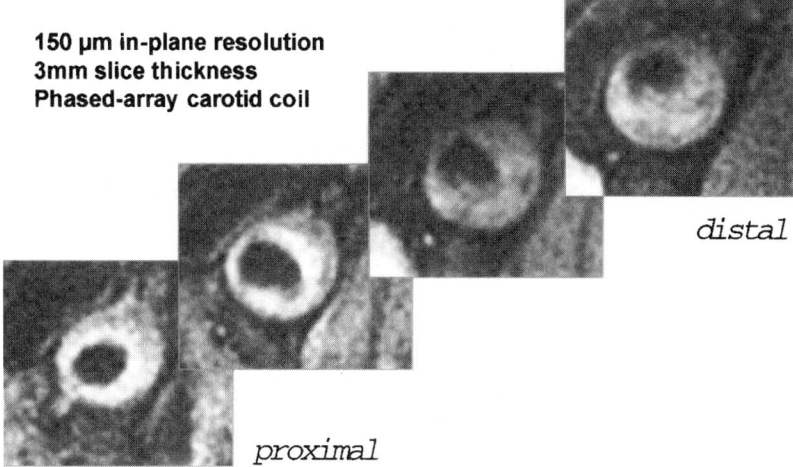

FIGURE 4. High-resolution MR *in vivo* T2-weighted image of a patient with severe carotid atherosclerotic plaques using a specially designed phased-array carotid coil. The MR images of right internal carotid plaques are 3 mm thick, with an in-plane resolution of 150 μm, and are obtained using long echo train fast spin echo imaging with "velocity-selective" flow suppression.

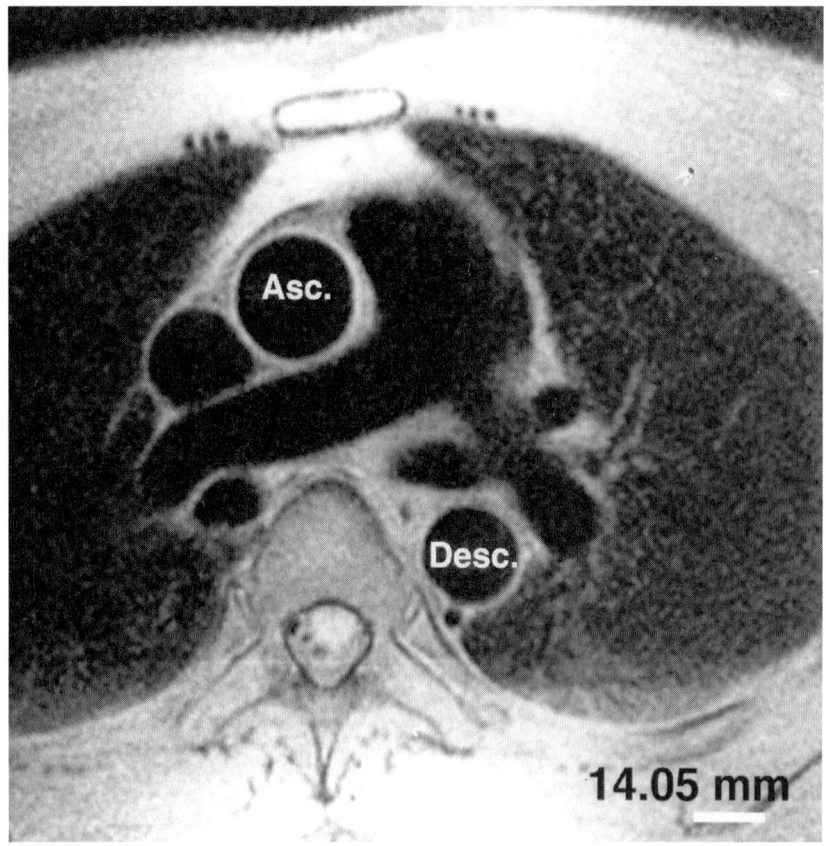

FIGURE 5. *In vivo* double inversion-recovery, fast spin-echo, proton-density weighted magnetic resonance image from a normal subject. Blood flow is suppressed and therefore the lumen is dark. The aortic wall of the ascending (Asc.) and descending (Desc.) aorta are clearly seen.

slice thickness was 3–5 mm. Transverse images of the lumen and wall of the proximal and distal segments of the right coronary, and the proximal segments of the left anterior descending arteries were obtained in 12 subjects. The images demonstrated excellent flow suppression, high contrast, and low signal-to-noise in the coronary arteries. Images of normal coronary wall showed a uniform hyperintense thin ring. The mean normal coronary wall thickness was 0.75 mm. MR images of plaques in coronary arteries with >40% stenosis by coronary x-ray angiography showed atherosclerotic plaques 3–5 mm in maximal wall thickness. FIGURE 8 shows an *in vivo* MR image of a patient with a plaque in the LAD. In conclusion, this study showed that the wall of human coronaries can be imaged *in vivo* using optimized fast spin echo with flow suppression. We demonstrate for the first time high resolution *in vivo* imaging of human coronary atherosclerotic plaque. Coronary wall characterization by

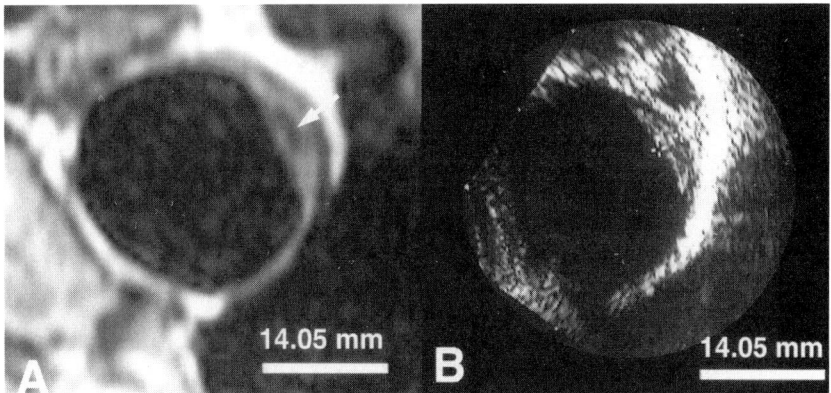

FIGURE 6. *In vivo* magnetic resonance image from a patient with a 4.5 mm thick plaque in the descending thoracic aorta: T2-weighted (**A**) with the corresponding transesophageal echocardiography (TEE) image (**B**). The MR images show an example of an AHA type Va plaque with a dark area in the center (*arrow*) identified on the T2-weighted image as a lipid-rich core (**A**). The lipid-rich core is separated from the lumen by a fibrous cap. Plaque characterization was based on the information obtained from T1-, proton-density-, and T2- weighted MR images. The MR images are 5 mm thick with an in-plane spatial resolution of 800 µm.

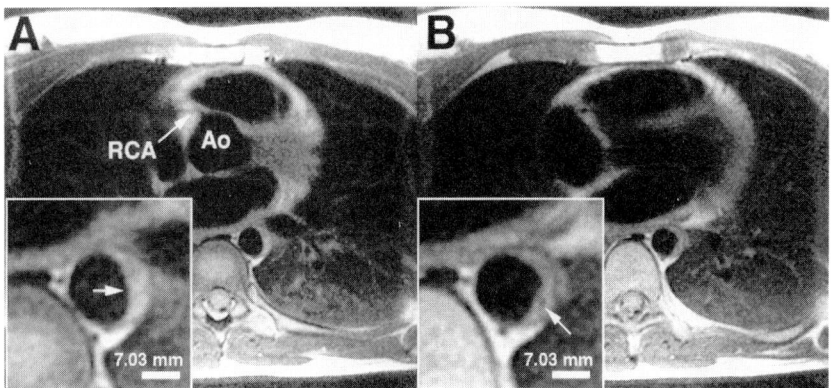

FIGURE 7. T2-weighted magnetic resonance (MR) images from a patient with severe diffuse disease in the descending thoracic aorta. The plaques are different in appearance and characteristics from one location to another. Plaque characterization was based on the information obtained from T1-, proton-density-, and T2-weighted MR images. The inserts in each panel represent magnified views of the descending thoracic aorta. (**A**) Type Vc (fibrocellular) plaque. (**B**) Lipid-rich plaque (type Va). MR images are 5 mm thick and acquired with no interslice gap, and displayed cephalad (**A**) to caudal (**B**). The origin of the right coronary artery (RCA) is clearly seen taking off from the aortic root (Ao).

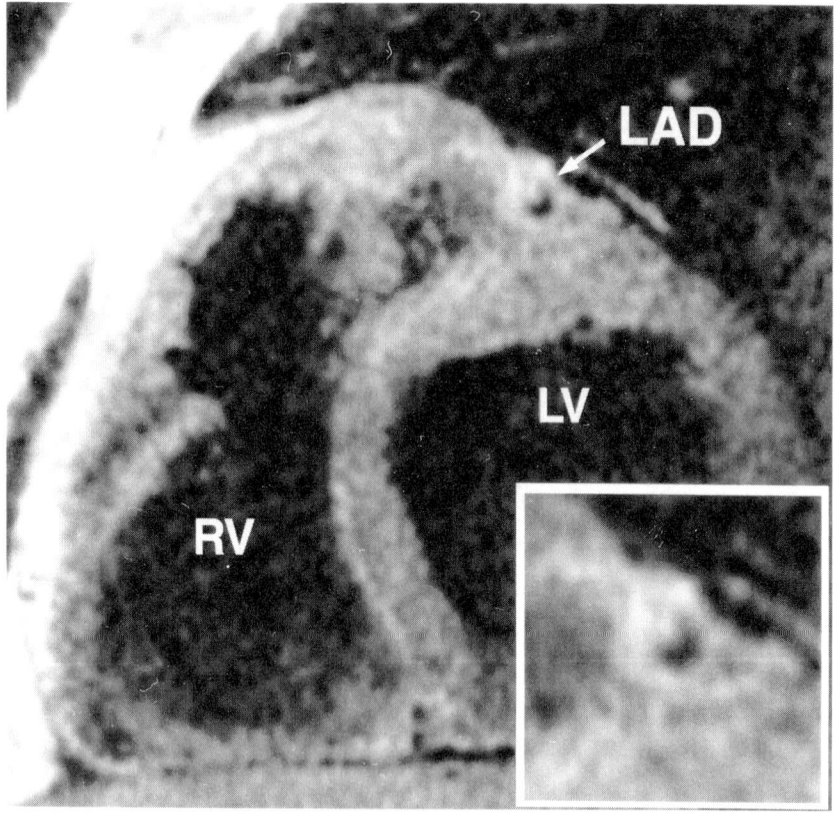

FIGURE 8. *In vivo* MRI cross-sectional image of a patient with a plaque (arrow) in the left anterior descending artery (LAD). The insert represents magnified view of the LAD plaque. The MR images are 3 mm thick with an in-plane spatial resolution of 750 µm, and are acquired during a suspended respiration (<16 sec) using long echo train fast spin echo imaging with "velocity-selective" flow suppression. RV = right ventricle. LV = left ventricle.

MR may be used for the detection of vulnerable coronary plaques that are susceptible to rupture and thrombosis.

CONCLUSIONS

The assessment of atherosclerotic plaques by imaging techniques is essential for the identification of vulnerable plaques. Several invasive and noninvasive imaging techniques are available to assess atherosclerotic disease vessels. Most of these techniques are strong in identifying the morphological features of the disease, such as lumenal diameter and stenosis or wall thickness, and in some cases provide an assessment of the relative risk associated with the atherosclerotic disease. These imaging techniques are ineffective in determining whether the plaques are unstable and vulnerable to thrombosis and proliferation. *In vivo*, high-resolution, multi-contrast MR imaging holds the best promise of non-invasively imaging vulnerable plaques, characterizing plaques in terms of lipid and fibrous content, and identifying the presence of thrombus or calcium in all arteries including the coronary arteries. MR allows serial evaluation assessment of the progression and/or regression of atherosclerosis over time. Application of MR imaging opens up whole new areas for diagnosis, prevention, and treatment (e.g., lipid-lowering drug regimens) of atherosclerotic disease.

ACKNOWLEDGMENTS

The authors are grateful for the stimulating discussions with Drs. John T. Fallon, Juan J. Badimon, Gerard T. Luk-Pat, Steve G. Worthley, Gerard Helft, Meir Shinnar, and Jean Francois Toussaint. We also acknowledge the help of Drs. John T. Fallon and Juan Gilberto Aguinaldo in manuscript review and suggestions.

REFERENCES

1. FUSTER, V., Z.A. FAYAD & J.J. BADIMON. 1999. Acute coronary syndromes: biology. Lancet **353** (Suppl 2): SII5–SII9.
2. ROSS, R. 1999. Atherosclerosis—an inflammatory disease. N. Engl. J. Med. **340:** 115–126.
3. FUSTER, V. 1994. Lewis A. Conner Memorial Lecture. Mechanisms leading to myocardial infarction: insights from studies of vascular biology. Circulation **90:** 2126–2146.
4. STARY H.C., A.B. CHANDLER, R.E. DINSMORE, V. FUSTER, S. GLAGOV, W. INSULL, JR., M.E. ROSENFELD, C.J. SCHWARTZ, W.D. WAGNER & R.W. WISSLER. 1995. A definition of advanced types of atherosclerotic lesions and a histological classification of atherosclerosis. A report from the Committee on Vascular Lesions of the Council on Arteriosclerosis, American Heart Association. Circulation **92:** 1355–1374.
5. STARY, H.C., A.B. CHANDLER, S. GLAGOV, J.R. GUYTON, W. INSULL, JR., M.E. ROSENFELD, S.A. SCHAFFER, C.J. SCHWARTZ, W.D. WAGNER & R.W. WISSLER. 1994. A definition of initial, fatty streak, and intermediate lesions of atherosclerosis. A report from the Committee on Vascular Lesions of the Council on Arteriosclerosis, American Heart Association. Circulation **89:** 2462–2478.
6. RICHARDSON, P.D., M.J. DAVIES & G.V. BORN. 1989. Influence of plaque configuration and stress distribution on fissuring of coronary atherosclerotic plaques. Lancet **2:** 941–944.
7. FERNANDEZ-ORTIZ, A., J.J. BADIMON, E. FALK, V. FUSTER, B. MEYER, A. MAILHAC, D. WENG, P.K. SHAH & L. BADIMON. 1994. Characterization of the relative thrombogenicity of atherosclerotic plaque components: implications for consequences of plaque rupture. J. Am. Coll. Cardiol. **23:** 1562–1569.
8. AMBROSE, J.A. 1996. Angiographic correlations of advanced coronary lesions in acute coronary syndromes. *In* Syndromes of Atherosclerosis: correlations of clinical imaging and pathology. V. Fuster, Ed: 105–122. Futura Publishing Company, Inc. Armonk, NY.
9. DINSMORE, R.E. & S.M. RIVITZ. 1996. Imaging techniques in carotid and peripheral vascular disease. *In* Syndromes of Atherosclerosis: correlations of clinical imaging and pathology. V. Fuster, Ed: 277–289. Futura Publishing Company, Inc. Armonk, NY.
10. KOHLER, T.R. 1996. Imaging of carotid artery lesions: a surgeon's view. *In* Syndromes of Atherosclerosis: correlations of clinical imaging and pathology. V. Fuster, Ed: 205–233. Futura Publishing Company, Inc. Armonk, NY.

11. NISSEN S.E., A.C. DE FRANCO, E.M. TUZCU & D.J. MOLITERNO. 1995. Coronary intravascular ultrasound: diagnostic and interventional applications. Coron. Artery Dis. **6:** 355–367.
12. GE, J., F. CHIRILLO, J. SCHWEDTMANN, G.R. HAUDE, D. BAUMGART, V. SHAH, C. VON BIRGELEN, S. SACK, H. BOUDOULAS & R. ERBEL. 1999. Screening of ruptured plaques in patients with coronary artery disease by intravascular ultrasound. Heart **81:** 621–627.
13. UCHIDA, Y., F. NAKAMURA, T. TOMARU, T. MORITA, T. OSHIMA, T. SASAKI, S. MORIZUKI & J. HIROSE. 1995. Prediction of acute coronary syndromes by percutaneous coronary angioscopy in patients with stable angina. Am. Heart J. **130:** 195–203.
14. THIEME, T., K.D. WERNECKE, R. MEYER, E. BRANDENSTEIN, D. HABEDANK, A. HINZ, S.B. FELIX, G. BAUMANN & F.X. KLEBER. 1996. Angioscopic evaluation of atherosclerotic plaques: validation by histomorphologic analysis and association with stable and unstable coronary syndromes. J. Am. Coll. Cardiol. **28:** 1–6.
15. HEISS, G., A.R. SHARRETT, R. BARNES, L.E. CHAMBLESS, M. SZKLO & C. ALZOLA. 1991. Carotid atherosclerosis measured by B-mode ultrasound in populations: associations with cardiovascular risk factors in the ARIC study. Am. J. Epidemiol. **134:** 250–256.
16. WEINBERGER, J., S. AZHAR, F. DANISI, R. HAYES & M. GOLDMAN. 1998. A new noninvasive technique for imaging atherosclerotic plaque in the aortic arch of stroke patients by transcutaneous real-time B-mode ultrasonography: an initial report. Stroke **29:** 673–676.
17. WEINBERGER, J., L. RAMOS, J.A. AMBROSE & V. FUSTER. 1988. Morphologic and dynamic changes of atherosclerotic plaque at the carotid artery bifurcation: sequential imaging by real time B-mode ultrasonography. J. Am. Coll. Cardiol. **12:** 1515–1521.
18. AGATSTON, A.S., W.R. JANOWITZ, F.J. HILDNER, N.R. ZUSMER, M. VIAMONTE, JR. & R. DETRANO. 1990. Quantification of coronary artery calcium using ultrafast computed tomography. J. Am. Coll. Cardiol. **15:** 827–832.
19. CALLISTER, T.Q., P. RAGGI, B. COOIL, N.J. LIPPOLIS & D.J. RUSSO. 1998. Effect of HMG-CoA reductase inhibitors on coronary artery disease as assessed by electron-beam computed tomography. N. Engl. J. Med. **339:** 1972–1978.
20. SOILA, K., P. NUMMI, T. EKFORS, M. VIAMONTE, JR. & M. KORMANO. 1986. Proton relaxation times in arterial wall and atheromatous lesions in man. Invest. Radiol. **21:** 411–415.
21. MAYNOR, C.H., H.C. CHARLES, R.J. HERFKENS, S.A. SUDDARTH & G.A. JOHNSON. 1989. Chemical shift imaging of atherosclerosis at 7.0 Tesla. Invest. Radiol. **24:** 52–60.
22. PEARLMAN, J.D., J. ZAJICEK, M.B. MERICKEL, C.S. CARMAN, C.R. AYERS, J.R. BROOKEMAN & M.F. BROWN. 1988. High-resolution ^{1}H NMR spectral signature from human atheroma. Magn. Reson. Med. **7:** 262–279.
23. MOHIADDIN, R.H., D.N. FIRMIN, S.R. UNDERWOOD, A.K. ABDULLA, R.H. KLIPSTEIN, R.S. REES & D.B. LONGMORE. 1989. Chemical shift magnetic resonance imaging of human atheroma. Br. Heart J. **62:** 81–89.
24. VINITSKI, S., P.M. CONSIGNY, M.J. SHAPIRO, N. JANES, S.N. SMULLENS & M.D. RIFKIN. 1991. Magnetic resonance chemical shift imaging and spectroscopy of atherosclerotic plaque. Invest. Radiol. **26:** 703–714.
25. GOLD, G.E., J.M. PAULY, G.H. GLOVER, J.C. MORETTO, A. MACOVSKI & R.J. HERFKENS. 1993. Characterization of atherosclerosis with a 1.5-T imaging system. J. Magn. Reson. Imaging **3:** 399–407.
26. ALTBACH, M.I., M.A. MATTINGLY, M.F. BROWN & A.F. GMITRO. 1991. Magnetic resonance imaging of lipid deposits in human atheroma via a stimulated-echo diffusion-weighted technique. Magn. Reson. Med. **20:** 319–326.
27. TOUSSAINT, J.F., J.F. SOUTHERN, V. FUSTER & H.L. KANTOR. 1994. ^{13}C-NMR spectroscopy of human atherosclerotic lesions. Relation between fatty acid saturation, cholesteryl ester content, and luminal obstruction. Arterioscler. Thromb. **14:** 1951–1957.
28. TOUSSAINT, J.F., J.F. SOUTHERN, V. FUSTER & H.L. KANTOR. 1995. T2-weighted contrast for NMR characterization of human atherosclerosis. Arterioscler. Thromb. Vasc. Biol. **15:** 1533–1542.
29. KAUFMAN, L., L.E. CROOKS, P.E. SHELDON, W. ROWAN & T. MILLER. 1982. Evaluation of NMR imaging for detection and quantification of obstructions in vessels. Invest. Radiology **17:** 554–560.

30. HERFKENS, R.J., C.B. HIGGINS, H. HRICAK, M.J. LIPTON, L.E. CROOKS, P.E. SHELDON & L. KAUFMAN. 1983. Nuclear magnetic resonance imaging of atherosclerotic disease. Radiology **148:** 161–166.
31. MARTIN, A.J., A.I. GOTLIEB & R.M. HENKELMAN. 1995. High-resolution MR imaging of human arteries. J. Magn. Reson. Imaging **5:** 93–100.
32. MERICKEL, M.B., S. BERR, K. SPETZ, T.R. JACKSON, J. SNELL, P. GILLIES, E. SHIMSHICK, J. HAINER, J.R. BROOKEMAN & C.R. AYERS. 1993. Noninvasive quantitative evaluation of atherosclerosis using MRI and image analysis. Arterioscler. Thromb. **13:** 1180–1186.
33. MERICKEL, M.B., C.S. CARMAN, J.R. BROOKEMAN, J.P.D. MUGLER, M.F. BROWN & C.R. AYERS. 1988. Identification and 3-D quantification of atherosclerosis using magnetic resonance imaging. Comput. Biol. Med. **18:** 89–102.
34. YUAN, C., J.S. TSURUDA, K.N. BEACH, C.E. HAYES, M.S. FERGUSON, C.E. ALPERS, T.K. FOO & D.E. STRANDNESS. 1994. Techniques for high-resolution MR imaging of atherosclerotic plaque. J. Magn. Reson. Imaging **4:** 43–49.
35. VON INGERSLEBEN, G., U.P. SCHMIEDL, T.S. HATSUKAMI, J.A. NELSON, D.S. SUBRAMANIAM, M.S. FERGUSON & C. YUAN. 1997. Characterization of atherosclerotic plaques at the carotid bifurcation: correlation of high-resolution MR imaging with histologic analysis—preliminary study. Radiographics **17:** 1417–1423.
36. TOUSSAINT, J.F., G.M. LAMURAGLIA, J.F. SOUTHERN, V. FUSTER & H.L. KANTOR. 1996. Magnetic resonance images lipid, fibrous, calcified, hemorrhagic, and thrombotic components of human atherosclerosis *in vivo*. Circulation **94:** 932–938.
37. YUAN, C., M.P. SKINNER, E. KANEKO, L.M. MITSUMORI, C.E. HAYES, E.W. RAINES, J.A. NELSON & R. ROSS. 1996. Magnetic resonance imaging to study lesions of atherosclerosis in the hyperlipidemic rabbit aorta. Magn. Reson. Imaging **14:** 93–102.
38. SKINNER, M.P., C. YUAN, L. MITSUMORI, C.E. HAYES, E.W. RAINES, J.A. NELSON & R. ROSS. 1995. Serial magnetic resonance imaging of experimental atherosclerosis detects lesion fine structure, progression and complications *in vivo*. Nature Med. **1:** 69–73.
39. SHINNAR, M., J.T. FALLON, S. WEHRLI, M. LEVIN, D. DALMACY, Z.A. FAYAD, J.J. BADIMON, M. HARRINGTON, E. HARRINGTON & V. FUSTER. 1999. The diagnostic accuracy of ex vivo magnetic resonance imaging for human atherosclerotic plaque characterization. Arterioscler. Thromb. Vasc. Biol. **19:** 2756–2761.
40. TOUSSAINT, J.F., J.F. SOUTHERN, V. FUSTER & H.L. KANTOR. 1997. Water diffusion properties of human atherosclerosis and thrombosis measured by pulse field gradient nuclear magnetic resonance. Arterioscler. Thromb. Vasc. Biol. **17:** 542–546.
41. MOODY, A.R., S. ALLDER, G. LENNOX, J. GLADMAN & P. FENTEM. 1999. Direct magnetic resonance imaging of carotid artery thrombus in acute stroke. Lancet **353:** 122–123.
42. MOODY, A.R., J.G. POLLOCK, A.R. O'CONNOR & M. BAGNALL. 1998. Lower-limb deep venous thrombosis: direct MR imaging of the thrombus. Radiology **209:** 349–355.
43. YUAN, C., C. PETTY, K.D. O'BRIEN, T.S. HATSUKAMI, J.F. EARY & B.G. BROWN. 1997. *In vitro* and *in situ* magnetic resonance imaging signal features of atherosclerotic plaque-associated lipids. Arterioscler. Thromb. Vasc. Biol. **17:** 1496–1503.
44. FAYAD, Z.A., J.T. FALLON, M. SHINNAR, S. WEHRLI, H.M. DANSKY, M. POON, J.J. BADIMON, S.A. CHARLTON, E.A. FISHER, J.L. BRESLOW & V. FUSTER. 1998. Noninvasive *in vivo* high-resolution magnetic resonance imaging of atherosclerotic lesions in genetically engineered mice. Circulation **98:**1541–1547.
45. FAYAD, Z.A., T.J. CONNICK & L. AXEL. 1995. An improved quadrature or phased-array coil for MR cardiac imaging. Magn. Reson. Med. **34:** 186–193.
46. HAYES, C.E., C.M. MATHIS & C. YUAN. 1996. Surface coil phased arrays for high-resolution imaging of the carotid arteries. J. Magn. Reson. Imaging **6:** 109–112.
47. FAYAD, Z.A., N. TAMANA, J.J. BADIMON, M. GOLDMAN, J. WEINBERGER, J.T. FALLON, G. AGUINALDO, M. SHINNAR, J.H. CHESEBRO & V. FUSTER. 1998. In-vivo MR characterization of plaques in the thoracic aorta. Circulation **98:** I-515.
48. EDELMAN, R.R., D. CHIEN & D. KIM. 1991. Fast selective black blood MR imaging. Radiology **181:** 655–660.
49. FAYAD, Z.A., T. NAHAR, J.T. FALLON, M. GOLDMAN, A.G. AGUINALDO, J.J. BADIMON & V. FUSTER. 1999. *In vivo* MR characterization of human aortic atherosclerotic plaques. Proc. Int. Soc. Magn. Reson. Med. **1:** 80.

50. SHINNAR, M., R. GALLO, Z.A. FAYAD, J.T. FALLON, A. PADUREAN, S.N. KONSTADT, D. MOSKOWITZ, J. ABELA, J.J. BADIMON & V.F. FUSTER. 1998. *In vivo* magnetic resonance imaging of post angioplasty coronary vessel wall lesion in pigs. J. Am. Coll. Cardiol. **33:** 339A.
51. WORTHLEY, S.G., G. HEFT, V. FUSTER, Z.A. FAYAD, O. RODRIGUEZ, J.T. FALLON, A.G. ZAMAN & J.J. BADIMON. 1999. In vivo high-resolution MR non-invasively defines coronary lesion size and composition in a porcine model. Circulation **100:** I-521.
52. FAYAD, Z.A., V. FUSTER, J.T. FALLON, S. SHARMA, T. JAYASUNDERA, S.G. WORTHLEY, G. HELFT, G. AGUINALDO & J.J. BADIMON. 1999. Human coronary atherosclerotic wall imaging using in vivo high resolution MR. Circulation **100:** I-520–521.

Questions and Answers

UNIDENTIFIED: What are you doing to improve the resolution of the MRI technique?

FAYAD: This technology relies on two things. Like any other technology, imaging relies on hardware. Also, there is a lot of power in MRI technology, in terms of the software; the way that you acquire the data, and how you minimize motion. We combined hardware and software techniques that we adopted from studies of the brain and other vessels as well as new techniques more specifically for the plaques. In the future, we may find some specific magnets that would be totally dedicated to cardiovascular imaging. At this time, they are actually dedicated to the brain and the spine, not to the heart. We are working on such a device.

UNIDENTIFIED: Masanori Aikawa showed some posters here on regression of atherosclerosis with cholesterol lowering. He also imaged the animals by MR and showed the utility of the MR technique for following the regression. So it is a very promising technique.

FAYAD: We have a rabbit model, a pig model, a rat model, and, obviously, the mouse model. We are using this not only in the animal, but also trying to do it clinically. As you said, it is really a very powerful technique in terms of serial imaging. It probably is going to reduce the number of animals you need. When we do serial imaging at this time where you group animals, you try to increase the numbers because you are imaging two different groups. With MRI it has been shown with some studies looking at global function of the heart that you actually need a smaller sample because you have a more accurate measurement technique.

Signaling Angiogenesis via p42/p44 MAP Kinase Cascade

GILLES PAGÈS, JULIE MILANINI, DARREN E. RICHARD, EDURNE BERRA, EMMANUEL GOTHIÉ, FRANCESC VIÑALS, AND JACQUES POUYSSÉGUR[a]

Centre de Biochimie, CNRS-UMR 6543, Université de Nice, Parc Valrose, 06108 Nice, France

ABSTRACT: Vascular endothelial growth factor (VEGF), a potent agonist secreted by virtually all cells, controls migration and division of vascular endothelial cells. Disruption of one VEGF allele in mice has revealed a dramatic lethal effect in early embryogenesis, suggesting a key role in vasculogenesis. We analyzed the regulation of VEGF mRNA in normal and transformed CCL39 fibroblasts and then dissected the VEGF promoter to identify the signaling pathway(s) controlling the activation of this promoter in response to growth factors, oncogenes, and hypoxic stress. We demonstrated that the p42/p44 MAP kinase signaling cascade controls VEGF expression at least at two levels. In normoxic conditions, MAPKs activate the VEGF promoter at the proximal (-88/-66) region where Sp-1/AP-2 factors bind. Activation of p42/p44 MAPKs is sufficient to turn on VEGF mRNA. At low O_2 tension, hypoxia inducible factor-1α (HIF-1α), a limiting factor rapidly stabilized and phosphorylated, plays a key role in the expression of several genes including VEGF. We demonstrated that p42/p44MAPKs stoichiometrically phosphorylate HIF-1α *in vitro* and that HIF-1–dependent VEGF gene expression is strongly enhanced by the exclusive activation of p42/p44MAPKs. Finally, we demonstrated that the regulation of p42/p44MAPK activity is critical for controlling proliferation and growth arrest of vascular endothelial cells at confluency. These results point to at least three major targets of angiogenesis where p42/p44 MAP kinases exert a determinant action.

INTRODUCTION

Angiogenesis is a fundamental physiological process by which new blood vessels are formed.[1,2] One of the most widely described mechanisms controlling the neovascularization associated with pathological processes[3] is the increased secretion of multiples growth factors[4–8] and cytokines[9,10] by "stressed cells" (by inflammation and psoriasis, for example) or nutrient-deprived tumor cells. Among growth factors, two major classes have been characterized: acid and basic FGF of the FGF family[4,5] and vascular endothelial growth factor, VEGF, a new family of secreted growth factors structurally related to PDGF (40% homology at the amino acid level).[6–8] VEGF, also described as a permeability factor, stimulates endothelial cell migration and prolifera-

---

[a]Address for correspondence: Jacques Pouysségur, Centre de Biochimie, CNRS-UMR 6543, Université de Nice, Parc Valrose, 06108 Nice, France. Voice: 33-492-07-64- 30; fax: 33-492-07-64-32

pouysseg@unice.fr

tion *in vitro* and has angiogenic activity *in vivo*.[11,12] Different isoforms of 121, 165, 189, and 206 amino acids resulted from alternative splicing of the same gene.[13] Virtually all tissues and cell types express VEGF mRNA. This expression is particularly elevated in highly vascularized tissue and in tumor-derived cell lines.[14] The importance of VEGF and VEGF-induced signaling was elegantly demonstrated by genetic inactivation of either one single VEGF allele[15,16] or each VEGF receptor subtype, VEGF-R1 and VEGF-R2[17,18] (see Ref. 19 for review). In all three cases, mouse development is dramatically stopped at a very early stage because of a failure in blood vessel development. Recently, another VEGF receptor specific for the VEGF 165 isoform was described. It is identical to neuropilin-1, a receptor for the collapsin/semaphorin family which mediates neuronal cell guidance.[20] Gene disruption of other receptors specific for blood or lymphatic vessels (Tie-1 and 2 and VEGF receptor-3) highlights their importance during embryogenesis.[21,22] Deprivation of oxygen during cell culture, which mimicks the necrotic hypoxic regions in solid tumors, induces VEGF mRNA expression by both an increase in the rate of transcription but also by stabilization of its mRNA.[23–25] Transcription of the VEGF gene following hypoxia is triggered through increased synthesis of the hypoxia-inducible factor-1 (HIF-1). HIF-1 is an heterodimer composed by HIF-1α and HIF-1β.[26] Whereas HIF-1β is constitutively expressed, the synthesis of HIF-1α is upregulated upon hypoxia and rapidly degraded by the proteasome following reoxygenation.[27,28]

Here we report that MAP kinase signaling, a conserved module for transducing cell surface signals to the nucleus, controls angiogenesis at least at two levels. At the level of the VEGF promoter it enhances transcription via direct phosphorylation of HIF-1α and by promoting the recruitment of the Sp1/AP2 complex. At the level of vascular endothelial cells, it controls cell-cycle entry.

VEGF mRNA but not VEGF-B and VEGF-C Are Regulated by Growth and Oncogenic Factors in CCL 39 Cells

Under normoxic conditions, exponential cultures of the Chinese hamster lung fibroblast cell line, CCL39 or its derivative PS 200, express barely detectable levels of VEGF mRNA (FIG. 1). Serum stimulation of growth-arrested CCL39 (data not shown) or PS 200 cells (FIG. 1) triggers the induction of VEGF mRNA. However, this expression is strongly elevated in cells transformed either with polyoma virus, Ha-Ras (Ras Val^{12})[29] or a constitutive active form of MAP kinase kinase (MKK1 SS/DD).[30] At least, four isoforms that correspond to the spliced variants described[13] detectably hybridize to a mouse VEGF probe. FIGURE 1 shows that in the polyoma virus, Ha-Ras, or MKK1 SS/DD transformed cells, the different VEGF mRNA isoforms are expressed at a level approximately ten times greater than that of control cells. This overexpression is particularly prominent for the clone 5c, which overexpressed Ha-Ras.[29] For each of the cell lines tested, FCS was able to increase the amount of VEGF mRNA, although in transformed cells the basal level was extremely elevated. However, this is not the case for cells expressing MKK1 SS/DD and isolated from a tumor produced in nude mice (T. MKK1 SS/DD). Interestingly, these cells were shown to be fully independent of serum growth factors.[30] This could explain the inability of serum to further modify the elevated level of VEGF mRNA in

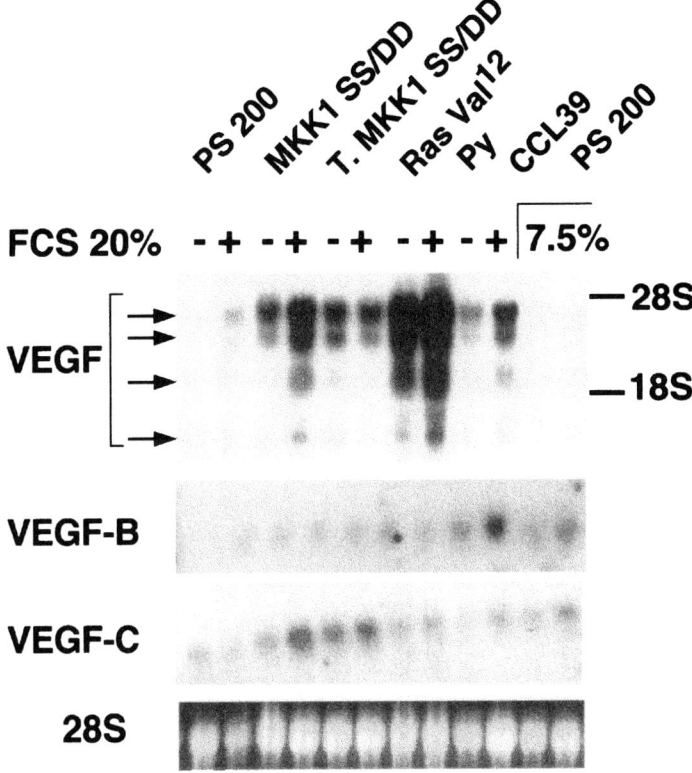

FIGURE 1. Expression of VEGF in resting, serum-stimulated, and transformed cells. 20 μg of total RNA isolated from cells transformed by Ras Val,[12] Polyoma virus (Py), constitutively active MAP kinase kinase (MKK1 SS/DD) or from T. MKK1 SS/DD cells recovered from nude mice[19] were analyzed by Northern blot in comparison with control cells (PS 200). Cells were serum deprived for 16 h (−) then stimulated with 20% FCS for 3 h (+). RNA isolated from exponentially growing normal cells were loaded as controls (CCL39, PS200 7.5%). The blot was hybridized with probes corresponding to VEGF, VEGF-B, and VEGF-C. Ethidium bromide coloration of 28S ribosomal RNA is shown as loading control.

these tumor cells. In the different cell lines tested, the other members of the VEGF family, VEGF-B and VEGF-C, are constitutively expressed showing that both genes are not tightly regulated via growth or oncogenic factors even if VEGF-C seems to be upregulated in MKK1 SS/DD transformed cells.

p42/p44 MAP Kinase Cascade Specifically Induces VEGF mRNA Expression in Raf-1:ER Expressing Cell

To further examine the contribution of the Ras/p42/p44 MAP kinase pathway in VEGF expression, we have chosen a cell line expressing an estradiol-inducible Raf-

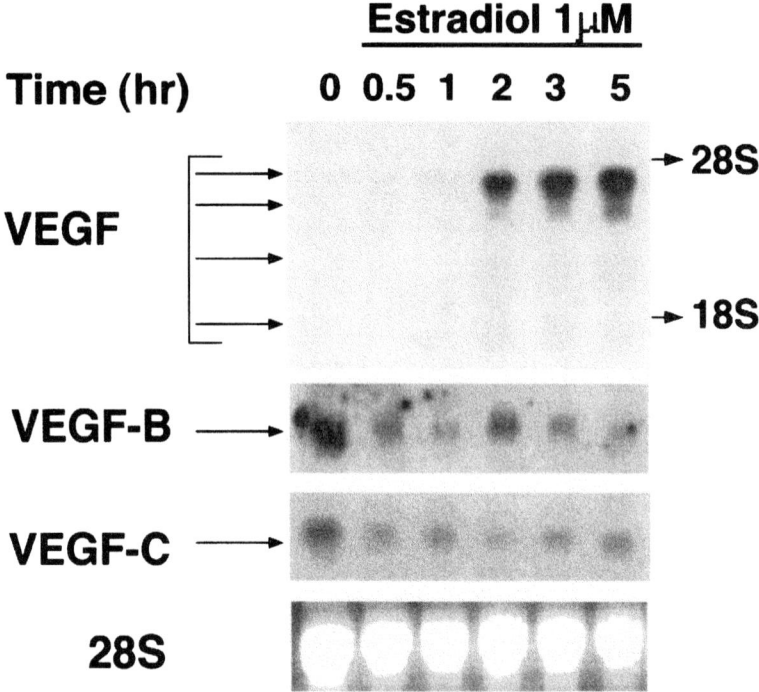

FIGURE 2. Regulation of expression of VEGF in Raf-1:ER expressing cells. 20 μg of RNA isolated from quiescent or estradiol-stimulated Raf-1:ER cells (1 μM) for the times indicated were analyzed by Northern blot for expression of VEGF, VEGF-B, and VEGF-C. As described in FIGURE 1, 28S ribosomal RNA is shown as loading control.

1 (Raf-1:ER cells).[31–33] In this case, the p42/p44 MAP kinase activity is rapidly activated by estradiol, eliminating the contribution of the SAP kinase cascade (p38MAPK/ JNK)[34–36] and the PI3 kinase cascade,[37,38] which are generally activated by serum or constitutively active Ras. Raf-1:ER expressing cells were serum-deprived for 16 h and then stimulated by the addition of estradiol for the times indicated. FIGURE 2 shows that VEGF transcripts are expressed at a detectable level after 2 h and are maximally expressed after 3 h of estradiol stimulation, the expression was sustained for up to five hours. A longer exposure of the blot shows detectable transcripts after only 30 min of stimulation (data not shown) and the expression of the three other spliced variants revealed in FIGURE 1. This rapid induction is compatible with the kinetics of activation of p42/p44 MAP kinases in these cells.[33] The expression of VEGF-B and VEGF-C mRNA species are not modified by estradiol treatment, confirming that activation of the p42/p44 MAP kinase pathway does not play any role in controlling their expression in these cells.

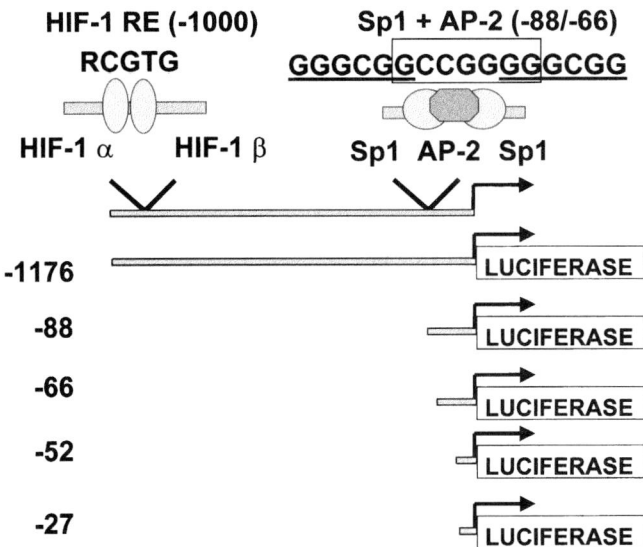

FIGURE 3. Description of the VEGF promoter. Shown are the different domains of the promoter: the proximal region containing overlapping AP-2 and Sp1 consensus binding sites and distal region containing the HIF-1 binding region. Also shown are the promoter constructs used in transient transfection assays described in FIGURE 4.

Characterization of the p42/p44 MAP Kinase Pathway Responsive Region of the VEGF Promoter

Since we suspected that the upregulation observed before was exerted at the transcriptional level, we constructed and analyzed the activities of different regions of the VEGF promoter. FIGURE 3 shows the detailed structure of the VEGF promoter and the different constructs used in transfection assays. The human, mouse, and rat VEGF promoter contains binding sites for AP-2, Sp1, or Sp1-related factors[13,39–42] in addition to binding sites for AP-1[43] and HIF-1,[24,39] which regulate the transcription of the gene during hypoxia.[44] Here, we compare the activities of the −1176, −88, −66, −52, and −27/+54 constructs in the presence or absence of MKK1 SS/DD localize the p42/p44 MAP kinase pathway–responsive element. FIGURE 4 shows that while the −1176 and −88/+54 constructs displayed constitutive baseline activity, which was increased by cotransfection with MKK1 SS/DD by a factor of 3.3 and 4.6, respectively, analysis of the −66, −52, and −27/+54 constructs showed a loss of both basal and MKK 1 SS/DD transcriptional activation. These results suggest that sequences between −88 and −66 are absolutely required for basal and p42/p44 MAP kinase–dependent pathway stimulated promoter activity. The loss of both basal and stimulated transcriptional activity could reflect a truncation of transcription factor binding sites in the −88/+54 construct that can regulate the overall activity of the promoter.

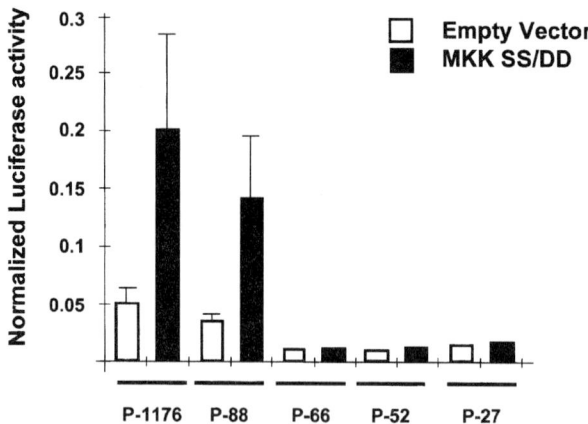

FIGURE 4. Identification of a p42/p44 MAP kinase pathway responsive region between −88 and −66 of the VEGF gene promoter by 5′ deletional analysis. CCL39 cells were transfected with 250 ng of the −88/+54, −66/+54, −52/+54, and −27/+54 in the presence or absence of 200 ng of expression vector coding for constitutive active MEK 1 (MKK1 SS/DD). In all cases 100 ng of an expression vector coding for β-galactosidase was co-transfected to normalize for transfection efficiency. Sixteen hours after the transfection, the cells were rinsed with PBS and grown in medium supplemented with 7.5% FCS for 48 hours. The cells were then lysed and luciferase activity measured. The results correspond to three different experiments. Each data point is the mean of triplicate determinations.

Cooperative Effects of AP-2 and Sp1 in MKK1 SS/DD Stimulation of VEGF Promoter

We have investigated whether the p42/p44 MAP kinase pathway induced VEGF mRNA levels by directly activating AP-2 or Sp1, whose binding sites are present between −88 and −66. FIGURE 3 shows that within this region there exists two putative binding sites for Sp1 and one for AP-2. These sites are conserved between human, mouse, and rat promoters.[39–42] Therefore, the intact −88/+54 construct or a construction with point mutations in the AP-2, both Sp1, or the three binding sites were transfected in exponentially growing cells and activation of the VEGF promoter was analyzed by luciferase assay. The response to the p42/p44 MAP kinase module was assessed by co-expression of constitutive active MKK1. FIGURE 5 shows that mutations of the AP-2 or both Sp1 putative binding sites done individually do not significantly modify basal and MKK1 SS/DD stimulated promoter activity. However, a combined mutation of AP-2 and both Sp1 binding sites dramatically decreases basal and MKK1 SS/DD–dependent transcriptional activation. This result suggests a cooperative effect of AP-2 and Sp1 for maximal transcriptional activation of the VEGF promoter.

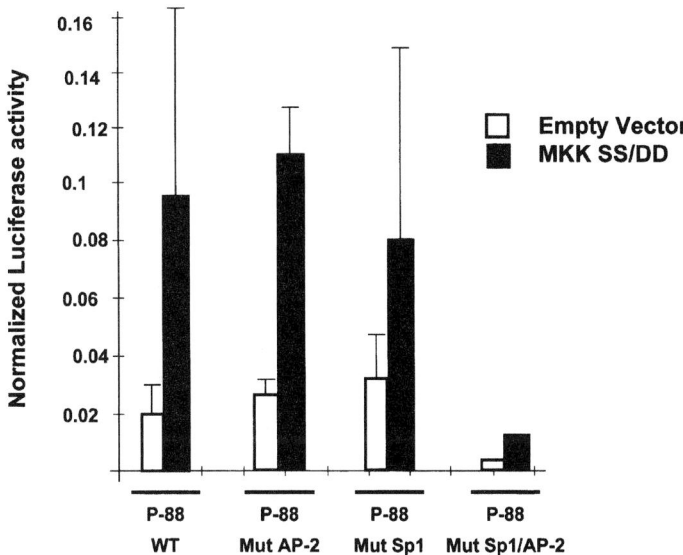

FIGURE 5. Cooperation of Sp1 and AP-2 for VEGF promoter activation. CCL39 cells were transfected with 250 ng of the −88/+54 promoter containing or not a mutation for AP-2, both Sp1, or the three binding sites in the presence or absence of 200 ng of expression vector coding for active MEK 1 (MKK1 SS/DD). In all cases 100 ng of an expression vector coding for β-galactosidase was co-transfected in order to normalize for transfection efficiency. Sixteen hours after the transfection, the cells were rinsed with PBS and grown in medium supplemented with 7.5% FCS for 48 hours. The cells were then lysed and luciferase activity measured. The results correspond to three different experiments. Each data point is the mean of triplicate determinations.

p42/p44 MAP Kinase Pathway Controls the Binding Activity of Nuclear Protein Extracts to the −88/−66 VEGF Promoter Region in Raf-1:ER Cells

In order to confirm the specific role of AP-2 and Sp1 transcription factors in the regulation of the VEGF promoter, we utilized a double-stranded probe encompassing the −88/−66 bp region in EMSAs experiments. FIGURE 6 shows four constitutive DNA binding complexes in resting or in estradiol-stimulated Raf-1:ER cells (complexes a, B, c, D; see lanes 1 and 6 of FIG. 6). To demonstrate that either Sp1 or AP-2 is present in at least the large complex B, we performed supershift experiments. Indeed, Sp1 antibodies supershifted part of complex B formed with extracts from resting cells or estradiol-stimulated cells (data not shown). Similarly, AP-2 antibodies supershifted part of complex B with extracts from estradiol-stimulated cells.[45] This supershift, however, is more evident in the presence of Sp1 neutralizing oligonucleotides. The binding specificity of the complexes formed was determined by exclusive competition with an excess of identical unlabeled DNA (FIG. 6). Under resting conditions, DNA binding of complexes a, B, and c are clearly inhibited by either Sp1− or AP-2–specific oligonucleotides (FIG. 6, compare lane 1 or 5 with

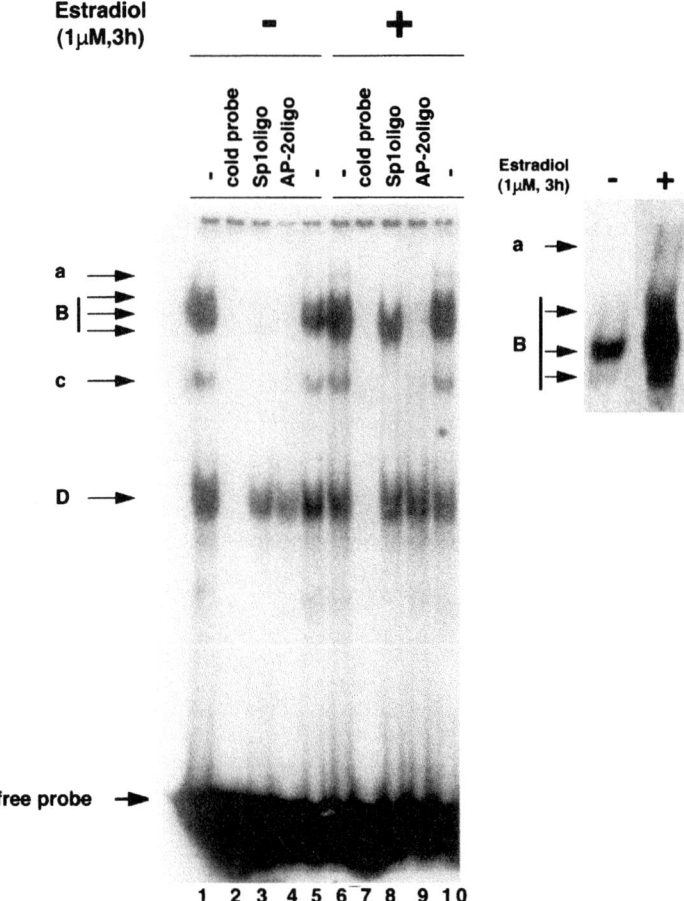

FIGURE 6. Identification of AP-2 and Sp1 transcription factors in the p42/p44 MAP kinase pathway–inducible DNA binding complex. EMSAs with nuclear extracts of untreated (lanes 1–5) or estradiol-stimulated (lanes 6–10) Raf-1:ER cells in the absence (lanes 1, 5, 6, and 10) or the presence of excess unlabeled probe (lanes 2 and 7) or excess of double-stranded Sp1 consensus oligonucleotides (lanes 3 and 8) or excess of doubled-stranded AP-2 consensus oligonucleotides (lanes 4 and 9). Formation of specific complexes is indicated on the left (a, B, c, and D). Competitor was used at a concentration of 100 molar excess. An enlargement of complexes a and B upon resting or stimulated conditions is shown on the right of the figure.

lanes 3 and 4). However, a remarkable change is observed when p42/p44 MAP kinase was specifically stimulated with estradiol. Nuclear extracts of cells stimulated for 3 h with estradiol show a strong increase in the binding of complex B. This is seen in FIGURE 6, where complex B is better resolved and enlarged. Another striking change occurs when binding is inhibited with a 100-fold excess of Sp1 oligonucleotides (FIG. 6, compare lanes 3 and 8). Under stimulated conditions, complex B resists the competition with the Sp1 oligonucleotides, reflecting that more proteins are bound and/or have a higher affinity. The same result is observed when AP-2 oligonucleotides are used as a competitor, even in this case the labeling of the resistant complex B is less intense. Altogether, these data clearly demonstrate that Sp1 and AP-2 transcription factors bind to the −88/−66 region of the VEGF promoter and that p42/p44 MAP kinase activity plays a key role in controlling the VEGF promoter activity via these sites.

We then focused our attention on another mechanism that also takes place in development and in the primary tumor neovascularization: hypoxia. In this case, another distal region of the VEGF promoter is regulated by fixation of HIF-1 (FIG. 3). We examined if the highly phosphorylated protein HIF-1α, an essential component of the HIF-1 complex, could be a target of p42/p44 MAPK.

p42/p44 MAPK Activation Induces HIF-1α Phosphorylation in Quiescent CCL 39 cells

To analyze whether p42/p44 MAP Kinases can phosphorylate HIF-1α, we performed SDS-PAGE mobility shift experiments with whole cell extracts from serum-deprived Raf-1:ER cells stimulated or not with estradiol. As seen in FIGURE 7(A) when quiescent Raf-1:ER cells are incubated in hypoxic conditions for 3 h, HIF-1α is induced and migrated as a single band at approximately 104 kD. When these cells

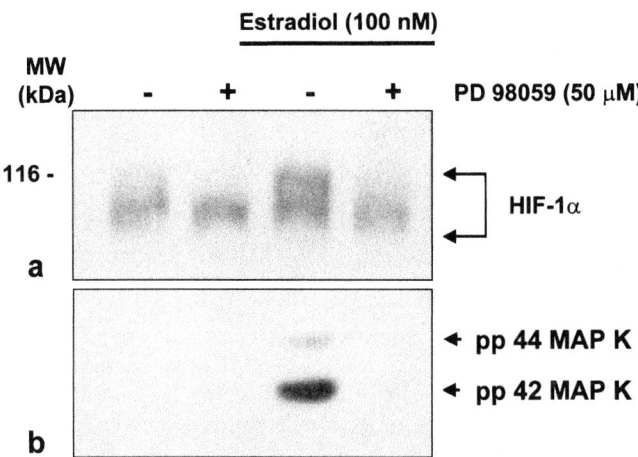

FIGURE 7. p42/p44 MAPK activation induces HIF-1α phosphorylation *in vivo*. CCL39 cells stably expressing the Raf-1:ER chimera (Raf-1:ER cells) were FCS-starved for 24 h before 3 h of hypoxia. Thirty min before the end of the hypoxic period, Raf-1:ER cells were stimulated with 100 nM estradiol for the times indicated. For inhibition with PD 98059, after the first 3 h of the hypoxic period, Raf-1:ER cells were preincubated for 30 min with 50 μM PD 98059, then stimulated with 100 nM estradiol for 30 min. Whole cell extracts (50 μg) were analyzed by SDS-PAGE (7.5% gel) and immunoblotting using an anti–HIF-1α antiserum (**A**) or an anti–phospho-p44/p42 MAPK polyclonal antibody (**B**).

were treated with estradiol for 30 min before the end of the 3 h hypoxic period, a form of HIF-1α appeared at 116 kD. Induction of p42/p44 MAPK activity can be seen with the phospho-specific anti p42/p44 MAPK antibody (FIG. 7, B). Essentially the same results were obtained using another stimulus shown to activate p42/p44 MAPK, 10% FCS (data not shown). Furthermore, this shift was inhibited by treatment of cells with the specific p42/p44 pathway inhibitor, PD 98059. Also, when the shifted form at 116 kD was treated with a non-specific protein phosphatase, HIF-1α completely migrated as the lower molecular weight form at 104 kD. Taken together, these results strongly suggest that HIF-1α is phosphorylated *in vivo* by p42/p44 MAPK. The possible implications of this phosphorylation are currently under investigation. However, we feel that this growth factor–mediated phosphorylation can cooperate with the hypoxic signal to modify HIF-1–mediated transcriptional activity.[46]

Enforcing Persistent Activation of p42/p44 MAPK Restores Growth-Signaling Events at Confluence

We then analyzed the status of p42/p44 MAP kinase activity in endothelial cells, one of the major targets of VEGF action. We observed that p42/p44 MAP kinase is very difficult to activate in confluent endothelial cells, which correspond to its poor proliferative capacity. In order to evaluate the importance of p42/p44 MAPK activity, we constructed 1G11 endothelial cells stably expressing the estradiol-inducible Raf-1 (Raf-1:ER cells). This chimera, as described earlier, can be activated by estradiol or its derivative tamoxifen. Thus we demonstrated that the combination of FCS and tamoxifen allows a more sustained p42/p44 MAPK activation in confluent cells.[47] This "forced" increment in p42/p44 MAPK activity alone is sufficient to promote a maximal entry of confluent cells in the cell cycle measured by BrdU incorporation or thymidine incorporation (FIG. 8). These results highlight the key role of the p42/p44 MAPK module in the regulation of endothelial cells proliferation, a notion that was previously firmly established in fibroblasts.[48]

CONCLUSION

In this study, we focused our attention on two different mechanisms of VEGF signaling. The first one concerns the regulation of expression of the VEGF itself. We show that it is upregulated in cells transformed by constitutive active members of the p42/p44 MAPK module, i.e., Ras and MEK. This first observation was confirmed by using a specific method to induce this signaling pathway, i.e., the Raf:ER chimera, which can be switched on by addition of estradiol or its derivative, tamoxifen. Thus, the simple activation of this chimera is sufficient to induce a high and sustained activation of p42/p44 MAPK, which results in an upregulation of VEGF gene transcription. We also demonstrated that this transcriptional activation is mediated by the recruitment of AP-2 and Sp1 transcription factors on the proximal region of the VEGF promoter. This upregulation of the promoter is probably the first response encountered in the transformed cells of primary tumors. Then as hypoxic phenomenon occurs in the core of primary tumors, the HIF-1 transcription factor could contribute to accentuate the VEGF gene transcription by fixation on a more distal region of the VEGF promoter. The p42/p44 MAPK also have an important role in such regulation

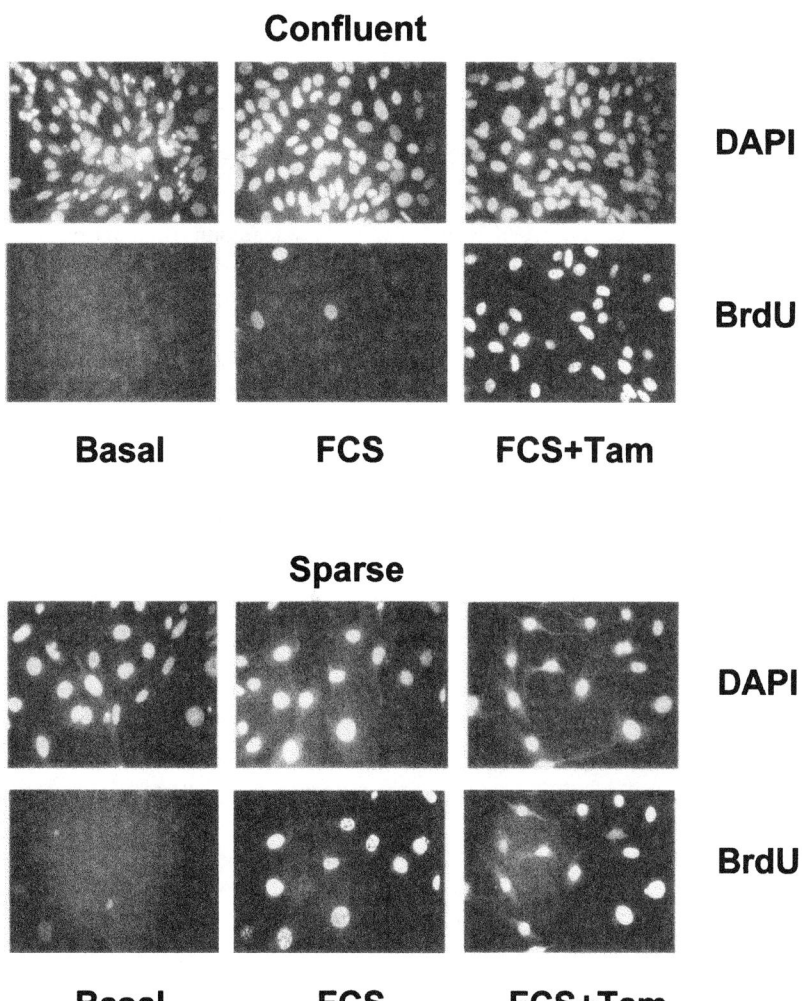

FIGURE 8. Enforced long-term activation of p42/p44 MAPK induces cell-cycle reentry of confluent endothelial cells. Nontransfected parental 1G11 or 1G11-Raf-1:ER cells were grown under conditions promoting sparseness or confluence and serum deprived for 24 hours. Cells were stimulated or not (basal) with 20% FCS (FCS) or 1 µM tamoxifen plus 20% FCS (FCS + Tam) for 24 hours. During the last 4 h, cells were labeled with BrdU. DNA synthesis was assessed by immunodetection of cells that had incorporated BrdU. Nuclei were stained with DAPI.

by phosphorylating HIF-1α, one of the limiting partners of HIF-1. We also demonstrated that the exclusive activation of the p42/p44 MAPK module (by stimulating the Raf:ER cells with estradiol) is sufficient to induce HIF-1–dependent VEGF expression. Finally, the key role of p42/p44 MAPK activation was further illustrated in vascular endothelial cells, one of the primary targets of VEGF action. We demonstrated that p42/p44 MAPK activity is low in confluent endothelial cells, a situation encountered in normal blood vessels. On the contrary, p42/p44 MAPK activity is higher in sparse cells, a condition that mimicks the neovascularization of solid tumors or the repair process of wound healing. We also demonstrated that it is possible to force cell-cycle reentry of confluent endothelial cells by an increased and sustained activation of p42/p44 MAPK. Such a situation could be encountered at the proximity of primary tumors when angiogenic factors (FGF, VEGF) stimulate the endothelial cells p42/p44 MAPK module following interaction with their receptors. Altogether, these data pointed out the importance of the p42/p44 MAPK signaling module in controlling different steps of the angiogenic program.

REFERENCES

1. FOLKMAN, J. et al.1971. Isolation of a tumor factor responsible for angiogenesis. J. Exp. Med. **133:** 275–288.
2. MUTHUKKARUPPAN, V. & R. AUERBACH. 1979. Angiogenesis in the mouse cornea. Science **205:** 1416–1418.
3. HANAHAN, D. & J. FOLKMAN. 1996. Patterns and emerging mechanisms of the angiogenic switch during tumorigenesis. Cell **86:** 353–364.
4. BASILICO, C. & D. MOSCATELLI. 1992. The FGF family of growth factors and oncogenes. Adv. Cancer Res. **59:** 115–165.
5. FOLKMAN, J. & Y. SHING. 1992. Angiogenesis. J. Biol. Chem. **267:** 10931–10934.
6. LEUNG, D.W. et al. 1989. Vascular endothelial growth factor is a secreted angiogenic mitogen. Science **246:** 1306–1309.
7. BREIER, G. & W. RISAU. 1996. The role of vascular endothelial growth factor in blood vessel formation. Trends Cell. Biol. **6:** 454–456.
8. RISAU, W. 1997. Mechanisms of angiogenesis. Nature **386:** 671–674.
9. COZZOLINO, F. et al. 1993. Interferon alpha and interleukin-2 synergistically enhance basic fibroblast growth factor synthesis and induce release, promoting endothelial cell growth. J. Clin. Invest. **91:** 2504–2512.
10. TOI, M., A.L. HARRIS & R. BICKNELL. 1991. Interleukin-4 is a potent mitogen for capillary endothelium. Biochem. Biophys. Res. Commun. **174:** 1287–1293.
11. FERRARA, N. & W.J. HENZEL. 1989. Pituitary follicular cells secrete a novel heparin-binding growth factor specific for vascular endothelial cells. Biochem. Biophys. Res. Commun. **161:** 851–858.
12. SHWEIKI, D. et al. 1992. Vascular endothelial growth factor induced by hypoxia may mediate hypoxia-initiated angiogenesis. Nature **359:** 843–945.
13. TISCHER, E. et al. 1991. The human gene for vascular endothelial growth factor. J. Biol. Chem. **266:** 11947–11954.
14. BERSE, B. et al. 1992. Vascular permeability factor (vascular endothelial growth factor) gene is expressed differentially in normal tissues, macrophages and tumors. Mol. Biol. Cell. **3:** 211–220.
15. CARMELIET, P. et al. 1996. Abnormal blood vessel development and lethality in embryos lacking a single VEGF allele. Nature **380:** 435–439.
16. FERRARA, N. et al. 1996. Heterozygous embryonic lethality induced by targeted inactivation of the VEGF gene. Nature **380:** 439–442.
17. SHALABY, F. et al. 1995. Failure of blood-island formation and vasculogenesis in Flk-1 deficient mice. Nature **376:** 62–66.
18. FONG, G.H. et al. 1995. Role of Flt-1 receptor tyrosine kinase in regulating the assembly of vascular endothelium. Nature **376:** 66–70.
19. NEUFELD, G. et al. 1999. Vascular Endothelial Growth Factor (VEGF) and its receptors. FASEB J. **13:** 9–22.

20. SOKER, S. et al. 1998. Neuropilin-1 is expressed by endothelial and tumor cells as an isoform-specific receptor for vascular endothelial growth factor. Cell **92:** 735–745.
21. SATO, T.N. et al. 1995. Distinct roles of the receptor tyrosine kinase Tie-1 and Tie-2 in blood vessels. formation. Nature **376:** 70–74.
22. DUMONT, D.J. et al. 1998. Cardiovascular failure in mouse embryos deficient in VEGF receptor 3. Science **282:** 946–949.
23. FINKENZELLER, G., A. TECHNAU & D. MARME. 1995. Hypoxia-induced transcription of the vascular endothelial growth factor gene is independent of functional AP-1 transcription factor. Biochem. Biophys. Res. Commun. **208:** 432–439.
24. IKEDA, E. et al. 1995. Hypoxia-induced transcriptional activation and increased mRNA stability of vascular endothelial growth factor in C6 glioma cells. J. Biol. Chem. **270:** 19761–19766.
25. LEVY, A.P., N.S. LEVY & M.A. GOLDBERG. 1996. Post-transcriptional regulation of vascular endothelial growth factor by hypoxia. J. Biol. Chem. **271:** 2746–2753.
26. WANG, G.L. & G.L. SEMENZA. 1995. Purification and characterization of hypoxia-inducible factor 1. J. Biol. Chem. **270:** 1230–1237.
27. SALCEDA, S. & J. CARO. 1997. Hypoxia inducible factor 1 alpha protein is rapidly degraded by the ubiquitin-proteasome system under normoxic conditions. J. Biol. Chem. **272:** 22642–22647.
28. HUANG, L.E. et al. 1998. Regulation of hypoxia-inducible factor 1alpha is mediated by an O_2^- dependent degradation domain via the ubiquitin-proteasome pathway. Proc. Natl. Acad. Sci. USA **95:** 7987–7992.
29. SEUWEN, K., A. LAGARDE & J. POUYSSÉGUR. 1988. Deregulation of hamster fibroblast proliferation by mutated ras oncogenes is not mediated by constitutive activation of phosphoinositide-specific phospholipase C. EMBO J. **7:** 161–168.
30. BRUNET, A., G. PAGÈS & J. POUYSSÉGUR. 1994. Constitutively active mutants of MAP kinase kinase (MEK1) induce growth factor-relaxation and oncogenicity when expressed in fibroblasts. Oncogene **9:** 3379–3387.
31. SAMUELS, M.L., J.M. WEBER & M. MCMAHON. 1993. Conditional transformation of cells and rapid activation of the mitogen-activated protein kinase cascade by an estradiol-dependent human raf-1 protein kinase. Mol. Biol. Cell. **13:** 6241–6252.
32. SAMUELS, M.L. & M. MCMAHON. 1994. Inhibition of platelet-derived growth factor and epidermal growth factor mediated mitogenesis and signalling in 3T3 cells expressing delta Raf-1:ER, an estradiol-regulated form of Raf-1. Mol. Biol. Cell. **14:** 7855–7866.
33. LENORMAND, P., M. MCMAHON & J. POUYSSÉGUR. 1996. Oncogenic Raf-1 activates p70 S6 kinase via mitogen-activated protein kinase-independent pathway. J. Biol. Chem. **271:** 15762–15768.
34. HAN, J. et al. 1994. A MAP kinase targeted by endotoxin and hyperosmolarity in mammalian cells. Science **265:** 808–811.
35. GALCHEVA-GARGOVA, Z. et al. 1994. An osmosensing signal transduction pathway in mammalian cells. Science **265:** 806–808.
36. DERIJARD, B. et al. 1995. Independent human MAP-kinase signal transduction pathways defined by MEK and MKK isoforms. Science **267:** 682–685.
37. RODRIGUEZ-VICIANA, P. et al. 1994. Phosphatidylinositol-3-OH kinase as a target of Ras. Nature **370:** 527–532.
38. KODAKI, T. et al. 1994. The activation of phosphatidyl 3-kinase by Ras. Curr. Biol. **4:** 798–806.
39. LEVY, A.P. et al. 1995. Transcriptional regulation of the rat vascular endothelial factor gene by hypoxia. J. Biol. Chem. **270:** 13333–13340.
40. KADONAGA, J.T. et al. 1987. Isolation of cDNA encoding transcription factor Sp-1 and functional analysis of the DNA binding domain. Cell **51:** 1079–1090.
41. HAGEN, G. et al. 1992. Cloning by recognition site screening of two novel GT box binding proteins: a family of Sp1 related genes. Nucl. Acids Res. **20:** 5519–5525.
42. SHIMA, D.T. et al. 1996. The mouse gene for vascular endothelial growth factor. Genomic structure, definition of the transcriptional unit, and characterization of the transcriptional and post-transcriptional regulatory sequences. J. Biol. Chem. **271:** 3877–3883.

43. ANGEL, P. *et al.* 1987. Phorbol ester-inducible genes contain a common cis element recognized by a TPA-modulated trans-acting factor. Cell **49:** 729–739.
44. FORSYTHE, J.A. *et al.* 1996. Activation of vascular endothelial growth factor gene transcription by hypoxia-inducible factor 1. Mol. Cell. Biol. **16:** 4604–4613.
45. MILANINI, J. *et al.* 1998. p42/p44 MAP kinase module plays a key role in the transcriptional regulation of vascular endothelial growth factor gene in fibroblasts. J. Biol. Chem. **273:** 18165–18172.
46. RICHARD, D.E. *et al.* 1999. p42/p44 MAP kinases phosphorylate hypoxia inducible factor 1 alpha (HIF-1α) and enhance the transcriptional activity of HIF-1. J Biol. Chem. **274:** 32631–32638.
47. VINALS, F. & J. POUYSSÉGUR. 1999. Confluence of vascular endothelial cells induces cell cycle exit by inhibiting p42/p44 Mitogen-Activated protein kinase activity. Mol. Cell. Biol. **19:** 2763–2772.
48. PAGÈS, G. *et al.* 1993. Mitogen-activated protein kinases $p42^{mapk}$ and $p44^{mapk}$ are required for fibroblast proliferation. Proc. Natl. Acad. Sci. USA **90:** 8319–8323.

Properties of Two VEGF Receptors, Flt-1 and KDR, in Signal Transduction[a]

YASUFUMI SATO,[b,c] SHINICHI KANNO,[b] NOBUYUKI ODA,[b] MAYUMI ABE,[b] MIKITO ITO,[d] KENYA SHITARA,[d] AND MASABUMI SHIBUYA[e]

[b]Department of Vascular Biology, Institute of Development, Aging and Cancer, Tohoku University, Sendai, Japan

[d]Tokyo Research Laboratories, Kyowa Hakko Kogyo Co., Machida, Japan

[e]Department of Genetics, Institute of Medical Science, University of Tokyo, Tokyo, Japan

ABSTRACT: The properties of two VEGF receptors, Flt-1 and KDR, in the signal transduction of VEGF in human umbilical vein endothelial cells (HUVECs) were investigated by using two newly developed blocking monoclonal antibodies (mAbs) against Flt-1 and KDR. VEGF stimulated the expression of transcription factor Ets-1 as well as matrix metalloproteinase-1 (MMP-1) and Flt-1 in HUVECs. The KDR/Flt-1 heterodimer and the KDR homodimer mediate the expression of Ets-1, MMP-1, and Flt-1. VEGF also stimulated DNA synthesis and migration of HUVECs. DNA synthesis is mediated by the same signaling system as the expression of Ets-1. In contrast, cell migration is regulated by two distinct signaling systems. The Flt-1 homodimer is required for actin reorganization. The KDR/Flt-1 heterodimer and the KDR homodimer are required for the assembly of vinculin in focal adhesion plaque by regulating the phosphorylation of focal adhesion kinase (FAK) and paxillin.

INTRODUCTION

Vascular endothelium is a continuous monolayer of endothelial cells (ECs) lining the inner surface of blood vessels. ECs are normally quiescent and play an important role in maintaining the integrity of blood vessels. However, they have the ability to form neo-vessels. Angiogenesis is a process by which new blood vessels are formed from pre-existing ones and it is a fundamental process in reproduction and development. The vascular system is the first functional organ that develops in the vertebrate embryo. The vasculature of the entire body is formed via two distinctive processes: vasculogenesis and angiogenesis (see Ref. 1 for review). The initial process of vascular development is vasculogenesis. In this process, EC precursors (so-called hemangioblasts or angioblasts of mesoderm origin) differentiate into ECs and form a primitive vascular plexus. In the subsequent process of angiogenesis, neovessels form from extant primitive vessels and branch to the entire body. In the adult, phys-

---

[a]This work was supported by a Grant-in-Aid for Scientific Research on Priority Areas from the Japanese Ministry of Education, Science, Sports and Culture.

[c]Address for correspondence: Yasufumi Sato, Department of Vascular Biology, Institute of Development, Aging and Cancer, Tohoku University, Sendai, 980-8575 Japan. Voice: 81-22-717-8532; fax: 81-22-717-8533.

y-sato@idac.tohoku.ac.jp

iological angiogenesis is observed only in a few restricted places, such as in the endometrium and the ovarian follicle, and this process is normally transient. However, persistent angiogenesis appears to play a crucial role in pathological states such as solid tumors, diabetic retinopathy, rheumatoid arthritis, and atherosclerosis.

Angiogenesis is controlled by the balance of angiogenic factors and angiogenesis inhibitors. A number of angiogenic factors have been identified to date. Among them, vascular endothelial growth factor (VEGF), a dimeric endothelial cell–specific growth factor, is thought to play a principal role by stimulating migration and proliferation of ECs and the expression of angiogenesis-related genes in ECs. In addition, VEGF increases vascular permeability, exerts procoagulant activity via the induction of tissue factor, and promotes the expression of VCAM-1 and ICAM-1 in ECs (see Ref. 2 for review). VEGF is mainly synthesized by cells surrounding ECs and acts on ECs as a paracrine factor. At least four species of VEGF can be produced as 121, 165, 189, and 206 amino acid forms as a result of alternative splicing.[3–6] VEGF binds to two receptor-type tyrosine kinases, Flt-1 (VEGF receptor-1)[7] and KDR/Flk-1 (VEGF receptor-2),[8] and to membrane protein neuropilin-1, which does not contain a tyrosine kinase domain.[9] Flk-1 is the murine homologue of human KDR, which shares 85% homology with KDR.[10] Both Flt-1 and KDR/Flk-1 have seven immunoglobulin-like domains in the extracellular domain, a single transmembrane region, and a consensus tyrosine kinase domain in the intracellular domain, which is interrupted by a kinase-insert domain. Flt-1 has a higher affinity for VEGF with dissociation constant (K_d) values of approximately 10–20 pM,[7] while the K_d of KDR is approximately 75–125 pM.[11] It has been shown that Flt-1 and KDR/Flk-1 have distinct functions in vascular development in embryos. Flk-1 knockout mice, which die by embryonic day 8.5 (E8.5), lack both ECs and hematopoietic cells.[12] In contrast, Flt-1 knockout mice, which also die around E8.5, have abundant ECs, but the ECs do not assemble into functional vessels.[13] In spite of these observations in knockout mice, the properties of KDR/Flk-1 and Flt-1 in the signal transduction of VEGF in differentiated ECs is largely unknown.

We investigated the roles of two VEGF receptors in human umbilical vein endothelial cells (HUVECs) by using newly developed blocking monoclonal antibodies (mAbs) against Flt-1 and KDR. VEGF induces the expression of various angiogenesis-related genes in ECs. Here, we observed that VEGF induced the expression of transcription factor Ets-1, matrix metalloproteinase-1 (MMP-1), KDR, and Flt-1 in HUVECs. Ets-1 is the product of the *c-ets-1* gene and is composed of 450 amino acids. It is a prototype of the Ets family transcription factors. We have previously demonstrated that Ets-1 is induced in ECs in response to angiogenic growth factors—not only VEGF but also bFGF.[14,15] Ets-1 regulates angiogenesis by inducing matrix metalloproteinase-1 (MMP-1), MMP-3, MMP-9, urokinase-type plasminogen activator (u-PA), and integrin β3 in ECs as target genes.[14,16] In addition, the promoter of Flt-1 contains Ets binding motifs and the expression of Flt-1 is regulated by Ets family transcription factors.[17] The induction of Ets-1 was augmented as early as 2 h after the addition of VEGF to the medium, whereas those of MMP-1 and Flt-1 were augmented at 4 h (FIG. 1). In contrast, the expression of KDR was unchanged by the treatment with VEGF. VEGF-mediated induction of Ets-1, as well as those of MMP-1 and Flt-1, was partially (10 μg/ml) or completely (30 μg/ml) inhibited by anti-KDR mAb, whereas anti–Flt-1 mAb (1 μg/ml) exhibited no inhibition (FIG. 1). In-

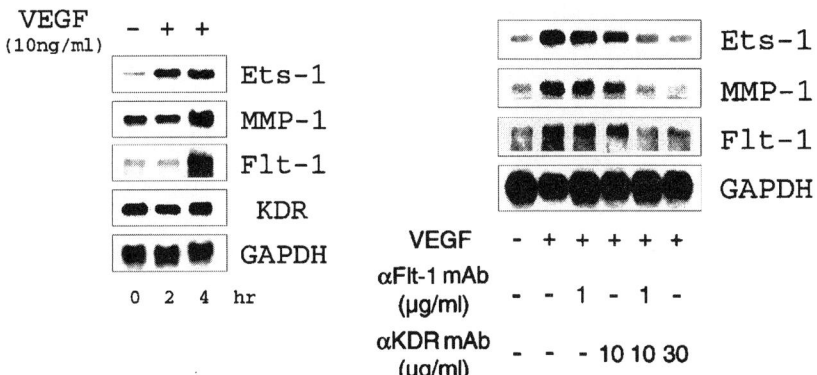

FIGURE 1. The dimers of KDR/KDR and KDR/Flt-1 regulated the expression of ets-1, MMP-1, and Flt-1 transcripts. HUVECs were left untreated or exposed to indicated concentrations of anti–Flt-1 mAb and/or anti–KDR mAb 15 min before the addition of VEGF. After the cultures were incubated with or without 10 ng/ml of VEGF for 4 h, total RNA was extracted and Northern blotting for ets-1, MMP-1, and Flt-1 transcripts was performed. VEGF induced ets-1, MMP-1, and Flt-1 in HUVECs. Ets-1 was induced as early as 2-h incubation with VEGF, while Flt-1 and MMP-1 were induced by 4-h incubation. KDR was not induced by VEGF. Anti-KDR mAb inhibited VEGF-stimulated induction of angiogenesis-related genes partially (10 μg/ml) or completely (30 μg/ml), whereas anti–Flt-1 mAb (1 μg/ml) had no effect.

terestingly, the combination of anti–Flt-1 mAb (1 μg/ml) and anti-KDR mAb (10 μg/ml) almost completely inhibited VEGF-mediated induction of Ets-1, MMP-1, and Flt-1. The combined effect of mAbs appeared to be due to KDR/Flt-1 heterodimerization,[18] and that the KDR homodimer and the KDR/Flt-1 heterodimer but not the Flt-1 homodimer transduced the signals of VEGF for the induction of Ets-1. VEGF stimulated DNA synthesis of HUVECs and is mediated by the same signaling system as the expression of Ets-1.[18]

VEGF stimulated the migration of HUVECs. In contrast to DNA synthesis and Ets-1 expression, 1 μg/ml of anti–Flt-1 mAb completely inhibited VEGF-stimulated migration of HUVECs, whereas anti-KDR mAb (up to 30 μg/ml) showed 50% inhibition.[18] VEGF elicited actin reorganization and vinculin assembly in focal adhesion plaque of HUVECs. Anti–Flt-1 mAb completely abrogated actin reorganization, but failed to affect vinculin assembly. Conversely, anti-KDR mAb inhibited vinculin assembly, but failed to affect actin reorganization. VEGF induced phosphorylation of FAK and paxillin.[18] Anti–Flt-1 mAb exhibited no effect on phosphorylation of FAK or paxillin, whereas anti-KDR completely inhibited phosphorylation of FAK and paxillin.[18] Therefore, Flt-1–mediated signal regulates actin reorganization, whereas KDR–mediated signal regulates vinculin assembly, both of which are required for cell migration.

FIGURE 2 summarizes the properties of Flt-1 and KDR. Our results clearly demonstrate that KDR and Flt-1 are both required for the signal transduction of VEGF effects in human vascular ECs of primary culture. However, Flt-1 lacking the tyrosine kinase domain has recently been shown to be sufficient for the normal devel-

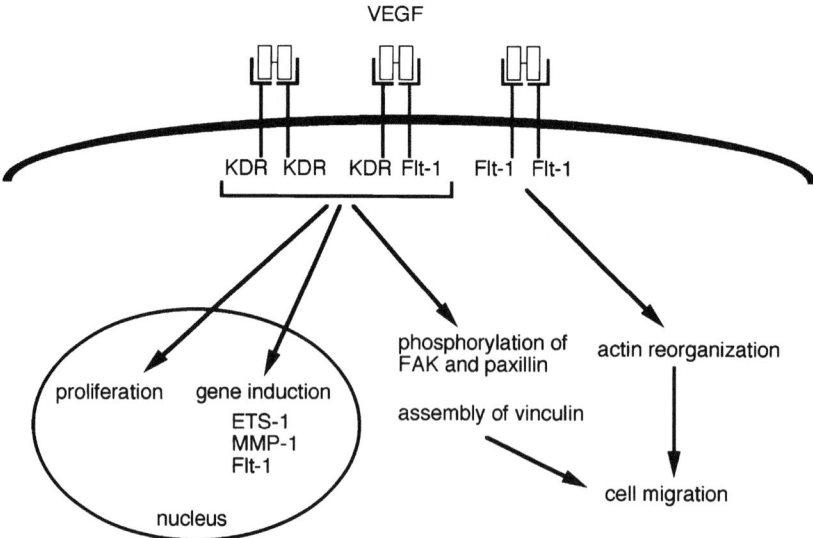

FIGURE 2. The intracellular signal transduction of VEGF-mediated effects in HUVECs. VEGF elicited dimers of KDR/KDR, KDR/Flt-1, and Flt-1/Flt-1. The dimers of KDR/KDR and KDR/Flt-1 mediated the signals for DNA synthesis, gene induction, phosphorylation of FAK and paxillin, and vinculin assembly. In contrast, the dimer of Flt-1/Flt-1 regulated cell migration via actin reorganization.

opment of vasculature in the murine embryo.[19] This discrepancy raises several questions. Is kinase-negative Flt-1 really negative in terms of the signal transduction? The signal transduction systems of ECs in those mice expressing tyrosine kinase–negative Flt-1 need to be determined. It is possible that some other signaling molecules may associate with tyrosine kinase–negative Flt-1. Alternately, the role of Flt-1 in ECs of developing vasculature in embryo and in postnatal and adult differentiated ECs may not be identical. In any case, our present results provide important information for understanding the function of two VEGF receptors in human differentiated endothelial cells.

REFERENCES

1. RISAU, W. 1997. Mechanisms of angiogenesis. Nature **386:** 671–674.
2. FERRARA, N. & T. DAVIS-SMYTH. 1997. The biology of vascular endothelial growth factor. Endocr. Rev. **18:** 4–25.
3. LEUNG, D.W., G. CACHIANWS, W.J. KUANG, D.V. GOEDDEL & N. FERRARA. 1989. Vascular endothelial growth factor is a secreted angiogenic mitogen. Science **246:** 1306–1309.
4. KECK, P.J., S.D. HAUSER, G. KRIVI, K. SANZO, T. WARREN, J. FEDER & D.T. CONNOLLY. 1989. Vascular permeability factor, an endothelial cell mitogen related to PDGF. Science **246:** 1309–1312.

5. TISCHER, E., R. MITCHELL, T. HARTMANN, M. SILVA, D. GOSPODAROWICZ, J. FIDDES & J. ABRAHAM. 1991. The human gene for vascular endothelial growth factor. J. Biol. Chem. **266:** 11947–11954.
6. HOUCK, K.A., N. FERRARA, J. WINER, G. CACHIANES, B. LI & D.W. LEUNG. 1991. The vascular endothelial growth factor family: identification of a fourth molecular species and characterization of alternative splicing of RNA. Mol. Endocrinol. **5:** 1806–1814.
7. DE VRIES, C., J.A. ESCOBEDO, H. UENO, K. HOUCK, N. FERRARA & L.T. WILLIAMS. 1992. The fms-like tyrosine kinase, a receptor for vascular endothelial growth factor. Science **255:** 989–991.
8. QUINN, T.P., K.G. PETERS, C. DE VRIES, N. FERRARA & L.T. WILLIAMS. 1993. Fetal liver kinase 1 is a receptor for vascular endothelial growth factor and is selectively expressed in vascular endothelium. Proc. Natl. Acad. Sci. USA **90:** 75339
9. SOKER, S., S. TAKASHIMA, H.Q. MIAO, G. NEUFELD & M. KLAGSBRUN. 1998. Neuropilin-1 is expressed by endothelial and tumor cells as an isoform-specific receptor for vascular endothelial growth factor. Cell **92:** 735–745.
10. MATTHEWS, W., C.T. JORDAN, M. GAVIN, N.A. JENKINS, N.G. COPELAND & I.R. LEMISCHKA. 1991. A receptor tyrosine kinase cDNA isolated from a population of enriched primitive hematopoietic cells and exhibiting close genetic linkage to c-kit. Proc. Natl. Acad. Sci. USA **88:** 9026–9030.
11. TERMAN, B.I., M.E. DOUGHER-VERMAZEN, D. CARRION, D.C. DIMITROV, D. ARMELLINO, D. GOSPODAROWICZ & P. BOHLEN. 1992. Identification of the KDR tyrosine kinase as a receptor for vascular endothelial cell growth factor. Biochem. Biophys. Res. Commun. **187:** 1579–1586.
12. SHALABY, F., J. ROSSANT, T.P. YAMAGUCHI, M. GERTSENSTEIN, X.F. WU, M.L. BREIMAN & A.C. SCHUH. 1995. Failure of blood-island formation and vasculogenesis in Flk-1-deficient mice. Nature **376:** 62–66.
13. FONG, G.H., J. ROSSANT, M. GERTSENSTEIN & M.L. BREITMAN. 1995. Role of the Flt-1 receptor tyrosine kinase in regulating the assembly of vascular endothelium. Nature **376:** 66–70.
14. IWASAKA, C., K. TANAKA, M. ABE & Y. SATO. 1996. Ets-1 regulates angiogenesis by inducing the expression of urokinase-type plasminogen activator and matrix metalloproteinase-1 and the migration of vascular endothelial cells. J. Cell. Physiol. **169:** 522–531.
15. TANAKA, K., N. ODA, C. IWASAKA, M. ABE & Y. SATO. 1998. Induction of Ets-1 in endothelial cells during reendothelialization after denuding injury. J. Cell. Physiol. **176:** 235–244.
16. ODA, N. *et al.* 1999. ETS-1 converts endothelial cells to the angiogenic phenotype by inducing the expression of matrix metalloproteinases and integrinbeta3. J. Cell. Physiol. **178:** 121–132.
17. WAKIYA, K., A. BEGUE, D. STEHELIN & M. SHIBUYA. 1996. A cAMP response element and an Ets motif are involved in the transcriptional regulation of flt-1 tyrosine kinase (vascular endothelial growth factor receptor 1) gene. J. Biol. Chem. **271:** 30823–30828.
18. KANNO, S., N. ODA, M. ABA, Y. TERAI, M. ITO, K. SHITARA, K. TABAYASHI, M. SHIBUYA & Y. SATO. 2000. Roles of two VEGF receptors, Flt-1 and KDR, in the signal transduction of VEGF effects in human vascular endothelial cells. Oncogenes (In press.)
19. HIRATSUKA, S., O. MINOWA, J. KUNO, T. NODA & M. SHIBUYA. 1998. Flt-1 lacking the tyrosine kinase domain is sufficient for normal development and angiogenesis in mice. Proc. Natl. Acad. Sci. USA **95:** 9349–9354.

Questions and Answers

F.W. LUSCINSKAS (*Brigham and Women's Hospital, Boston, MA, USA*): Can you tell us to what epitopes your antibodies bind?

SATO: The epitope of the binding site is already characterized and it is located in the first and second immunoglobulin domain. We are now preparing another manuscript to show that the specific epitope of the monoclonal antibody recognizes the first and the second immunoglobulin domain.

LUSCINSKAS: Have you had an opportunity to visualize as a cell biology experiment where the receptors go if you signal to the KDR-1 versus the other receptor with your antibodies? Can you follow the localization, did they go to the nucleus or not depending on which receptors you allow to be ligated?

SATO: We did not do those experiments.

P. CARMELIET (*Flanders Interuniversity Institute of Biotechnology, Leuven, Belgium*): What is the molecular weight of the receptor-1 and receptor-2?

SATO: Flt-1 is a little bit smaller than KDR and it seems that Flt-1 is approximately 210 and KDR is 230.

CARMELIET: Maybe I missed it on your slides, but did you show that you really have one molecule, I mean heterodimerization? Might you not just have picked up KDR and then the other one separately?

SATO: In that experiment we did not crosslink, so we just did IP and Western, using their different antibodies. If we use anti–Flt-1 for the IP and anti-KDR for the Western, we only show band.

CARMELIET: But if they just sit together, forming a large complex or something?

SATO: In the SDS page, they dissociate. We did not crosslink.

CARMELIET: Have you looked at the effect of the heterodimers of VEGF and PlGF or if you give them both separately together as homodimers? Do you see any effect then, especially because you suggest the heterodimerization of the receptors?

SATO: It is a good point, but we have not had an opportunity to do those experiments.

G. GARCIA-CARDENA (*Brigham and Women's Hospital, Boston, MA, USA*): Nitric oxide has been involved in the downstream effects of VEGF. For example, it causes edema and hypotension in some of the collateral experiments or limb ischemic experiments. Have you looked at nitric oxide release *in vivo* or *in vitro*, using your antibodies? Can you block nitric oxide release without blocking cell migration? That would be a fantastic tool for a lot of things.

SATO: We have not done it yet.

S. MORI (*Chiba University, Chiba, Japan*): I would like to ask one question about the downstream effects of Flt-1 homodimers. You showed that migration was stimulated by Flt-1 homodimers and there was a report that the p38 is involved in the migration process stimulated by the VEGF. Do you have data about this?

SATO: Yes, we have data. It seems that the Flt-1 homodimer transduces the signal by a p38 MAP kinase and that regulates actin organization. In case of KDR-KDR homodimer or KDR-Flt heterodimer, there is activation of MAP ERK 1/2 to cross the MAP kinase. Also, our data suggest that the ERK 1/2 is not the major player for the migration. Our results indicated that both signals are required for cell adhesion, the other signal.

MORI: According to your data, are Ets-1 as well as actin assembly required for cell migration?

SATO: It is required. So if you block the KDR, there is a 50% reduction of cell migration. What I am saying is that there are two systems; one is the engine, the other is the wheel. If you break the engine, the car cannot move; and if you break the wheel, the car can move, but very, very slowly.

J. POUYSSÉGUR (*Center de Biochemie-CRNS, Nice, France*): I was very interested in the aspect of heterodimerization. Do you think that the homodimer KDR is better than the heterodimer flt-1/KDR? You mentioned the work of people who have done this expression of KDR versus flt-1 in the porcine aortic cells. I just wanted to know whether they mentioned, when you introduce the flt-1, did they get higher sensitivity for mitogenicity when KDR is present? This would be an argument that the heterodimer is perhaps more potent for mitogenicity than the homodimer KDR.

SATO: I understand your point, but at this moment we can't distinguish those homodimers and heterodimers. We need another tool to induce only the heterodimer or only the homodimer.

Regulation of Angiogenesis by Controlling VEGF Receptor

SEI-ITSU MUROTA,[a] MITSUE ONODERA, AND IKUO MORITA

Section of Cellular Physiological Chemistry, Graduate School, Tokyo Medical and Dental University, 1-5-45, Yushima, Bunkyo-ku, Tokyo 113-8549, Japan

ABSTRACT: The endothelial cells cultured in collagen gel caused upregulation of KDR expression, which resulted in an increase in tube formation. Endothelial cells exposed to high glucose (33 mmol/l) for 30 days increased the tube formation induced by VEGF, but not by serum and bFGF. Immunohistochemical study showed that KDR expression was upregulated by the high-glucose treatment. The endothelial cells treated with 0.5 ~ 5 µg/ml eicosapentaenoic acid (EPA, 20:5, n-3) for 48 h displayed a dose-dependent suppression of tube formation, VEGF-induced proliferation, and activation of p42/p44 MAP kinase but not bFGF-induced ones. Pretreatment with arachidonic acid (20:4, n-6) and docosahexaenoic acid (22:6, n-3) did not show such effects. The expression of KDR was downregulated by the EPA pretreatment. The bone is the richest tissue in microvessel networks except for the liver. Osteoblasts produced VEGF and some factor(s) that could induce KDR upregulation in endothelial cells and could enhance tube formation. These results lead to the speculation that the regulation of KDR expression as well as VEGF production is deeply involved in angiogenesis under various conditions.

INTRODUCTION

The growth signal of vascular endothelial growth factor (VEGF) is transferred through its specific tyrosine kinase receptor, KDR. VEGF production is known to be regulated by various substances and conditions in several tissues and cells. By contrast, the regulation of KDR remains unknown. Therefore, in this paper we examined the nature of KDR regulation. Endothelial cells in culture were examined for the relationship between their tube-forming activity and KDR expression.

Angiogenesis is an important pathophysiological event occurring in various kinds of disorders, such as inflammation, wound repair, solid tumor growth, and proliferative diabetic retinopathy. To treat these disorders, it is necessary to discover the mechanism of angiogenesis and thus control neovascularization. Until today, some *in vivo* assay systems using the corneal micropocket, the transparent chamber, and chick embryo chorioallantoic membrane, for example, have been used for evaluation of neovascularization. However, the reliance on these *in vivo* assay systems alone is troubling. The obtained results must be viewed with some suspicion because we cannot completely eliminate the possibility of nonspecific neovascularization due to inflammation. Any substance can, more or less, induce inflammation if it is tested in

---

[a]Address for correspondence: Sei-itsu Murota, Voice: 81-3-5803-5574; fax: 81-3-5803-0212. murocell@dent.tmd.ac.jp

any of these *in vivo* models. Subsequently, the induced inflammation can produce various kinds of chemical mediators, including angiogenic substances such as PGE_2. Therefore, even if neovascularization is observed in such *in vivo* models, we cannot be sure that the induced neovascularization is surely caused by the substance itself. For this reason we established an *in vitro* assay system capable of evaluating angiogenesis.[1,2] By using this *in vitro* assay system we obtained a good correlation between KDR expression and tube-forming activity of endothelial cells.

EXPERIMENTAL METHODS

Endothelial cells were examined on their tube-forming activity by the *in vitro* type I collagen gel method.[1–3] KDR expression was quantified by immunofluorescence image analysis.[4]

RESULTS AND DISCUSSION

EPA-Pretreated Endothelial Cells Show Downregulation of KDR Expression

We examined the effects of some polyunsaturated fatty acids on the tube formation. Endothelial cells were cultured with a medium supplemented with one of three polyunsaturated fatty acids, namely eicosapentaenoic acid (EPA), arachidonic acid, and docosahexaenoic acid (DHA). After 48 h, fatty acid composition in the cellular phospholipid fraction of each culture was analyzed. EPA treatment caused a significant increase (more than 20-fold) in the EPA content in the phospholipid fraction in the cells. Similarly, arachidonic acid treatment and DHA treatment caused significant increases in the arachidonic acid content and the DHA content in the phospholipid fraction in each culture, respectively.[3]

We then examined tube-forming activity of these polyunsaturated fatty acid–pretreated cells. In the EPA-pretreated endothelial cells, tube-forming activity was significantly suppressed. On the other hand, arachidonic acid pretreatment caused a significant increase in the tube-forming activity of the cells, while DHA pretreatment was essentially inactive.[3] The EPA pretreatment did not affect the production of PGE_2 and PGI_2 in the cells at all. The inhibitory effect of the EPA treatment on tube formation was dependent on the dose of EPA in the pretreatment.

To figure out why the EPA-pretreated endothelial cells lost their angiogenic activity, we examined their response to growth factors. The control cells responded well to VEGF and increased cell number almost twofold within four days, while the EPA-pretreated cells responded very little to VEGF. On the other hand, there was no difference between the two groups in the response to bFGF, though the response was not as large. The lack of response to VEGF was specific to EPA-pretreated cells. Cells pretreated with arachidonic acid and DHA responded normally to VEGF and in number similarly to the control cells.[4]

Since the VEGF signal is transferred through MAP kinase, we next examined the effect of VEGF on MAP kinase activity in endothelial cells. In the control cells, VEGF treatment caused a big increase in the MAP kinase activity, while in the EPA-pretreated endothelial cells, the VEGF-induced MAP kinase activation was very

TABLE 1. Culture in collagen gel caused upregulation of KDR expression, followed by increased cell number in response to VEGF in endothelial cells ($N = 4$)

	Culture in plastic dish	Culture in collagen gel
KDR expression[a] (% of control)	45.1 ± 1.3 (100)	88.5 ± 0.7 (196)
Cell number[b]	1.8-fold	3.6-fold

[a]Immunofluorescence intensity (×1,000).
[b]Increased cell number during two days of VEGF (10 ng/ml) treatment.

much limited. Yet when exposed to bFGF, the EPA-pretreated cells responded normally and increased the MAP kinase activity to the same extent as the control cells.[4]

Examination of VEGF receptor expression showed that EPA pretreatment caused significant downregulation of KDR expression.[4]

Upregulation of KDR Is Seen under Various Conditions in Endothelial Cells

Since we found that the EPA pretreatment caused downregulation of KDR in endothelial cells, we next determined under what conditions upregulation of KDR occurs.

During the course of the investigation, we found that endothelial cells regulate their own angiogenesis by controlling their VEGF receptor expression, which happens under various conditions.

First of all, we found KDR was upregulated in endothelial cells when they are cultured in collagen. In a sandwich culture condition[1,2] endothelial cells are surrounded by collagen molecules. In this environment endothelial cells expressed more KDR than control cells, which were cultured in ordinary plastic dishes. Due to the upregulation of KDR, the endothelial cells cultured in the collagen gel responded well to VEGF and increased more in cell number than those cultured in ordinary plastic dishes (TABLE 1).

Hyperglycemia is one of the risk factors of microangiopathy in diabetes mellitus. Therefore, we next examined the effect of high glucose treatment on KDR expression in endothelial cells.

A 30-day culture of endothelial cells in a medium containing 33 mM glucose caused upregulation of KDR. VEGF treatment caused further upregulation of KDR in the long-term, high-glucose culture, but not in the control culture. Due to the upregulation of KDR, the endothelial cells in the long-term, high-glucose culture responded very well to VEGF and increased tube formation to almost double the control culture (TABLE 2). Short-term treatment, i.e., only for three days, of endothelial cells with high glucose was essentially inactive (data not shown). The results suggest that long-term exposure to high glucose is necessary for endothelial cells to upregulate KDR expression.

When endothelial cells were cultured with a conditioned medium of osteoblasts, a remarkable increase in the KDR expression was evident, suggesting that there maybe some factor in the osteoblast-conditioned medium that enables endothelial cells to upregulate their KDR expression. Due to the upregulation of KDR, the endothelial cells cultured in the osteoblast-conditioned medium responded well to VEGF and increased tube formation to almost double the control culture (TABLE 3).

TABLE 2. Long-term, high-glucose treatment effects[a]

	Control	Glucose	Glucose + VEGF[b]
KDR expression[c] (% of control)	106 ± 8.6 (100)	152 ± 12 (143)	251 ± 5.5 (237)
Tube length $(mm/mm^2) \times 10^{-2}$ (% of control)	4.31 ± 0.13 (100)	4.12 ± 0.06 (96)	15.95 ± 0.13 (370)

[a]Long-term (30 days) treatment of endothelial cells with high-dose glucose (33 mM) caused upregulation of KDR expression, followed by increased tube formation in response to VEGF ($N = 4$).
[b]10 ng/ml for four days.
[c]Immunofluorescence intensity (×1,000).

TABLE 3. Effects of osteoblast-conditioned medium on KDR expression and tube formation[a]

	Control medium	Osteoblast-conditioned medium	Osteoblast-conditioned medium + VEGF[b]
KDR expression[c] (% of control)	60.0 ± 1.6 (100)	140 ± 10 (233)	—
Tube length $(mm/mm^2) \times 10^{-2}$ (% of control)	3.3 ± 0.5 (100)	31.5 ± 1.9 (955)	92.0 ± 7.5 (2,788)

[a]Culture in the osteoblast-conditioned medium caused upregulation of KDR expression, followed by increased tube formation in response to VEGF in endothelial cells ($N = 4$).
[b]10 ng/ml for four days.
[c]Immunofluorescence intensity per cell (×1,000).

The mechanisms of the up- and downregulation of KDR expression in endothelial cells under such conditions as described above still remain unknown. However, it is known that there are two NFκB sites, three AP-2 sites, and five SP-1 sites in the promoter region of the human KDR gene. Our preliminary data showed that EPA pretreatment caused suppression of NFκB activation in endothelial cells. This may be associated with the downregulation of KDR expression in the EPA-pretreated endothelial cells. Regarding the upregulation of KDR in collagen cultures, it may be speculated that the signal is transferred through cell adhesion molecule, since there is a paper showing that VEGF causes upregulation of the $\alpha_v\beta_3$ in cultured endothelial cells.

Regarding the upregulation of KDR under the long-term, high-glucose culture, it may partly be due to advanced glycosylation endproducts (AGE), which are produced nonenzymatically during the long-term culture in a high concentration of glucose. Because our preliminary experiments showed that the addition of AGE to the culture medium caused upregulation of KDR expression in endothelial cells within just three days.

Regarding the upregulation of KDR expression in endothelial cells cultured in the osteoblast-conditioned medium, there is a possibility that the VEGF produced by osteoblasts may cause a positive feedback of KDR expression.

REFERENCES

1. NAKAO-HAYASHI, J., H. ITO, T. KANAYASU, N. ASUWA, I. MORITA, T. ISHII & S. MUROTA. 1991. Effects of glucose on migration, proliferation and tube formation by vascular endothelial cells. Virch. Archiv. B Cell. Pathol. **60:** 245–252.
2. KANAYASU, T., J. NAKAO-HAYASHI, N. ASUWA, I. MORITA, T. ISHII, H. ITO & S. MUROTA. 1989. Leukotriene C_4 stimulates angiogenesis in bovine carotid artery endothelial cells in vitro. Biochem. Biophys. Res. Commun. **159:** 572–578.
3. KANAYASU, T., I. MORITA, J. NAKAO-HAYASHI, C. FUJISAWA, H. ITO & S. MUROTA. 1991. Eicosapentaenoic acid inhibits in vitro angiogenesis via inhibition of vascular endothelial cell proliferation. Lipids **26:** 271–276.
4. YANG, S., I. MORITA & S. MUROTA. 1998. Eicosapentaenoic acid attenuates vascular endothelial growth factor-induced proliferation via inhibiting FLK-1 receptor expression in bovine carotid artery endothelial cells. J. Cell. Physiol. **176:** 342–349.

Questions and Answers

J.H. CAMPBELL (*University of Queensland, Brisbane, Australia*): The collagen that you are sandwiching your cell between, does it matter what type of collagen you use? Which type did you use? Is it an effect of the collagen itself or is it simply the fact that you are creating a microenvironment for the endothelial cells?

MUROTA: It was type I collagen, and the VEGF receptor expression was modulated by environmental factors, but also, as you suggested, by the geometry of the culture conditions. There are both possibilities. In the case of collagen, the mechanism of upregulation of collagen is still unknown, but maybe the collagen acts through an integrin like $\alpha_v\beta_3$.

Y. SATO (*Tohoku University, Sendai, Japan*): You showed the induction of KDR. Have you ever checked whether it is at the transcriptional level or the translational level? Have you done Northern blotting or Western blotting?

MUROTA: Such experiments will be done in the near future.

SATO: For the induction of KDR by the osteoblast culture medium, what is the physiological role?

MUROTA: We were speculating that one of the factors may be VEGF. We know already that osteoblasts produce VEGF. It might include the basic FGF, but we don't have the evidence. There is a report that VEGF induces KDR upregulation, so maybe they act in a positive feedback way.

SATO: Where the osteoclasts in the bone exist, is there active angiogenesis?

MUROTA: Yes, bone is the richest tissue in the body with regard to angiogenesis, except for the liver.

M.A. GIMBRONE (*Brigham and Women's Hospital, Boston, MA, USA*): I would like to get back to the question of what the signal is in the matrix that may be inducing tube formation. A number of years ago, Elisabetta Dejana, when she was visiting with us on a minisabbatical, did some very interesting experiments showing that there were in fact integrin receptors that could bind vitronectin on the apical membrane of a polarized endothelial monolayer. In other words, when you put an endothelial cell down, there is a top and a bottom normally in culture and we think the same is true *in vivo*. She demonstrated, in fact, by surface iodination and fractionation of the surfaces that the apical membrane was perfectly competent to bind matrix proteins. In your model you were forcing that binding by making the sandwich. Have you done a "half-sandwich" in which you grow the endothelial cells on the vitrogen gel, do not superimpose the top monolayer, and examine the VEGF receptor induction in responsiveness, etc.?

MUROTA: I have not done a "half-sandwich" culture, but we did mix the culture with collagen gel, and we got a beautiful upregulation of KDR.

GIMBRONE: So the hypothesis I would propose is that the polarity interruption by allowing matrix to bind to the apical membrane in the differentiated phenotype is the switch that enables the formation of an angiogenic tube.

MUROTA: I think you are right.

Y. YAMAMOTO (*Kanazawa University, Kanazawa, Japan*): You showed that longer exposures to glucose, but not short exposure, induce KDR and potentiate tube formation. Is it possible that glycation rather than glucose itself accounts for this?

MUROTA: We have done that experiment already. One of the mechanisms that we are thinking of is that the advanced glycation endproduct (AGE) plays a role. We added AGE directly to the culture and it upregulated KDR in only three days. So I think that the AGE plays a very important role in this.

YAMAMOTO: What do you think is the major factor responsible for the osteoblast-derived conditioned medium effects?

MUROTA: We still don't know. We are thinking VEGF and maybe basic FGF are candidates.

YAMAMOTO: I have a comment related to Dr. Sato's question about the occurrence of osteoblasts. To my knowledge, in some circumstances pericytes that are neighbors to endothelial cells can trans-differentiate into osteoblasts, such as under hypoxia or exposure to VEGF. The latter circumstance is what we have observed. Osteoblast-conditioned-medium–like effect can occur *in vivo*, and the major molecule responsible for that may be osteopontin, whose major effect on the vasculature has recently been well documented.

MUROTA: Thank you for your comment.

S. MORI (*Chiba University, Chiba, Japan*): I have a question about the mechanism of high glucose–enhanced KDR expression. Did you check the glucosamine in your promoter assay? Because many of the glucosamine response elements contain SP-1 sites, as does the VEGF promoter.

MUROTA: Thank you. We have not checked it yet.

Transcriptional Regulation of Smooth Muscle Phenotypic Modulation

RYOZO NAGAI,[a–c] KEIKO KOWASE,[b] AND MASAHIKO KURABAYASHI[b]

[a]*Department of Cardiovascular Medicine, University of Tokyo, Graduate School of Medicine, Tokyo, Japan*

[b]*The Second Department of Internal Medicine, Gunma University School of Medicine*

ABSTRACT: Phenotypic modulation of vascular smooth muscle cell plays a pivotal role in the development of vascular pathology, such as atherosclerosis and restenosis after angioplasty. We have identified the zinc finger protein BTEB2 as a DNA binding protein that regulates the nonmuscle myosin heavy chain (SMemb) promoter. BTEB2 is expressed in fetal aorta but not in adult aorta and is induced in the neointima in response to vascular injury. BTEB2 also activates a number of vascular disease–associated genes, such as tissue factor, PAI-1 (plasminogen activator inhibitor-1), and Egr-1 gene. We have further isolated and characterized the human BTEB2 gene. Functional studies using 5′-deletion and site-directed mutation constructs demonstrated that phorbol ester induces Egr-1, which can activate the BTEB2 promoter through binding to −32 from the transcription start site. These results suggest that phenotypic modulation of vascular smooth muscle cells occurring in response to mitogen stimulation may be mediated by BTEB2 through Egr-1 induction.

INTRODUCTION

Vascular smooth muscle cells (SMCs) display two distinct phenotypes depending on the growth condition both *in vivo* and *in vitro*.[1,2] Phenotypic modulation of vascular SMCs plays a critical role in the development of vascular pathology, such as atherosclerosis and restenosis after percutaneous transcatheter coronary angioplasty (PTCA).[3,4] Among many differences between these two phenotypes are the cytoskeletal organization, ability to synthesize growth factors, and their receptors and extracellular matrices.[5,6] Because phenotypic modulation of SMCs involves a cascade of events in which different genes are turned on and off in a regulated manner, one approach to studying the pathogenesis of vascular disease is to analyze the regulatory mechanisms of gene expression that distinguish the two phenotypes.[4]

Smooth muscle myosin heavy chain is one of the most extensively characterized molecules that distinguish neointimal SMCs from medial SMCs.[7–12] We have identified at least three different isoforms of myosin heavy chains expressed in vascular SMC.[13] SM1 and SM2 are generated from a single gene through an alternative splicing of the 3′ exons and represent a differentiation marker of contractile type SMCs. SMemb, also known as an NMHC-B, is encoded by a distinct gene and represents an undifferentiation marker of vascular SMC.[7,14]

---

[c]Address for correspondence: Ryozo Nagai, M.D., Department of Cardiovascular Medicine, University of Tokyo Graduate School of Medicine, 7-3-1 Hongo, Bunkyo, Tokyo 113-8859. Voice: 03-5800-6526; fax 03-3815-2087.

In this study, we tried to elucidate the mechanisms that allow the SMemb gene to be transcriptionally active in a certain set of tissues.

MATERIALS AND METHOD

Cell Culture

C2/2 cells, a cell line derived from rabbit aortic smooth muscle cells, were cultured in Dulbecco's modified Eagle's medium (DMEM, GIBCO) with 5% fetal calf serum. COS-7 cells were cultured in DMEM with 10% fetal calf serum.

South Western Screening of C2/2 cDNA Library

The C2/2 cell cDNA library in the expression vector λgt11 was screened with the five-times repeated fragment of the −115 to −85 SMemb promoter as a probe, using the procedure of Singh and colleagues.[15] One of the positive clones selected was used as a probe of second screening with a rabbit fetal aortic cDNA library. The probe was radiolabeled using a random primed DNA labeling kit (Amersham). Positive clones were subcloned into the EcoRI site of pBluescript (Stratagene). The insert cDNA was sequenced by the dideoxy-chain termination method in denatured double-stranded plasmid.

Electrophoretic Mobility Shift Assay

In each gel mobility shift assay, 1 μg of GST-BTEB2 fusion protein was used. Annealed double-stranded oligonucleotides synthesized by Nippon Bio-Service were [α-^{32}P]-labeled by a fill-in reaction of Klenow fragments. The binding reaction was preincubated for 20 min at room temperature in a total volume of 20 μl containing 10 mM Tris HCl at pH 7.5, 50 mM NaCl, 0.5 mM DTT, 10% glycerol, 0.05% NP-40, 2 μg of poly(dI-dC) as a nonspecific competitor, and GST-BTEB2 fusion protein. After addition of about 1.0–2.0×10^{-4} cpm of the labeled probe, the reaction was incubated for an additional 20 min at room temperature and analyzed in a 5% polyacrylamide nondenaturing gel in low ionic strength buffer at 4°C

DNA Transfection and Luciferase Assay

Reporter plasmids for luciferase assay by deletion mutagenesis in SMemb promoter were prepared as: wild type 5′ deletion construct at −105 bp, −99 bp, −89 bp, and −36 bp of SMemb promoter sequence, which were named Del-105, Del-99, Del-89, and Del-36, respectively. In addition, reporter plasmids with mutation in SMemb promoter were prepared as: pGVm1, pGVm2, pGVm3, pGVm4, which contained a cluster of mutated nucleotides at −105 to −101, −100 to −96, −95 to −91, and −90 to −85, respectively. DNA transfection was performed by the modified calcium phosphate–DNA coprecipitation method. Transfected cell cultures were harvested for nuclear extract preparation 48 h after transfection. Cell extracts were prepared by luciferase assay kit, and luciferase activities were measured by the Lumat LB9501 luminometer (Berthold).

RNase Protection Assay

The 274 nt EcoRI/SacI 5′-region fragment from rabbit BTEB2 cDNA clone was subcloned into EcoRI/SacI site of pBluescript II SK(−) (Stratagene). After linearizing the plasmid DNA by digestion with HindIII, the RNA probe was synthesized with T3 RNA polymerase and [α-^{32}P]UTP by procedures of the Riboprobe Gemini System II kit (Promega). Five micrograms of total RNA were hybridized with the RNA probe. RNase protection assay was carried out using procedures of the Ribonuclease Protection Assay Kit (Ambion). The probe and protected fragments were analyzed on a denaturing urea-5% polyacrylamide gel.

Isolation and Sequencing Analysis of the Human BTEB2 Gene

Human placenta genomic library (Stratagene, San Diego, CA) was screened with a 657 bp cDNA probe containing the full length of the coding region of rabbit BTEB2 cDNA.[16] After three rounds of screening, four positive clones were isolated. One of these clones was selected for restriction enzyme and Southern blot analysis. The DNA fragment containing the 5′ end of the BTEB2 gene was identified by hybridizing the membranes with a 290 bp human BTEB2 cDNA probe containing the published 5′-untranslated region[16] and used for further restriction enzyme mapping and nucleotide sequencing.

Promoter-Luciferase Vector Chimeric Construct of BTEB2 Gene

The BTEB2 promoter-luciferase reporter genes were constructed by cloning a XbaI-SacII fragment that corresponded to nucleotides −2300 to +236 relative to the transcriptional start site into pGVB (PicaGene, Nippon Gene). The serial deletion constructs were prepared as follows; ApaI-SacII fragment (nucleotide +236 to −363) and SacI-SacII (nucleotide +236 to −67) fragments were cloned into the corresponding sites of the pGVB, and resultant plasmids were designated as −363Luc and −67Luc, respectively. The reporter plasmids of −32Luc and −32mutLuc were constructed by inserting the DNA fragments spanning −32 and +236 into pCR2.1 Vector (Invitrogen), and KpnI-HindIII fragments were cloned into the corresponding sites of the pGVB, respectively.

RESULTS

We isolated and characterized BTEB2, which recognizes the *cis*-acting regulatory element within the SMemb gene, by southwestern screening of a cDNA expression library prepared from C2/2 cells.[14,17] Sequence comparisons showed rabbit BTEB2 to be highly homologous to the human BTEB2 (FIG. 1). As shown in FIGURE 2, BTEB2 is a member of a family of Krüppel-like transcription factors to which GKLF, EKLF, and LKLF also belong (FIG. 2).[18] This family of transcription factors has been implicated in the regulation of tissue-specific gene expression.[19,20] EKLF was conclusively demonstrated to represent a CACCC-binding protein that controls the β-globin gene. LKLF and GKLF are preferentially expressed in lung and gut, respectively.

To determine the regulation of BTEB2 expression in aorta, we analyzed the BTEB2 mRNA levels in developing rabbit aorta. BTEB2 mRNA was more abundant in fetal and 2-week-old aortas in comparison to adult aortas. In addition, the immu-

```
        1          10         20         30         40         50         60         70         80         90        100
Rabbit  ATGCCAGTTCTACAAACCAGACAGCAGTGATGGACACTCTCAATGTTTCTATGTCACCCCCATGGCCTGAGCCCCATGGCCTGAGCCCATGGCACACACCTCTGCCGTTCCAC
        M  P  S  S  T  N  Q  T  A  V  M  D  T  L  N  V  S  M  S  A  A  M  A  G  L  N  T  H  T  S  A  V  P  Q
Human   M  P  S  S  T  N  Q  T  A  A  M  D  T  L  N  V  S  M  S  A  A  M  A  G  L  N  T  H  T  S  A  V  P  Q
                                 -CA-                   -T--                                  -T--        -T--  -G-
                   110        120        130        140        150        160        170        180        190        200

        AGACTGCAATGAAACAGTTCCAGGGCATGCCCCCTGCACATACACAATGCCAAGTCAGTTCTGCCACAACAGGCCACTTACTTTCCCCATCACCACC
        T  A  M  K  Q  F  Q  G  M  P  P  C  T  Y  T  M  P  S  Q  F  L  P  Q  Q  A  T  Y  F  P  P  S  P  P
        T  A  V  K  Q  F  Q  G  M  P  P  C  T  Y  T  M  P  S  Q  F  L  P  Q  Q  A  T  Y  F  P  P  S  P  P
             -G-                                                                               -G-
           210        220        230        240        250        260        270        280        290        300

        GAGCTCAGAGCCTGGAAGTCCTGATAGACAAGCAGAGATGCTCCAGAATTTAACCCCACCGCCATCCTATGCTGCTACCATTGCTTCCAAGCTGGCAATT
        S  S  E  P  G  S  P  D  R  Q  A  E  M  L  Q  N  L  T  P  P  S  Y  A  A  T  I  A  S  K  L  A  I
        A---                                -A-                       -T-                       -A---   -T-A---
           310        320        330        340        350        360        370        380        390        400

        CACAATCCAAATTTACCTGCCACCCTGCCAGTCAATTCGCAAAACATCCAACCCGTCAGATACAATAGAAGGAGTAACCCCGACCTGGAGAAACGCCGCA
        H  N  P  N  L  P  A  T  L  P  V  N  S  Q  N  I  Q  P  V  R  I  Y  N  R  R  S  N  P  D  L  E  K  R  R  I
        H  N  P  N  L  P  T  T  L  P  V  N  S  Q  N  I  Q  P  V  R  I  Y  N  R  R  S  N  P  D  L  E  K  R  R  I
                       -CA-              -T--C--A-                      -T--                                     -A---
           410        420        430        440        450        460        470        480        490        500

        TCCATTACTGCGATTACCCTGGCTGCACAAAAGTTTATACAAAGTCTCTCATTAAAAGCTCACCTGAGGACTCACCTGGTGAGAGCCGTACAAGTG
        H  Y  C  D  Y  P  G  C  T  K  V  Y  T  K  S  S  H  L  K  A  H  L  R  T  H  T  G  E  K  P  Y  K  C
        H  Y  C  D  Y  P  G  C  T  K  V  Y  T  K  S  S  H  L  K  A  H  L  R  T  H  T  G  E  K  P  Y  K  C
             -C-                -T--                           -C-                                  -A---
           510        520        530        540        550        560        570        580        590        600

        CACCTGGGAAGGCTGCGACTGGAGGTTCGCGCGCTCCGAGAGCTGACTCGCCACTACCGGAAGCACACCGGCGCCAAGCCCTTCCAGTGCGGGGTGTGC
        T  W  E  G  C  D  W  R  F  A  R  S  D  E  L  T  R  H  Y  R  K  H  T  G  A  K  P  F  Q  C  G  V  C
        T  W  E  G  C  D  W  R  F  A  R  S  D  E  L  T  R  H  Y  R  K  H  T  G  A  K  P  F  Q  C  G  V  C
        T---                           -A--G--T--         -C---                         -A---
           610        620        630        640        650        660

        AACCGCAGCTTCTCACGCTCGGACCACCTGGCCCTGCACATGAAGCGGCACCAGAACTGA
        N  R  S  F  S  R  S  D  H  L  A  L  H  M  K  R  R  H  Q  N  *
        N  R  S  F  S  R  S  D  H  L  A  L  H  M  K  R  H  Q  N  *
                         -G-          -T--A---         -T--A---
```

DNA Seq. homology: 93.6%
AA. Seq. homology: 98.6%

FIGURE 1. Nucleotide and deduced amino acid sequences of rabbit and human BTEB2 cDNA. Similarities of the nucleotide and amino acid sequences between rabbit and human are 93.6% (618/660) and 98.6% (216/219), respectively.

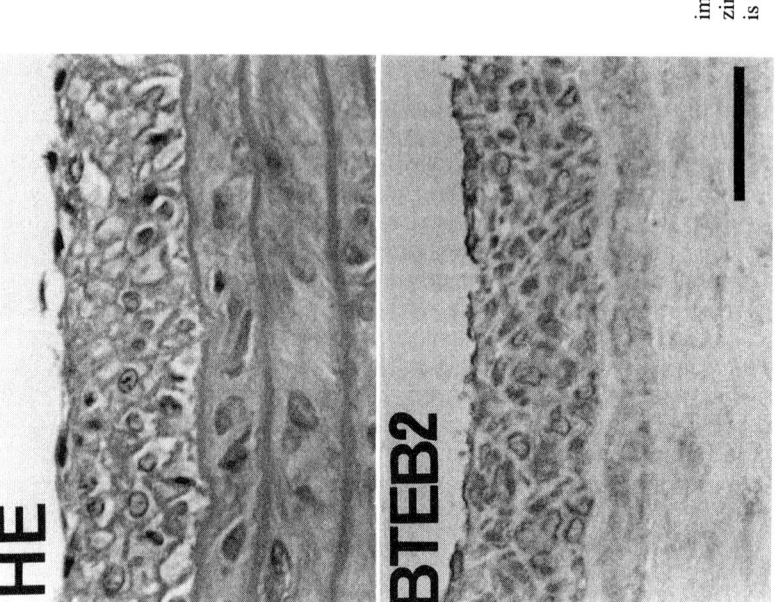

FIGURE 2. Structure of BTEB2. (*Left*) SMemb is expressed in neointima formed after balloon angioplasty in rabbit. (*Right*) BTEB2 contains three zinc-finger motifs that are involved in DNA binding. Transactivation domain is found in amino terminus of zinc finger domain.

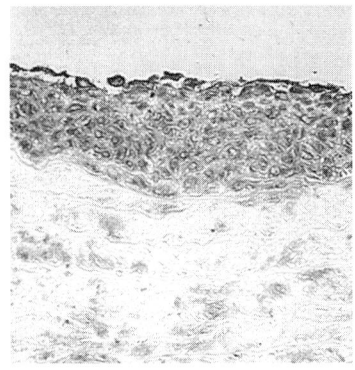 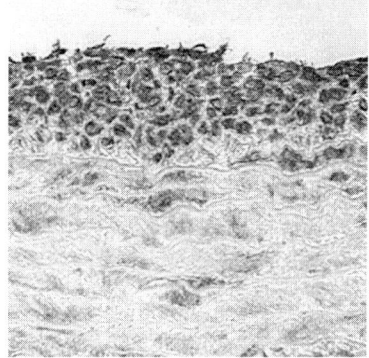

BTEB2 **Egr-1**

FIGURE 3. Expression of BTEB2 and Egr-1 after balloon injury. Rabbit aortic sections were stained with anti-BTEB2 or Egr-1. BTEB2 and Egr-1 were coexpressed in neointima 4 weeks after balloon injury.

nohistochemistry indicated that BTEB2 protein is markedly increased in neointima after balloon injury in rabbit aorta (FIG. 3). These data led us to hypothesize that BTEB2 plays a role in phenotypic modulation of vascular SMC. To test that, we cotransfected BTEB2 expression plasmid with a variety of reporter genes. As shown in FIGURES 4 and 5, BTEB2 induced the promoter activity of not only SMemb but also tissue factor, PAI-1, and Egr-1 genes. Tissue factor and PAI-1 are known to play a key role in the development of atherosclerosis.[21] Egr-1, one of the immediate early response genes, has recently been shown to be important for the inducible expression of platelet-derived growth factor-A and -B chain, vascular endothelial cell growth factor (VEGF), and basic fibroblast growth factor (bFGF).[22]

To determine the molecular mechanisms underlying this induction, we tried to identify the regulatory mechanisms of BTEB2 expression. We have cloned the promoter region of the human BTEB2 gene and identified *cis*-elements and *trans*-acting factors that govern the transcription of BTEB2 in vascular SMCs. Most notably, BTEB2 promoter contains a consensus sequence of Egr-1 binding site at −32 and gel shift assays demonstrate that this site is occupied by Egr-1. Incubation of the SMC nuclear extracts with anti–Egr-1 antibody clearly supershifted the complex. Transient transfection assays indicated that Egr-1 overexpression increased BTEB2 promoter activity and deletion of the sequence attenuated this inducibility (data not shown).

DISCUSSION

Our previous studies indicated that the SMemb gene in arterial wall is almost exclusively expressed in proliferating vascular smooth muscle cells in neointima, which develop in atherosclerosis and after balloon injury of aorta. In this study, we

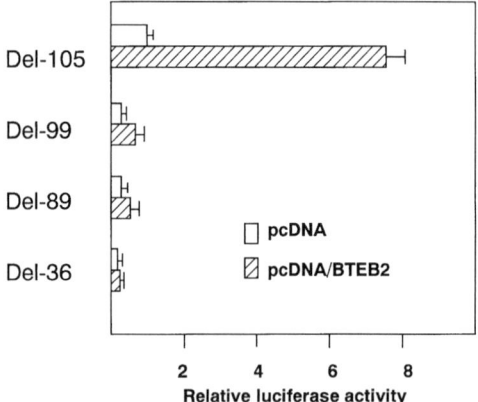

FIGURE 4. Effects of BTEB2 on SMemb promoter activity. The 5′-deletion analysis was carried out by using the constructs Del-105, Del-99, Del-89, and Del-36. COS7 cells were transfected with luciferase reporter constructs containing various lengths of the 5′-flanking region of the rabbit SMemb gene along with either empty vector or BTEB2 expression vector. In the bar graph, results are shown as relative luciferase activities normalized with protein concentration of the cell lysate and are shown by the relative value to the activity of the Del-105 without BTEB2.

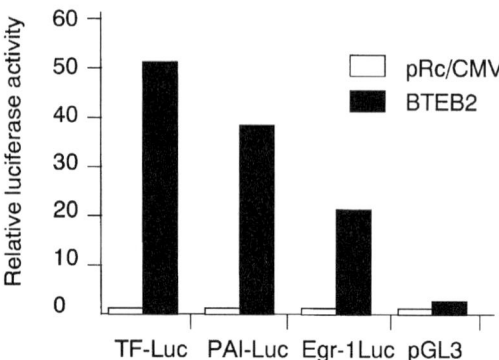

FIGURE 5. Activation of vascular disease–associated genes by BTEB2. BTEB2 expression plasmid was cotransfected with indicated reporter genes. Promoter of either tissue factor (TF), PAI-1, or Egr-1 was activated by BTEB2 expression vector.

have cloned a cDNA encoding BTEB2, a member of the zinc finger family of transcription factors, by using the southwestern screening method in which we employed a *cis*-acting regulatory element within the mouse SMemb gene as a hybridization probe. Major findings in this study were: (1) BTEB2 expression is downregulated in aorta during development—BTEB2 expression was clearly detected in fetal aorta but barely detected in adult aorta; (2) BTEB2 is expressed in neointima, which developed in response to balloon injury and the expression profiles are similar to that of SMemb expression; (3) BTEB2 can activate the SMemb promoter as assessed by transient transfection of SMemb-luciferase reporter plasmid into C2/2 cells; (4) BTEB2 also induces the promoter activity of tissue factor, PAI-1 or Egr-1, whose expression is known to be activated in vascular disease; and (5) BTEB2 gene is activated by growth stimulation through Egr-1 induction. These results suggest that BTEB2 is one of the transcription factors mediating the smooth muscle phenotypic modulation that occurs during the development of vascular disease.

We demonstrated that the 5'-flanking region of the BTEB2 gene harbors functional Egr-1 binding sites. Further, we indicated that BTEB2 mRNA levels were increased in response to phorbol ester (PMA) stimulation, which activates protein kinase C pathways. PMA-induced BTEB2 expression seems to be mediated through MEK1-Erk pathways as judged from the results that MEK1 inhibitor PD98059 significantly blocked this induction (data not shown). This was supported by the transient transfection experiments in which MEK1 expression construct activated BTEB2 promoter. Taken together, our data suggest that transcription of the BTEB2 gene is regulated by signal transduction pathways activated by growth promoting factors.

CONCLUSION

In conclusion, the functional data taken together with the DNA binding data support the hypothesis that the response of the BTEB2 promoter to PMA is mediated by Egr-1. Taking into account that the time course of the induction of BTEB2 by PMA is long-lasting compared with that of Egr-1, the findings in the present study may represent one of the molecular mechanisms underlying sustained activation of many genes in phenotypically modulated SMC subsequent to the activation of early response genes, including Egr-1.

REFERENCES

1. AIKAWA, M. *et al.* 1995. Phenotypic modulation of smooth muscle cells during progression of human atherosclerosis as determined by altered expression of myosin heavy chain isoforms. Ann. N.Y. Acad. Sci. **748:** 578–585.
2. OWENS, G.K. 1995. Regulation of differentiation of vascular smooth muscle cells. Physiol. Rev. **75:** 487–517.
3. ROSS, R. 1995. Cell biology of atherosclerosis. Annu. Rev. Physiol. **57:** 791–804.
4. DZAU, V.J. *et al.* 1993. Vascular biology and medicine in the 1990s: scope, concepts, potentials, and perspectives. Circulation **87:** 705–719.
5. FRID, M.G. *et al.* 1992. Phenotypic changes of human smooth muscle cells during development: late expression of heavy caldesmon and calponin. Dev. Biol. **153:** 185–193.
6. MIANO, J.M. *et al.* 1994. Smooth muscle myosin heavy chain exclusively marks the smooth muscle lineage during mouse embryogenesis. Circ. Res. **75:** 803–812.
7. NAGAI, R. *et al.* 1989. Identification of two types of smooth muscle myosin heavy chain isoforms by cDNA cloning and immunoblot analysis. J. Biol. Chem. **264:** 9734–9737.
8. KAWAMOTO, S. & R.S. ADELSTEIN. 1991. Chicken nonmuscle myosin heavy chains: differential expression of two mRNAs and evidence for two different polypeptides. J. Cell Biol. **112:** 915–924.
9. SIMONS, M. *et al.* 1991. Human nonmuscle myosin heavy chains are encoded by two genes located on different chromosomes. Circ. Res. **69:** 530–539.

10. BABIJ, P., C. KELLY & M. PERIASAMY. 1991. Characterization of a mammalian smooth muscle myosin heavy-chain gene: complete nucleotide and protein coding sequence and analysis of the 5′ end of the gene. Proc. Natl. Acad. Sci. USA **88:** 10676–10680.
11. MIANO, J.M. *et al.* 1994. Smooth muscle myosin heavy chain exclusively marks the smooth muscle lineage during mouse embryogenesis. Circ. Res. **75:** 803–812.
12. WATANABE, M. *et al.* 1996. Tandem elements of CCTCCC are required for the cell-type-specific expression of the mouse smooth muscle myosin heavy chain gene (SM1/2) promoter. Circ. Res. **78:** 978–989.
13. KURO-O, M. *et al.* 1989. Developmentally regulated expression of vascular smooth muscle myosin heavy chain isoforms. J. Biol. Chem. **264:** 18272–18275.
14. MANABE, I. *et al.* 1997. Isolation of the embryonic form of smooth muscle myosin heavy chain (SMemb/NMHC-B) gene and characterization of its 5′-flanking region. Biochem. Biophys. Res. Commun. **239:** 598–605.
15. SINGH, H. *et al.* 1988. Molecular cloning of an enhancer binding protein: isolation by screening of an expression library with a recognition site DNA. Cell **52:** 415–423.
16. SOGAWA, K. *et al.* 1993. cDNA cloning and transcriptional properties of a novel GC box-binding protein, BTEB2. Nucl. Acids Res. **21:** 1527–1532.
17. WATANABE, N. *et al.* 2000. BTEB2, a Krüppel-like transcription factor, regulates expression of the SMemb/non-muscle myosin heavy chain B (SMemb/NMHC-B) gene. Circ. Res. **85:** 182–191.
18. CHEN, X. & J.J. BIEKER. 1996. Erythroid Kruppel-like factor (EKLF) contains a multi-functional transcriptional activation domain important for inter- and intramolecular interactions. EMBO J. **15:** 5888–5896.
19. MILLER, I.J. & J.J. BIEKER. 1993. A novel, erythroid cell-specific murine transcription factor that binds to the CACCC element and is related to the Kruppel family of nuclear proteins. Mol. Cell. Biol. **13:** 2776–2786.
20. SHIELDS, J.M., R.J. CHRISTY & V.W. YANG. 1996. Identification and characterization of a gene encoding a gut-enriched Kruppel-like factor expressed during growth arrest. J. Biol. Chem. **271:** 20009–20017.
21. SCHNEIDERMAN, J. *et al.* 1992. Increased type 1 plasminogen activator inhibitor gene expression in atherosclerotic human arteries. Proc. Natl. Acad. Sci. USA **89:** 6998–7002.
22. KHACHIGIAN, L.M. *et al.* 1996. Egr-1-induced endothelial gene expression: a common theme in vascular injury. Science **271:** 1427–1431.

Questions and Answers

P. LIBBY (*Brigham and Women's Hospital, Boston, MA, USA*): That is a wonderful model, sticking with the problem and following it up in a progressive way over a sustained period of time. You made a convincing case that in vascular injury the BTEB2 and HEX are involved. Have you had a chance to look in atherosclerotic lesions and at some of the risk factors for atherosclerosis per se, such as lipoproteins or modified lipoproteins as regulators of these transcription factors?

NAGAI: No, I have not examined that yet.

A.W. CLOWES (*University of Washington, Seattle, WA, USA*): I was very interested in your studies on retinoic acid—that you could inhibit the induction of BTEB2. Have you looked at any other factors, such as TGF-β or anything known to inhibit smooth muscle cell growth?

NAGAI: We have examined only the tissue factor gene.

P. CARMELIET (*Flanders Interuniversity, Institute of Biotechnology, Leuven, Belgium*): When endothelial cells form tubes during angiogenesis, they gradually become surrounded by smooth muscle cells and later by pericytes. Which form is expressed? Do you have information before birth, during development?

NAGAI: The SMemb is relatively selectively expressed in smooth muscle cells.

CARMELIET: Is that early on in the smooth muscle cell precursor also, or not?

NAGAI: Smooth muscle precursor should express SMemb.

CARMELIET: Is that also true during pathological angiogenesis, like myocardial vascularization?

NAGAI: Yes, it also is the case for BTEB2 or HEX.

CARMELIET: HEX was, I thought, originally found and identified in endothelial cells. Do you know anything about HEX expression in pathological angiogenesis, like in tumors or in myocardial revascularization?

NAGAI: Yes, they are positive during angiogenesis in tumors, even in smooth muscle cells, not only in endothelial cells.

Y. SATO (*Tohoku University, Sendai, Japan*): If you block the effect of BTEB2 by using the dominant negative molecule or antisense CDN can you inhibit transformation?

NAGAI: We once tried using antisense oligo, but we have not succeeded. One reason may be that BTEB2 expression is so abundant in cultured smooth muscle cells that, maybe, we could not inhibit it completely. We are now making adenoviral antisense of BTEB2. That should give us some answers.

SATO: You showed on the gel analysis of BTEB2, using the SMemb promoter, that there are two bands: a higher band and a lower band. By using the competition assay, both bands disappeared. You showed that the higher band is BTEB2. What is the lower band?

NAGAI: Both bands disappeared in the presence of anti-BTEB2.

SATO: Both bands disappeared following antibody?

NAGAI: Right, maybe two bands are formed with anti-BTEB2 protein. SP-1 seems to bind to this region as well.

G. GARCIA-CARDEÑA (*Brigham and Women's Hospital, Boston, MA, USA*): In terms of the expression of either of the myosins or the BTEB2 and HEX, have you looked at the different lineages of the smooth muscle, namely neural crest–derived or mesangial cell or arterial versus venous?

NAGAI: Yes. We looked at it, and the neural crest–derived cells became positive for BTEB2 after differentiation into precursors of smooth muscle cells.

GARCIA-CARDEÑA: In smooth muscle cells from arteries and from veins, do you have the myosins and BTEB2 present or is it specific for only some of the vascular beds?

NAGAI: They both express BTEB2.

Blood Vessels from Bone Marrow[a]

JULIE H. CAMPBELL,[b] JOHNNY L. EFENDY, CHIH- LU HAN,
AND GORDON R. CAMPBELL

*Centre for Research in Vascular Biology, Department of Anatomical Sciences,
The University of Queensland, Brisbane, Queensland, 4072 Australia*

> ABSTRACT: Lengths of silastic tubing were inserted into the peritoneal cavity of rats or rabbits. By two weeks the free-floating implants had become covered by a capsule consisting of several layers of "macrophage"-derived myofibroblasts and collagen matrix overlaid by a single layer of mesothelial cells. The tubing was removed from the harvested implant and the tissue everted. This now resembled an artery with an inner lining of mesothelial cells (the "intima"), a "media" of myofibroblasts, and an outer collagenous "adventitia." The tube of living tissue was grafted by end-to-end anastomoses into the transected carotid artery or abdominal aorta of the same animal in which the tissue had been grown, where it remained patent for four months and developed structures resembling elastic lamellae. The myofibroblasts developed a high volume fraction of myofilaments and became responsive to contractile and relaxing agents similar to smooth muscle cells of the adjacent artery wall.

Segments of mammary artery, saphenous vein, or synthetic prostheses are commonly used to bypass regions of coronary arteries compromised by atherosclerotic lesions. However, none of these biological and synthetic grafts is ideal. Autologous mammary artery and saphenous vein are flexible, viable, non-thrombogenic, and compatible, but mammary artery may not always be the proper size or length and saphenous vein may have varicose degenerative alterations that can lead to aneurysm formation when transplanted to a high pressure arterial site. Synthetic vascular prostheses, such as Dacron fabric grafts and expanded polytetrafluoroethylene (ePTFE), perform reasonably satisfactorily in high flow, low resistance conditions, but these materials are not suitable for small caliber arterial reconstructions since they are foreign bodies and blood coagulation can occur on the luminal surface and result in occlusion.

Studies carried out first by others[1] then ourselves[2,3] showed that a small foreign body (plastic disc, boiled liver, agar, gelatin, egg white, filter membranes, and boiled blood clot) introduced into the peritoneal cavity of the rat, rabbit, or mouse initiates

---

[a]This work was supported in part by a grant from the National Health and Medical Research Council of Australia and by a post-graduate award (J.L.E.) from The University of Queensland. It is the subject of Australian Provisional Patent Application No. PP5422/98 filed August 21, 1998 with extra data added December 22, 1998 (PP7859/98).

[b]Address for correspondence: Julie H. Campbell, Centre for Research in Vascular Biology, Department of Anatomical Sciences, the University of Queensland, Brisbane, Queensland, 4072 Australia. Voice: 61-7-33654658; fax: 61-7-33657261.
julie.campbell@mailbox.uq.edu.au

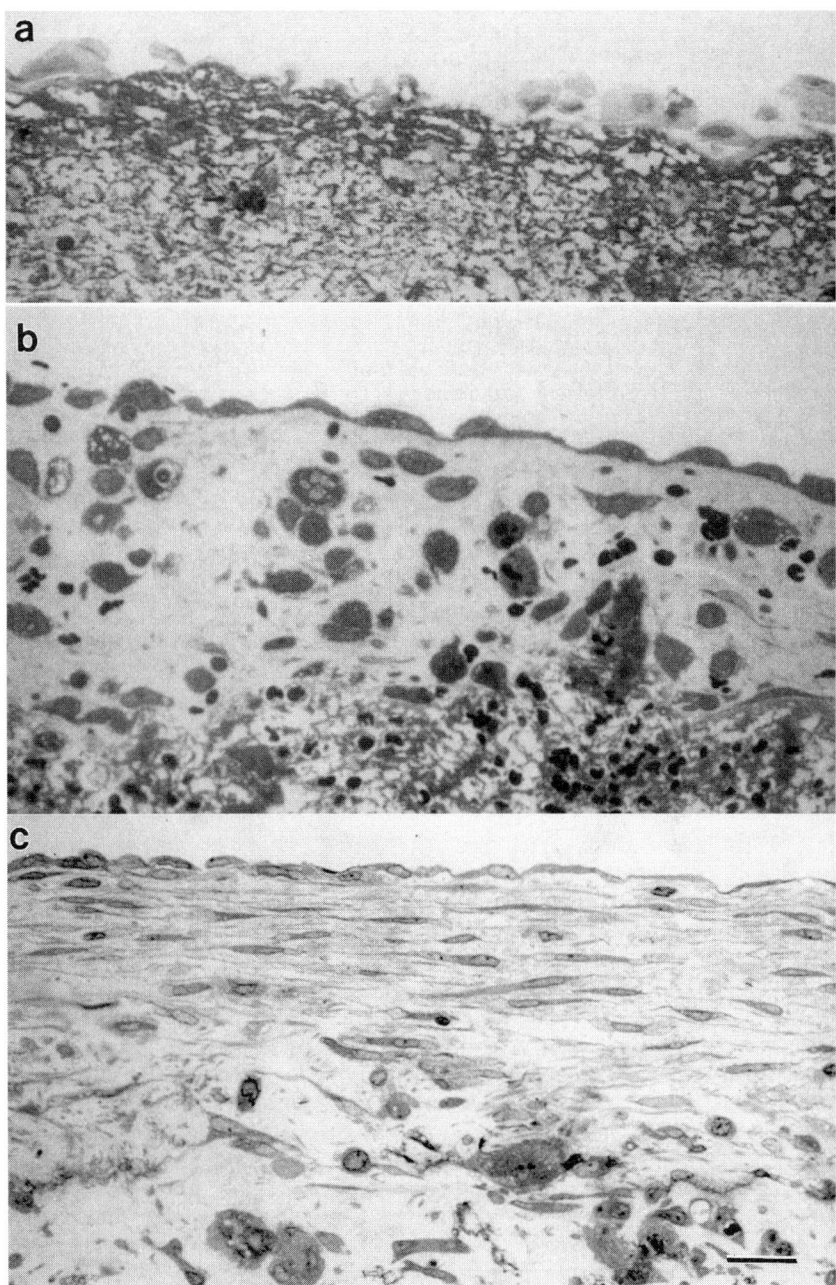

FIGURE 1. Semi-thin sections of the developing granulation tissue wall around boiled blood clots in the peritoneal cavity of the rat, stained with toluidine blue. (**a**) Day 3. (**b**) Day 7, bar = 45 μm. (**c**) Day 14, bar = 60 μm.

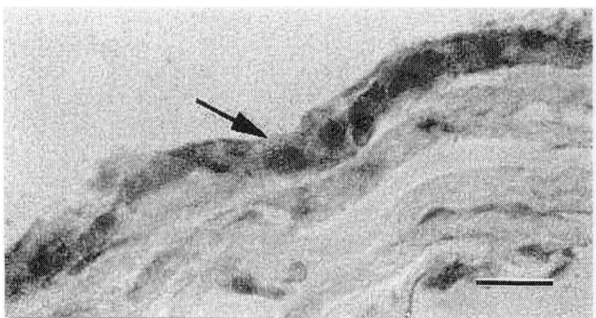

FIGURE 2. Section of granulation tissue tube freshly harvested from the peritoneal cavity of the rat stained with von Willebrand factor, indicating that the capsule is lined by mesothelial cells (*arrow*). Bar = 30 µm.

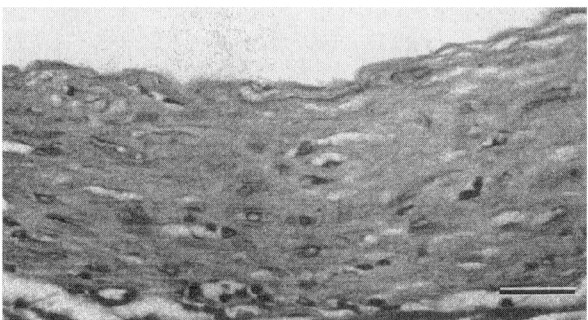

FIGURE 3. Section of a tube of granulation tissue after 14 days growth in the peritoneal cavity of a rat. Hematoxylin and eosin stain. Bar = 60 µm.

an inflammatory response with a resultant capsule of granulation tissue covered by a layer of mesothelium (FIG. 1). We considered that this process could be utilized to develop a tube of living myofibroblasts and matrix lined by non-thrombogenic mesothelial cells for use as an autologous vascular substitute.

Four pieces of silastic tubing were placed in the peritoneal cavity of each of 30 rats and 20 rabbits. The tubing was 10 mm long by 3 mm outer diameter (rat) or 20 mm long by 5 mm outer diameter (rabbit). Two weeks after implantation the animals were anesthetized and the tubing removed. Any implants that were not free-floating in the peritoneal fluid were discarded. The silastic tubing was carefully removed from the free-floating implants with little to no damage to the living tissue, and segments of one tube of tissue from each animal processed for light microscopy, immunohistochemistry,[4] and transmission electron microscopy.[5] It was observed that a layer of connective tissue had developed close to the silastic tubing and this, in turn, was covered by several layers of cell-rich granulation tissue. Mesothelial cells, which stained for von Willebrand factor,[6] formed the outer lining of the myofibroblast capsule (FIG. 2). Most importantly, the tube-like structure could be easily everted such that the mesothelium now lined the lumen. This created a hollow tube that mimicked the structure of a normal blood vessel, with an inner "endothelium" (mesothelium in this case), "media" of smooth muscle–like cells, and outer "adventitia" of connective tissue (FIG. 3). The volume fraction of myofilaments (V_{vmyo}) in cells of the rat tube was $35.7 \pm 1.6\%$ compared with $63.7 \pm 5.7\%$ ($p < 0.05$) for smooth muscle cells in the aorta of the same animals.

Another length of living granulation tissue, trimmed, everted and with the silastic tubing discarded, was transplanted into the abdominal aorta (rat) or common carotid artery (rabbit) of the animal in whose peritoneal cavity it had been grown (autologous transplant). To accomplish this, two vascular clamps were placed on the area above and below the transplant site. The vessel was resected and the elastic recoil of the artery left a gap of 5–10 mm between the cut ends. The graft was aligned with this gap and two stay sutures (9–0 silk) placed at each anastomosis to orient the graft and the artery and to facilitate the placing of other sutures. Suturing at the distal anastomosis was done first, followed by the proximal anastomosis. A total of eight interrupted sutures were placed at each end. Four more interrupted sutures (Ethicon 9–0) were then placed to fill the intervals between them. The grafts were not preclotted, nor were heparin or spasmolytics administered, in order to test the non-thrombogenicity of the mesothelial lining.

When suturing was completed, the distal clamp was released to allow the graft to fill with blood under low pressure, and then the proximal clamp released to allow blood flow under full arterial pressure through the graft. A graft was deemed successful at the time of operation if it was fully dilated and pulsating. Unsuccessful grafts were limp and flaccid, with no detectable pulse. The wound was irrigated with saline solution and closed with Dexon 4–0 sutures. The animals had free access to standard food and water. Rats were sacrificed at 1, 1.5, 2, 3, and 4 months ($N = 6$ per group) and rabbits at 1, 2, 3, and 4 months ($N = 5$ per group).

The overall patency of the transplants in both the rat and rabbit at the different time points was 63%, a rate that is likely to be improved greatly by the inclusion of heparin at the time of surgery. These transplants possessed a normal, intact wall with a strong pulse. Mesothelium (or migrated endothelium) comprised the inner lining. A large amount of extracellular matrix on the outer surface contributed to an increased thickness of the transplants and cells of the media stained for α-smooth muscle actin (FIG. 4) and smooth muscle myosin. By 6 weeks after transplantation, the tissue responded by contraction to 100 mmol/l potassium chloride and 10^{-4} mmol/l phenylephrine and relaxed in response to 10^{-5} mol/l acetylcholine.[7] By 3 months the V_{vmyo} of the cells in the rat transplants was $58.7 \pm 1.4\%$, which was not significantly different from that of smooth muscle cells in the rat aorta ($63.7 \pm 5.7\%$).

To determine the origin of the contractile myofibroblasts in the implants, six female C57BL/6 mice expressing the Ly5.2 antigen on the surface of their hemopoietic cells were X-irradiated to destroy bone marrow then immediately transfused with 10^6 nucleated bone marrow cells taken from the femur and tibia of a congenic strain of male mice expressing the Ly5.1 allelle on their hemopoietic cells. By 4 weeks, all six female mice had successful donor engraftment of >80% and had four small pieces (3 mm × 0.5 mm outer diameter) of silastic tubing placed in their peritoneal cavity. After 2 weeks, by which time a capsule of granulation tissue had formed around the tubing, the grafts were removed and those that had remained free-floating were processed. Immunohistochemistry revealed that the cells of the granulation tissue stained positively for α-smooth muscle actin. Transmission electron microscopy showed that these cells

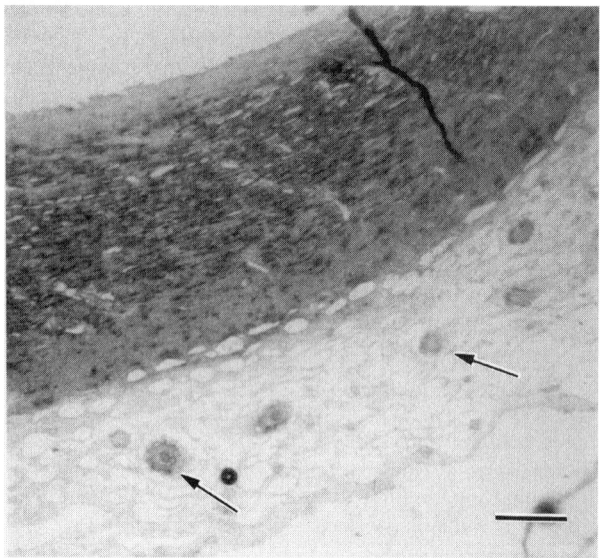

FIGURE 4. Section of granulation tissue, 4 months after transplantation (by end-to-end anastomoses) into the abdominal aorta of the same animal in which the tissue was grown, stained with biotinylated antibody to α-smooth muscle actin (1A4). Note the development of an "adventitia" on the outer surface with vasa vasora (*arrows*). Bar = 50 µm.

were elongated with a folded nucleus and had cytoplasm filled with contractile filaments and synthetic organelles, characteristic of myofibroblasts or developing smooth muscle cells. During the early stages of capsule formation, the rounded cells stained with fluoresceinated antibodies to Ly5.1, but this was lost by 2 weeks when the cells had differentiated to elongated cells containing contractile filaments. However, *in situ* hybridization with a Y-chromosome probe showed that more than half of the myofibroblasts were derived from the male donor and thus from bone marrow–derived peritoneal "macrophages" within the female host.[8]

Our studies have thus shown that tubes of granulation tissue can be grown within an animal's own peritoneal cavity from peritoneal "macrophages" and mesothelial cells. The tubes of living granulation tissue, lined with an anticoagulant surface, can be used successfully as an autologous arterial transplant where they remain patent for at least four months with the constituent cells becoming more smooth muscle–like and responding to contractile agents and an "endothelium"-dependent relaxing agent (acetylcholine). If this new type of vascular graft material can be reproduced in the human, it may open new perspectives in the field of arterial reconstructive surgery.

REFERENCES

1. RYAN, G.B. *et al* 1973. Myofibroblasts in an avascular fibrous tissue. Lab. Invest. **29:** 197–206.
2. CAMPBELL, G.R. & G.B. RYAN. 1983. Origin of myofibroblasts in the avascular capsule around free-floating intraperitoneal blood clots. Pathol. **15:** 253–264.

3. MOSSE, P.R.L. *et al.* 1985. A comparison of the avascular capsule surrounding free floating intraperitonal blood clots in mice and rabbits. J. Pathol. **17:** 401–407.
4. ROLFE, B.E. *et al.* 1995. T-lymphocytes affect smooth muscle cell biology. Arterioscler. Thromb. **15:** 1204–1210.
5. MANDERSON, J.A. & G.R. CAMPBELL. 1986. Venous response to endothelial denudation. J. Pathol. **18:** 77–87.
6. MORGANTI, M. *et al.* 1996. Detection of minimal but significant amount of von Willebrand factor in human omentum mesothelial cell cultures. Biomed. Pharmacother. **50:** 369–372
7. CAMPBELL, J.H. *et al.* 2000. A novel vascular graft grown within the recipient's own peritoneal cavity. Circ. Res. **85:** 1173–1178.
8. EFENDY, J.L. 1999. Granulation tissue of haemopoietic origin as a vascular graft. Ph.D. thesis, University of Queensland, Australia.

Endothelial Dysfunction, Hemodynamic Forces, and Atherogenesis[a]

MICHAEL A. GIMBRONE, JR.,[b] JAMES N. TOPPER,[c] TOBI NAGEL,[d] KEITH R. ANDERSON, AND GUILLERMO GARCIA-CARDEÑA

Vascular Research Division, Department of Pathology, Brigham and Women's Hospital and Harvard Medical School, Boston, Massachusetts 02115-5817, USA

ABSTRACT: Phenotypic modulation of endothelium to a dysfunctional state contributes to the pathogenesis of cardiovascular diseases such as atherosclerosis. The localization of atherosclerotic lesions to arterial geometries associated with disturbed flow patterns suggests an important role for local hemodynamic forces in atherogenesis. There is increasing evidence that the vascular endothelium, which is directly exposed to various fluid mechanical forces generated by pulsatile blood flow, can discriminate among these stimuli and transduce them into genetic regulatory events. At the level of individual genes, this regulation is accomplished via the binding of certain transcription factors, such as NFκB and Egr-1, to shear-stress response elements (SSREs) that are present in the promoters of biomechanically inducible genes. At the level of multiple genes, distinct patterns of up- and downregulation appear to be elicited by exposure to steady laminar shear stresses versus comparable levels of non-laminar (e.g., turbulent) shear stresses or cytokine stimulation (e.g., IL-1β). Certain genes upregulated by steady laminar shear stress stimulation (such as eNOS, COX-2, and Mn-SOD) support vasoprotective (i.e., anti-inflammatory, anti-thrombotic, anti-oxidant) functions in the endothelium. We hypothesize that the selective and sustained expression of these and related "atheroprotective genes" in the endothelial lining of lesion-protected areas represents a mechanism whereby hemodynamic forces can influence lesion formation and progression.

VASCULAR ENDOTHELIUM: A CENTRAL COMPONENT IN THE ATHEROSCLEROTIC DISEASE PROCESS

The involvement of vascular endothelium in disease processes such as atherosclerosis has been recognized since the time of Virchow,[1] but mechanistic insight into the pathobiology of this tissue has developed only recently, largely as a result of the application of modern cellular and molecular biological techniques.[2] We now appreciate

---

[a]This research was supported primarily by grants from the National Heart, Lung and Blood Institute (P01-HL36028, R37-HL51150, P50-HL56985) and a sponsored research agreement with the Brigham and Women's Hospital from Millennium Pharmaceuticals, Inc. (Cambridge, MA).

[b]Address for correspondence: Michael A. Gimbrone, Jr., Vascular Research Division, Department of Pathology, Brigham and Women's Hospital, 221 Longwood Avenue, Boston, MA 02115. Voice: 617-732-5901; fax: 617-732-5933.

mgimbrone@rics.bwh.harvard.edu

[c]Current address: Falk Cardiovascular Research Center, Stanford University School of Medicine, 300 Pasteur Drive, Stanford CA 94305.

[d]Current address: Genentech, 1 DNA Way, MS 34, So. San Francisco, CA 94080-4990.

that the single-cell thick lining of the circulatory system is, in fact, a vital organ whose health is essential to normal vascular physiology and whose dysfunction can be a critical factor in the pathogenesis of vascular disease. It has been our laboratory's working concept that the vascular endothelium is a dynamically mutable interface, whose structural and functional properties are responsive to a variety of stimuli, both local and systemic, and further that its phenotypic modulation to a dysfunctional state can constitute a pathogenic risk factor for vascular diseases. In the arterial wall, certain consequences of endothelial dysfunction are directly related to the pathogenesis of atherosclerosis and its complications.[3] These consequences include altered vascular reactivity and vasospasm; altered intimal permeability to lipoproteins; enhanced mononuclear leukocyte recruitment and intimal accumulation as foam cells; altered vascular cell growth regulation and survival (e.g., decreased endothelial regeneration, increased smooth muscle cell proliferation, enhanced susceptibility to apoptosis); and altered hemostatic/fibrinolytic balances (favoring thrombin generation, and platelet and fibrin deposition). Pathophysiological stimuli of arterial endothelial dysfunction that are especially relevant to atherogenesis include activation by cytokines and bacterial products; infection by bacteria, viruses, and other pathogens; stimulation by advanced glycation endproducts (AGEs) generated in diabetes and with aging; chronic exposure to hyperhomocysteinemia and/or hypercholesterolemia; and accumulation of oxidized lipoproteins and their components (e.g., lysophosphatidylcholine) within the vessel wall. In addition to these biochemical stimuli, it is now clear that various biomechanical forces, generated by the pulsatile flow of blood through the branched arterial vasculature, can also influence the structure and function of endothelial cells and even modulate their expression of pathophysiologically relevant genes.[5–7]

The possibility that hemodynamic forces can act directly as pathophysiologic stimuli for endothelial dysfunction provides a conceptual rationale for the long-standing observation that the earliest lesions of atherosclerosis characteristically develop in a non-random pattern, the geometry of which correlates with branchpoints and other regions of altered blood flow.[8–10] In this brief review, we provide an update of ongoing studies in our laboratory focused on the molecular mechanisms involved in the regulation of endothelial gene expression by biomechanical forces, and the new insights they have provided into the pathogenesis of atherosclerosis.

HEMODYNAMICS AND VESSEL WALL BIOLOGY

The pulsatile flow of blood through the branched tubular array of the arterial vasculature generates various types of hemodynamic forces—wall shear stresses, hydrostatic pressures, and cyclic strains—that can impact vessel wall biology. As the cellular layer in direct contact with blood, the endothelium bears the frictional forces (wall shear stresses) imparted by the flow of this viscous flow. Blood flow patterns can vary in complexity from the relatively uniform (time-averaged) well-developed laminar flow (with corresponding wall shear stresses in the range of 5–15 dynes/cm^2), that occur in the unbranched portions of medium-sized muscular arteries, to the complex disturbed laminar flow patterns (involving regions of flow separation, recirculation, and reattachment) that result in significant temporal and spatial gradients of wall shear stress over relatively short distances.[11–14] The latter disturbed laminar flow patterns occur near branch points, bifurcations, and major curves—arterial geometries that are typically associated with the earliest appearance (and subsequent progression) of atherosclerotic lesions. In contrast, the unbranched, tubular portions of arteries that carry uniform laminar flow are relatively protected from atherogenesis (at least in the early stages of lesion formation). For many years, the common wisdom therefore held that low shear areas (e.g., the complex geometries in which the time-averaged fluctuations in wall shear stresses were numerically small, due to forward-reverse flow cycles) were especially atherosclerosis-prone,[15] whereas high shear areas were relatively atherosclerosis-protected (see Refs. 14 and 16 for discussion). Indeed, this nonrandom pattern of atherosclerotic lesion development holds true not only for various experimental models (dietary and/or genetic), across multiple animal species (monkeys, rabbits, pigs, rodents), but also for the natural history of this disease in humans.[9,10,16–18]

A number of *in vivo* observations suggest that hemodynamic forces can alter endothelial structure and function.[19–24] These include the demonstration of increased macromolecular permeability, lipoprotein accumulation, endothelial cell damage and repair, leukocyte adhesion molecule expression, and mononuclear leukocyte recruitment near branch points and bifurcations, as well as the localization of ellipsoidal endothelial cell (and nuclear) shape and axial alignment (in the direction of flow) to laminar flow regions, and the disruption of this orderly pattern in regions of disturbed flow. In addition, experimental alterations of vascular architecture (e.g., surgical coarctation and shunts) have been shown to result in both acute and chronic vessel wall changes that appear to be (at least in part) endothelium dependent. In the presence of hypercholesterolemia, these surgically modified vascular geometries can develop lesions that resemble atherosclerosis. Taken together, these *in vivo* observations are consistent with a direct, or indirect, effect of one or more hemodynamic stimuli on endothelial function/dysfunction in the context of atherogenesis.

Evidence of the direct action of hemodynamic forces on endothelial structure and function has come primarily from *in vitro* studies, in which cultured monolayers of human- and animal-derived vascular endothelial cells have been subjected to defined fluid mechanical stimulation, under well-controlled experimental conditions. Utilizing a modified cone and plate viscometer, in the early 1980s, our group observed that unidirectional steady laminar shear stresses could induce time- and force-dependent cell-shape and alignment changes in cultured endothelial monolayers, which was reversible upon the cessation of flow.[24–26] These shear-induced changes were accompanied by reorganization of actin-containing stress fibers, as well as other cytoskeletal components, thus mimicking the morphology of aortic endothelium *in vivo*. Further studies by our group, and several others, have also documented a variety of changes in the metabolic and synthetic activities of endothelial cells in response to defined biomechanical forces, including the production of prostacyclin, growth factors, coagulation and fibrinolytic components, extracellular matrix components, and vasoactive mediators.[5,27] Some of these more acute, shear-induced changes appear to involve regulation at the level of rate-limiting enzymes or substrate availability (e.g., arachidonic acid release by calcium-sensitive phospholipases and NO production by nitric oxide synthase). However, in the case of delayed responses, in which *de novo* protein synthesis is occurring, transcriptional upregulation of gene expression appears to be stimulated as a direct consequence of exposure to fluid mechanical forces.

MECHANISMS OF ENDOTHELIAL GENE REGULATION BY BIOMECHANICAL FORCES

In vitro studies have demonstrated that the application of physiological levels of laminar shear stress to cultured monolayers of endothelial cells can modulate the expression of a broad spectrum of pathophysiologically relevant genes including: growth factors, such as PDGF-A and PDGF-B; transforming growth factor-β; fibrinolytic factors, such as tPA; and adhesion molecules, such as ICAM-1 and VCAM-1.[6,7] The force-dependencies and kinetic profiles for these various genes show qualitatively different patterns, suggesting that the molecular mechanisms linking an externally applied force to genetic regulatory events in the nucleus are complex. These patterns could reflect a complex interplay of stimuli and responses at several levels, including intracellular second messenger pathways, transcriptional activators and inhibitors, and post-transcriptional effects at the mRNA and/or protein level. To experimentally dissect the molecular mechanisms involved in the biomechanical regulation of endothelial genes, we have utilized a well-characterized cone-plate flow apparatus to expose confluent monolayers of cultured human umbilical vein (HUVEC) or bovine aorta to shear stress (e.g., 5–10 dynes/cm^2). We have analyzed gene expression by various techniques (e.g., Northern blotting, transfection of shear-responsive reporter gene constructs, nuclear run-on assays, and differential display of expressed transcripts). Initially, we studied individual genes (e.g., PDGF-A, PDGF-B, ICAM-1) as molecular model systems, focusing on the analysis of their promoters and interacting transcriptional factors. More recently, we have begun to analyze the patterns of multiple endothelial genes that are responding in a coordinated fashion to different types of biomechanical stimuli.[28]

Early studies in our group, by Resnick and colleagues,[29] focused on the transcriptional regulation of the human PDGF-B gene, which had previously been shown to be shear-sensitive at the level of steady-state mRNA. Nuclear run-on assays confirmed increased transcriptional activity after one hour of flow exposure, and a reporter gene (consisting of a 1.3 kb fragment of the human PDGF-B promoter, coupled to chloramphenicol acyltransferase), when transfected into BAEC monolayers exposed to laminar shear stress, registered several-fold increased expression compared to "no flow" controls. Through the use of 5′ nested deletional mutations of the PDGF-B promoter, shear responsiveness was localized to a relatively short region situated near the transcriptional start site (position −153 to −101). Oligonucleotide probes spanning this region then were used in gel-shift assays of nuclear extracts from large samples (10^7 cells) of both static and laminar shear stress–stimulated endothelial monolayers. A specific, shear-inducible DNA–nuclear protein complex was consistently observed, which localized to a 12 bp portion within the shear-responsive region. Mutational analysis defined a 6 bp core-binding sequence, GAGACC, which was termed the "shear-stress response element" or SSRE. Nuclear protein–DNA binding events could be demonstrated with probes based on this SSRE as early as 30 minutes after the onset of flow, and thus were consistent with the kinetics and transcriptional activation of the intact endothelial PDGF-B gene, as demonstrated by nuclear run-on analysis. Hybrid promoters consisting of this core-binding sequence (GAGACC) coupled with a non–shear-sensitive reporter gene construct were activated by shear stress, thus demonstrating that the SSRE motif was sufficient to confer shear-responsiveness. Interestingly, computer analysis of gene sequence databases reveals that there was conservation of the sequence across species (human, murine, feline) within the PDGF-B promoter, suggesting that this mechanism of genetic response to biomechanical stimulation in endothelial cells has been conserved in this gene over many years of evolution.

Further studies have also identified other positive and negative SSREs, in addition to the original SSRE motif identified in the PDGF-B promoter. These include: a TRE (AP-1) site in the human monocyte chemotactic protein-1 (MCP-1) promoter, Egr-1/SP1 binding sites in the PDGF-A promoter, and SP1/Egr-1 binding sites in the proximal promoter of the tissue factor gene. Each appear to mediate shear-induced upregulation of these genes.[30–33] In addition, negative SSREs had been mapped in the promoters of other genes, such as VCAM-1 (an AP-1 consensus sequence in the proximal promoter), which appear to mediate downregulation in response to a shear-stress stimulus.[34]

In parallel with these promoter analyses, considerable attention has also been focused on the influence of biomechanical forces on the expression and activation of various known transcription factors. For example, certain immediate-early response genes, such as c-fos and Egr-1, whose encoded proteins function as transactivating factors, are directly and rapidly induced by shear-stress stimulation in vascular endothelial cells.[31,36] Other transcriptional factors, such as the NFκB system, show their typical pattern of activation (cytoplasmic-to-nuclear translocation) immediately following the onset of shear-stress stimulus.[35] Studies in our group have demonstrated that NFκB components (p50, p65) can interact directly with the SSRE motif in the human PDGF-B promoter, thus promoting further insight into the transduction mechanisms involved in shear-induced gene expression. Interestingly, these SSREs appear to function in a context-specific manner, such that an element that can mediate a transcriptional response to shear-stress stimulation in the context of one promoter might not do so in the context of another, unrelated, promoter. Thus, these sequence elements appear to function in a manner analogous to promoter elements that mediate transcriptional responses to various humoral stimuli, such as growth factors and cytokines.[28] As discussed below, recent studies of novel genes transcriptionally regulated by biomechanical stimulation in endothelial cells have led to the discovery of new transcription factors.

At the present time, considerable attention is being focused on the fundamental question of the identity, location, and mechanisms of action of endothelial flow-sensitive mechanotransducers. Several distinct molecules (e.g., cell-surface ion channels, various receptor-associated G-proteins, and members of the mitogen-activated and stress-activated protein kinase cascades) are rapidly activated in response to fluid shear stresses applied to the endothelial cell surface.[27,37] In addition, cellular organelles, such as the cytoskeleton, plasma-membrane caveoli, lateral cell-cell junctional proteins, basal focal adhesion complexes, and even the lipid bilayer of the plasma membrane, also appear to be participating in shear-induced endothelial responses.[27,38,39] Finally, various second messengers, including ionized cytosolic calcium, intracellular lipid products of the polyphosphoinositide pathway, and nitric oxide, are generated in the context of flow stimulation. As discussed by Davies,[27] the challenges to understand the interaction of these spatially and temporally disparate components in the dynamic interplay of the endothelial cell's response to biomechanical stimulation are in sorting out where transmission becomes transduction, as well as cause-effect relationships.

IMPLICATIONS OF COMPLEX FLOW PATTERNS FOR ENDOTHELIAL GENE REGULATION

The endothelial cells lining the branched tubular array of the arterial vasculature are subjected to a broad spectrum of flow patterns depending upon their location. Studies by several laboratories, including our own, using different *in vitro* model systems clearly indicate that endothelial cells can sense differences in the temporal and/or spatial characteristics of flow and translate these biomechanical stimuli into different biological responses. For example, steady laminar flow appears to enhance endothelial survival by suppressing apoptosis,[40,41] whereas turbulent flow can trigger endothelial cell division.[42] Differences in the temporal properties of laminar flow stimulation, generated by instantaneous (impulse) versus gradual (ramp) application of the same final level of shear stress, can elicit very different responses in endothelial gene expression.[39] Similarly, oscillatory versus steady laminar flows elicit marked differences in the pattern of adhesion molecule expression in cultured endothelium.[43] To focus more specifically on the effects of spatial gradients in shear stress on endothelial biology, DePaola and colleagues[44] developed an *in vitro* model system that generates large gradients in shear stress over the relatively small dimensions of a cultured endothelial monolayer, thus mimicking the spatial pattern of flow separation (with reversal), reattachment, and flow recovery associated with arterial bifurcations *in vivo*. Using this *in vitro* spatial disturbed-flow model, dramatic differences in endothelial cell shape, migration, and proliferation have been demonstrated in association with this disturbed flow, as compared with uniform laminar flow.[44,45] In addition, significant differences in endothelial expression of connexin43 at the level of mRNA and protein, and concomitant changes in cell-cell communication via gap junctions, also have been correlated with the presence of shear stress gradients in this model.[46] Recent studies suggest that these *in vitro* observations may indeed have a counterpart *in vivo*.[47] Most recently, Nagel and coworkers[14] have demonstrated that endothelial cell monolayers exhibit significant spatial heterogeneity in the nuclear localization of certain critical transcription factors, including NFκB, Egr-1, c-jun, and c-fos, and that these differences correspond to the local shear stress gradient. Taken together, these studies thus strongly suggest that spatial gradients in wall shear stress, in contrast to absolute shear stress magnitudes (*cf.* Ref. 15) can be important determinants of endothelial responses at the level of gene regulation. Further studies are needed to elucidate the potential interplay of both temporal and spatial fluctuations in the biomechanical regulation of endothelial gene expression and, ultimately, to correlate these stimuli with the endothelial phenotypes actually observed in different *in vivo* biomechanical environments.

HOW MIGHT FLOW-INDUCED ENDOTHELIAL PHENOTYPIC MODULATION CONTRIBUTE TO ATHEROGENESIS *IN VIVO*?

To more systematically address the question of modulation of endothelial phenotype by biomechanical stimulation, our laboratory has turned to high-throughput molecular biological strategies.[28,48] Specifically, we have used a reverse transcription–polymerase chain reaction–based high-throughput differential display of transcripts to compare the patterns of genes that are upregulated or downregulated in cultured human endothelial cells in response to physiological levels of steady laminar shear stress, a comparable level of turbulent (nonlaminar) shear stress, and a soluble cytokine stimulus (IL-1β) at a maximally effective concentration.[48] This approach has revealed distinctive patterns of endothelial gene expression not previously appreciated, including a set of genes that appear to be upregulated in a sustained fashion by steady laminar shear stress, but not by turbulent shear stress. Certain of these differentially regulated transcripts encode known endothelial genes of relevance to atherogenesis, such as eNOS (the endothelial isoform of nitric oxide synthase), COX-2 (the inducible isoform of cyclooxygenase), and Mn-SOD (manganese-dependent superoxide dismutase). These endothelial genes encode enzymes that exert potent anti-thrombotic, anti-adhesive, anti-proliferative, anti-inflammatory, and anti-oxidant effects, both within the endothelial lining and in interacting cells, such as platelets, leukocytes, and vascular smooth muscle. The biological consequences of these steady laminar shear upregulated endothelial genes thus would be predicted to be vasoprotective or anti-atherogenic.[2,7,8]

Given the well-established observation that uniform laminar shear stresses are characteristically associated with atherosclerotic lesion–protected arterial geometries *in vivo*, these molecular biological observations have led us to hypothesize that this type of biomechanical stimulation acts to chronically upregulate the expression of a subset of "athero-protective genes" in endothelial cells, which then act locally in the lesion-protected areas to offset the effects of systemic risk factors, such as hypercholesterolemia, hyperhomocysteinemia, hyperglycemia (diabetes), and hypertension. The coordinated and selective upregulation of athero-protective genes by uniform laminar shear stress is thus a possible mechanistic link between the local hemodynamic milieu, endothelial gene expression, and early events in atherogenesis. This working hypothesis, of course, does not exclude the potential direct action of complex disturbed laminar flows, such as occur in lesion-prone arterial geometries, as stimuli for the expression of pro-atherogenic genes (e.g., adhesion molecules, growth factors, cytokines).[2,7,8]

Critical testing of this "athero-protective gene hypothesis" will depend upon refinement of both *in vitro* and *in vivo* fluid mechanical models and a validation of candidate athero-protective genes in the setting of human vascular pathobiology. The development of reliable methods for linear amplification of transcripts from small numbers of cells and their analysis by cDNA micro-arrays or analogous genome-scale technologies should hold much promise in this regard. Application of these comprehensive and relatively unbiased methods of molecular analysis to endothelial cells subjected to experimentally defined flow conditions will add significantly to our understanding of the dynamic range of biomechanically induced phenotypic modulation. Ultimately, the extension of this method of analysis to endothelial phenotype in the natural disease context should provide valuable new insights into the links between endothelial dysfunction, hemodynamic forces, and atherogenesis.

ACKNOWLEDGMENTS

The authors wish to acknowledge the past and present members of the Vascular Research Division at the Brigham and Women's Hospital for their conceptual input and experimental collaboration in the original studies summarized here, and also the long-standing collaboration of Professor C.F. Dewey and his colleagues in the Fluid Mechanics Laboratory at the Massachusetts Institute of Technology. Finally, we would like to dedicate this chapter to the memory of Dr. Russell Ross.

REFERENCES

1. VIRCHOW, R. 1856. Der ateromatose Prozess der Arterien. Wien Med. Wochenshr. **6:** 825–841.
2. GIMBRONE, M.A., JR. & J.N. TOPPER. 1998. Biology of the Vessel Wall: Endothelium. *In* Molecular Basis of Heart Diseases. K.R. Chien, Ed: 331–348. Harcourt Brace & Co. Troy, MO.
3. GIMBRONE, M.A., JR. *et al.* 1997. Hemodynamics, endothelial gene expression and atherogenesis. Ann. N.Y. Acad. Sci. **811:** 1–11.
4. ROSS, R. 1999. Atherosclerosis—An Inflammatory Disease (a review). N. Engl. J. Med. **340**(2): 115–126.
5. RESNICK, N. & M.A. GIMBRONE, JR. 1995. Hemodynamic forces are complex regulators of endothelial gene regulation (a review). FASEB J. **9:** 874–882.
6. GIMBRONE, M.A. JR., T. NAGEL & J.N. TOPPER. 1997. Biomechanical activation: an emerging paradigm in endothelial adhesion biology. Perspectives Series: Cell Adhesion in Vascular Biology. J. Clin. Invest. **99**(8): 1809–1813.
7. TOPPER, J.N. & M.A. GIMBRONE, JR. 1999. Hemodynamics and endothelial phenotype: new insights into the modulation of vascular gene expression by fluid mechanical stimuli. *In* Endothelium and Mechanical Forces. P. Lelkes, Ed.: 207–219. Harwood Academic Publishers. London.
8. GIMBRONE, M.A., JR. 1999. Foreword. *In* Endothelium and Mechanical Forces. P. Lelkes, Ed.: VII–IX. Harwood Academic Publishers. London.
9. CORNHILL J.F. & M.R. ROACH. 1976. A quantitative study of the localization of atherosclerotic lesions in the rabbit aorta. Atherosclerosis **23:** 489–501.
10. GLAGOV, S. *et al.* 1988. Hemodynamics and atherosclerosis: insights and perspectives gained from studies of human arteries. Arch. Pathol. Lab. Med. **112:** 1018–1031.
11. GIDDENS, D.P., C.K. ZARINS & S. GLAGOV. 1993. The role of fluid mechanics in the localization and detection of atherosclerosis. J. Biomech. Eng. **115:** 588–594.
12. KARINO, T. 1986. Microscopic structure of disturbed flows in the arterial and venous systems, and its implication in the localization of vascular diseases. Int. Angiol. **5:** 297–313.
13. FRIEDMAN, M.H., V. O'BRIEN & L.W. EHRLICH. 1975. Calculations of pulsatile flow through a branch: implications for the hemodynamics of atherogenesis. Circ. Res. **36:** 277–285.
14. NAGEL, T. *et al.* 1999. Vascular endothelial cells respond to spatial gradients in fluid shear stress by enhanced activation of transcription factors. Arterioscler. Thromb. Vasc. Biol. In press.
15. CARO, C.G., J.M. FITZ-GERALD & R.C. SCHROTER. 1971. Atheroma and arterial wall shear. Observations, correlations, and proposal of a shear dependent mass transfer mechanism for atherogenesis. Proc. Royal Soc. London (B) **177:** 109–159.
16. WOLF, N. 1982. Haemodynamic factors and plaque formation. *In* Pathology of Atherosclerosis. Ch. 9: 187–215. Butterworth Scientific. London.
17. PATHOBIOLOGICAL DETERMINANTS OF ATHEROSCLEROSIS IN YOUTH (PDAY) RESEARCH GROUP. 1993. Natural history of aortic and coronary atherosclerotic lesions in youth; findings from the PDAY study. Arterioscler. Thromb. Vasc. Biol. **13:** 1291–1298.
18. NAKASHIMA, Y. *et al.* 1994. ApoE-deficient mice develop lesions of all phases of atherosclerosis throughout the arterial tree. Arterioscler. Thromb. Vasc. Biol. **14:** 133–140.
19. NEREM, R.M., M.J. LEVESQUE & J.F. CORNHILL. 1981. Vascular endothelial morphology as an indicator of blood flow. J. Biochem. Eng. **103:** 172–178.
20. LANGILLE, B.L. & F. O'DONNELL. 1986. Reductions in arterial diameter produced by chronic decreases in blood flow are endothelium-dependent. Science **231:** 405–407.
21. JORIS, I., T. ZAND & G. MAJNO. 1982. Hydrodynamic injury of the endothelium in acute aortic stenosis. **106:** 394–408.

22. WALPOLA, P.L. et al. 1995. Expression of ICAM-1 and VCAM-1 and monocyte adherence in arteries exposed to altered shear stress. Arterioscler. Thromb. Vasc. Biol. **15:** 2–10.
23. ZAND, T. et al. 1999. Lipid deposition in rat aortas with ultraluminal hemispherical plug stenosis: a morphological and biophysical study. Amer. J. Pathol. **155**(1): 85–92.
24. BUSSOLARI, S.R., C.F. DEWEY, JR. & M.A. GIMBRONE, JR. 1982. Apparatus for subjecting living cells to fluid shear stress. Rev. Sci. Instrum. **53**(12): 1851–1854.
25. DEWEY, C.F., JR. et al. 1981. The dynamic response of vascular endothelial cells to fluid shear stress. J. Biomech. Eng. **103:** 177–185.
26. REMUZZI, A. et al. 1984. Orientation of endothelial cells in shear fields in vitro. Biorheology **21:** 617–630.
27. DAVIES, P.F. 1995. Flow-mediated endothelial mechanotransduction. Physiol. Rev. **75:** 519–560.
28. TOPPER, J.N. & M.A. GIMBRONE, JR. 1999. Blood flow and vascular gene expression: fluid shear stress as a modulator of endothelial phenotype. Molec. Med. Today **5**(1): 40–46.
29. RESNICK, N. et al. 1993. Platelet-derived growth factor B chain promoter contains a cis-acting fluid shear-stress-responsive element. Proc. Natl. Acad. Sci. USA **90:** 4591–4595.
30. SHYY, J.Y.J. et al. 1995. The cis-acting phorbol ester 12-O-tetradecanoylphorbol-13-acetate-responsive element is involved in shear stress-induced monocyte chemotactic protein 1 gene expression. Proc. Natl. Acad. Sci. USA **92:** 8069–8073.
31. KHACHIGIAN, L.M. et al. 1997. Egr-1 is activated in endothelial cells exposed to fluid shear stress and interacts with a novel shear-stress response element in the PDGF A-chain promoter. Arterioscler. Thromb. Vasc. Biol. **17:** 2280–2286.
32. MALEK, A.M. & S. IZUMO. 1994. Molecular aspects of signal transduction of shear stress in the endothelial cell (editorial review). J. Hypertens. **12:** 989–999.
33. LIN, M.C. et al. 1997. Shear stress induction of the tissue factor gene. J. Clin. Invest. **15:** 737–744.
34. KORENAGA, R. et al. 1997. Negative transcriptional regulation of the VCAM-1 gene by fluid shear stress in murine endothelial cells. Am. J. Physiol. **273:** C1506–C1515.
35. KHACHIGIAN, L.M. et al. 1995. Nuclear factor-κB interacts functionally with the platelet-derived growth factor B-chain shear-stress-response-element in vascular endothelial cells exposed to fluid shear stress. J. Clin. Invest. **96**(2): 1169–1175.
36. HSIEH, J.-.J, N.-Q. LI & J.A. FRANGOS. 1993. Pulsatile and steady flow induces c-fos expression in human endothelial cells. J. Cell. Physiol. **154:** 143–151.
37. TRAUB, O. & B.C. BERK. 1998. Laminar shear stress: mechanisms by which endothelial cells transduce an atheroprotective force. Arterioscler. Thromb. Vasc. Biol. **18:** 677–685.
38. DAVIES, P.F., T. MUNDEL & K.A. BARBEE. 1995. A mechanism for heterogeneous endothelial responses to flow in vivo and in vitro. J. Biomech. **28:** 1553–1560.
39. FRANGOS, J.A. & X.P. BAO. 1997. NO regulated PDGF-A and MCP-1 expression induced by temporal gradients in shear stress in human endothelial cells. Jpn. J. Pharmacol. **75:** 31.
40. DIMMELER, S. et al. 1996. Shear stress inhibits apoptosis of human endothelial cells. FEBS Lett. **399:** 71–74.
41. GARCIA-CARDEÑA, G. et al. 2000. Distinct mechanical stimuli differentially regulate the P13K/Akt survival pathway in endothelial cells. Ann. N.Y. Acad. Sci. This volume.
42. DAVIES, P.F. et al. 1986. Turbulent fluid shear stress induces vascular endothelial cell turnover in vitro. Proc. Natl. Acad. Sci. USA **83:** 2114–2117.
43. CHAPPELL, D.C. et al. 1998. Oscillatory shear stress stimulates adhesion molecule expression in cultured human endothelium. Circ. Res. **82:** 532–539.
44. DEPAOLA, N. et al. 1992. Vascular endothelium responds to fluid shear stress gradients. Arterioscler. Thromb. **12:** 1254–1257.
45. TARDY, Y. et al. 1997. Shear stress gradients remodel endothelial monolayers in vitro via a cell proliferation-migration-loss cycle. Arterio. Thromb. Vasc. Biol. **17:** 3102–3106.

46. DePaola, N. et al. Spatial and temporal regulation of gap junction Connexin43 in vascular endothelial cells exposed to controlled disturbed flows *in vitro*. Proc. Natl. Acad. Sci. USA **96:** 3154–3159.
47. Gabriels, J.E. & D.L. Paul. 1998. Connexin43 is highly localized to sites of disturbed flow in rat aortic endothelium but connexin37, and connexin40 are more uniformly distributed. Circ. Res. **83:** 636–643.
48. Topper, J.N. et al. 1996. Identification of vascular endothelial genes differentially responsive to fluid mechanical stimuli: cyclooxygenase-2, manganese superoxide dismutase, and endothelial cell nitric oxide synthase are selectively up-regulated by steady laminar shear stress. Proc. Natl. Acad. Sci. USA **93:** 10417–10422.

Questions and Answers

G.K. Hansson (*Karolinska Hospital, Stockholm, Sweden*): This kind of experimental design, an unbiased analysis of gene expression that you showed, should permit an analysis of how these different factors interact. For instance, how will a certain biomechanical milieu affect the response to a biochemical stimulus, let's say in a certain disturbed flow, for example.

Gimbrone: We have spent almost a year now retooling to do this type of high through-put analysis of multiple, interacting stimuli. Differential display lends itself very nicely initially to acquiring a lot of data, but then you spend a lot of time, since you don't know the sequence of each band in the differential display gels. We are now moving to cDNA array transcriptional profiling, where each dot of the 5,000 plus on a given array will have information content. Differential display is great for gene discovery, but it is not as useful for describing the behavior of multiple known genes. Transcriptional profiling is the method of choice.

P. Ganz (*Brigham and Women's Hospital, Boston, MA, USA*): You showed a number of genes that were regulated by either laminar or turbulent flow, but, in your early slides, you also showed a time course for laminar shear showing that some genes go up for a few hours and then they come down. Therefore, I wonder, for those of us who are older than four or six hours, in whom something may have gone up and already returned to baseline, what is the *in vivo* translation of these experiments? Also, specifically, for COX-2, have you shown this protein in vascular endothelium *in vivo*?

Gimbrone: The immunostaining that I showed for mouse aorta actually was COX-2 protein. The endothelium is uniformly stained except around the ostia. Regarding the temporal patterns of gene expression, you are asking a very important question. All these *in vitro* models are a change from something to something else. The static culture condition is very non-physiologic; it is not the way an endothelial cell normally lives. It is not until you precondition under shear and then change from that more physiologically relevant baseline that you may actually be able to see the interplay of multiple components. So the issue of the "set-point" of the cell is very important. For MnSOD, COX-2, and eNOS, as long as you apply laminar shear, they remain upregulated, they do not downregulate. That also appears to be true *in vivo*.

Ganz: Are there differences in vascular beds not explained simply by differences in laminar flow?

Gimbrone: Yes, almost certainly. But practically, we are often limited by the availability of good reagents (e.g., antibodies) to demonstrate these differences *in vivo*. You saw the nice work earlier with antibodies to human receptors for VEGF and how revealing that was. In our own studies with BSC-2, SMAD-6, and SMAD-7, and now with the mouse and human data on COX-2, we are beginning to get some insight into vascular bed differences.

P. CARMELIET (*Flanders Interuniversity, Institute of Biotechnology, Leuven, Belgium*): In your list of target genes, I am missing some receptors as well as some angiogenic factors, or receptors for angiogenic factors. Nevertheless, embryonic vascular development is highly influenced by flow. Do you have any insights?

GIMBRONE: I agree with your point. There will be more data forthcoming.

CARMELIET: Is there anything known on the role of turbulence or disturbed laminar flow in terms of tumor angiogenesis?

GIMBRONE: I have been instructed by my fluid-mechanical engineering colleagues that the definition of turbulence is very precise; likewise the definition of disturbed laminar flow is very precise. The size of the vessel that one can model and actually measure flow is a practical limitation. In the mouse aorta, we do not know the near-wall environment, in terms of laminar versus disturbed flow, because it is extraordinarily hard to measure or model flows in that tiny structure, and I am talking about the aorta, let alone the capillary. In general, the wall shears are very low by the time you get down to the capillary level. I do not think turbulence can exist in the microvascular bed.

A.R. TALL (*Columbia University, New York, NY, USA*): The one thing that is not apparently explained by your findings today is how the cytoskeleton might change, mediating the change in the shape of the cell. One expects that it may also be involved in sensing changes in flow. Do you have any insights into how this is mediated?

GIMBRONE: Peter Davies, at the University of Pennsylvania, has done elegant studies on the role of the cytoskeleton as a potential sensing organ for biomechanical deformation and I refer you to his recent work. Years ago, when he was in our group, we also did some measurements of ionized calcium transients that are evoked by changes in shear in the endothelial cell. In fact, shear can be a very important short-term regulator of ionized calcium flux, MAP kinase pathways, and integrin-dependent adhesion to the extracellular matrix—all of which may participate in flow sensing.

Role of the Vascular NADH/NADPH Oxidase System in Atherosclerosis

MITSUHIRO YOKOYAMA,[a] NOBUTAKA INOUE, AND SEINOSUKE KAWASHIMA

First Department of Internal Medicine, Kobe University School of Medicine, 5-2, 7-chome, Kusunoki-cho, Chuo-ku, Kobe 650-0017 Japan

ABSTRACT: It is apparent that vascular tissues can produce reactive oxygen species, including the superoxide anion, and that their increased production can contribute to altered control of vasomotor tone and atherosclerosis. The NADH/NADPH oxidase system, which includes a 22 kD subunit (p22 phox), is the major source of superoxide production in vascular tissues. The superoxide radical oxidizes LDL and oxidized LDL is shown to be a key component in atherogenesis. Superoxide anion inactivates the NO radical, an anti-atherogenic molecule. Lysophosphatidylcholine, which accumulates during oxidative modification of LDL, has multiple effects on vascular cells, including cell proliferation, migration, apoptosis, and gene expression. Lysophosphatidylcholine stimulates superoxide production in endothelial cells through the NADH/NADPH oxidase–dependent mechanism. To investigate the expression of p22 phox in normal and atherosclerotic coronary arteries, samples were obtained from autopsy and examined using immunohistochemistry. In normal vessels, weak positive staining of p22 phox was detectable only in the adventitial layer. In contrast, strong immunoreactivity for p22 phox was present in atherosclerotic lesions around lipid core and shoulder regions. P22 phox was localized in the macrophages, fibroblasts, endothelial cells, and some smooth muscle cells which was identified by immunofluorescence double staining. The genetic analysis of the p22 phox gene by restriction fragment length polymorphism (RFLP) for control subject and patients with coronary artery disease revealed that the prevalence of the TC+TT genotype of the C242T polymorphism of the p22 phox gene in control subjects was significantly more frequent than in coronary artery disease patients, indicating that the mutation of the p22 phox gene might reduce the susceptibility for coronary artery disease, which is independent of other coronary risk factors. These observations suggest that oxidative stress, mainly via the NADH/NADPH oxidase system in the vasculature, may play an important role in the pathogenesis of atherosclerosis.

INTRODUCTION

Nitric oxide (NO) is a principal molecule involved in the anti-atherosclerotic properties of the endothelium.[1] NO prevents the development of atherosclerosis by inhibiting monocyte and neutrophil adhesion to the endothelium, platelet adhesion,

---

[a]Address for correspondence: Mitsuhiro Yokoyama, First Department of Internal Medicine, Kobe University School of Medicine, 5-2, 7-chome, Kusunoki-cho, Chuo-ku, Kobe 650-0017, Japan. Voice: 81-78-382-5840; fax: 81-78-382-5858.
yokoyama@med.kobe-u.ac.jp

and aggregation. It also inhibits vascular smooth muscle cell proliferation and migration as well as oxidative modification of LDL.[2] The endothelium-derived (ED) NO–mediated vasorelaxation is known to be impaired in subjects with coronary risk factors such as hypercholesterolemia, diabetes, and smoking.[3,4]

Recently it has become evident that reactive oxygen species, including superoxide (O_2^-) anion, can be produced in vascular cells and that they contribute to stimulation of smooth muscle cell growth, inactivation of EDNO, oxidation of LDL, and endothelial cell injury (damage) (FIG. 1).[5] Therefore, superoxide anion is considered a pro-atherogenic molecule involved in the pathogenesis of atherosclerosis. The production of these reactive oxygen species is increased in pathophysiological conditions such as atherosclerosis, hypertension, and diabetes.

Thus, the imbalance between NO and O_2^- is critical to initiate and continue the atherosclerotic process.

OXIDATIVE STRESS IN VASCULAR ENDOTHELIAL CELLS

Vascular cells, including smooth muscle cells, endothelial cells, and macrophages, are capable of producing superoxide anion from a variety of enzymatic sources, including xanthine/xanthine oxidase, NADH/NADPH oxidase, lipoxygenase, cyclooxygenase, and nitric oxide synthase.

To clarify the sources of superoxide production in basal vascular endothelial cells, we measured the superoxide production in intact bovine aortic endothelial cells (BAEC) grown on microcarrier beads, using the lucigenin chemiluminescence method.[7] Diphenyliodonium (DPI, 100 μM), an inhibitor of flavoproteins including the phagocytic NADPH oxidase, attenuated O_2^- production in intact BAEC. However, oxypurinol (100 μM), an inhibitor of xanthine oxidase; rotenone (30 μM), an inhibitor of mitochondrial electron transport; indomethacin (10 mM), an inhibitor of cyclooxygenase; and 5,8,11,14-eicosatetraynic acid (ETYA, 50 μM), an inhibitor of lipoxygenase, all had no significant effect. Tiron (10 mM), a scavenger of O_2^-, potently inhibited O_2^- production. Lactate (10 mM), which increased intracellular NADH via lactic dehydrogenase, stimulated O_2^- production.

Next, the effects of lysophosphatidylcholine (LPC), a major biological constituent of oxidized LDL, on O_2^- production in BAEC were examined.[8,9] Treatment of BAEC with LPC (5 μg/ml) for 2 h enhanced O_2^- production, whereas phosphatidylcholine did not have significant effect. The increase in O_2^- production caused by LPC was dependent on concentration and time. This effect of LPC was reversed with DPI treatment to nearly basal levels.

There are several indications that phosphorylation by protein kinase C (PKC) is required for the assembly and activation of neutrophil NADH/NADPH oxidase. Lysophosphatidylcholine also is known to stimulate PKC. We then examined the effects of PKC inhibitors on O_2^- production in BAEC. Both PKC inhibitors, GF 109203 (5 μM) and Ro 318220 (10 μM), did not inhibit LPC-enhanced O_2^- production, although these inhibitors were effective in preventing phorbol ester (PMA)–stimulated O_2^- production. The protein tyrosine kinases are known to mediate signal transduction and cellular functions, so we tested the effects of tyrosine kinase inhibitors, genistein (75 μM) and herbimycin (1 μM). Both tyrosine kinase inhibitors markedly attenuated LPC-enhanced O_2^- production.

These data indicate that the basal production of superoxide anion in BAEC is mainly mediated by the NADH/NADPH oxidase system and that LPC enhances O_2^- production through this enzyme system in a PKC-insensitive and tyrosine kinase–sensitive manner.

The majority of data regarding O_2^- production in vessels and vessel homogenates is based on measurements of the intensity of lucigenin-enhanced chemiluminescence. The validity of these data was recently questioned, because lucigenin itself increased formation of O_2^- in the presence of enzymes capable of providing a one-electron reduction of lucigenin, such as NO synthase and xanthine/xanthine oxidase. We therefore performed electron spin resonance (ESR) spectroscopy with a spin trap shown to detect OH^- with a high sensitivity and specificity.

The spin trap agent was dimethyl-1-pyroline-N-oxide (DMPO). ESR spectrum measurement was carried out in a suspension of bovine aortic endothelial cells. Under control conditions, few ERS signals for OH radicals were detected, whereas lysophosphatidylcholine (10 µg/ml) markedly increased vascular OH radical signals. LPC produced OH radicals in a time-dependent manner. LPC-induced OH radicals were abolished by DPI (10 µM) treatment. Thus, we could confirm our lucigenin data using ESR spectroscopic method.

NADH/NADPH OXIDASE AND CORONARY ARTERY DISEASE

During the past several years, it has become evident that both the endothelium and smooth muscle cells contain membrane-bound oxidases that utilize NADH and NADPH as substrates for electron transfer to molecular oxygen. These oxidases have similarities to neutrophil NADPH oxidase in that they possess flavin-binding and heme-binding regions. Four components of neutrophil NADPH oxidase have been fully characterized. Two of them, the gp91 phox and p22 phox subunits, are membrane-bound, whereas the others, p47 phox and p67 phox, are present in the cytosol. A common component of neutrophil oxidase and vascular smooth muscle oxidase is p22 phox. Dr. Kathy Griendling at Emory University has cloned the p22 phox of vascular smooth muscle cells, which has high homology with neutrophil p22 phox.[10–12]

Polymorphism of the NADH/NADPH Oxidase p22 phox Gene in Patients with Coronary Artery Disease[13]

There are four types of polymorphism of p22 phox gene, namely C242T, G508A, C549T, and A640G. C242T polymorphism of the p22 phox substitutes histidine-72 by tyrosine located in the potential heme-binding site. A640G polymorphism is located in the 3′ untranslated region. However, the clinical significance of these polymorphisms has never been examined. We examined whether these polymorphisms are associated with risk of coronary artery disease by restriction fragment length polymorphism (RFLP) method in 201 cases with significant coronary artery stenosis (≥75%) and 201 control subjects. Three genotypes, CC homozygotes (wild type), TC heterozygotes, and TT homozygotes (mutant type), in the C242T polymorphism were separated by RFLP. The distribution of genotypes and the frequency of alleles of C242T polymorphism are summarized in TABLES 1 and 2. The T allele frequen-

TABLE 1. Prevalence of genotypes and allele frequencies of the NADH/NADPH oxidase *p22 phox* polymorphism

Genotype	Control subjects	Case patients	p
C242T polymorphism			
CC, N (%)	148 (73.6)	173 (86.1)	.002
TC+TT, N (%)	53 + 0 (26.4)	26 + 2 (13.9)	
T allele frequency	0.13	0.08	
A640G polymorphism			
AA, N (%)	42 (20.9)	36 (17.9)	NS
AG+GG, N (%)	79 + 80 (79.1)	83 + 82 (82.1)	
G allele frequency	0.59	0.61	

TABLE 2. Odds ratio of C232T polymorphism and major coronary risk factors

	Odds ratio	95% CI	p
TT+TC	0.49	0.28–0.87	0.15
Smoking status	2.36	1.52–3.67	.0001
Hypercholesterolemia	2.19	1.23–3.90	.0079
Diabetes status	5.05	2.71–9.45	.0001
Hypertension	2.22	1.33–3.73	.0023

cies in control subjects and CAD patients were 0.13 and 0.08, respectively, and the prevalence of the TC+TT genotypes was significantly more frequent in control subjects than in coronary artery disease patients. In contrast, the allele frequency of A640G polymorphism was not different between control subjects and case patients. The odds ratio of the TC+TT versus the CC genotype of the C242T polymorphism between CAD patients and control subjects was 0.49. The association of this polymorphism with CAD was statistically significant and independent of the A640G polymorphism and other risk factors (smoking, hyperlipidemia, hypertension, and diabetes) when subjected to logistic regression analysis. Thus, the mutation of the heme-binding site of the p22 phox gene may reduce susceptibility to coronary artery disease. Our observations suggest that C242T polymorphism of the p22 phox is a novel genetic marker that has a protective effect on coronary risk.

p22 phox Expression in Human Coronary Artery[14]

Using human coronary artery sections from autopsied cases ($N = 11$), the expression of p22 phox was examined with immunohistochemistry, immunofluorescence double staining, and Western blotting. All sections were examined by hematoxylin-eosin stain and classified into non-atherosclerotic coronary arteries without thickening or with only mild and diffuse intimal thickening (21 segments) and atherosclerotic coronary arteries (47 segments).

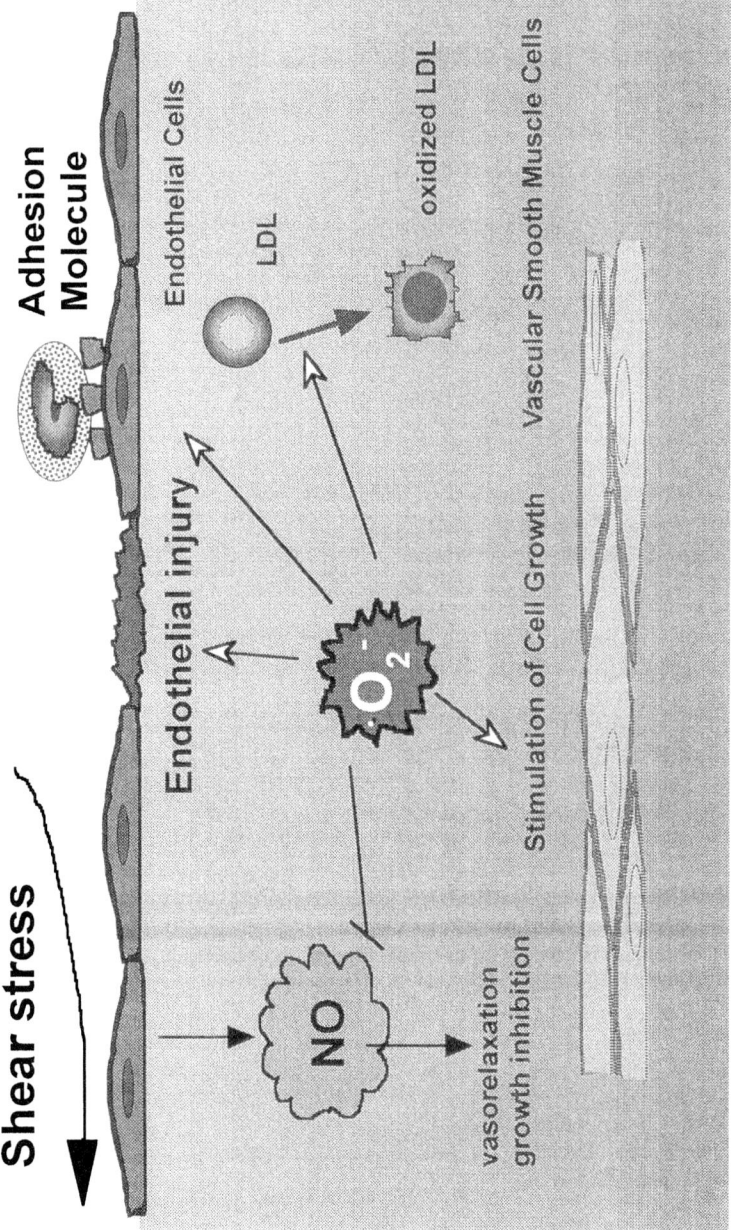

FIGURE 1.

In non-atherosclerotic coronary arteries, weakly positive immunoreactivity of p22 phox was observed clearly in the adventitia. The expression of p22 phox was scarcely detectable in the endothelium, neointima, or media. The cells expressing p22 phox in the adventitia were fibroblasts, because they were positive for anti-prolyl 4-hydroxylase antibody by double staining. In atherosclerotic coronary arteries, various histopathological changes were observed, including advanced atheromatous lesions (such as fibrous and lipid-rich plaques) and hypercellular lesions. The immunoreactivity of p22 phox was detectable throughout the vessel wall. p22 phox was expressed not only in the adventitia but also in the neointima, media, and endothelium. In hypercellular lesions, the expression of p22 phox was intense in accumulating cells. In advanced atheromatous lesions, strong p22 phox–positive immunoreactivity was detected in neointimal macrophages and smooth muscle cells. Interestingly intense localized expression of p22 phox was observed in macrophages accumulating at the border of atheromatous plaques. There was little stain, however, in the center of the lipid core.

To identify cell types of p22 phox–expressing cells, immunofluorescence double staining was performed. Most of the p22 phox–expressing cells in hypercellular lesions were positive for CD68. Some of the p22 phox–expressing cells in atheromatous lesions were positive for alpha-actin. These results suggested that macrophages and some smooth muscle cells accumulating in atheromatous lesions might acquire the ability to express p22 phox during the progression of atherosclerosis. p22 phox–expressing cells in adventitia were positive for a marker of fibroblasts (prolyl-4-hydroxylase). p22 phox–expressing cells in the endothelium were positive for von Willebrand factor, a marker of endothelial cells. Western blotting of p22 phox using anti–human p22 phox antibody was carried out in non-atherosclerotic and atherosclerotic coronary segments. p22 phox was detectable in both segments, but it was more pronounced in atherosclerotic than in non-atherosclerotic segments.

CONCLUSION

Vascular cells are capable of producing superoxide anion mainly through the NADH/NADPH oxidase system. Coronary risk factors, such as atherogenic lipids, hypertension, and smoking, are known to induce oxidative stress in the vasculature.

NADH/NADPH oxidase p22 phox might play an important role in the pathogenesis of atherosclerotic coronary artery disease via enhancing O_2^- production. Thus, the balance between NO radical, an anti-atherogenic molecule, and O_2^- radical, a pro-atherogenic molecule, is critically important to maintain functional homeostasis in the vascular cells.

ACKNOWLEDGMENTS

We thank our colleagues Doctors Saori Takeshita, Hiroshi Azumi, Yoshiyuki Rikitake, Ken-ichi Hirata, Yoshitake Hayashi, and Hiroshi Itoh for their contribution to the work in our laboratory summarized above and Ms. Taeko Isono for preparation of the manuscript.

REFERENCES

1. LLOYD-JONES, M.D. & K.D. BLOCH. 1996. The vascular biology of nitric oxide and its role in atherogenesis. Annu. Rev. Med. **47:** 365–375.
2. RIKITAKE, Y. et al. 1998. Inhibitory effect of inducible type nitric oxide synthase on oxidative modification of low density lipoprotein by vascular smooth muscle cells. Atherosclerosis **136:** 51–57.
3. HIRATA, K. et al. 1992. Impaired vasodilatory response to atrial natriuretic peptide during atherosclerosis progression. Arterioscler. Thromb. **12:** 99–105.
4. KANAZAWA, K. et al. 1996. Endothelial constitutive nitric oxide synthase protein and mRNA increased in rabbit atherosclerotic aorta despite impaired endothelium-dependent vascular relaxation. Am. J. Pathol. **148:** 1945–1956.
5. INOUE, N. et al. 1998. Stretch force on vascular smooth muscle cells enhances oxidation of LDL via superoxide production. Am. J. Physiol. **274:** H1928–H1932.
6. COX, D.A. & M.L. COHEN. 1996. Effects of oxidized low density lipoprotein on vascular contraction and relaxation: Clinical and pharmacological implications in atherosclerosis. Pharmacol. Rev. **48:** 3–19.
7. TAKESHITA, S. et al. 1999. Lysophosphatidylcholine enhances superoxide anions production via the NADH/NADPH oxidase system in cultured bovine aortic endothelial cells. Submitted for publication.
8. YOKOYAMA, M. et al. 1992. Lysophosphatidylcholine: essential role in the inhibition of endothelium-dependent vasorelaxation by oxidized low density lipoprotein. Biochem. Biophys. Res. Commun. **168:** 301–308.
9. INOUE, N. et al. 1992. Lysophosphatidylcholine inhibits bradykinin-induced phosphoinositide hydrolysis and calcium transients in cultured bovine aortic endothelial cells. Circ. Res. **71:** 1410–1421.
10. GRIENDLING, K.K. et al. 1993. Angiotensin II stimulates NADH/NADPH oxidase activity in cultured vascular smooth muscle cells. Circ. Res. **74:** 1141–1148.
11. FUKUI, T. et al. 1995. Cytochrome b-558 α subunit cloning and expression in rat aortic smooth muscle cells. Biochim. Biophys. Acta **1231:** 215–219.
12. USHI-FUKAI, M. et al. 1996. p22^{phox} is a critical component of the superoxide-generating NADH/NADPH oxidase system and regulates angiotensin II-induced hypertrophy in vascular smooth muscle cells. J. Biol. Chem. **271:** 23317–23321.
13. INOUE, N. et al. 1998. Polymorphism of the NADH/NADPH oxidase p22phox gene in patients with coronary artery disease. Circulation **97:** 135–137.
14. AZUMI, H. et al. 1999. Expression of NADH/NADPH oxidase p22^{phox} in human coronary artery. Circulation **100:** 1494–1498.

Questions and Answers

M.A. GIMBRONE (*Brigham and Women's Hospital, Boston, MA, USA*): The pattern of the expression of p22 phox in the lesions is very reminiscent of something that can be activated by a locally generated cytokine or perhaps other substances. Has that been examined? Is p22 phox a cytokine-inducible gene in macrophages, smooth muscle cells, or endothelial cells?

YOKOYAMA: There is no information at all. We have never examined it by stimulating the cytokines.

GIMBRONE: Does lysophosphatidylcholine regulate the expression of that gene?

YOKOYAMA: We would like to try.

GIMBRONE: On the poster from your group about the glutathione peroxidase induction by laminar shear, I noticed that you are growing the bovine aortic endothelial cells on microcarrier beads to do your LPC experiments. Have you ever put those beads in a flow chamber with the cells on them and to see if lysophosphatidylcholine's ability to induce these various changes in the endothelium via superoxide is different in the preconditioned flow–exposed endothelium?

YOKOYAMA: Not yet.

Molecular Basis of Angiogenesis
Role of VEGF and VE-Cadherin

PETER CARMELIET[a] AND DESIRE COLLEN

Center for Transgene Technology and Gene Therapy, Flanders Interuniversity, Institute for Biotechnology, KU Leuven, Leuven, B-3000, Belgium

> ABSTRACT: The formation of new blood vessels (angiogenesis) is essential for embryonic development and contributes to the pathogenesis of numerous disorders. In contrast, insufficient angiogenesis may lead to tissue ischemia and failure. The recent discovery of novel angiogenic molecules has initiated efforts to improve tissue perfusion via therapeutic angiogenesis. However, rational design of such treatment strategies mandates a better understanding of the molecular mechanisms of angiogenesis. In this brief review, the role of a prime angiogenic candidate, namely vascular endothelial growth factor (VEGF) and its homologues, in physiological and pathological angiogenesis will be discussed with particular attention to myocardial ischemia and heart failure. In addition, a novel interaction between the junctional protein vascular endothelial-cadherin (VE-cadherin) and VEGF, essential for the endothelial survival function of VEGF, will be reviewed.

DEVELOPMENT OF A FUNCTIONAL VASCULATURE

Blood vessels form via vasculogenesis and angiogenesis. The former process involves differentiation of precursor stem cells to endothelial cells, which subsequently assemble into vessels,[1] whereas the latter implicates growth of endothelial sprouts via budding of individual angioblasts or endothelial cells from preexisting capillaries. Vasculogenesis results in the formation of a primitive vascular network, which subsequently expands and remodels via angiogenesis in a more mature vasculature, comprising large vessels branching into smaller capillaries. Vessels in the embryo form initially via vasculogenesis and subsequently via angiogenesis, whereas new vessels in the adult predominantly develop via angiogenesis. Although endothelial cells have attracted most of the attention in angiogenesis research, they, alone, are unable to complete a mature, functional vascular network—the end result of angiogenesis. Periendothelial mural cells (smooth muscle cells in large vessels, pericytes in small vessels, and cardiomyocytes in the heart) exhibit a wide variety of functions). They protect new blood vessels, which initially consist of endothelial cells alone, against hemodynamic or traumatic rupture and provide hemostatic control. They inhibit proliferation and induce differentiation of endothelial cells. They determine barrier function as macrophage-like scavengers.[2] Initiation of vessel sprouting requires loosening of

---

[a]Address for correspondence: P. Carmeliet, M.D., Ph.D., Center for Transgene Technology and Gene Therapy, Campus Gasthuisberg, Herestraat 49, University of Leuven, Leuven, B-3000, Belgium. Voice: 32-16-34-57-72; fax: 32-16-34-59-90.
peter.carmeliet@med.kuleuven.ac.be

mural cells from their resident site, which allows endothelial cells to start proliferating and migrating. In addition, mural cells contribute to the remodeling and maturation of new blood vessels: during an initial plasticity window, endothelial-lined vessels undergo hyperoxia-induced vascular pruning, but once these endothelial channels are covered by mural cells, they become resistant to regression.[4,5] The vasomotor and viscoelastic properties of mural wall around endothelial cells accommodate rapid changes in blood flow or pressure. Furthermore, reperfusion of ischemic tissues (including the heart) depends not only on endothelial growth in new capillaries (true angiogenesis) but, probably more important, on enlargement and remodeling of preexisting arterioles during collateral growth (arteriogenesis).[6]

VASCULAR ENDOTHELIAL GROWTH FACTOR

Vascular endothelial growth factor (VEGF), unlike other known angiogenic factors, has a unique combination of properties: (1) it is produced by cells in close proximity to endothelial cells[7]; (2) it is secreted and exerts a direct and largely restricted effect on endothelial cells via interaction with cellular receptors VEGF receptor-2 (VEGFR-2) and VEGF-receptor-1 (VEGFR-1)[8]; (3) it induces a pleiotropic response allowing endothelial cells to proliferate, to migrate, to assemble into tubes, to survive, and to increase their permeability[9–11]; (4) its expression is highly regulated by hypoxia, providing a physiological feedback mechanism to accommodate insufficient tissue oxygenation by promoting blood vessel formation[12]; and (5) it is a potent growth factor since its over- or under-expression significantly affects blood vessel formation *in vivo*.[13,14] The restricted expression of VEGF and its receptors in the vascular network during embryogenesis suggests a role for these molecules in vascular development.[7,15] In contrast to the minimal levels of VEGF gene expression in most adult tissues, VEGF expression is detectable in adult kidney, possibly implicating a role in the maintenance of blood vessels and/or in endothelial fenestration.[10,11] VEGF expression can be induced in a variety of cell types during myocardial ischemia,[12] atherosclerosis,[16] diabetic and ischemic retinopathy,[9] tumorigenesis,[17] arthritis, psoriasis, and wound healing,[18] suggesting that the VEGF:VEGF receptor gene family is implicated in pathological neovascularization. VEGF (gene) therapy is currently being tested to improve ischemic heart disease and peripheral limb vasculopathy.[19]

Targeted inactivation of a single *VEGF* allele resulted in haplo-insufficiency with embryonic lethality due to abnormal blood vessel development around 9 days of gestation.[13,14,20] The dorsal aorta had a smaller lumen, sprouting of vessels was reduced, and connections of large blood vessels with the heart appeared abnormal. In the yolk sac and placenta, only an irregular plexus of enlarged capillaries was present. Blood vessel development was more affected in homozygous VEGF-deficient embryos, generated by aggregation of homozygous VEGF-deficient embryonic stem cells with tetraploid embryos, than in heterozygous VEGF-deficient embryos. These data suggest a tight gene dose–dependent relationship and production of only minimally required VEGF levels during development. Taken together, VEGF is not essential for initial differentiation of angioblasts to early endothelial cells, but threshold levels of VEGF appear to be required for further blood vessel formation. Conditional inactivation of the *VEGF* gene or administration of soluble VEGFR-1/IgG chimeric VEGF antagonists at birth resulted in impaired postnatal vascular development and endothelial survival, leading to increased mortality, stunted body growth, and impaired organ development (in particular liver, heart, and renal failure).[21]

INTERACTION BETWEEN VEGF AND VE-CADHERIN

Endothelial cells are linked to each other by tight- and adherens-type junctions. The latter are formed by transmembrane calcium-dependent adhesive proteins, called cadherins.[22] VE-cadherin is only found at endothelial adherens junctions[23] and interacts, via its cytoplasmic tail, with three proteins of the *armadillo* family, called β-catenin, plakoglobin, and p120. Beta-catenin and plakoglobin anchor cadherins to the cortical actin cytoskeleton.[24] The extracellular domain of VE-cadherin mediates initial cell adhesion, whereas the cytosolic tail is required for interaction with the cytoskeleton and junctional strength. VE-cadherin may also be implicated in cell differentiation, growth, and migration.[25] The extracellular adhesive domain and the intracellular β-catenin binding region of VE-cadherin participate in density-dependent inhibition of endothelial growth.[26] Indirect evidence suggests that cadherins transfer intracellular signals but the intracellular mediators remain unknown. Cadherins may bind β-catenin and plakoglobin, thereby decreasing the cytoplasmic pool of free β-catenin. The latter can translocate to the nucleus and affect gene transcription via binding of high mobility group (HMG) transcription factors.[27] Instead, β-catenin, bound to cadherins, cannot bind to HMG transcription factors. Cadherins may also participate in signaling by clustering signaling molecules and growth factor receptors. In the mouse, VE-cadherin is expressed in hemangioblasts from day 7.5 of gestation (E7.5) onwards[28] and, thereafter, constitutively in all endothelial cells.

In order to define the role of VE-cadherin and of its binding to β-catenin in intracellular signaling, mice were generated that lacked a functional *VE-cadherin* gene (VEC$^{-/-}$), that expressed a mutant *VE-cadherin* gene lacking the β-catenin–binding cytoplasmic tail by introducing a stop codon in front of the 82 carboxyterminal residues, interacting with β-catenin (VEC$^{\delta C/\delta C}$), or that did not express detectable VE-cadherin levels because of an intronic *neomycin phosphotransferase* (*neo*) gene (VEC$^{neo/neo}$).[29] Surprisingly, all three strains died at E9.5 due to vascular insufficiency. VEC$^{+/+}$ and mutant embryos were indistinguishable at E8.0, e.g., immediately after onset of angioblast formation. By E8.25–8.5, angioblasts in both wild type and mutant embryos differentiated to endothelial cells, which became assembled in primitive vessels within the embryo and yolk sac, indicating that initial vasculogenesis occurred after loss/truncation of VE-cadherin. However, by E8.5, certain vessels in mutant embryos had a minimal or even no lumen whereas others were dilated. In mutant embryos, endothelial cells in the yolk sac formed channels that started to disconnect from each other at their branches, whereas endocardial cells detached from each other and laid scattered in the ventricular cavity. The lack of yolk sac–derived red blood cells inside E8.5 wild-type embryos indicated that the vitello-embryonic circulation was not yet established. Vascular defects in mutant VE-cadherin embryos were more severe beyond E8.75–E9.0, when the primitive vascular network in wild-type embryos expands via sprouting angiogenesis and remodels in a branching network of large and small vessels. Endothelial cells throughout the entire vasculature progressively became disconnected from each other and exhibited numerous gaps, detached from their underlying basement membrane and laid scattered inside the lumen. Several of these endothelial cells were apoptotic. Sprouting of intersomitic vessels and remodeling into a network of large and small branches were impaired in mutant embryos and yolk sacs, often resulting in irregular, dilated vessels. Other vessels were present as cords with a minimal lumen, contained few disconnected and scattered endothelial cells, progressively disconnected from each other at branches, thereby inducing stagnating blood lakes, or regressed. Beyond E9.25, vessels in mutant VE-cadherin embryos regressed, disintegrated, and collapsed, causing circulatory insufficiency and progressive necrosis. Thus, normal VE-cadherin function is not or only minimally required for assembly into a primitive capillary plexus (vasculogenesis) but it is essential for subsequent expansion, maturation, branching, and remodeling into a network of veins and arteries of different sizes (angiogenesis) and prevention of vascular regression.

Loss or truncation of VE-cadherin did not affect endothelial differentiation or proliferation, but impaired endothelial survival. When immortalized wild-type and mutant endothelial cells were cultured in the absence of serum, mutant endothelial cells exhibited increased apoptosis. Notably, the endothelial survival factor VEGF rescued survival of wild-type but not mutant endothelial cells. In contrast, basic fibroblast growth factor (bFGF) rescued endothelial survival regardless of the presence or absence of VE-cadherin. Notably, intravenous injection of VE-cadherin antibodies in adult wild-type mice also caused apoptosis of mature endothelial cells. VEGF is a survival factor for endothelial cells via activation of VEGFR-2 and subsequent signaling of PI3-kinase.[30] PI3-kinase inhibitors blocked VEGF-mediated survival of wild-type endothelial cells, but did not affect apoptosis of mutant endothelial cells when cultured in the absence of serum. Coimmunoprecipitation experiments revealed an association between VE-cadherin, β-catenin, PI3-kinase, and VEGFR-2 in wild-type but not mutant cells. VEGF increased phosphorylation of Akt in HUVEC cells treated with VE-cadherin antibodies. Thus, a multicomponent complex comprising VE-cadherin, β-catenin, VEGFR-2, and PI3-kinase is required for the endothelial survival function of VEGF-A through activation of Akt. Disruption of this complex by truncation of VE-cadherin (which abolishes association with β-catenin) or by VE-cadherin antibodies (which prevents clustering of VE-cadherin) renders endothelial cells refractory to the VEGF survival signal.

Taken together, neither VE-cadherin nor the stabilization of the adherens-type junctions, which depend on the interaction of the VE-cadherin tail with the cytoskeleton, are required for initial assembly of endothelial cells *in vivo*, possibly because of the minimal hemodynamic stress before onset of the circulation and/or to the presence of other adhesive molecules at interendothelial contacts. The vascular defects in older mutant embryos are attributable to increased endothelial apoptosis, due to an inability of VE-cadherin–deficient cells to respond to the survival activity of VEGF. Once endothelial cells are assembled and organized in primitive vessels, subsequent remodeling and pruning of the primitive vascular labyrinth requires endothelial apoptosis. VE-cadherin is not essential during initial vessel assembly but it does regulate endothelial apoptosis during the second phase of angiogenesis. Interestingly, the role of VE-cadherin is specific for VEGF and not for bFGF, a pleiotropic factor that also affects non-endothelial cells, thereby rendering the VEGF/VE-cadherin response highly restricted to endothelial cells.

ISCHEMIC CARDIOMYOPATHY AND CARDIAC FAILURE IN MICE EXPRESSING A SINGLE VEGF$_{120}$ ISOFORM

The mouse *VEGF* gene is alternatively transcribed in at least three isoforms (VEGF$_{120}$, VEGF$_{164}$, VEGF$_{188}$). VEGF$_{120}$ is diffusible in the extracellular milieu, whereas the longer isoforms display an increased binding to heparan sulfate–rich matrix.[10,11,33] These isoforms have been reported to differ in their mitogenicity, chemotactic properties, receptor binding characteristics, and tissue-specific expression.[33–36] It remains, however, controversial whether the isoforms differ in specificity, potency, or quality for their role in normal, pathologic, or therapeutic angiogenesis *in vivo*.[33,37–39] Nevertheless, current gene therapy protocols use VEGF$_{120}$ or VEGF$_{164}$ indiscriminately for improvement of tissue ischemia.

Mice expressing solely VEGF$_{120}$ (VEGF$^{120/120}$ mice) were generated using the Cre/*lox*P system to remove exons 6 and 7, which encode basic domains that are only present in VEGF$_{164}$ and/or VEGF$_{188}$. A fraction of homozygous VEGF$_{120}$ embryos died shortly after birth. The remainder of these mutant mice gained less weight, became lethargic, and died before 14 days after birth of cardiac failure. Indeed, VEGF$^{120/120}$ mice exhibited depressed left ventricular (LV) systolic pressure, contractility and relaxation, spontaneous arrhythmia, and had enlarged systolic and diastolic LV diameters.

In wild-type mice, the number of capillaries and coronary vessels increased during the first three postnatal weeks three- and tenfold, respectively, to match the increasing metabolic demands of the hypertrophying cardiomyocytes. In contrast, the capillary density did not change in VEGF$^{120/120}$ mice, resulting in larger intercapillary distances, increased myocyte-to-capillary ratios, and impaired oxygen delivery. The angiogenic defects (as well as the ischemia) were most pronounced in the subendomyocardium, consistent with previous observations that angiogenic sprouting occurs in an epi- to endocardial gradient.[40] Capillaries in VEGF$^{120/120}$ hearts were also more irregular, tortuous, and dilated, suggesting immature vessel remodeling. Hearts from VEGF$^{120/120}$ mice contained fewer coronary vessels and reduced smooth muscle coverage, possibly related to the reduced levels of PDGF-B and its receptor type-β (molecules involved in smooth muscle recruitment[41]).

The vascular defects in myocardial angiogenesis in VEGF$^{120/120}$ mice resulted in myocardial ischemia, as evidenced by a >80% reduction of myocardial blood flow, by ST-segment depressions and T-wave inversions at rest and dramatic ST-segment elevations upon respiratory stress, by signs of severe hypoxia in the subendomyocardium causing upregulation of hypoxia-inducible genes, and by abnormal propagation of the electrical pulse as a result of connexin43 uncoupling. Thus, VEGF$^{120/120}$ mice exhibited many features of ischemic cardiomyopathy observed in patients. In addition, the VEGF$^{120/120}$ mouse model may well be the first animal model of ischemic heart disease with signs of hibernation, i.e., contractile dysfunction with sarcomere rarefication but preservation of ATP stores, glycogen storage, nuclear distortion, expression of fetal genes.[42,44]

The present data indicate that VEGF$_{120}$ by itself is insufficient for normal angiogenesis. Since *VEGF$_{120}$* mRNA levels in VEGF$^{120/120}$ mice were comparable to the three VEGF isoforms in VEGF$^{+/+}$ mice, the various VEGF isoforms may exert different biological functions, for example by binding to different receptors.[33] Interestingly, expression of the $VEGF_{164}$-specific receptor neuropilin-1[33] was reduced in $VEGF^{120/120}$ mice. The various VEGF isoforms may also affect angiogenesis by a different spatial localization, as $VEGF_{164}$ and $VEGF_{188}$ isoforms bind more avidly to heparan sulfate–rich extracellular matrix, thereby affecting endothelial differentiation,[45] stabilization, or remodeling.[38] Alternatively, some of the vascular defects (e.g., the tortuosity and enlargement) may be related to the increased levels of $VEGF_{120}$ in $VEGF^{120/120}$ mice as compared to wild-type mice, as overexpression of $VEGF_{120}$ induces irregular, dilated vessels.[38] Surprisingly, VEGF also influenced the formation of smooth muscle cell–surrounded coronary arteries. This could be a direct effect of VEGF on smooth muscle cells or an indirect effect on production of recruitment factors such as platelet-derived growth factor-B.[41]

$VEGF_{120}$ and $VEGF_{165}$ appear to be used non-discriminatively for angiogenic gene therapy, in part because their role during angiogenesis *in vivo* was unknown. The severe angiogenic defects in $VEGF^{120/120}$ mice illustrate the functional complementarity of the VEGF isoforms in angiogenesis, and suggest that specific VEGF isoforms may be important for an optimal angiogenic response *in vivo*. Ongoing efforts to generate and phenotype mice that exclusively express $VEGF_{164}$ or $VEGF_{188}$, or a selective combination, will be useful to further unravel their distinct angiogenic role. Apart from constituting useful tools to assess which of the specific VEGF isoforms can optimally rescue angiogenic defects, $VEGF^{120/120}$ mice might also be used as a source of ischemic tissues to discover novel candidate genes involved in the myocardial response to ischemia or to test the possible therapeutic benefit of cardioprotective drugs.

HYPOXIC REGULATION OF VEGF-MEDIATED ANGIOGENESIS

Formation of blood vessels is triggered by reduced supply of oxygen and nutrients, occurring when intercapillary distances exceed 100 μm (i.e., exceeding three to seven cell layers). Hypoxia is an important regulator of VEGF expression.[12] Hypoxic regulation of VEGF gene expression is mediated by a family of hypoxia-inducible transcription factors (HIF) including HIF-1β (or the arylhydrocarbon receptor nuclear translocator; ARNT), HIF-1α, and HIF-2α. They mediate the response to hypoxia, hypoglycemia, insulin, and IGF-1 by binding to hypoxia-response promoter elements within a range of physiological oxygen concentrations (0.5–20%).[46–50] In addition, hypoxia upregulates expression of VEGF by improving its translation and stabilizing its transcripts.[51,52] The von Hippel Lindau (VHL) tumor suppressor gene product suppresses, whereas the RNA-binding HuR protein destabilizes expression of VEGF during normoxia.[51,52] Deficiency of these hypoxia regulators results in embryonic lethality due to defective angiogenesis, despite normal vasculogenesis. This suggests that the initial steps of vascular development are not critically regulated by oxygen but that subsequent vascular remodeling becomes dependent on oxygen levels.[53–57] Transgenic mice harboring a mutant *VEGF* gene in which the hypoxia-response element for HIF-1 was deleted are viable but exhibit impaired hypoxia-driven angiogenesis (unpublished observations). Tumors deficient in HIF-1β or HIF-1α failed to develop vascularized tumors and lacked hypoxic induction of VEGF expression.[55,58,59] Despite severe hypoxia, HIF-1α–deficient tumors exhibited uncontrolled growth, due to refractoriness to hypoxic apoptosis and growth suppression.[59] Hypoxia-inducible factors and hypoxia-response elements are currently being used for angiogenic gene therapy during ischemic conditions.

VEGF HOMOLOGUES

More recently, other VEGF-related factors have been identified. Homo- or heterodimerization of these ligands may determine their biological specificity.[60] Placental growth factor (PLGF) is expressed in the placenta and, to a lesser extent, in the heart, lung, and thyroid gland.[61] PLGF binds only to VEGFR-1 and causes intracellular signaling in endothelial cells and trophoblasts that is distinct from that of VEGF.[62,63] Three alternatively transcribed *PLGF* mRNAs have been identified in man, of which PLGF-2 contains additional 21 basic amino acid residues,[64–66] has affinity for extracellular matrix components, and binds neuropilin-1.[67] Although PLGF homodimers may cause endothelial proliferation and migration *in vitro* and induce vascular permeability and angiogenesis *in vivo*, PLGF might also affect these responses via interaction with VEGF.[60,62,63,65,68–72] Furthermore, different combinations of PLGF/VEGF heterodimers may provide distinct angiogenic signals.[72,73] PLGF may also affect the angiogenic response indirectly by stimulating monocyte recruitment.[74] Notably, hypoxia does not affect or even slightly decreases PLGF expression,[72,75] but significantly affects formation of PLGF/VEGF heterodimers.[72,73] PLGF may also affect angiogenesis indirectly by stimulating monocyte recruitment.[74] Deficiency of PLGF in transgenic mice did not affect physiological angiogenesis during embryogenesis or neonatal growth, but impaired angiogenesis during a variety of pathological conditions (unpublished observations in collaboration with G. Persico and colleagues, Naples, Italy). Despite its high expression in placenta[76] and signaling via VEGFR-1 in trophoblasts,[63] PLGF-deficient mice were fertile. The role of PLGF in pathological angiogenesis remains unknown.

VEGF-B has similar endothelial mitogenic potency as VEGF, binds VEGFR-1, and is primarily expressed in developing myocardium and to a lesser extent in developing muscle, bone, pancreas, adrenal gland and in the smooth muscle cells in large vessels.[77–79] VEGF-B is coexpressed and able to heterodimerize with VEGF, but is not regulated by hypoxia. It remains largely cell-associated, possibly providing spatial cues to outgrowing endothelial cells, or acting as a releasable pool to induce endothelial cell regeneration after injury. Recent data suggest that VEGF-B–deficient mice develop normally and are healthy, but display subtle cardiac defects (U. Eriksson and colleagues, personal communication).

VEGF-C (also called VEGF-related factor, VEGF-2) binds VEGFR-3 in its mature form and VEGFR-2 with a lower affinity in its incompletely processed form. It stimulates migration and proliferation of endothelial cells *in vitro* and *in vivo*,[80–84] and inhibits PDGF-stimulated smooth muscle cell migration.[85] In the adult, it is most abundantly expressed in the heart, placenta, lung, kidney, muscle, ovary, and small intestine.[81] VEGF-C and VEGFR-3 may initially be involved in development of the venous system, as suggested by their embryonic expression pattern.[80,81,86] Loss of VEGFR-3 causes embryonic lethality due to defective angiogenesis,[87] whereas VEGF-C improves ischemic limb revascularization[88] and stimulates *in vivo* angiogenesis.[82] VEGF-C and VEGFR-3 also regulate lymphangiogenesis, as suggested by their expression in lymphatic vessels[80,81,86,89] and by the hyperplasia of lymphatic vessels in mice overexpressing VEGF-C or embryos treated with VEGF-C.[90,91]

VEGF-D, originally isolated from c-fos knockout mouse fibroblasts,[92] is induced by c-fos and is more abundant in serum-starved quiescent cells.[92] *In vivo*, VEGF-D is expressed in the lung, heart, small intestines, lung, anterior pituitary, kidney, liver, and skin.[93] VEGF-D is a ligand for VEGFR-2 and VEGFR-3 and a mitogen for endothelial cells.[94] Although the structural similarities between VEGF-C and VEGF-D suggest similar functions, their expression patterns differ and the precise role of VEGF-D in vascular development and pathological angiogenesis remains unknown.

VEGF Receptors

Receptor tyrosine kinases that bind VEGF homologues with different specificity and affinity have been identified: VEGFR-1 (Flt1) binds VEGF and PLGF; VEGFR-2 (Flk1) binds VEGF, VEGF-C, and VEGF-D; and VEGFR-3 (Flt4) binds VEGF-C and VEGF-D.[33] In addition, the semaphorin receptors neuropilin-1 and neuropilin-2 are low-affinity surface-associated receptors that selectively bind $VEGF_{165}$ and PLGF-2.[33] Neuropilin-1 appears to function as a VEGFR-2 coreceptor, assisting binding of $VEGF_{165}$ and potentiating its biological effects.[35] However, it is unclear whether neuropilin-1 also functions as a coreceptor for VEGFR-1.[33] Heparan sulfates may regulate the interaction and biological activity of VEGF with its receptors. VEGFR-1 and VEGFR-2 have overlapping, yet distinct temporo-spatial expression patterns during embryogenesis.[15,95] Both receptors are present in primitive endothelial cells and subsequently, in most capillaries in developing organs. In all these tissues VEGF is expressed by adjacent cells, suggesting paracrine regulation of VEGF-dependent blood vessel formation. VEGFR-2 induces intracellular signaling and mediates endothelial proliferation, migration, survival, and vascular permeability.[30,80,96] The importance of VEGFR-2 for vascular development was revealed by the embryonic lethality around 10 days of gestation due to complete absence of organized blood vessels in embryos lacking VEGFR-2.[97] More recent analysis of chimeric VEGFR-2–deficient mice indicated a cell-autonomous requirement for VEGFR-2 in endothelial cell differentiation.[98] In addition, VEGFR-2 is expressed on hemangioblasts (the common precursor of endothelial and hematopoietic cells)[99,100] and may be implicated in their migration to sites of angiogenesis.[97] The observation that VEGF deficiency did not result in a similar phenotype as VEGFR-2 deficiency may suggest the involvement of other VEGF-related ligands or rescue by maternal VEGF. VEGFR-2 inhibitor studies have amply demonstrated the importance of this receptor for pathological angiogenesis.[101,102]

The role of VEGFR-1 in vessel formation remains more enigmatic. VEGFR-1 is a functional receptor for trophoblasts mediating nitric oxide release,[103] and for monocytes/macrophages, mediating expression of tissue factor, chemotaxis, and transmigration through endothelial cells. In endothelial cells, it mediates proliferation but not migration in response to VEGF, possibly because it does not activate MAP kinase.[33,74] This is further exemplified by the mitogenic properties of VEGF mutants unable to bind VEGFR-1.[34] Although PLGF homodimers only bind VEGFR-1, it remains to be determined whether induction of endothelial proliferation and migration *in vitro* and vascular permeability and angiogenesis *in vivo* depend on interaction with VEGFR-1 or, in addition or instead, on an interaction with

VEGF, possibly via heterodimerization. A soluble VEGFR-1 has been identified, but its *in vivo* function remains unknown.[104] The second Ig-like domain of VEGFR-1 contains critical determinants required for interaction with VEGF and PLGF.[105] Loss of VEGFR-1 results in embryonic lethality around 10 days of gestation: despite the presence of numerous differentiated endothelial cells, the latter failed to form an organized vascular network and assembled in abnormally large and fused vessels.[106] These findings suggest a possible role of VEGFR-1 in contact inhibition of endothelial cell growth or in endothelial cell assembly. The rather unexpected finding that VEGFR-1 lacking the tyrosine kinase domain is sufficient for normal vascular development in mice questions the role of this receptor as a signaling tyrosine kinase and may suggest that it performs its role in angiogenesis primarily as a ligand-binding molecule.[107]

VEGFR-3 is expressed in the early embryo in blood vessels, in particular in certain veins. Subsequently, it becomes restricted to sites of lymphangiogenesis and is currently one of the most specific markers of lymphatic vessels in normal and pathologic conditions. Loss of VEGFR-3 did not prevent vasculogenesis and angiogenic sprouting, but impaired remodeling of the expanding embryonic vasculature, suggesting that this receptor is involved in development of the vascular system before its role in lymphangiogenesis.[87] The role of neuropilin-1 in vascular development is suggested by findings of cardiovascular failure in neuropilin-1–deficient embryos,[108] and excess capillaries and blood vessels, dilatation of vessels, and malformed hearts in chimeric mice overexpressing neuropilin-1.[109] However, the precise role of neuropilin-1 and neuropilin-2 in pathological angiogenesis remains to be determined.

ACKNOWLEDGMENTS

The authors are grateful to the members of the Center for Transgene Technology and Gene Therapy and to all external collaborators who contributed to these studies.

REFERENCES

1. RISAU, W. 1997. Mechanisms of angiogenesis. Nature **386:** 671–674.
2. HIRSCHL, K.K. & P.A. D'AMORE. 1996. Pericytes in the microvasculature. Cardiovasc. Res. **32:** 687–698.
3. SIMS, D.E., F.N. MILLER, A. DONALD & M.A. PERRICONE. 1990. Ultrastructure of pericytes in early stages of histamine-induced inflammation. J. Morph. **206:** 333–342.
4. JAIN, R.K. *et al.* 1998. Endothelial cell death, angiogenesis, and microvascular function after castration in an androgen-dependent tumor: role of vascular endothelial growth factor. Proc. Natl. Acad. Sci. USA **95:** 10820–10825.
5. BENJAMIN, L.E., I. HEMO & E. KESHET. 1998. A plasticity window for blood vessel remodelling is defined by pericyte coverage of the preformed endothelial network and is regulated by PDGF- B and VEGF. Development **125:** 1591–1598.
6. SCHAPER, W. & W.D. ITO. 1996. Molecular mechanisms of coronary collateral vessel growth. Circ. Res. **79:** 911–919.
7. BREIER, G., M. CLAUSS & W. RISAU. 1995. Coordinate expression of vascular endothelial growth factor receptor-1 (flt-1)and its ligand suggests a paracrine regulation of murine vascular development. Dev. Dyn. **204:** 228–234.
8. TERMAN, B.I. & M. DOUGHER VERMAZEN. 1996. Biological properties of VEGF/VPF receptors. Cancer Metastasis Rev. **15:** 159–163.

9. KLAGSBRUN, M. & P.A. D'AMORE. 1996. Vascular endothelial growth factor and its receptors. Cytokine Growth Factor Rev. **7:** 259–270.
10. FERRARA, N. & T. DAVIS-SMYTH. 1997. The biology of vascular endothelial growth factor. Endocrine Rev. **18:** 4–25.
11. DVORAK, H.F., L.F. BROWN, M. DETMAR & A.M. DVORAK. 1995. Vascular permeability factor/vascular endothelial growth factor, microvascular hyperpermeability, and angiogenesis. Am. J. Pathol. **146:** 1029–1039.
12. DOR, Y. & E. KESHET. 1997. Ischemia-driven angiogenesis. Trends Cardiovasc. Med. **7:** 289–294.
13. CARMELIET, P. *et al.* 1996. Abnormal blood vessel development and lethality in embryos lacking a single vascular endothelial growth factor allele. Nature **380:** 435–439.
14. FERRARA, N. *et al.* 1996. Heterozygous embryonic lethality induced by targeted inactivation of the VEGF gene. Nature **380:** 439–442.
15. YAMAGUCHI, T.P., D.J. DUMONT, R.A. CONLON, M.L. BREITMAN & J. ROSSANT. 1993. flk-1, an flt-related receptor tyrosine kinase is an early marker for endothelial cell precursors. Development **118:** 489–498.
16. KUZUYA, M. *et al.* 1995. Induction of angiogenesis by smooth muscle cell-derived factor: possible role in neovascularization in atherosclerotic plaque. J. Cell. Physiol. **164:** 658–667.
17. PLATE, K.H. & W. RISAU. 1995. Angiogenesis in malignant gliomas. Glia **15:** 339–347.
18. FRANK, S. *et al.* 1995. Regulation of vascular endothelial growth factor expression in cultured keratinocytes. Implications for normal and impaired wound healing. J. Biol. Chem. **270:** 12607–12613.
19. ISNER, J.M. & A. TAKAYUKI. 1998. Therapeutic angiogenesis. Front. Biosci. **3:** 49–69.
20. CARMELIET, P. & D. COLLEN. 1997. Insights into vascular biology via targeted gene inactivation and adenovirus-mediated gene transfer of the plasminogen system in Coronary Restenosis. *In* Genetics to Therapeutics. G.Z. Feuerstein, Ed.: 225–240. Marcel Dekker, Inc. New York.
21. GERBER, H.P. *et al.* 1999. VEGF is required for growth and survival in neonatal mice. Development **126:** 1149–1159.
22. HYNES, R.O. 1992. Specificity of cell adhesion in development: the cadherin superfamily. Curr. Opin. Genet. Dev. **2:** 621–624.
23. LAMPUGNANI, M.G. *et al.* 1992. A novel endothelial-specific membrane protein is a marker of cell-cell contacts. J. Cell Biol. **118:** 1511–1522.
24. GUMBINER, B.M. 1996. Cell adhesion: the molecular basis of tissue architecture and morphogenesis. Cell **84:** 345–357.
25. DEJANA, E. 1996. Endothelial adherens junctions: implications in the control of vascular permeability and angiogenesis. J. Clin. Invest. **98:** 1949–1953.
26. CAVEDA, L. *et al.* 1996. Inhibition of cultured cell growth by vascular endothelial cadherin (cadherin-5/VE-cadherin). J. Clin. Invest. **98:** 886–893.
27. BEHRENS, J. *et al.* 1996. Functional interaction of beta-catenin with the transcription factor LEF-1. Nature **382:** 638–642.
28. BREIER, G. *et al.* 1996. Molecular cloning and expression of murine vascular endothelial-cadherin in early stage development of cardiovascular system. Blood **87:** 630–641.
29. CARNALITY, P. *et al.* 1999. Targeted deficiency or cytosolic truncation of the VE-cadherin gene in mice impairs VEGF-mediated endothelial survival and angiogenesis. Cell **98:** 147–157.
30. GERBER, H.P. *et al.* 1998. Vascular endothelial growth factor regulates endothelial cell survival through the phosphatidylinositol 3′-kinase/Akt signal transduction pathway. Requirement for Flk-1/KDR activation. J. Biol. Chem. **273:** 30336–30343.
31. GERBER, H.P., V. DIXIT & N. FERRARA. 1998. Vascular endothelial growth factor induces expression of the antiapoptotic proteins Bcl-2 and A1 in vascular endothelial cells. J. Biol. Chem. **273:** 13313–13316.
32. NUNEZ, G. & L. DEL PESO. 1998. Linking extracellular survival signals and the apoptotic machinery. Curr. Opin. Neurobiol. **8:** 613–618.
33. NEUFELD, G., T. COHEN, S. GENGRINOVITCH & Z. POLTORAK. 1999. Vascular endothelial growth factor (VEGF) and its receptors. FASEB J. **13:** 9–22.

34. KEYT, B.A. *et al.* 1996. The carboxyl-terminal domain (111–165) of vascular endothelial growth factor is critical for its mitogenic potency. J. Biol. Chem. **271:** 7788–7795.
35. SOKER, S., S. TAKASHIMA, H.Q. MIAO, G. NEUFELD & M. KLAGSBRUN. 1998. Neuropilin-1 is expressed by endothelial and tumor cells as an isoform-specific receptor for vascular endothelial growth factor. Cell **92:** 735–745.
36. BASIC, M., N.A. EDWARDS & M.J. MERRILL. 1995. Differential expression of vascular endothelial growth factor (vascular permeability factor) forms in rat tissues. Growth Factors **12:** 11–15.
37. TAKESHITA, S. *et al.* 1996. Gene transfer of naked DNA encoding for three isoforms of vascular endothelial growth factor stimulates collateral development *in vivo*. Lab. Invest. **75:** 487–501.
38. CHENG, S.Y., M. NAGANE, H.S. HUANG & W.K. CAVENEE. 1997. Intracerebral tumor-associated hemorrhage caused by overexpression of the vascular endothelial growth factor isoforms VEGF121 and VEGF165 but not VEGF189. Proc. Natl. Acad. Sci. USA **94:** 12081–12087.
39. TOKUNAGA, T. *et al.* 1998. Vascular endothelial growth factor (VEGF) mRNA isoform expression pattern is correlated with liver metastasis and poor prognosis in colon cancer. Br. J. Cancer **77:** 998–1002.
40. TOMANEK, R.J. 1996. Formation of the coronary vasculature: a brief review. Cardiovasc. Res. **31:** E46–51.
41. HIRSCHI, K.K., S.A. ROHOVSKY & P.A. D'AMORE. 1998. PDGF, TGF-beta, and heterotypic cell-cell interactions mediate endothelial cell-induced recruitment of 10T1/2 cells and their differentiation to a smooth muscle fate [published erratum appears in J. Cell Biol. 1998. **141(5):**1287.]. J. Cell Biol. **141:** 805–814.
42. VANOVERSCHELDE, J.L.J. *et al.* 1997. Chronic myocardial hibernation in humans. From bedside to bench. Circulation **95:** 1961–1971.
43. KLONER, R.A., R. BOLLI, E. MARBAN, L. REINLIB & E. BRAUNWALD. 1998. Medical and cellular implications of stunning, hibernation and preconditioning. An NHLBI workshop. Circulation **97:** 1848–1867.
44. BORGERS, M. 1997. Pathologic findings in chronic hibernating myocardium. *In* Stunning, Hibernation, and Preconditioning: Clinical pathophysiology of myocardial G.R. Hendrickx, S.F. Vatner & W. Wijns, Eds.: 287–306. Lippincott-Raven Publishers. Philadelphia.
45. RISAU, W. 1998. Development and differentiation of endothelium. Kidney Int. Suppl. **67:** S3–6.
46. O'ROURKE, J.F. *et al.* 1997. Hypoxia response elements. Oncol. Res. **9:** 327–332.
47. RATCLIFFE, P.J., J.F. O'ROURKE, P.H. MAXWELL & C.W. PUGH. 1998. Oxygen sensing, hypoxia-inducible factor-1 and the regulation of mammalian gene expression. J. Exp. Biol. **201:** 1153–1162.
48. SEMENZA, G.L. *et al.* 1998. Hypoxia-inducible factor 1: From molecular biology to cardiopulmonary physiology. Chest **114:** 40S–45S.
49. WENGER, R.H. & M. GASSMANN. 1997. Oxygen(es) and the hypoxia-inducible factor-1. Biol Chem **378:** 609–616.
50. ZELZER, E. *et al.* 1998. Insulin induces transcription of target genes through the hypoxia-inducible factor HIF-1alpha/ARNT. EMBO J. **17:** 5085–5094.
51. LEVY, N.S., S. CHUNG, H. FURNEAUX & A.P. LEVY. 1998. Hypoxic stabilization of vascular endothelial growth factor mRNA by the RNA-binding protein HuR. J. Biol. Chem. **273:** 6417–6423.
52. MUKHOPADHYAY, D., B. KNEBELMANN, H.T. COHEN, S. ANANTH & V.P. SUKHATME. 1997. The von Hippel-Lindau tumor suppressor gene product interacts with Sp1 to repress vascular endothelial growth factor promoter activity. Mol. Cell. Biol. **17:** 5629–5639.
53. MALTEPE, E., J.V. SCHMIDT, D. BAUNOCH, C.A. BRADFIELD & C.M. SIMON. 1997. Abnormal angiogenesis and responses to glucose and oxygen deprivation in mice lacking the protein ARNT. Nature **386:** 403–407.
54. IYER, N.V. *et al.* 1998. Cellular and developmental control of O_2 homeostasis by hypoxia- inducible factor 1 alpha. Genes Dev. **12:** 149–162.
55. RYAN, H.E., J. LO & R.S. JOHNSON. 1998. HIF-1 alpha is required for solid tumor formation and embryonic vascularization. EMBO J. **17:** 3005–3015.

56. KOZAK, K.R., B. ABBOTT & O. HANKINSON. 1997. ARNT-deficient mice and placental differentiation. Dev. Biol. **191:** 247–306.
57. GNARRA, J.R. *et al.* 1997. Defective placental vasculogenesis causes embryonic lethality in VHL-deficient mice. Proc. Natl. Acad. Sci. USA **94:** 9102–9107.
58. WOOD, S.M., J.M. GLEADLE, C.Q. PUGH, O. HANKINSON & P. RATCLIFFE. 1996. The role of the aryl hydrocarbon receptor nuclear transporter (ARNT) in hypoxic induction of gene expression. J. Biol. Chem. **271:** 15117–15123.
59. CARMELIET, P. *et al.* 1998. Role of HIF-1alpha in hypoxia-mediated apoptosis, cell proliferation, and tumor angiogenesis. Nature **394:** 485–490.
60. DISALVO, J. *et al.* 1995. Purification and characterization of a naturally occurring vascular endothelial growth factor:placenta growth factor heterodimer. J. Biol. Chem. **270:** 7717–7723.
61. PERSICO, M.G., V. VINCENTI & T. DIPALMA. 1999. Structure, expression and receptor-binding properties of placenta growth factor (PlGF). Curr. Top. Microbiol. Immunol. **237:** 31–40.
62. LANDGREN, E., P. SCHILLER, Y. CAO & L. CLAESSON-WELSH. 1998. Placenta growth factor stimulates MAP kinase and mitogenicity but not phospholipase C-gamma and migration of endothelial cells expressing Flt 1. Oncogene **16:** 359–367.
63. DESAI, J., V. HOLT-SHORE, R.J. TORRY, M.R. CAUDLE & D.S. TORRY. 1999. Signal transduction and biological function of placenta growth factor in primary human trophoblast. Biol. Reprod. **60:** 887–892.
64. MAGLIONE, D., V. GUERRIERO, G. VIGLIETTO, P. DELLI BOVI & M.G. PERSICO. 1991. Isolation of a human placenta cDNA coding for a protein related to the vascular permeability factor. Proc. Natl. Acad. Sci. USA **88:** 9267–9271.
65. ZICHE, M. *et al.* 1997. Placenta growth factor-1 is chemotactic, mitogenic, and angiogenic. Lab. Invest. **76:** 517–531.
66. CAO, Y., W.R. JI, A. ROSIN & Y. CAO. 1997. Placenta growth factor: identification and characterization of a novel isoform generated by RNA alternative splicing. Biochem. Biophys. Res. Commun. **235:** 493–498.
67. MIGDAL, M. *et al.* 1998. Neuropilin-1 is a placenta growth factor-2 receptor. J. Biol. Chem. **273:** 22272–22278.
68. BIRKENHAGER, R. *et al.* 1996. Synthesis and physiological activity of heterodimers comprising different splice forms of vascular endothelial growth factor and placenta growth factor. Biochem. J. **316:** 703–707.
69. PARK, J.E., H.H. CHEN, J. WINER, K.A. HOUCK & N. FERRARA. 1994. Placenta growth factor. Potentiation of vascular endothelial growth factor bioactivity, *in vitro* and *in vivo*, and high affinity binding to Flt-1 but not to Flk-1/KDR. J. Biol. Chem. **269:** 25646–25654.
70. SAWANO, A., T. TAKAHASHI, S. YAMAGUCHI, M. AONUMURA & M. SHIBUYA. 1996. Flt-1 but not KDR/Flk-1 tyrosine kinase is a receptor for placenta growth factor, which is related to vascular endothelial growth factor. Cell Growth Differ. **7:** 213–221.
71. HAUSER, S. & H.A. WEICH. 1993. A heparin-binding form of placenta growth factor (PlGF-2) is expressed in human umbilical vein endothelial cells and in placenta. Growth Factors **9:** 259–268.
72. CAO, Y. *et al.* 1996. Heterodimers of placenta growth factor/vascular endothelial growth factor: endothelial activity, tumor cell expression, and high affinity binding to Flk-1/KDR. J. Biol. Chem. **271:** 3154–3162.
73. CAO, Y., P. LINDEN, D. SHIMA, F. BROWNE & J. FOLKMAN. 1996. *In vivo* angiogenic activity and hypoxia induction of heterodimers of placenta growth factor/vascular endothelial growth factor. J. Clin. Invest. **98:** 2507–2511.
74. CLAUSS, M. 1998. Functions of the VEGF receptor-1 (FLT-1) in the vasculature. Trends Cardiovasc. Med. **8:** 241–245.
75. VIGLIETTO, G. *et al.* 1995. Upregulation of vascular endothelial growth factor (VEGF) and downregulation of placenta growth factor (PlGF) associated with malignancy in human thyroid tumors and cell lines. Oncogene **11:** 1569–1579.
76. CLARK, D.E., S.K. SMITH, D. LICENCE, A.L. EVANS & D.S. CHARNOCK-JONES. 1998. Comparison of expression patterns for placenta growth factor, vascular endothelial

growth factor (VEGF), VEGF-B and VEGF-C in the human placenta throughout gestation. J. Endocrinol. **159:** 459–467.
77. OLOFFSON, B. *et al.* 1996. Vascular endothelial growth factor B, a novel growth factor for endothelial cells. Proc. Natl. Acad. Sci. USA **93:** 2576–2581.
78. AASE, K. *et al.* 1999. Localization of VEGF-B in the mouse embryo suggests a paracrine role of the growth factor in the developing vasculature. Dev. Dyn. **215:** 12–25.
79. OLOFSSON, B. *et al.* 1998. Vascular endothelial growth factor B (VEGF-B) binds to VEGF receptor-1 and regulates plasminogen activator activity in endothelial cells. Proc. Natl. Acad. Sci. USA **95:** 11709–11714.
80. JOUKOV, V. *et al.* 1996. A novel vascular endothelial growth factor, VEGF-C, is a ligand for the Flt4 (VEGFR-3) and KDR (VEGFR-2) receptor tyrosine kinases. EMBO J. **15:** 290–298.
81. KUKK, E. *et al.* 1996. VEGF-C receptor binding and pattern of expression with VEGFR-3 suggests a role in lymphatic vascular development. Development **122:** 3829–3837.
82. CAO, Y. *et al.* 1998. Vascular endothelial growth factor C induces angiogenesis *in vivo*. Proc. Natl. Acad. Sci. USA **95:** 14389–14394.
83. LEE, J. *et al.* 1996. Vascular endothelial growth factor-related protein: a ligand and specific activator of the tyrosine kinase receptor Flt4. Proc. Natl. Acad. Sci. USA **93:** 1988–1992.
84. TAIPALE, J. *et al.* 1999. Vascular endothelial growth factor receptor-3. Curr. Top. Microbiol. Immunol. **237:** 85–96.
85. JING-SHAN, H. *et al.* 1997. A novel regulatory function of proteolytically cleaved VEGF-2 for vascular endothelial and smooth muscle cells. FASEB J. **11:** 498–504.
86. KAIPAINEN, A. *et al.* 1995. Expression of the fms-like tyrosine kinase 4 gene becomes restricted to lymphatic endothelium during development. Proc. Natl. Acad. Sci. USA **92:** 3566–3570.
87. DUMONT, D.J. *et al.* 1998. Cardiovascular failure in mouse embryos deficient in VEGF receptor-3. Science **282:** 946–949.
88. WITZENBICHLER, B. *et al.* 1998. Vascular endothelial growth factor-C (VEGF-C/VEGF-2) promotes angiogenesis in the setting of tissue ischemia. Am. J. Pathol. **153:** 381–394.
89. LYMBOUSSAKI, A. *et al.* 1998. Expression of the vascular endothelial growth factor C receptor VEGFR-3 in lymphatic endothelium of the skin and in vascular tumors. Am. J. Pathol. **153:** 395–403.
90. JELTSCH, M. *et al.* 1997. Hyperplasia of lymphatic vessels in VEGF-C transgenic mice. Science **276:** 1423–1425.
91. OH, S.J. *et al.* 1997. VEGF and VEGF-C: specific induction of angiogenesis and lymphangiogenesis in the differentiated avian chorioallantoic membrane. Dev. Biol. **188:** 96–109.
92. ORLANDINI, M., L. MARCONCINI, R. FERRUZZI & S. OLIVIERO. 1996. Identification of a c-fos-induced gene that is related to the platelet-derived growth factor/vascular endothelial growth factor family [corrected; erratum to be published]. Proc. Natl. Acad. Sci. USA **93:** 11675–11680.
93. AVANTAGGIATO, V., M. ORLANDINI, D. ACAMPORA, S. OLIVIERO & A. SIMEONE. 1998. Embryonic expression pattern of the murine figf gene, a growth factor belonging to platelet-derived growth factor/vascular endothelial growth factor family. Mech. Dev. **73:** 221–224.
94. ACHEN, M.G. *et al.* 1998. Vascular endothelial growth factor D (VEGF-D) is a ligand for the tyrosine kinases VEGF receptor 2 (Flk1) and VEGF receptor 3 (Flt4). Proc. Natl. Acad. Sci. USA **95:** 548–553.
95. DUMONT, D.J. *et al.* 1995. Vascularization of the mouse embryo: a study of flk-1, tek, tie, and vascular endothelial growth factor expression during development. Dev. Dyn. **203:** 80–92.
96. SEETHARAM, L. *et al.* 1995. A unique signal transduction from FLT tyrosine kinase, a receptor for vascular endothelial growth factor VEGF. Oncogene **10:** 135–147.
97. SHALABY, F. *et al.* 1995. Failure of blood-island formation and vasculogenesis in Flk-1-deficient mice. Nature **376:** 62–66.

98. SHALABY, F., J. HO, W.L. STANFORD et al. 1997. A requirement for Flk-1 in primitive and definitive hematopoiesis and vasculogenesis. Cell **89:** 981–990.
99. CHOI, K., M. KENNEDY, A. KAZAROV, J.C. PAPADIMITRIOU & G. KELLER. 1998. A common precursor for hematopoietic and endothelial cells. Development **125:** 725–732.
100. EICHMANN, A. et al. 1997. Ligand-dependent development of the endothelial and hemopoietic lineages from embryonic mesodermal cells expressing vascular endothelial growth factor receptor 2. Proc. Natl. Acad. Sci. USA **94:** 5141–5146.
101. WITTE, L. et al. 1998. Monoclonal antibodies targeting the VEGF receptor-2 (Flk1/KDR) as an anti-angiogenic therapeutic strategy. Cancer Metastasis Rev. **17:** 155–161.
102. MACHEIN, M.R., W. RISAU & K.H. PLATE. 1999. Antiangiogenic gene therapy in a rat glioma model using a dominant-negative vascular endothelial growth factor receptor 2. Hum. Gene Ther. **10:** 1117–1128.
103. KHALIQ, A. et al. 1996. Localisation of placenta growth factor (PlGF) in human term placenta. Growth Factors **13:** 243–250.
104. CLARK, D.E. et al. 1998. A vascular endothelial growth factor antagonist is produced by the human placenta and released into the maternal circulation. Biol. Reprod. **59:** 1540–1548.
105. DAVIS-SMYTH, T., H. CHEN, J. PARK, L.G. PRESTA & N. FERRARA. 1996. The second immunoglobulin-like domain of the VEGF tyrosine kinase receptor Flt-1 determines ligand binding and may initiate a signal transduction cascade. EMBO J. **15:** 4919–4927.
106. FONG, G.H., J. ROSSANT, M. GERTSENSTEIN & M.L. BREITMAN. 1995. Role of the Flt-1 receptor tyrosine kinase in regulating the assembly of vascular endothelium. Nature **376:** 66–70.
107. HIRATSUKA, S., O. MINOWA, J. KUNO, T. NODA & M. SHIBUYA. 1998. Flt-1 lacking the tyrosine kinase domain is sufficient for normal development and angiogenesis in mice. Proc. Natl. Acad. Sci. USA **95:** 9349–9354.
108. KITSUKAWA, T. et al. 1997. Neuropilin-semaphorin III/D-mediated chemorepulsive signals play a crucial role in peripheral nerve projection in mice. Neuron **19:** 995–1005.
109. KITSUKAWA, T., A. SHIMONO, A. KAWAKAMI, H. KONDOH & H. FUJISAWA. 1995. Overexpression of a membrane protein, neuropilin, in chimeric mice causes anomalies in the cardiovascular system, nervous system and limbs. Development **121:** 4309–4318.

Questions and Answers

M.A. GIMBRONE (*Brigham and Women's Hospital, Boston, MA, USA*): Is there any co-localization of the VEGF-R1 or VEGF-R2 with VE-cadherin at the lateral cell junctions?

CARMELIET: Yes. There is co-localization of these molecules (in particular VEGF-R2), by immunofluorescence in cultured cells, as well as *in vivo* by immunoelectron microscopy.

GIMBRONE: Is that relationship different in the resting monolayering compared with a sprouting or activated monolayer? In other words, does ligand modulate co-localization?

CARMELIET: All the studies *in vitro* have been done on cell monolayers that are making close contacts. We don't know the situation in sprouting vessels or migrating vessels.

Y. SATO (*Tohoku University, Sendai, Japan*): You did not find any abnormality in vasculogenesis, perhaps indicating that there is another adhesion molecule playing a role during this process.

CARMELIET: Or, that it does not play a major role. Vasculogenesis occurs at the time before the onset of flow; although the heart is beating, there is no blood flow. In the yolk sac, for example, there is no connection with the embryo, so there are no real hemodynamic forces. So either it does not play an essential role, or it is not needed.

SATO: But even in a stem cell system there is no segregation.

CARMELIET: I have no explanation for that except that this is an artificial system. We also have looked at another system where we culture yolk sacs. If you just culture a blastocyst in high serum, the yolk sac will develop with the vasculature but the embryo will degenerate. Also, in that system we see that, initially, vessels can assemble in the absence of blood flow. Subsequently they deteriorate.

SATO: There is a paper suggesting that VCAM-1 can play a role in cell adaptation. And there is also a paper about β-cadherin-2, which is isolated from the heart. Have you checked those other adhesion molecules?

CARMELIET: VCAM-1 seems to be expressed at the same level. All markers that we have looked at (e.g., VEGF receptors and tie-2 receptors) are at normal levels in the mutants. So the differentiation program *per se* does not seem to be affected.

SATO: You showed that VEGF cannot protect from apoptosis, whereas the FGF somehow was protective. Can you explain that?

CARMELIET: I wish that I could.

SATO: There is a paper showing that angiopoietin-I, which is the ligand of the tie-2 receptor, is also anti-apoptotic. Have you ever checked angiopoietin-I for this?

CARMELIET: No, but this is a good question. The beauty of this system is that you have cross-talk between two endothelial cell–specific factors, and angiopoietin may not be exclusively operating on endothelial cells.

SATO: You showed that the PI3-kinase is associated with the VEGF type 2 receptor, but there is no motif for the binding of the tie-2. We have data that the PI3-kinase is associated with the tie receptor.

CARMELIET: We found references in the literature that there is. Also, we found receptor 3 co-localized in the junction; it is not involved in the process of endothelial cell survival.

J.J. POUYSSÉGUR (*Centre de Biochimie-CNRS, University of Nice, France*): Concerning the observation that, in your knockout model, VEGF cannot protect against apoptosis compared to FGF. I would propose another mechanism that I think could be the string between the two receptors for the signaling via the MAP kinase cascade. As I briefly mentioned to you, you can completely protect against apoptosis induced in many cells by growth factor deprivation or by integrin disengagement. All of this can be suppressed simply by activating the p42/p44 MAP kinase. So it should be possible to determine whether VEGF and FGF have a different strength for MAP kinase activation. If this is correct, we can map MAP kinase constitutively with the VE-cadherin promoter. So by expression you should completely protect the phenotype by just turning on the signal for MAP kinase.

CARMELIET: Our data certainly do not exclude any other intercellular signaling mechanism. What this shows is actually the β-catenin. It was believed that the association of β-catenin with junctional proteins is just removing it from a pool that could be used for signaling via the WNT pathway. What these data show is that there is an alternative mechanism, but certainly they do not exclude other cross-talk.

D.J. LOSKUTOFF (*Scripps Research Institute, La Jolla, CA, USA*): Thinking about your middle cerebral artery ligation model, it certainly does not make any sense that you get a smaller infarct in the absence of TPA, and a larger one in the absence of PAI-1, but absence of plasminogen and α_2-antiplasmin certainly seems consistent with what we know. Have you tried to rescue any of these phenotypes in fibrin/fibrinogen-deficient mice?

CARMELIET: No. As I said, these mice are not available to us.

Annexin II and Regulation of Cell Surface Fibrinolysis

KATHERINE A. HAJJAR[a] AND SUCHITRA S. ACHARYA

Departments of Pediatrics and Medicine, Weill Medical College of Cornell University, New York, New York 10021, USA

ABSTRACT: The regulated function of the fibrinolytic system is fundamental to the solubilization of fibrin-containing thrombi and to a number of other biologic processes. In recent years, several receptors, which serve to localize proteolytic activity on the cell surface, have been identified on endothelial cells, blood cells, neuronal cells, and tumor cells. One such receptor is annexin II, a calcium- and phospholipid-binding protein that serves as a profibrinolytic coreceptor for tissue plasminogen activator and plasminogen on endothelial cells. Accumulating evidence suggests that impaired cell surface fibrinolytic assembly could lead to progressive atherothrombotic disease. In addition, dysregulation of annexin II expression in acute promyelocytic leukemia is an important mechanism for the bleeding diathesis associated with this malignancy.

INTRODUCTION

The fibrinolytic system represents an orderly cascade of proteolytic reactions culminating in the generation of the serine protease plasmin.[1] Plasmin is not only responsible for clearance of fibrin from the intravascular space, but may also modify fibrin and other substrates in the extravascular environment. In recent years it has become apparent that this system may assemble on cell surfaces that provide a protected environment for the preservation of proteolytic activity. Plasminogen and its activators are known to interact with receptors expressed on a variety of cell types including endothelial cells, macrophages, neuronal cells, and some tumor cells. It is not yet clear what role these interactions may play *in vivo* in maintaining intravascular as well as extravascular homeostasis. However, several clues derived from *in vitro* studies indicate that dysfunctional fibrinolytic assembly may predispose to atherothrombotic vascular disease.

ANNEXIN II–MEDIATED ASSEMBLY OF PLASMINOGEN AND T-PA

Endothelial cells are thought to play a key role in intravascular plasmin generation *in vivo*. They synthesize and secrete the two major forms of plasminogen activator, tissue plasminogen activator (t-PA) and urokinase,[2] and release the physiological inhibitor of these activators, plasminogen activator inhibitor type-1.[3]

---

[a]Address for correspondence: Katherine A. Hajjar, Departments of Pediatrics and Medicine, Weill Medical College of Cornell University, Box 45, 300 York Avenue, New York, NY 10021. Voice: 212-746-2034; fax: 212-746-8809.

In addition, cultured human umbilical vein endothelial cells bind both plasminogen and t-PA in a concentration-dependent manner (K_d 310 nM and B_{max} 1,400,000 sites per cell, and K_d 18 nM and B_{max} 815,000 sites per cell, respectively).[4,5] These binding interactions preserve catalytic efficiency and apparently protect plasmin and t-PA from their inhibitors, thus potentially modulating hemostatic and thrombotic events at the blood vessel surface.

Endothelial cell membranes contain a major non-fibrin plasminogen and t-PA binding protein, which is oriented on the outer face of the membrane. This M_r ~36,000 protein specifically binds radiolabeled t-PA as well as plasminogen (K_d 30 nM, B_{max} 650 fmol/well and K_d 114 nM, B_{max} 495 fmol/well, respectively).[6,7] The isolated t-PA/plasminogen binding site is resistant to reduction and preserves the capacity for plasmin generation. These studies provide support for the hypothesis that plasminogen and t-PA can assemble on the endothelial cell surface in a manner that enhances cell surface plasmin generation.

Sequence analysis of two internal peptides from the putative endothelial cell tPA/plasminogen co-receptor identified the protein as an analog of the calcium- and phospholipid-binding protein, annexin II.[8] The full-length cDNA, derived by polymerase chain reaction, revealed complete identity with the published sequence for the heavy chain of human annexin II,[9] and the ligand-precipitated receptor immunoreacted specifically with a monoclonal antibody to annexin II.[8] Expression of annexin II in 293 cells transfected with the cDNA conferred the ability to bind plasminogen (K_d 114 nM; B_{max} 347,000 sites per cell) as well as t-PA (K_d 48 nM; B_{max} 380,000 sites per cell). In addition, when human umbilical vein endothelial

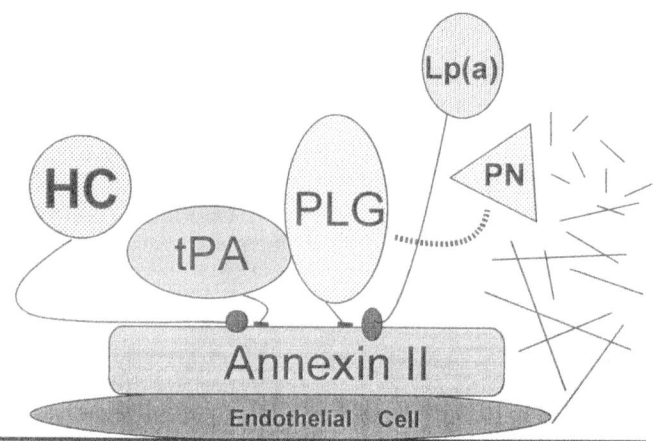

FIGURE 1. Annexin II dysfunction in atherosclerosis—potential mechanisms. The calcium-dependent, phospholipid-binding protein, annexin II, is expressed as a peripheral component of the outer leaflet of the endothelial cell plasma membrane. Homocysteine (HC) derivatizes the "tail" domain of annexin II (*solid circle*), rendering it incompetent for t-PA binding. Lipoprotein(a) [Lp(a)] competes with plasminogen (PLG) for its binding site (*solid oval*) within the "core" domain, inhibiting plasminogen binding. Thus, either HC or Lp(a) may impair t-PA/plasminogen assembly, thereby reducing constitutive generation of plasmin (PN).

cells were treated with phosphorothioated antisense oligonucleotides representing bases 4 through 24 of the annexin II cDNA, binding of both plasminogen and t-PA was reduced by 40% and 50%, respectively. Sense and missense oligonucleotides had no significant effect on binding. Similarly, polyclonal antibody to annexin II, but not annexin I, blocked 40–50% of ligand binding to the same cells. These data suggested that annexin II contributes a major proportion of plasminogen and t-PA binding sites on the surface of cultured endothelial cells.

Annexin II is a widely distributed, highly conserved, M_r 36,000 peripheral membrane protein expressed abundantly on endothelial cells, monocyte/macrophages, early myeloid cells, and some tumor cells.[1] All 20 known annexins consist of a conserved "core" domain (M_r 30,000–40,000), which imparts phospholipid-binding capacity, and a variable amino terminal "tail" domain (M_r 3,000–6,000) through which specialized functions are acquired.[10,11] Extracellular annexin II has been reported to participate in a number of processes localized to the cell surface. These include tumor cell interaction with hepatic sinusoidal endothelial cells,[12] endothelial cell and glioma cell adhesion to matrix via tenascin C,[13,14] trafficking of IgG in the placenta,[15] and docking of cytomegalovirus on the surface of endothelial cells.[16,17]

On endothelial cells, annexin II is expressed as a peripheral membrane protein.[18] Although it lacks a classical signal peptide, annexin II is constitutively translocated to the endothelial cell surface within 16 hours of its biosynthesis where it appears to constitute 4–5% of the total cellular pool. Exogenous ^{125}I-labeled annexin II bound to EGTA-treated endothelial cells with high affinity (K_d 49 nM) in a calcium-dependent manner (I_{50} 3 μM). Peptides mimicking the classical "annexin repeat" (KGXGT) blocked its interaction with the endothelial cell. Recombinant annexin II bearing the calcium-binding site substitution D161A of repeat 2 failed to compete with binding of the wild-type protein to the cell surface, whereas E246A and D321A mutants involving calcium-binding sites of repeats 3 and 4, competed effectively. These data indicate that annexin II interacts with cell surface phospholipid via a high affinity calcium-dependent binding site located within annexin repeat 2 of the core domain.

In further studies, purified native annexin II had a profound effect on the efficiency of t-PA-dependent plasminogen activation.[19] Kinetic analyses revealed that annexin II conferred an ~60-fold increase in catalytic efficiency upon t-PA-dependent activation of either Glu-PLG or Lys-PLG. This effect required lysine-binding sites of plasminogen, as it was 90–95% abrogated in the presence of the lysine analog ε-aminocaproic acid or by treatment of annexin II by carboxypeptidase B, indicating a carboxyl terminal lysine-dependent mechanism. In addition, this effect was specific for t-PA, because urokinase-mediated plasminogen activation was not affected by annexin II. Thus, annexin II is fibrin-like in its ability to independently bind both t-PA and plasminogen, its enhancement of plasmin generation, and its specificity for t-PA in contrast to u-PA.

ANNEXIN II BINDING DOMAINS FOR PLASMINOGEN AND T-PA

Not unlike its binding to fibrin, plasminogen assembly on annexin II appears to require receptor modification or "activation" by means of a carboxyl terminal cleavage event.[8] In transfection analyses, expression of the K307T mutant, in which the dibasic sequence K307-R308 is altered, led to a dramatic reduction in binding of plasminogen.[8] Thus, processing of annexin II by a plasmin-like protease at or near the cell surface appears to expose a carboxyl terminal lysine residue (K307), thus fostering plasminogen binding. The identity of the relevant plasmin-like protease is unknown. The K307T mutant of annexin II expressed on 293 cells failed to bind plasminogen. On the other hand, the K328I mutant bound this ligand in a manner equivalent to the wild type. Binding of PLG to both the wild-type and the K328I mutant was eliminated following pretreatment of 293 cells with carboxypeptidase B, an agent that removes carboxyl terminal lysine and arginine residues. Others have reported that p11, a polypeptide that forms a heterotetramer with annexin II monomer, may contribute significantly to plasminogen binding.[20,21]

T-PA binding to immobilized native annexin II monomer was inhibited by intact fluid phase recombinant annexin II, but not by its core fragment (Gly^{25}–Asp^{339}).[22] These data implicated the tail domain in the t-PA interaction. Two overlapping peptides derived from the tail domain (residues 2–13: STVHEILCKLSL and residues 8–19: LCKLSLEGDHST), but not a third peptide (residues 14–25: EGDHSTPPSAYG), blocked binding of t-PA to the intact recombinant monomer. A hexapeptide reflecting the region of overlap (residues 7–12: LCKLSL) also blocked 95% of binding of t-PA to annexin II (I_{50} 208 µM), whereas a related peptide (LGKLSL) which lacked C^9, had no effect on binding. When four different cysteine mutants of annexin II were expressed in 293 cells (C9G, C113G, C262G, C335G), only C9G failed to support binding. These data localize the t-PA binding of annexin II to the tail domain (residues 7–12) and highlight the importance of C^9 in the binding interaction.

ANNEXIN II FUNCTION AND ATHEROGENESIS

Annexin II function may be diminished in certain atherogenic states (FIG. 1). Lipoprotein(a) [Lp(a)] is an atherogenic lipoprotein particle that contains the plasminogen-like apolipoprotein(a)[23] bound to low density lipoprotein. In *in vitro* studies, Lp(a) inhibited plasminogen binding, as well as plasmin generation, at the cell surface.[24] Like unlabeled PLG, purified Lp(a) and recombinant apo(a) both blocked binding of labeled PLG to cultured endothelial cells, while neither LDL nor Lp(–), the reductively cleaved particle from which apo(a) had been removed, inhibited this interaction. Further, competitive binding experiments confirmed that the highly atherogenic low-density lipoprotein-like particle, Lp(a), competes with plasminogen for binding to annexin II.[7] In direct binding studies, recombinant labeled apo(a) showed saturable equilibrium binding to endothelial cells (K_d 259 nM; B_{max} 2,200,000 sites per cell). In a fluorogenic assay based on hydrolysis of the synthetic plasmin substrate D-Val-Leu-Lys-aminofluoromethylcoumarin, Lp(a) had no effect on t-PA–dependent plasminogen activation in the fluid phase, whereas the same reaction was reduced by 93% in association with endothelial cells. Since Lp(a) was shown to accumulate within atherosclerotic lesions, these findings provided a potential link between impaired cell surface fibrinolytic potential and progressive atherosclerosis.

Homocysteine is a thiol-containing amino acid intermediate that accumulates in hereditary deficiencies of cystathionine β-synthase, methionine synthase, or methyltetrahydrofolate reductase, or in dietary deficiencies of folate, B_6, or B_{12}.[25] Homocysteinemia is epidemiologically associated with occlusive vascular disease due to both thromboembolism and atherosclerosis.[26] The mechanistic basis for this association is unclear.

Recent studies suggest that binding of t-PA to cultured endothelial cells and to endothelial cell membrane–derived annexin II is inhibited by homocysteine.[27] Preincubation of endothelial cells with nontoxic levels of homocysteine selectively and specifically reduced the number of available t-PA binding sites by 65% with a concomitant decrease in t-PA catalytic activity. Interestingly, homocysteine had no effect on plasminogen binding. No change in affinity for t-PA or plasminogen and no change in the maximal number of plasminogen binding sites were observed. Cell surface expression of annexin II was indistinguishable in homocysteine-treated cells as compared with control cells. However, binding of t-PA to annexin II derived from membrane extracts of homocysteine-treated endothelial cells was sharply reduced while plasminogen binding to the same protein remained intact. These data suggest that homocysteine may perturb endothelial cell function, thus promoting a prothrombotic state at the surface of the blood vessel wall.

Homocysteine appears to disable the t-PA–binding tail domain of annexin II.[22] In studies utilizing recombinant annexin II monomer, electrospray ionization mass spectrometry indicated that homocysteine physically alters the receptor, increasing its mass by 135 ± 4 daltons. By tandem mass spectrometric analysis of a tryptic digest of homocysteine-treated annexin II, this increase was explained by derivatization of a single cysteine residue (C9) within the amino terminal t-PA binding domain. A disulfide-mediated complex between homocysteine and annexin II was also demonstrated in cultured endothelial cells that were metabolically labeled with [^{35}S]-homocysteine. Modification of annexin II by micromolar concentrations of homocysteine was associated with a dose- and time-related reduction in t-PA binding. Interestingly, the I_{50} for inhibition of t-PA binding to annexin II was ~11 µM, a value close to the upper limit of normal for homocysteine in plasma (~14 µM). Thus, inhibition of t-PA–annexin II assembly on the endothelial cell, and subsequent reduction in plasmin generation, could underlie the prothrombotic/proatherogenic state associated with homocysteine *in vivo*.

OVEREXPRESSION OF ANNEXIN II AND BLEEDING IN ACUTE PROMYELOCYTIC LEUKEMIA

Acute promyelocytic leukemia (APL), a subset of myelogenous leukemia, is generally associated with the t(15;17) translocation and a severe coagulopathy.[28,29] The t(15;17) breakpoint disrupts two genes, a putative transcription factor (*PML*) and a nuclear retinoid receptor (RARα), and results in a chimeric protein, PML-RARα, that blocks differentiation. Although several factors probably contribute to the bleeding disorder, recent evidence suggests that primary fibrinolysis may play a major role. Leukemia cells from APL patients expressed high levels of annexin II.[30] T(15;17)-positive APL cells stimulated cell surface t-PA–dependent plasmin generation twice as efficiently as t(15;17)-negative cells. This pathologic increase was eliminated in the presence of anti-annexin II IgG, and induced upon transfection of t(15;17)-negative cells with annexin II cDNA. T(15;17)-positive APL cells displayed abundant annexin II protein and mRNA, which disappeared through a transcriptional mechanism within 3–5 days of treatment with the differentiating agent all-*trans*-retinoic acid (ATRA). Dysregulation of annexin II expression in APL cells is accompanied by accelerated t-PA–dependent plasmin production. Annexin II expression in APL cells is subject to modulation by ATRA and may represent an important mechanism for hemorrhage.

FUTURE DIRECTIONS

The extent to which annexin II directs cell surface plasmin generation *in vivo* is unclear. In particular, it will be important to discern whether defects or dysfunction in annexin II–mediated fibrinolytic assembly can be documented in individuals with thrombotic disease or atherosclerosis. Animal models to study the physiologic function of annexin II will be central to this endeavor. In future studies, the effects of homocysteine and lipoprotein(a) on annexin II function will need to be examined in both animal models and human subjects.

REFERENCES

1. HAJJAR, K.A. 1998. The molecular basis of fibrinolysis. *In* Hematology of Infancy and Childhood. D.G. Nathan & S.H. Orkin, Eds.: 1557–1573. W.B. Saunders Co. Philadelphia.
2. LEVIN, E.G. & D.J. LOSKUTOFF. 1982. Cultured bovine endothelial cells produce both urokinase and tissue-type plasminogen activators. J. Cell Biol. **94:** 631–636.
3. LOSKUTOFF, D.J. & T.S. EDGINGTON. 1977. Synthesis of a fibrinolytic activator and inhibitor by endothelial cells. Proc. Natl. Acad. Sci. USA **74:** 3903–3907.
4. HAJJAR, K.A., P.C. HARPEL, E.A. JAFFE & R.L. NACHMAN. 1986. Binding of plasminogen to cultured human endothelial cells. J. Biol. Chem. **261:** 11656–11662.
5. HAJJAR, K.A., N.M. HAMEL, P.C. HARPEL & R.L. NACHMAN. 1987. Binding of tissue plasminogen activator to cultured human endothelial cells. J. Clin. Invest. **80:** 1712–1719.
6. HAJJAR, K.A. & N.M. HAMEL. 1990. Identification and characterization of human endothelial cell membrane binding sites for tissue plasminogen activator and urokinase. J. Biol. Chem. **265:** 2908–2916.
7. HAJJAR, K.A. 1991. The endothelial cell tissue plasminogen activator receptor: specific interaction with plasminogen. J. Biol. Chem. 266: 21962–21970.
8. HAJJAR, K.A., A.T. JACOVINA & J. CHACKO. 1994. An endothelial cell receptor for plasminogen and tissue plasminogen activator: I. Identity with annexin II. J. Biol. Chem. **269:** 21191–21197.
9. HUANG, K., B.P. WALLNER, R.J. MATTALIANO, R. TIZARD, C. BURNE, A. FREY, C. HESSION, P. MCGRAY, L.K. SINCLAIR, E.P. CHOW, J.L. BROWNING, K.L. RAMACHANDRAN *et al.* 1986. Two human 35 kd inhibitors of phospholipase A2 are related to substrates of pp60 v-src and of the epidermal growth factor receptor/kinase. Cell **46:** 191–199.
10. RAYNAL, P. & H.B. POLLARD. 1994. Annexins: the problem of assessing the biologic role for a gene family of multifunctional calcium- and phospholipid-binding proteins. Biochim. Biophys. Acta **1197:** 63–93.
11. SWAIRJO, M.A. & B.A. SEATON. 1994. Annexin structure and membrane interactions: A molecular perspective. Ann. Rev. Biophys. Biomol. Struct. **23:** 193–213.
12. TRESSLER, R.J., T.V. UPDYKE, T.J. YEATMAN & G.L. NICOLSON. 1993. Extracellular annexin is associated with divalent cation-dependent tumor cell adhesion of metastatic RAW 117 large-cell lymphoma cells. J. Cell. Biochem. **53:** 265–276.
13. CHUNG, C.Y. & H.P. ERICKSON. 1994. Cell surface annexin II is a high affinity receptor for the alternatively spliced segment of tenascin-C. J. Cell Biol. **126:** 539–548.

14. CHUNG, C.Y., J.E. MURPHY-ULLRICH & H.P. ERICKSON. 1996. Mitogenesis, cell migration and loss of focal adhesion induced by tenascin-C interacting with its cell surface receptor, annexin II. Mol. Biol. Cell. **7:** 883–892.
15. KRISTOFFERSEN, E.K. & R. MATRE. 1996. Surface annexin II on placental membranes of the fetomaternal interface. Am. J. Reprod. Immunol. **36:** 141–149.
16. WRIGHT, J.F., A. KUROSKY, E.L.G. PRYZDIAL & S. WASI. 1995. Host cellular annexin II is associated with cytomegalovirus particles isolated from cultured human fibroblasts. J. Virol. **69:** 4784–4791.
17. BOLD, S., M. OHLIN, W. GARTEN & K. RADSAK. 1996. Structural domains involved in human cytomegalovirus glycoprotein B-mediated cell-cell fusion. J. Gen. Virol. **77:** 2297–2302.
18. HAJJAR, K.A., C.A. GUEVARA, E. LEV, K. DOWLING & J. CHACKO. 1996. Interaction of the fibrinolytic receptor, annexin II, with the endothelial cell surface: essential role of endonexin repeat 2. J. Biol. Chem. **271:** 21652–21659.
19. CESARMAN, G.M., C.A. GUEVARA & K.A. HAJJAR. 1994. An endothelial cell receptor for plasminogen/tissue plasminogen activator: II. Annexin II-mediated enhancement of t-PA-dependent plasminogen activation. J. Biol. Chem. **269:** 21198–21203.
20. KASSAM, G., K.S. CHOI, J. GHUMAN, H.M. KANG, S.L. FITZPATRICK, T. ZACKSON, S. ZACKSON, M. TOBA, A. SHINOMIYA & D.M. WAISMAN. 1998. The role of annexin II tetramer in the activation of plasminogen. J. Biol. Chem. **273:** 4790–4799.
21. KASSAM, G., B.H. LE, K.S. CHOI, H.M. KANG, L.P. FITZPATRICK & D.M. WAISMAN. 1998. The p11 subunit of the annexin II tetramer plays a key role in the stimulation of t-PA-dependent plasminogen activation. Biochemistry **37:** 16958–16966.
22. HAJJAR, K.A., L. MAURI, A.T. JACOVINA, F. ZHONG, U.A. MIRZA, J.C. PADOVAN & B.T. CHAIT. 1998. Tissue plasminogen activator binding to the annexin II tail domain: direct modulation by homocysteine. J. Biol. Chem. **273:** 9987–9993.
23. MCLEAN, J.W., J.E. TOMLINSON, W.J. KUANG, D.L. EATON, E.Y. CHEN, G.M. FLESS, A.M. SCANU & R.M. LAWN. 1987. cDNA sequence of human apolipoprotein(a) is homologous to plasminogen. Nature **330:** 132–137.
24. HAJJAR, K.A., D. GAVISH, J. BRESLOW & R.L. NACHMAN. 1989. Lipoprotein(a) modulation of endothelial cell surface fibrinolysis and its potential role in atherosclerosis. Nature **339:** 303–305.
25. MUDD, H., H.L. LEVY & F. SKOVBY. 1995. Disorders of transsulfuration. *In* The Metabolic and Molecular Basis of Inherited Disease. C.R. Scriver, A.L. Beaudet, W.S. Sly & D. Valle, Eds.: 1279–1327. McGraw-Hill, Inc. New York.
26. MUDD, H., F. SKOVBY, H.L. LEVY, K.D. PETTIGREW, B. WILCKEN, R.E., PYERITZ, G. ANDREA, G.H.J. BOERS, I.L. BROMBERG, R. CERONE, B. FOWLER, H. GROBE *et al.* 1985. The natural history of homocystinuria due to cystathionine β-synthase deficiency. Am. J. Hum. Gen. **37:** 1–31.
27. HAJJAR, K.A. 1993. Homocysteine-induced modulation of tissue plasminogen activator to its endothelial cell membrane receptor. J. Clin. Invest. **91:** 2873–2879.
28. DOMBRET, H., M.L. SCROBOHACI, P. GHORRA, J.M. ZINI, M.T. DANIEL, S. CASTAIGNE & L. DEGOS. 1993. Coagulation disorders associated with acute promyelocytic leukemia: corrective effect of all-trans retinoic acid treatment. Leukemia **7:** 2–9.
29. DOMBRET, H., M.L. SCROBOHACI, M.T. DANIEL, J.M. MICLEA, S. CASTAIGNE, C. CHOMIENNE, P. FENAUX & L. DEGOS. 1995. In vivo thrombin and plasmin activities in patients with acute promyelocytic leukemia (APL): Effect of all-trans-retinoic acid (ATRA) therapy. Leukemia **9:** 19–24.
30. MENELL, J.S., G.M. CESARMAN, A.T. JACOVINA, M.A. MCLAUGHLIN, E.A. LEV & K.A. HAJJAR. 1999. Annexin II and bleeding in acute promyelocytic leukemia. N. Engl. J. Med. **340:** 994–1004.

The Fat Mouse
A Powerful Genetic Model to Study Hemostatic Gene Expression in Obesity/NIDDM

DAVID J. LOSKUTOFF,[a] KAZUHIKO FUJISAWA, AND FAHUMIYA SAMAD

*Department of Vascular Biology, The Scripps Research Institute,
La Jolla, California 92037, USA*

ABSTRACT: In this chapter, we summarize our studies on plasminogen activator inhibitor 1 (PAI-1), tissue factor, and transforming growth factor beta (TGF-β) expression in obesity, using genetically obese mice as a model. These studies emphasize the key role played by the adipocyte, a cell whose numbers, size, and metabolic activity are grossly altered in obesity/NIDDM. They also implicate multiple cytokines, hormones, and growth factors in the abnormal expression of these and perhaps other hemostatic genes by adipocytes in obesity/NIDDM. These studies demonstrate that tumor necrosis factor alpha (TNF-α) plays a central role in the expression of hemostatic genes in this disorder.

INTRODUCTION

Obesity is a major public health problem in Western societies with substantial economic consequences. For example, in the United States alone, more than 30% of the population is defined as clinically obese, and in that population, there is a steadily increasing risk for obesity-associated disorders including cardiovascular disease (CVD), hypertension, insulin resistance, and non–insulin-dependent diabetes mellitus (NIDDM).[1,2] In spite of the magnitude and cost of this problem, the molecular changes in obesity that promote these conditions are far from resolved. The fact that human obesity is a polygenic disorder with complex environmental and behavioral characteristics has made obesity research one of the more difficult areas of investigation in the medical sciences.[1,3] However, recent studies of genetically obese mice and rats have produced breakthroughs in several areas of obesity-related research, primarily because obesity in these animals appears to be monogenic (i.e., to result from mutations in single genes). In this regard, five different genes, all mapped to different chromosomal locations, have been shown to cause distinct syndromes of spontaneous obesity with severe insulin resistance in mice.[3] These include the obese (ob), diabetes (db), tubby (tub), lethal yellow (A[y]), and fat (fat) mutations. Genes encoding intercellular adhesion molecule 1 (ICAM-1) and the leukocyte integrin αMβ2 (Mac-1) also have been implicated in the regulation of adipose tissue mass.[4] These animal studies, together with studies of cultured adipocytes, have provided fundamental new information about

---

[a]Address for correspondence: Dr. David J. Loskutoff, The Scripps Research Institute, Department of Vascular Biology, 10550 N. Torrey Pines Road, VB-3, La Jolla, CA 92037. Fax: 619-784-7353.
loskutof@scripps.edu

the factors and cells that may be responsible for the altered hemostatic balance leading to increased cardiovascular risk in obesity/NIDDM. We have employed these animal and cell culture models to examine changes in the expression of plasminogen activator inhibitor 1 (PAI-1) and tissue factor (TF) and to begin to delineate the cytokine pathways that regulate their expression.

RESULTS

PAI-1 Expression and Regulation in the Adipose Tissue of Obese Mice

PAI-1 appears to be the primary physiological inhibitor of plasminogen activation in blood since it is the only PAI detected in complex with single-chain tissue PA (tPA) in carefully collected human plasma. Moreover, the second-order rate constant for its interaction with tPA and urokinase-like PA (uPA) (approximately 3.5 × 10^7 $M^{-1}s^{-1}$) is at least two orders of magnitude higher than that of other PAIs.[5–8] The normal concentration of PAI-1 protein in human plasma ranges from 6–80 ng/ml with the geometric mean at 24 ng/ml (the concentration of tPA is 5–10 ng/ml). Abnormalities in the concentration of PAI-1 are frequently associated with vascular disease. For example, the inhibitor is elevated in a variety of thrombotic conditions, including myocardial infarction and deep venous thrombosis (reviewed in Refs. 5–8). Elevated PAI-1 also correlates with thrombosis in animal models, and transgenic mice that overexpress PAI-1 have been reported to develop venous thrombosis.[9] On the other hand, the absence of PAI-1 in humans leads to life-long bleeding problems, presumably resulting from the development of a hyperfibrinolytic state (reviewed in Ref. 10). In this regard, disruption of the PAI-1 gene in mice is associated with a mild hyperfibrinolytic state as manifested by increased resistance to endotoxin-induced thrombosis.[9] Finally, neutralizing plasma PAI-1 activity with specific antibodies or by the use of PAI-1 inhibitors[8,11] enhances spontaneous or tPA-mediated thrombolysis. These observations emphasize that imbalances in the PA/PAI-1 ratio are likely to promote either thrombosis or bleeding. As summarized below, this balance is severely disturbed in obesity/NIDDM.

The possibility that the adipose tissue itself may directly contribute to the elevated expression of PAI-1 in obesity has recently gained considerable attention. Initial clues for such a hypothesis came from the observation that the adipose tissue of the mouse contained relatively high levels of PAI-1 mRNA.[12] Moreover, clinical studies demonstrated that weight loss due to surgical treatment, diet, etc., led to significantly reduced plasma PAI-1 levels in obese humans.[1,2,13,14] These findings were noteworthy not only because the adipose tissue was known to secrete a variety of proteins into blood,[3,15] but also because in obesity, the size and number of adipocytes, and thus the amount of adipose tissue mass, typically increases several-fold. Thus, in obesity the PAI-1 biosynthetic capacity of the adipose tissue may approach or even exceed that of other tissues.

We have employed genetically obese (ob/ob) mice[16–18] in an attempt to delineate the mechanisms that regulate PAI-1 in obesity. These mice produce an inactive, truncated form of the ob gene product leptin.[19] Leptin appears to be expressed and secreted by adipocytes in proportion to their triglyceride stores, and its levels in plasma correlates with the extent of obesity (reviewed in Ref. 3). We observed that plasma PAI-1 activity was approximately five- to sixfold higher in these mice than in their lean counterparts (TABLE 1), and that this elevation increased further as a function of age.[17] Importantly, PAI-1 gene expression was significantly elevated in the epididymal, subcutaneous, and brown adipose tissues of obese mice compared to the lean controls. Although there was a generalized increase in PAI-1 mRNA in other major organs as well, these effects were small compared to the increases in the fat. *In situ* hybridization studies of adipose tissues from obese mice demonstrated elevated PAI-1 mRNA in adipocytes, vascular smooth muscle cells, and occasional endothelial cells.[17] The key role of adipocytes in PAI-1 biosynthesis is emphasized by the demonstration that mature, fully differentiated 3T3-L1 adipocytes in culture produce significant levels of PAI-1 mRNA and protein.[16,20,21] Expression of PAI-1 mRNA also has been demonstrated in the visceral and subcutaneous fat of obese rats[20] and in adipose tissues from human subjects.[22] In both cases, omental tissue explants produced significantly more PAI-1 antigen than subcutaneous tissues from the same individuals, and in humans, cardiovascular risk is most closely correlated with android obesity.[1,13]

A variety of observations implicate specific hormones and/or cytokines in the increased expression of PAI-1 by adipose tissue in obesity. For example, the adipose tissue synthesizes TNF-α, and the expression of this cytokine is chronically elevated in adipose tissue from obese mice and humans.[3] The abnormal expression of TNF-α by adipose cells in obesity may interfere with certain aspects of insulin signaling, such as the tyrosine kinase activity of the insulin receptor, and thus contribute to insulin resistance and hyperinsulinemia (TABLE 1). Interestingly, TNF-α is known to stimulate PAI-1 biosynthesis by a variety of cultured cells and by many murine tissues *in vivo*.[7,8,12] Moreover, administration of TNF-α to lean mice significantly increased PAI-1 mRNA in adipocytes, in adventitial cells, and in vascular smooth muscle cells in the adipose tissues.[16] This pattern of PAI-1 expression is similar to the pattern of PAI-1 mRNA observed in the adipose tissues of obese mice. Again, the central role of the adipocyte is emphasized by the finding that TNF-α also induced PAI-1 expression in mature 3T3-L1 adipocytes.[16] Recent studies show that human adipose tissue explants also respond to exogenous TNF-α with increased PAI-1 mRNA and protein expression,[23] and that the addition of pentoxifylline (an inhibitor of TNF-α mRNA synthesis) decreased PAI-1 mRNA and protein. Taken together, these observations support the hypothesis that the chronic elevation in TNF-α that occurs locally in the adipose tissues in human and rodent obesity may act via an autocrine manner to stimulate PAI-1 biosynthesis by the adipocyte and other cells in the adipose tissue. This cytokine may thus contribute to the elevated plasma PAI-1 observed in obesity/NIDDM (TABLE 1).

Evidence in support of the view that insulin may play a role in the elevation of PAI-1 comes from observations that hyperinsulinemic NIDDM patients often display reduced fibrinolysis, possibly because of elevated plasma PAI-1.[13] Moreover, conditions that increase endogenous plasma insulin levels (e.g., a high calorie carbohydrate meal) are associated with increases in plasma PAI-1, while conditions that reduce endogenous insulin (e.g., fasting or by treatment with metformin or with troglitazone, an insulin-sensitizing agent) are associated with decreases in plasma PAI-1.[13,24] Direct administration of insulin into rabbits[25] and mice,[17] and into the forearm vascular bed of human volunteers,[26] significantly increased the level of plasma PAI-1. Although these observations suggest that insulin directly contributes to the elevated PAI-1 in obesity/NIDDM, a number of other human studies failed to demonstrate elevated plasma PAI-1 in response to acutely or chronically administered insulin (reviewed in Refs. 13 and 24). Thus, whereas some animal and clinical studies show a very strong correlation between insulin and plasma PAI-1, other studies are inconsistent and appear to depend upon the method of insulin increase, the metabolic state of the individual, and whether the patient is lean or obese. Although it is difficult to reconcile these differences, it is possible that sufficient levels of plasma insulin were not achieved in some of the human studies. It is also possible that long-term insulin treatment may suppress endogenous insulin and proinsulin secretion.[27,28] Another possibility is that proinsulin or proinsulin-split products rather than insulin per se are involved since NIDDM patients have an elevated basal ratio of plasma proinsulin to immunoreactive insulin, and the concentration of PAI-1 in the plasma of these patients correlates more with the concentration of proinsulin and des[31,32] proinsulin than with insulin.[28] Finally, recent observations raise the possibility that insulin resistance, rather than hyperinsulinemia, may be involved.[29] Obviously, further studies are required to resolve these apparent inconsistencies.

The results of animal studies were more consistent than the human studies and provide additional insights into underlying mechanisms. For example, in the rabbit, plasma PAI-1 antigen and liver PAI-1 mRNA were shown to increase slightly after administration of insulin or proinsulin.[25] Similarly, intraperitoneal administration of insulin to lean mice increased PAI-1 antigen in the plasma, and increased PAI-1 mRNA modestly (less than twofold) in a variety of tissues, including the liver.[17] However, the major effect of insulin on PAI-1 gene expression in the mouse was in the adipose tissues (five- to sevenfold increase), a tissue not examined in the rabbit. Thus, the adipose tissue may be the primary insulin-responsive tissue in the mouse, at least in terms of PAI-1. Insulin induced PAI-1 mRNA primarily in adipocytes,[17] and had no apparent effect on PAI-1 biosynthesis in large-vessel endothelial cells. These observations are consistent with the lack of response of cultured endothelial cells,[30] and indicate that the induction of PAI-1 by insulin in the adipose tissue is relatively specific for the adipocyte. In this respect, PAI-1 mRNA and antigen also were induced by insulin in cultured 3T3-L1 adipocytes, with the level of induction being considerably higher than that reported for other cell types.[17] Although insulin was shown to stimulate PAI-1 mRNA expression in cultured hepatocytes,[30,31] it had only modest effects on PAI-1 gene expression by murine liver.[17] These results point to the importance of the adipose tissue and the adipocytes within it, in insulin-mediated PAI-1 induction in obesity.

TGF-β Expression and Regulation in Obese Mice

The multifunctional cytokine TGF-β stimulates PAI-1 biosynthesis by a large variety of cultured cells.[7] Infusion of TGF-β into rabbits[32] and mice[12,18] dramatically increased plasma PAI-1 activity and induced PAI-1 mRNA in numerous tissues. In the mouse, the most TGF-β–responsive tissue, in terms of PAI-1, appeared to be the adipose tissue.[12,18] *In situ* hybridization analysis showed that TGF-β induced PAI-1 in smooth muscle cells and adipocytes, but not in large-vessel endothelial cells in the adipose tissue, in agreement with previous studies in the kidney.[7] TGF-β also stimulated PAI-1 gene expression in cultured mouse[18,21] and human[22] adipocytes. Our studies

TABLE 1. Alterations in the levels of hemostatic proteins expressed in 6-month-old obese mice

	ob/ob mice[a]		TNFR-deficient ob/ob mice[b]	
	Increase in plasma antigen	Increase in adipose tissue mRNA	Decrease in plasma antigen	Decrease in adipose tissue mRNA
PAI-1	6×	7×	2×	6×
TGF-β	–	3×	–	7×
Insulin	9×	–	2.5×	–
TF	–	2.5×	–	–

[a] For ob/ob mice, the change is compared to wild-type lean mice.
[b] For TNFR-deficient ob/ob mice, change is compared to ob/ob mice.

demonstrate that TGF-β therefore has the potential to be a major regulator of PAI-1, and perhaps other genes in obesity. One important question in this regard is whether TGF-β expression, like that of TNF-α, is elevated in obesity, a situation that would make these initial studies more meaningful. In fact, the level of TGF-β mRNA was significantly higher in the adipose tissue of both the ob/ob (TABLE 1) and db/db mice when compared to their lean counterparts.[18] This increase again was due to increased expression of TGF-β mRNA by mature adipocytes and stromal vascular cells.

Finally, experiments were performed to identify potential mechanisms that contribute to the chronically elevated levels of TGF-β associated with the adipose tissues of obese mice. As already discussed, both insulin and TNF-α are chronically elevated in the adipose tissue of insulin-resistant obese rodents and humans, and both stimulate PAI-1 biosynthesis. We thus asked whether TGF-β expression in the adipose tissue could be induced by either of these molecules.[18] We observed that intraperitoneal administration of TNF-α into lean mice induced TGF-β mRNA in the adipose tissue and caused a strong induction of TGF-β in cultured 3T3-L1 cells. These observations raise the possibility that the chronically elevated levels of TNF-α in the obese adipose tissue may act in an autocrine/paracrine manner and contribute to the elevated TGF-β mRNA expression in obesity. Insulin failed to increase TGF-β mRNA in adipose tissues of lean mice, even though the addition of insulin to cultured 3T3-L1 cells caused a modest elevation of TGF-β mRNA.

The increase in TGF-β gene expression in adipose tissue in obesity may have broad implications in the pathophysiology of obesity and its related complications. It is known that TGF-β inhibits *in vitro* proliferation of many cells. However, it stimulates the growth of fibroblasts, and has been shown to increase pre-adipocyte cell proliferation in many species (reviewed in Ref. 18). Thus, the augmented expression of TGF-β in the obese adipose tissue may increase adipocyte precursor cell proliferation, thereby contributing to the excessive cellularity of the fat deposits associated with the obese phenotype. Obesity and NIDDM are also associated with characteristic long-term complications, including microvascular kidney disease and atherosclerosis.[13,33] It is interesting to note in this regard that several investigators have reported overexpression of TGF-β in the glomeruli in human and experimental diabetes.[34,35]

TNF-α CONTRIBUTES TO THE ELEVATED PAI-1 AND TGF-β IN OBESE MICE

Our studies indicate that the mechanisms that lead to the elevated plasma PAI-1 levels observed in obesity and related NIDDM are complex and may involve multiple cytokines, hormones, and growth factors (FIG. 1). The fact that TNF-α, insulin, and TGF-β are elevated in obesity and induce PAI-1 in the plasma and adipose tissue of lean mice suggests the involvement of at least these three mediators in the regulation of PAI-1 in obesity. However, the relationship between these mediators and the elevated levels of PAI-1 is at present only correlative. Direct evidence requires further experiments employing specific inhibitors or neutralizing antibodies. We decided to investigate the effects of TNF-α in more detail since it seems to play such a central role in the altered metabolic activities associated with obesity (FIG. 1). For example, TNF-α clearly increases PAI-1 and induces TGF-β *in vivo* and in cultured adipocytes,[18] and it has been directly implicated in the insulin resistance and hyperinsulinemia associated with obesity (FIG. 1).[36–38] Both insulin and TGF-β induce PAI-1 *in vivo* and *in vitro* in cultured adipocytes. We observed that a 3-h intraperitoneal administration into obese mice of a hamster antibody that neutralizes mouse TNF-α decreased plasma PAI-1 levels significantly (by about 50%). Interestingly, the antibody had a more dramatic effect on PAI-1 mRNA in the adipose tissue of these obese mice, decreasing it almost to the levels of the lean animals. These initial experiments suggest that TNF-α contributes directly to the observed increase in PAI-1 associated with this condition. This conclusion is supported by studies using ob/ob mice that lack both the p55 and the p75 TNF-α receptors (TABLE 1).[39] As expected, the hyperinsulinemia improves considerably in these animals, with the plasma insulin levels decreasing by 50–60% (TABLE 1), although not to the levels of the con-

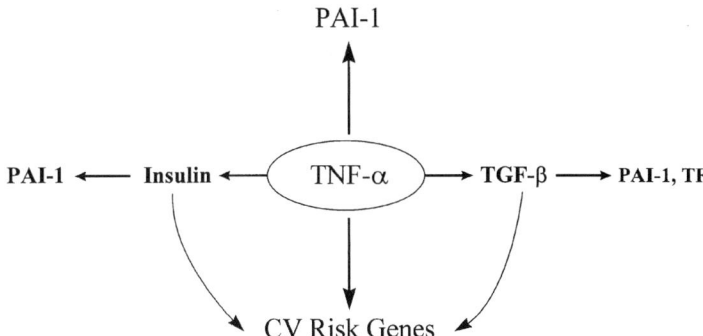

FIGURE 1. Regulation of PAI-1, TF, and TGF-β gene expression in obese mice. The transition from the lean to the obese state is associated with a chronic elevation in TNF-α expression by the adipose tissue. TNF-α is known to contribute to the insulin resistance/hyperinsulinemia associated with this condition, and insulin induces PAI-1 in adipose tissue. Our studies using TNF-α receptor–deficient mice[39] indicate that TNF-α also induces PAI-1 and TGF-β, and that TGF-β induces PAI-1 and TF. Thus, the increase in TNF-α appears to activate a cytokine cascade that in turn, induces PAI-1, TF, and possibly other hemostatic genes that may promote cardiovascular risk.

trol. Additionally, in obese mice lacking both TNF-α receptors, the plasma PAI-1 antigen levels are only about 50% of those of the obese controls, although again, not at the level of the lean mice. Moreover, in these TNF-α receptor–deficient ob/ob mice, PAI-1 and TGF-β mRNA in adipose tissue decreased almost to the levels of lean animals (TABLE 1). These studies thus clearly demonstrate that the chronic elevations in TNF-α in obese mice contribute to the hyperinsulinemia, elevated adipose tissue TGF-β mRNA, and elevated PAI-1 associated with this condition (FIG. 1). The fact that elimination of TNF-α or its receptors did not return the plasma PAI-1 levels to those of the lean controls suggest that other mediators may be involved. This possibility is under investigation.

TF EXPRESSION AND REGULATION IN OBESE MICE

Tissue factor (TF) serves as a cell surface receptor for the activation of factor VII and may be the major cellular initiator of the coagulation cascade.[9,40] A number of clinical studies have shown an increase in TF-mediated coagulation and in factor VII activity/antigen in obese and NIDDM patients.[41–43] To further investigate the relationship between TF and obesity, we compared the level of TF gene expression in a variety of tissues from lean and obese mice. TF mRNA levels were elevated in several tissues (including the brain, lung, kidney, heart, and adipose tissues) (TABLE 1)[44] from ob/ob mice when compared with their lean counterparts. The level of TF mRNA increased with age and the degree of obesity in all tissues of ob/ob mice, but not in the lean mice. In the adipose tissue, examination of TF mRNA by RT-PCR after collagenase digestion and differential centrifugation and by *in situ* hybridization, revealed enhanced expression primarily in adipocytes.[44] Experiments were performed to investigate the regulation of TF gene expression in this system. Although TNF-α and insulin stimulated TF gene expression in the adipose tissue, the effects were modest (≤ twofold) at best. TF mRNA expression also was induced by insulin in the kidney, brain, and lung, but again, the effects were modest. In contrast to these results, TGF-β proved to be a potent inducer of TF in the epididymal and subcutaneous fat of lean mice (six- to eightfold), and the primary responsive cell again appeared to be the adipocyte.[44] These results raise the possibility that the combination of increased procoagulant activity (due to increased TF) and decreased fibrinolytic activity (because of the high PAI-1) may contribute to the increased risk for fatal thrombosis in obesity/NIDDM (FIG. 1).

SUMMARY

In summary, obesity/NIDDM in the mouse is associated with increased procoagulant activity and decreased fibrinolytic potential. Unexpectedly, the adipocyte appears to play a central role in the hemostatic defects observed in murine and, perhaps, human obesity. Thus, the simple paradigm of adipocyte as merely a fat storage cell is rapidly evolving into one of this cell as metabolically active secretory cell that can alter the composition of the blood. Thus, the increased numbers and altered metabolic activities of adipocytes may play a critical role in changing the hemostatic balance in obesity, thereby contributing to cardiovascular complications associated with this condition. They do so both by abnormally expressing certain antifibrinolytic and/or procoagulant proteins like PAI-1, tissue factor, and perhaps other hemostatic proteins, and also by producing elevated levels of cytokines, like TNF-α and TGF-β, which may act in an autocrine and paracrine manner to alter gene expression in the adipose tissue and perhaps elsewhere (FIG. 1). Our data suggest that these changes, together with the increased insulin due to the compensatory hyperinsulinemia associated with this condition, contribute to the altered gene expression profile and increased cardiovascular risk in obesity/NIDDM.

REFERENCES

1. FINER, N. 1997. Obesity. Brit. Med. Bull. **53:** 229–450.
2. NIELSEN, S. & M.D. JENSEN. 1997. Obesity and cardiovascular disease: is body structure a factor? Curr. Opin. Lipidol. **8:** 200–204.
3. SPIEGELMAN, B.M. & J.S. FLIER. 1996. Adipogenesis and obesity: Rounding out the big picture. Cell **87:** 377–389.
4. DONG, Z.M., J.C. GUTIERREZ-RAMOS et al. 1997. A new class of obesity genes encodes leukocyte adhesion receptors. Proc. Natl. Acad. Sci. USA **94:** 7526–7530.
5. SPRENGERS, E.D. & C. KLUFT. 1987. Plasminogen activator inhibitors. Blood **69:** 381–387.
6. VAN MEIJER, M. & H. PANNEKOEK. 1995. Structure of plasminogen activator inhibitor 1 (PAI-1) and its function in fibrinolysis: An update. Fibrinolysis **9:** 263–276.
7. FEARNS, C., F. SAMAD et al. 1995:Synthesis and localization of PAI-1 in the vessel wall. *In* Vascular Control of Hemostasis. V.W.M. Van Hinsbergh, Ed.: 207–226. Harwood Academic Publishers. Amsterdam.
8. LAWRENCE, D.A. & D. GINSBURG. 1996. Gene expression and function of plasminogen activator inhibitor-1. *In* Fibrinolysis in Disease: Molecular and Hemovascular Aspects of Fibrinolysis. P. Glas-Greenwalt, Ed.: 21–29. CRC Press Inc. Boca Raton, FL.
9. CARMELIET, P. & D. COLLEN. 1997. Molecular genetics of the fibrinolytic and coagulation systems in haemostasis, thrombogenesis, restenosis and atherosclerosis. Curr. Opin. Lipidol. **8:** 118–125.
10. BRUCKERT, E., A. ANKRI et al. 1994. Relation between plasminogen activator inhibitor-1 and hepatic enzyme concentrations in hyperlipidemic patients. Thromb. Haemostas. **72:** 434–437.
11. FRIEDERICH, P.W., M. LEVI et al. 1997. Novel low-molecular-weight inhibitor of PAI-1 (XR5118) promotes endogenous fibrinolysis and reduces postthrombolysis thrombus growth in rabbits. Circulation **96:** 916–921.
12. SAWDEY, M.S. & D.J. LOSKUTOFF. 1991. Regulation of murine type 1 plasminogen activator inhibitor gene expression in vivo: Tissue specificity and induction by lipopolysaccharide, tumor necrosis factor-α, and transforming growth factor-β. J. Clin. Invest. **88:** 1346–1353.
13. JUHAN-VAGUE, I. & M.C. ALESSI. 1997. PAI-1, obesity, insulin resistance and risk of cardiovascular events. Thromb. Haemost. **78:** 656–660.
14. CALLES-ESCANDON, J., D. BALLOR et al. 1996. Amelioration of the inhibition of fibrinolysis in elderly, obese subjects by moderate energy intake restriction. Am. J. Clin. Nutr. **64:** 7–11.
15. AILHAUD, G., P. GRIMALDI et al. 1992. A molecular view of adipose tissue. Int. J. Obes. **16:** S17–S21.
16. SAMAD, F., K. YAMAMOTO et al. 1996. Distribution and regulation of plasminogen activator inhibitor-1 in murine adipose tissue in vivo: Induction by tumor necrosis factor-a and lipopolysaccharide. J. Clin. Invest. **97:** 37–46.
17. SAMAD, F. & D.J. LOSKUTOFF. 1996. Tissue distribution and regulation of plasminogen activator inhibitor-1 in obese mice. Mol. Med. **2:** 568–582.
18. SAMAD, F., K. YAMAMOTO et al. 1997. Elevated expression of transforming growth factor-b in adipose tissue from obese mice. Mol. Med. **3:** 37–48.

19. ZHANG, Y., R. PROENCA et al. 1994. Positional cloning of the mouse obese gene and its human homologue. Nature **372**: 425–432.
20. SHIMOMURA, I., T. FUNAHASHI et al. 1996. Enhanced expression of PAI-1 in visceral fat: Possible contributor to vascular disease in obesity. Nature Med. **2**: 800–803.
21. LUNDGREN, C.H., S.L. BROWN et al. 1996. Elaboration of type-1 plasminogen activator inhibitor from adipocyte—A potential pathogenetic link between obesity and cardiovascular disease. Circulation **93**: 106–110.
22. ALESSI, M.C., F. PEIRETTI et al. 1997. Production of plasminogen activator inhibitor 1 by human adipose tissue. Possible link between visceral fat accumulation and vascular disease. Diabetes **46**: 860–867.
23. CIGOLINI, M., M. TONOLI et al. 1999. Expression of plasminogen activator inhibitor-1 in human adipose tissue: A role for TNF-α. Atherosclerosis **143**: 81–90.
24. EHRMANN, D.A., D.J. SCHNEIDER et al. 1997. Troglitazone improves defects in insulin action, insulin secretion, ovarian steroidogenesis, and fibrinolysis in women with polycystic ovary syndrome. J. Clin. Endocrinol. Metab. **82**: 2108–2116.
25. NORDT, T.K., H. SAWA et al. 1995. Induction of plasminogen activator inhibitor type-1 (PAI-1) by proinsulin and insulin in vivo. Circulation **91**: 764–770.
26. CARMASSI, F., M. MORALE, L. FERRINI, G. DELL'OMO, M. FERDEGHINI, R. PEDRINELLI & F. DE NEGRI. 1999. Local insulin infusion stimulates expression of plasminogen activator inhibitor-1 and tissue-type plasminogen activator in normal subjects. Am. J. Med. **107**: 344–350.
27. JAIN, S.K., D.K. NAGI et al. 1993. Insulin therapy in type 2 diabetic subjects suppresses plasminogen activator inhibitor (PAI-1) activity and proinsulin-like molecules independently of glycaemic control. Diabetic Med. **10**: 27–32.
28. NAGI, D.K., T.J. HENDRA et al. 1990. The relationships of concentrations of insulin, intact proinsulin and 32-33 split proinsulin with cardiovascular risk factor in type 2 (non-insulin-dependent) diabetic subjects. Diabetologia **33**: 532–537.
29. LORMEAU, B., M.H. AUROUSSEAU et al. 1997. Hyperinsulinemia and hypofibrinolysis: Effects of short-term optimized glycemic control with continuous insulin infusion in Type II diabetic patients. Metabolism **46**: 1074–1079.
30. ALESSI, M.C., F. ANFOSSO et al. 1995. Up-regulation of PAI-1 synthesis by insulin and proinsulin in HEP G2 cells but not in endothelial cells. Fibrinolysis **9**: 237–242.
31. NORDT, T.K., D.J. SCHNEIDER et al. 1994. Augmentation of the synthesis of plasminogen activator inhibitor type-1 by precursors of insulin: A potential risk factor for vascular disease. Circulation **89**: 321–330.
32. FUJII, S. & B.E. SOBEL. 1990. Induction of plasminogen activator inhibitor by products released from platelets. Circulation **82**: 1485–1493.
33. ARRANTS, J. 1994. Hyperinsulinemia and cardiovascular risk. Heart Lung **23**: 118–122.
34. BORDER, W.A. 1994. Transforming growth factor-beta and the pathogenesis of glomerular diseases. Curr. Opin. Nephrol. Hypertens. **3**: 54–58.
35. SHARMA, K. & F.N. ZIYADEH. 1995. Hyperglycemia and diabetic kidney disease. The case for transforming growth factor-beta as a key mediator. Diabetes **44**: 1139–1146.
36. HOTAMISLIGIL, G.S., N.S. SHARGILL et al. 1993. Adipose expression of tumor necrosis factor-α: Direct role in obesity-linked insulin resistance. Science **259**: 87–91.
37. HOTAMISLIGIL, G.S., P. ARNER et al. 1995. Increased adipose tissue expression of tumor necrosis factor-α in human obesity and insulin resistance. J. Clin. Invest. **95**: 2409–2415.
38. HOTAMISLIGIL, G.S. & B.M. SPIEGELMAN. 1994. Tumor necrosis factor α: A key component of the obesity-diabetes link. Diabetes **43**: 1271–1278.
39. SAMAD, F., K.T. UYSAL, S.M. WIESBROCK, M. PANDEY, G.S. HOTAMISLIGIL & D.J. LOSKUTOFF. 1999. Tumor necrosis factor-α is a key component in the obesity-linked elevation of plasminogen activator inhibitor-1. Proc. Natl. Acad. Sci. USA (In press).
40. EDGINGTON, T.S., C.D. DICKINSON et al. 1997. The structural basis of function of the TF×VIIa complex in the cellular initiation of coagulation. Thromb. Haemostas. **78**: 401–405.
41. MEADE, T.W., V. RUDDOCK et al. 1993. Fibrinolytic activity, clotting factors and long-term incidence of ischaemic heart disease in the Northwick Park Heart Study. Lancet **342**: 1076–1079.

42. JUHAN-VAGUE, I., M.C. ALESSI et al. 1996. Thrombogenic and fibrinolytic factors and cardiovascular risk in non-insulin-dependent diabetes mellitus. Ann. Med. **28:** 371–380.
43. KARIO, K., T. MATSUO et al. 1995. Activation of tissue factor-induced coagulation and endothelial cell dysfunction in non-insulin-dependent diabetic patients with microalbuminuria. Arterioscler. Thromb. Vasc. Biol. **15:** 1114–1120.
44. SAMAD, F., M. PANDEY et al. 1998. Tissue factor gene expression in the adipose tissues of obese mice. Proc. Natl. Acad. Sci. USA **95:** 7591–7596.

Questions and Answers

G.K. HANSSON (*Karolinska Hospital, Stockholm, Sweden*): The production of TNF-α in the fat tissue of these mice would suggest that there might be some slight inflammation going on there. On the other hand, TGF-β would tend to downregulate some of these activities. Have you looked at whether, for example, you have leukocyte adhesion molecules expressed in microvascular endothelium?

LOSKUTOFF: It is curious that TNF-α was described initially as a cachectic molecule and here it is upregulated in obesity. But it is upregulated so slightly that you cannot detect it in the plasma. It is a sort of autocrine or paracrine kind of thing. You see it is made by the adipose tissue, and if you extract that adipose tissue, you could find it upregulated, but you really cannot measure it in blood.

HANSSON: That is a classic cytokine, isn't it—acting locally?

A.R. TALL (*Columbia University, New York, NY, USA*): Apparently there are patients with rheumatoid arthritis that are getting TNF receptor–soluble form as an antagonist to TNF-α action. I have heard it stated, but not actually read that such individuals do not show a change in the glucose or insulin level—a piece of evidence against the Spigelman hypothesis. Would there be any value in looking at PAI-1 levels in obese rheumatoid patients being treated in such a fashion?

LOSKUTOFF: I think that's asking for trouble—trying to interpret whatever you get there. I think the correlation with TNF is pretty good, at least in rodents.

P. CARMELIET (*Flanders Interuniversity, Institute of Biotechnology, Leuven, Belgium*): Have you challenged your mice with any kind of prothrombotic stimulus, for example, endotoxin injection locally into the footpad?

LOSKUTOFF: We have done that. One of the issues may be that these animals are in a compromised pre-thrombotic state—and it is really hard to do because those rodents are very resistant to thrombosis. But, in fact, we have done the experiment that Peter suggests, which is to see if their sensitivity to endotoxin is altered and, in fact, it is shifted by about tenfold.

CARMELIET: Can you speculate about the role of tissue factor that can be shed into the circulation?

LOSKUTOFF: Clearly, there is a lot of angiogenesis going on in adipose tissue. Both tissue factor and PAI-1 may have roles in this process that may not be related to their roles in coagulation and fibrinolysis. Perhaps there is an axis here that we should explore.

CARMELIET: Can you say something about the double-cross with PAI-1 knockouts?

LOSKUTOFF: We have done very little more than weigh these animals. There is no question that the PAI-1–deficient ob/ob mouse weighs less than the ob/ob mouse. But the lean PAI-1–deficient is a little bit smaller than the wild-type mouse as well. The obese mouse is sterile; so it takes a lot of work to get enough animals to characterize them. These animals get kidney disease, sclerosis of the kidney, and so we are trying to ask whether the absence of PAI-1 may protect in that setting.

H. YAMAMOTO (*Kanazawa University, Kanazawa, Japan*): Do all the ob/ob mice develop microvascular changes like diabetics?

LOSKUTOFF: I don't think so. It is very hard to get at the vascular system of these obese animals because they are so embedded in fat.

M.A. GIMBRONE (*Brigham and Women's Hospital, Boston, MA, USA*): The white adipose tissue is probably the highest density capillary endothelial bed in the body, maybe second to the lung. You did the classical fractionation where you float off the adipocytes and you look at them, while the stromal/vascular pellet goes down in the tube. In a few of the slides you showed us the pellet data, most of the time you did not. You showed us cross-sections and commented that it looked like it was adipocytes that were expressing PAI-1. How do you know that it is not the capillary endothelium, especially when activated by TNF?

LOSKUTOFF: The data that argue that it is not the capillary endothelium is that adipocytes themselves behave exactly the way I have told you. If we take those fractions and look for von Willebrand factor, for instance, there is no detectable von Willebrand factor in those floating cells. That is the best data.

GIMBRONE: You convinced me that the fat can express PAI-1, but I am asking the other question, what rules out the presence of PAI-1 in the activated fat pad endothelial cells?

LOSKUTOFF: I cannot rule that out. If we do the histology of what is in that fraction, there are still some immature lipid-laden adipocytes that come down.

GIMBRONE: One of the first sources, 25 years ago, for the attempt to culture microvascular endothelium happened to be epididymal fat pad and it was precisely this kind of enzymatic dissociation method that allowed people to culture out the endothelium. So I know that people can culture endothelial cells from fat pad. We have done it.

LOSKUTOFF: Right. The endothelium by *in situ* hybridization in the obese animal is in fact occasionally active. I would say that the capillaries are making it. If you are looking at the histology of fat, there are a number of nuclei there and you would be hard pressed, no matter how hard you look, to say this is absolutely an adipocyte and this is absolutely the nucleus of it. The only thing I can conclude is that the adipocytes certainly are a major part of this, and whether endothelial cells are as well, I just cannot know for sure.

Participation of Reactive Oxygen Intermediates in the Angiotensin II–Activated Signaling Pathways in Vascular Smooth Muscle Cells

TOMOSABURO TAKAHASHI, TAKAHIRO TANIGUCHI,[a] MASANORI OKUDA, AKIHIRO TAKAHASHI, SATORU KAWASAKI, KOJI DOMOTO, MASAKO TAGUCHI, YUICHI ISHIKAWA,[b] AND MITSUHIRO YOKOYAMA

Department of Internal Medicine (First Division), [b]Faculty of Health Science, Kobe University School of Medicine, Kobe 650-0017, Japan

INTRODUCTION

Angiotensin II (Ang II), the main peptide hormone of the renin-angiotensin system, has been known to play an important role in the development of various cardiovascular diseases in addition to its key regulatory role in the regulation of blood pressure and circulating volume.[1] Although Ang II is a potent hypertrophic factor for vascular smooth muscle cells (VSMC),[1] molecular mechanisms responsible for a growth-promoting action of Ang II have not been fully understood. Recent studies suggest that reactive oxygen intermediates (ROI) may function as second messengers in the intracellular signaling pathways that mediate cellular responses induced by growth factors and cytokines.[2] Therefore, we examined whether ROI were involved in Ang II–activated signaling pathways in cultured VSMC.

METHODS

Cultured VSMC were prepared from rat thoracic aorta by enzymatic dissociation as described previously.[3] Ras activity was analyzed by quantification of Ras-bound GDP and GTP as described previously.[3] MAP kinase activity was measured by a MAP kinase renaturation assay in myelin basic protein–containing polyacrylamide gels as described previously.[3] Tyrosine phosphorylation of paxillin was analyzed by immunoblotting of anti-paxillin immunoprecipitates with anti-phosphotyrosine antibody as described previously.[4] Protein synthesis was measured by [^{3}H]leucine incorporation into the trichloroacetic acid precipitable materials as described previously.[4]

---

[a]Address for correspondence: Takahiro Taniguchi, Department of Internal Medicine (First Division), Kobe University School of Medicine, 7-5-1 Kusuoki-cho, Chuo-ku, Kobe 650-0017, Japan. Voice: 8178-382-5111; fax: 8178-382-5858.
taniguch@med.kobe-u.ac.jp

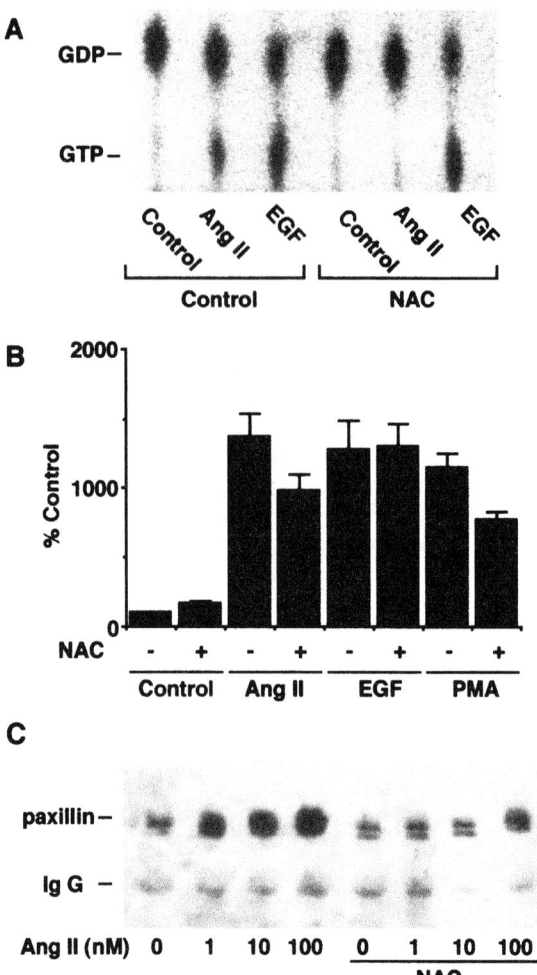

FIGURE 1. Effects of NAC on Ang II–activated signaling pathways. Cultured VSMC were pretreated for 4 h with or without 10 mM NAC. (**A**) Cells were then stimulated with 100 nM Ang II or 100 ng/ml EGF for 2 min. Ras activities were analyzed and positions of GDP and GTP are indicated. (**B**) Cells were stimulated with 100 nM Ang II, 100 ng/ml EGF, or 100 nM PMA for 5 min. MAP kinases activities were measured and expressed as the percentage of the unstimulated levels. (**C**) Cells were stimulated with the indicated concentrations of Ang II for 10 min and tyrosine phosphorylation of paxillin was analyzed.

RESULTS AND DISCUSSION

Effect of NAC on Ang II–Activated Signaling Pathways

To test for the possible involvement of ROI in Ang II–activated signaling pathways, we examined the effect of antioxidant *N*-acetylcysteine (NAC) on the signaling events induced by Ang II in VSMC. NAC is a thiol-based antioxidative agent that directly scavenges ROI and also increases the intracellular level of reduced glutathione (GSH). GSH is a hydroxy radical scavenger and a substrate of glutathione peroxidase that degrades H_2O_2.

We have previously reported that in VSMC, Ang II induces MAP kinases activation mainly via protein kinase C activation[5] and that Ras is also activated in response to Ang II,[3] but this activation of Ras is dispensable for Ang II–induced MAP kinases activation. As shown in FIGURE 1A, treatment of cells with 100 nM Ang II or 100 ng/ml epidermal growth factor (EGF) induced Ras activation as demonstrated by an increase in the GTP-bound active form of Ras. In cells pretreated with 10 mM NAC for 4 h, Ang II–induced Ras activation was almost completely inhibited, while EGF-induced Ras activation remained unchanged. Ang II as well as EGF also significantly stimulated kinase activities of MAP kinases (FIG. 1B). NAC inhibited Ang II–stimulated MAP kinase activity by approximately 30%, but did not affect EGF-stimulated MAP kinase activity. These results suggest that ROI participate in Ang II– but not EGF-induced Ras and MAP kinases activation in VSMC. Protein kinase C–activating phorbol ester, phorbol 12-myristate 13-acetate (PMA), also stimulated MAP kinases activity. This activation of MAP kinases by PMA was also inhibited by NAC by approximately 30%, suggesting that the inhibitory effect of NAC was not localized to the hormone receptor alone. Ang II transduces its signals not only to the nucleus but also to focal adhesions and stimulates tyrosine phosphorylation of a focal adhesion–associated protein, paxillin.[6] In accord with previously published results,[6] Ang II stimulated tyrosine phosphorylation of paxillin in a dose-dependent manner (FIG. 1C). And treatment with NAC resulted in a marked inhibition of Ang II–stimulated paxillin phosphorylation. Thus, ROI may be involved in the Ang II signals to the focal adhesions.

Effects of H_2O_2 on Signaling Pathways

If ROI are the signaling molecules that mediate the Ang II–induced signaling pathways, an increase in intracellular concentrations of ROI would be expected to mimic the effects of Ang II in these signaling events. Then, we examined the effect of direct exposure of cells with H_2O_2 on these signaling events. H_2O_2 is widely used as an experimental source of oxygen-derived free radicals, because it can readily cross the cell membrane and give rise to the highly reactive hydroxy radical.

Exposure of VSMC with 1 mM H_2O_2 did not affect the ratio of Ras-bound GTP in VSMC (Fig. 2A), but caused a significant MAP kinases activation (FIG. 2B). This activation was maximal at around 10 min. Taken together with the results from the experiments with NAC, it is suggested that ROI is necessary but not sufficient for Ang II–induced Ras activation and is sufficient and necessary for full activation of MAP kinases by Ang II in VSMC. One possible explanation for these results is that one or more signaling events besides ROI generation are critical for the induction of

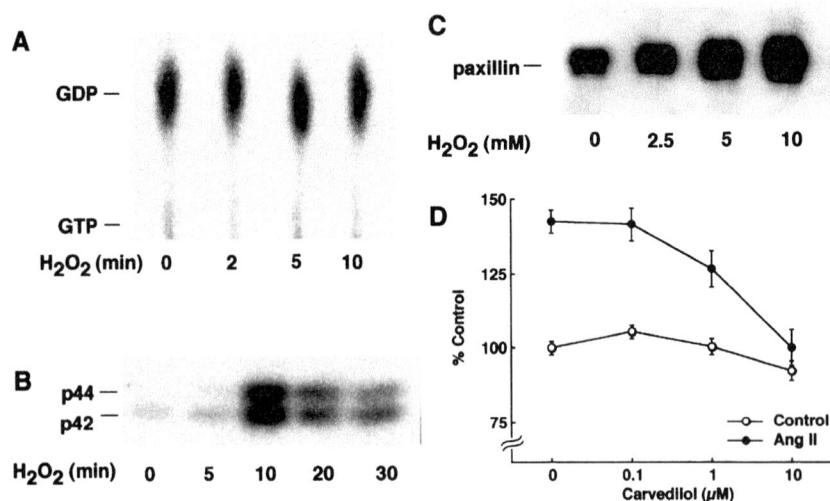

FIGURE 2. Effects of H_2O_2 on signaling pathways and effect of Carvedilol on Ang II–stimulated protein synthesis. (**A**) Cultured VSMC were treated with 1 mM H_2O_2 for various periods of time as indicated and Ras activities were analyzed. (**B**) Cells were treated with 1 mM H_2O_2 for various periods of time as indicated and MAP kinases activities were measured. (**C**) Cells were treated with the indicated concentrations of H_2O_2 for 10 min and tyrosine phosphorylation of paxillin was analyzed. (**D**) Cell were treated with or without the indicated concentrations of Carvedilol for 30 min prior to stimulation with 10 nM Ang II for 24 h. Protein synthesis was measured by [^{3}H]leucine incorporation.

Ras activation by Ang II, and ROI may function as only one of the parallel signaling intermediates mediating Ang II–induced MAP kinases activation. Tyrosine phosphorylation of paxillin was also significantly induced by treatment with H_2O_2 for 10 min (FIG. 2C) and this effect was concentration dependent. The concentration of H_2O_2 required for MAP kinase activation and paxillin phosphorylation is unlikely to be achieved in cells by physiological stimuli. However, ROI may be generated by Ang II at a site more proximal to the target, whereas the external added H_2O_2 diffuses indiscriminately. Therefore, these results suggested a possible involvement of ROI in Ang II–induced signaling pathways in VSMC.

Effect of Carvedilol on Ang II–Stimulated Protein Synthesis

In the final experiment, we assessed the effect of Carvedilol, which is an antihypertensive agent with antioxidative property, on Ang II–stimulated protein synthesis. Stimulation with Ang II resulted in approximately 1.4-fold increase in protein synthesis (FIG. 2D). Carvedilol dose-dependently inhibited Ang II–induced increase in protein synthesis and 10 µM of Carvedilol almost completely inhibited Ang II–stimulated increase in protein synthesis.

In conclusion, the results presented here suggest that ROI participate in Ang II–induced signal transduction pathways at multiple sites in VSMC and the relative contribution made by ROI to the intracellular signaling pathways varies among different mitogens even in the same cells. It seems likely that antioxidative agents may inhibit the development of vascular disease in which Ang II is implicated.

REFERENCES

1. GRIENDLING, K.K., B. LASSEGUE & R.W. ALEXANDER. 1996. Angiotensin receptors and their therapeutic implications. Annu. Rev. Pharmacol. Toxicol. **36:** 281–306.
2. LANDER, H.M. 1997. An essential role for free radicals and derived species in signal transduction. FASEB J. **11:** 118-124.
3. TAKAHASHI, T., Y. KAWAHARA, M. OKUDA, H. UENO, A. TAKESHITA & M. YOKOYAMA. 1997. Angiotensin II stimulates mitogen-activated protein kinases and protein synthesis by a Ras-independent pathway in vascular smooth muscle cells. J. Biol. Chem. **272:** 16018–16022.
4. TAKAHASHI, T., Y. KAWAHARA, M. OKUDA & M. YOKOYAMA. 1996. Increasing cAMP antagonizes hypertrophic response to angiotensin II without affecting Ras and MAP kinase activation in vascular smooth muscle cells. FEBS Lett. **397:** 89–92.
5. TSUDA, T., Y. KAWAHARA, Y. ISHIDA, M. KOIDE, K. SHII & M. YOKOYAMA. 1992. Angiotensin II stimulates two myelin basic protein/microtubule-associated protein 2 kinases in cultured vascular smooth muscle cells. Circ. Res. **71:** 620–630.
6. OKUDA, M., Y. KAWAHARA, I. NAKAYAMA, M. HOSHIJIMA & M. YOKOYAMA. 1995. Angiotensin II transduces its signal to focal adhesions via angiotensin II type 1 receptors in vascular smooth muscle cells. FEBS Lett. **368:** 343–347.

C-C and C-X-C Chemokines Trigger Firm Adhesion of Monocytes to Vascular Endothelium under Flow Conditions[a]

FRANCIS W. LUSCINSKAS,[b-d] ROBERT E. GERSZTEN,[d,e] EDUARDO A. GARCIA-ZEPEDA,[d,f] YAW-CHYN LIM,[c,d] MASAYUKI YOSHIDA,[g] HAN A. DING,[c] MICHAEL A. GIMBRONE, JR.,[c,d] ANDREW D. LUSTER,[d,f] AND ANTHONY ROSENZWEIG[d,e]

[c]*Vascular Research Division, Department of Pathology, Brigham and Women's Hospital, Boston, Massachusett 02115, USA*

[d]*Harvard Medical School, Boston, Massachusetts 02114, USA*

[e]*The Cardiovascular Research Center and Cardiology Division, Massachusetts General Hospital, Boston, Massachusetts 02114, USA*

[f]*Infectious Disease Unit, Massachusetts General Hospital, Boston, Massachusetts 02114, USA*

[g]*Molecular Genetics, Medical Research Institute, Tokyo Medical and Dental University, Tokyo, Japan*

INTRODUCTION

In experimental models of atherogenesis, a characteristic manifestation is the continued recruitment and accumulation in the arterial intima of mononuclear leukocytes (monocytes, lymphocytes, and foam cells) (reviewed in Ref. 14). It is widely recognized that the vascular endothelial lining plays an active and important role in this process of mononuclear leukocyte egress through induction and expression of surface adhesion molecules that can capture leukocytes under conditions of blood flow. During the past several years many investigators have contributed toward a working paradigm of leukocyte recruitment that can be represented conceptually as an overlapping cascade of adhesive interactions that is initiated by attachment of leukocytes to the apical endothelial surface and then followed by low velocity rolling, arrest, spreading, and diapedesis between two adjacent endothelial cells into tissues. The members of the selectin (E-, P-, and L-selectins) and immunoglobulin (VCAM-1) gene families interacting with their counterreceptors on leukocytes have been demonstrated to support leukocyte initial attachment, or tethering, and subsequent rolling interactions under flow conditions.[1,10,16] Once in contact with the apical surface, chemoattractants elaborated by the endothelium, including certain chemoat-

---

[a]This work supported by National Institutes of Health grants HL03348 (R.E.G.); HL54202, AI40970, and HL59521 (A.R.); HL36028 (M.A.G. and A.R.); and HL53993 (F.W.L.). A.R. is an Established Investigator of the American Heart Association.

[b]Address for correspondence: Francis W. Luscinskas, Ph.D., Vascular Research Division, 221 Longwood Avenue, Boston, MA 02115; Voice: 617-732-6004; fax: 617-732-5933.
fluscinskas@rics.bwh.harvard.edu

tractant cytokines, also known as chemokines,[12] trigger leukocyte integrins activation, resulting in stable arrest and ultimately transendothelial migration of the leukocyte via interactions with VCAM-1 and intercellular adhesion molecule-1 (ICAM-1). While the adhesion cascade has been well-characterized for blood neutrophils and lymphocytes, less information is available for monocytes.

In this brief report, we provide an overview of our recent efforts to understand the role of individual endothelial cell adhesion molecules, in particular VCAM-1 and E-selectin, and physiologically relevant endothelial-derived chemokines, in monocyte adhesive interactions with the vascular endothelium using an *in vitro* flow model.[2–4,9]

RESULTS AND DISCUSSION

To investigate the mechanisms of monocyte adhesion and stable arrest on endothelium, we have used recombinant adenovirus-5–containing specific endothelial adhesion molecules (VCAM-1 or E-selectin) to transduce human umbilical vein endothelial cell monolayers, a well-characterized model of vascular endothelium. Studies were conducted using an *in vitro* flow model consisting of a parallel-plate flow apparatus that generates physiologically relevant levels of two-dimensional laminar fluid shear stress[11,15] and a live-time phase-contrast microscopic video analysis system capable of measuring leukocyte–endothelial adhesive interactions on videotape offline.[6]

Our initial studies revealed that VCAM-1 can mediate initial attachment to vascular endothelium under flow, but VCAM-1–transduced monolayers alone supported much less monocyte firm adhesion than 6-h TNF-α–activated endothelial monolayers. Based on this result, we had previously predicted[3] that other signals expressed by activated endothelial cells could substantially enhance both monocyte initial attachment and firm adhesion on the apical endothelial cell surface under flow conditions. At an estimated fluid shear stress of 1.5 dynes/cm^2, the level of monocyte attachment to TNF-α–activated endothelium was more than that attachment to VCAM-1–transduced endothelial monolayers.[3,9] We then examined what effect the combination of both VCAM-1 and E-selectin would have on monocyte-endothelial adhesion. The expression of E-selectin with VCAM-1 significantly increased monocyte-endothelial interactions (data not shown), but the predominant type of interactions observed were monocyte rolling, rather than firm adhesion as we had observed previously with TNF-α–activated monolayers. To test whether a separate signal was required for stable adhesion, independent of adhesion molecules per se, we examined several relevant chemokines that had been implicated in monocyte recruitment in experimental models of atherogenesis.[12,14] Although previous studies had suggested a requirement for chemoattractant in leukocyte arrest,[7] this question had not been studied using intact endothelium expressing specific adhesion molecules under defined flow conditions and physiologically relevant chemokines.

The design of the flow assay was modified as follows. Various concentrations of chemokines were added to isolated monocytes perfused over E-selectin–transduced monolayers, as a model of selectin-mediated monocyte rolling. Monocyte rolling and firm adhesion was determined one minute before and one minute after addition of the chemokine. Monocyte chemoattractant protein-1 (MCP-1) at concentrations ≥ 250 pM converted virtually all rolling monocytes to firmly adherent cells within seconds. For comparison purposes, we found that MCP-4, a C-C chemokine that induces monocyte chemotaxis and Ca^{2+} transients, produced a modest increase in monocyte firm adhesion over a range of concentrations as high as 100 nM (data not shown). Surprisingly, IL-8, a C-X-C chemokine predominantly recognized as a chemoattractant of neutrophils and/or lymphocytes, at concentrations $\geq$ 2 nM triggered monocyte firm adhesion similar to that observed with MCP-1. In contrast, epithelial cell–derived neutrophil-activating peptide-78 (ENA-78), granulocyte chemotactic protein (GCP 2), and other C-X-C chemokines, interferon-γ–inducible protein-10 (IP-10) and platelet factor 4 (PF4), had essentially no effect on monocyte interactions in this assay. The effect of IL-8 on monocyte arrest was seen with recombinant chemokine obtained from two different sources (Peprotech, Edison, NJ, and R&D Systems, Minneapolis, MN) and was prevented by preincubation with a neutralizing mAb to IL-8.

The process of MCP-1 or IL-8 chemokine-induced monocyte arrest was detected by tracking individual monocytes in small randomly selected regions of interest (ROI) of the videotape of experiments using computer software. The computer software identified and monitored the movement of monocytes, frame-by-frame, for 3 to 5 seconds before and after chemoattractant activation. The history of individual monocytes, depicted in FIGURE 1 as white tails appended to each monocyte within the ROI (white box), was superimposed on the video image. In this way, we could show that monocytes rolling on E-selectin–transduced endothelial cell monolayers (FIG. 1, top left and right panels; cells with white tails) can be converted to firmly adherent cells after addition of MCP-1 (1 nM, bottom right panel; note, few monocytes have white tails) or IL-8 (2 nM IL-8, bottom left panel). Several other results suggest that the effect on adhesion was not due to *de novo* recruitment of other leukocytes, such as neutrophils, that might theoretically contaminate the monocyte preparations. First, the purity of the starting population of monocytes was confirmed both by flow cytometry and histochemical staining (FIG. 2). Elutriated monocytes were consistently > 91% pure (range 91–95%, N = 10) as assessed by CD14 expression by indirect immunofluorescence assay and flow cytometry, with essentially no lymphocytes (< 3%) (FIG. 2, left panel). In analysis with mAb that recognized C-X-C receptor 1 (CXCR1), CXCR2, the IL-8 receptors (FIG. 2, right panel) or CCR2, the predominant monocyte MCP-1 receptor (not shown), were abundantly expressed on elutriated human monocytes obtained from several blood donors, consistent with previous reports. In addition, histochemical analysis of endothelial cell coverslips recovered from the flow chamber after IL-8 or MCP-1 treatment were reviewed by clinical hematologists blinded to the treatment protocol. Specifically, the adherent leukocytes uniformly possessed the morphologic features of monocytes. The monocyte firm adhesion seen after IL-8 or MCP-1 treatment reflected the arrest of virtually all the previously rolling leukocytes, rather than recruitment of a different (newly arrived) population from the flow stream (FIG. 1). We conclude that both IL-8 and MCP-1 can have a dramatic effect on rolling monocytes and trigger rapid arrest of most monocytes interacting with E-selectin–expressing vascular endothelium. As reported in detail elsewhere, additional experiments revealed a partial role for α4β1- and β2-integrins in chemokine-induced monocyte arrest and a partial inhibition of arrest by pretreatment of monocytes with a combination of neutralizing mAb to CXCR1 and CXCR.[2]

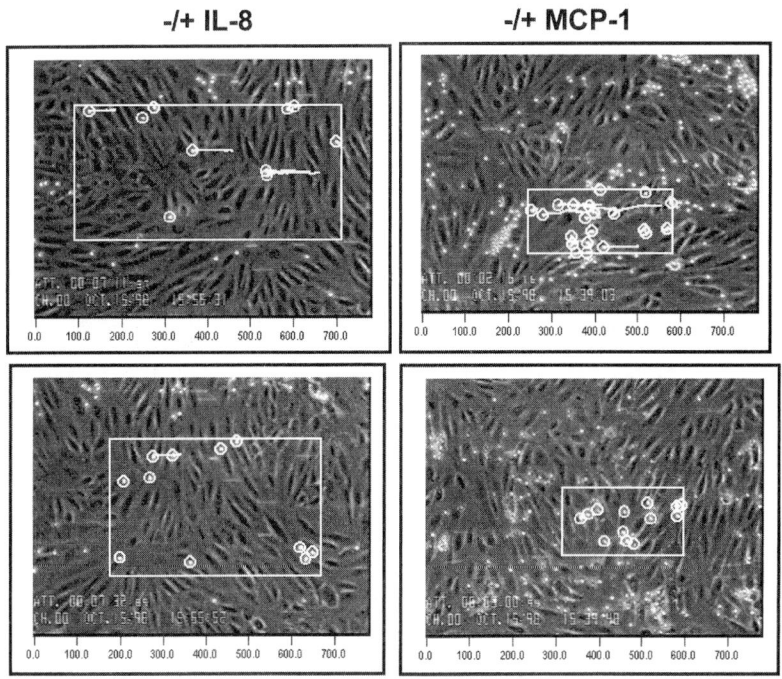

FIGURE 1. Computer-assisted analysis of IL-8 and MCP-1 triggered monocyte attachment to adenovirally transduced or cytokine-activated HUVEC. Endothelial monolayers were transduced with AdE-sel for 48 h before the experiment. The interaction of monocytes with these monolayers was studied at 2.0 dynes/cm^2. The indicated chemokine, either IL-8 or MCP-1, was added to the monocyte reservoir at room temperature and rolling monocytes in randomly selected regions of interest (ROI) were identified and monitored by customized software running under Windows95® for 3 to 10 sec before and after addition of the chemokine. ROI were selected for each videotape and the software used to identify and then track, frame-by-frame, each monocyte interacting with the apical surface. The x-y coordinates of each cell history were saved in a database and the cell history converted to an *x-y* plot and then superimposed on the last video frame analyzed (*white box*). This allows in register assignment of a cell history (*cells circled in white and with appended white tails*) to the correct monocyte in the video frame. MCP-1 (1 nM) and IL-8 (2 nM) converted virtually all monocyte rolling to firm adhesion. The *x*-axis is calibrated in μm.

SUMMARY

In summary, our findings indicate that specific chemokines that are elaborated by endothelial cells after cytokine or endotoxin activation[5,13] can play an essential role in monocyte recruitment beyond their chemoattractant activities. We show that this action is to translate initial monocyte tethering into firm adhesion via rapid leukocyte integrin activation. The *in vitro* model presented here provides a sensitive sys-

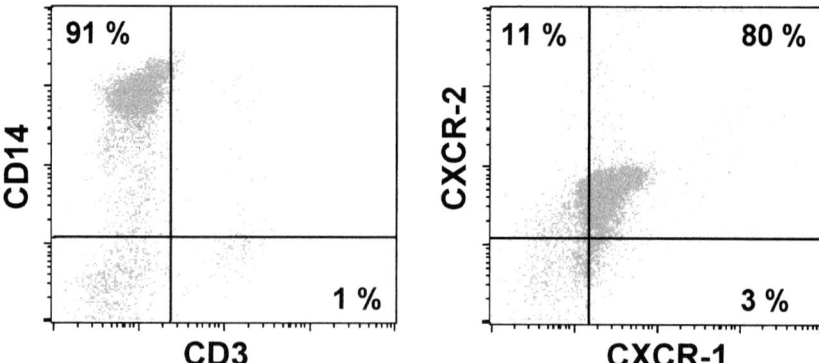

FIGURE 2. Flow cytometric analysis for surface expression of CD14, CD3, CXCR1, and CXCR2 on elutriated human monocytes. Isolated monocytes (3×10^5/tube) were subjected to flow cytometry with fluorescently labeled mAb to CD3 and CD14 (*left*), and CXCR1 and CXCR2 (*right*) as previously described for purified leukocytes. Surface expression of CXCR1 and CXCR2 on CD14-positive cells is shown (*right*) from one of six independent experiments.

tem for investigating the modulating ability of chemokines and reveals an important biological effect that is not predicted by results in simpler *in vitro* assays, such as measurement of calcium transients or chemotaxis.[2] The surprising finding that the C-X-C chemokine IL-8 can trigger monocyte firm adhesion to vascular endothelium suggests a potential role for this chemokine in monocyte recruitment and underscores the biological complexity of the chemokine family.

ACKNOWLEDGMENTS

The authors wish to thank Kay Case and Bill Atkinson of the Vascular Research Division at the Brigham and Women's Hospital for preparation of human endothelial cell cultures and the Blood Banks of both the Brigham and Women's Hospital and Massachusetts Hospital for providing single-donor platelet pheresis leukopacks from human volunteers blood donors. The technical assistance of Drs. Ling Li and Quifen Qui is greatly appreciated. We also thank Dr. Myron Cybulsky for providing the rabbit VCAM-1 cDNA and antibody Rb1/9, Dr. David Dichek for his help in construction of AdVCAM-1 and providing AdLacZ, Leukosite for providing antibody 2D7, Dr. Israel Charo for his thoughtful comments, Dr. Zareh N. Demirjian as well as other members of the MGH Clinical Hematology Laboratory for their review of leukocyte morphology, and Edward Marcus (EM Laboratories, Brighton, MA) for development of software used to track leukocytes in videotape and for generating the computer overlays used in FIGURE 1.

REFERENCES

1. BUTCHER, E.C. 1991. Leukocyte-endothelial cell recognition: three (or more) steps to specificity and diversity. Cell **67:** 1033–1036.
2. GERSZTEN, R.E., E. GARCIA-ZEPEDA, Y.-C. LIM, M. YOSHIDA, H. DING, M.A. GIMBRONE JR., A.D. LUSTER, F.W. LUSCINSKAS & A. ROSENZWEIG. 1999. MCP-1 and IL-8 trigger firm adhesion of monocytes to vascular endothelium under flow conditions. Nature **398:** 718–723.
3. GERSZTEN, R.E., Y.-C. LIM, H.T. DING, K. SNAPP, G.S. KANSAS, D.A. DICHEK, C. CABANAS, F. SANCHEZ-MADRID, M.A. GIMBRONE, JR., A. ROSENZWEIG & F.W. LUSCINSKAS. 1998. Adhesion of monocytes to VCAM-1 transduced human endothelial cells: Implications for atherogenesis. Circ. Res. **82:** 871–878.
4. GERSZTEN, R.E., F.W. LUSCINSKAS, H.T. DING, D.A. DICHEK, L.M. STOOLMAN, M.A. GIMBRONE, JR. & A. ROSENZWEIG. 1996. Adhesion of memory lymphocytes to vascular cell adhesion molecule-1-transduced human vascular endothelial cells under simulated physiological flow conditions in vitro. Circ. Res. **79:** 1205–1215.
5. GIMBRONE, M.A., JR., M.S. OBIN, A.F. BROCK, E.A. LUIS, P.E. HASS, C.A. HEBERT, Y.K. YIP, D.W. LEUNG, D.G. LOWE, W.J. KOHR, W.C. DARBONNE, K.B. BECHTOL & J.B. BAKER. 1989. Endothelial interleukin-8: a novel inhibitor of leukocyte-endothelial interactions. Science **246:** 1601–1603.
6. GOETZ, D.J., D.M. GREIF, J. SHEN & F.W. LUSCINSKAS. 1999. Cell-cell adhesive interactions in an *in vitro* flow chamber. Methods Mol. Biol. **96:** 137–145.
7. LAWRENCE, M.B. & T.A. SPRINGER. 1991. Leukocytes roll on a selectin at physiologic flow rates: distinct from and prerequisite for adhesion through integrins. Cell **65:** 1–20.
8. LIM, Y.C., L. HENAULT, A.J. WAGERS, G.S. KANSAS, F.W. LUSCINSKAS & A.H. LICHTMAN. 1999. Expression of functional selectin ligands on Th cells is differentially regulated by IL-12 and IL-4. J. Immunol. **162:** 3193–3201.
9. LIM, Y.C., K. SNAPP, G.S. KANSAS, R. CAMPHAUSEN, H. DING & F.W. LUSCINSKAS. 1998. Important contributions of P-selectin glycoprotein ligand-1-mediated secondary capture to human monocyte adhesion to P- selectin, E-selectin, and TNF-α-activated endothelium under flow in vitro. J. Immunol. **161:** 2501–2508.
10. LUSCINSKAS, F.W. & M.A. GIMBRONE, JR. 1996. Endothelial-dependent mechanisms in chronic inflammatory leukocyte recruitment. Annu. Rev. Med. **47:** 413–421.
11. LUSCINSKAS, F.W., G.S. KANSAS, H. DING, P. PIZCUETA, B.E. SCHLEIFFENBAUM, T.F. TEDDER & M.A. GIMBRONE, JR. 1994. Monocyte rolling, arrest and spreading on IL-4-activated vascular endothelium under flow is mediated via sequential action of L-selectin, β_1-integrins, and β_2-integrins. J. Cell Biol. **125:** 1417–1427.
12. LUSTER, A.D. 1998. Chemokines—chemotactic cytokines that mediate inflammation. N. Engl. J. Med. **338:** 436–445.
13. ROLLINS, B.J. & J.S. POBER. 1991. Interlukin-4 induces the synthesis and secretion of MCP-1/JE by human endothelial cells. Am. J. Pathol. **138:** 1315–1319
14. ROSS, R. 1999. Atherosclerosis—an inflammatory disease. N. Eng. J. Med. **340:** 115–126.
15. SHEN, J., F.W. LUSCINSKAS, A. CONNOLLY, C.F. DEWEY, M.A. GIMBRONE JR. & J. SHEN. 1992. Fluid shear stress modulates cytosolic free calcium in vascular endothelial cells. Am. J. Physiol. **262:** C384–390.
16. SPRINGER, T.A. 1994. Traffic signals for lymphocyte recirculation and leukocyte emigration: the multistep paradigm. Cell **76:** 301–314.

Distinct Mechanical Stimuli Differentially Regulate the PI3K/Akt Survival Pathway in Endothelial Cells

GUILLERMO GARCÍA-CARDEÑA, KEITH R. ANDERSON, LAURA MAURI, AND MICHAEL A. GIMBRONE, JR.[a]

Vascular Research Division, Department of Pathology, Brigham and Women's Hospital, Harvard Medical School, Boston, Massachusetts 02115, USA

INTRODUCTION

Vascular endothelial cells (EC) are among the longest-lived cells in the body and are quiescent in the normal adult mammal, except in the context of certain well-regulated physiologic processes (e.g., growth, female reproductive cycles) and pathophysiologic states (e.g., tumor progression, diabetic retinopathy).[1,2] As a result of their unique location, endothelial cells are constantly exposed to mechanical forces that can control endothelial cell biology and modulate vessel wall function.[3] Of these forces, wall shear stress, the tangential component of blood flow, has been implicated in the initiation and development of atherosclerosis. Wall shear stress is highly variable in magnitude, frequency, and direction in different regions of the vascular tree. Interestingly, the focal pattern of early atherosclerotic lesions, in human subjects and experimental animals, correlates with branch points, curvatures, and regions of altered blood flow.[4] Increased endothelial cell turnover is observed in these "lesion prone" areas,[5] suggesting an important link between local hemodynamics and endothelial cell survival. Recently, the intracellular signaling pathways by which growth factors promote cell survival began to be elucidated.[6] In several cell lines, the protection against apoptosis provided by growth factors is due to stimulation of the phosphatidylinositol-3-OH kinase (PI3K) pathway, which results in phosphorylation and activation of the protein kinase Akt (also known as protein kinase B, PKB), and subsequent phosphorylation of BAD and Caspase-9. These series of events ultimately result in cell survival.[7,8] Since laminar shear stress inhibits apoptosis of human endothelial cells *in vitro*[9] and these effects are in part mediated by Akt phosphorylation,[10] we explored the possibility that distinct mechanical stimuli namely, laminar shear stress and turbulent shear stress, may differentially regulate the PI3K/Akt pathway in endothelial cells.

---

[a]Address for correspondence: Dr. Michael A. Gimbrone, Jr., Vascular Research Division, Department of Pathology, Brigham and Women's Hospital, 221 Longwood Avenue, Boston, MA 02115. Voice: 617-732-5901; fax: 617-732-5933.
   gimbrone@bustoff.bwh.harvard.edu

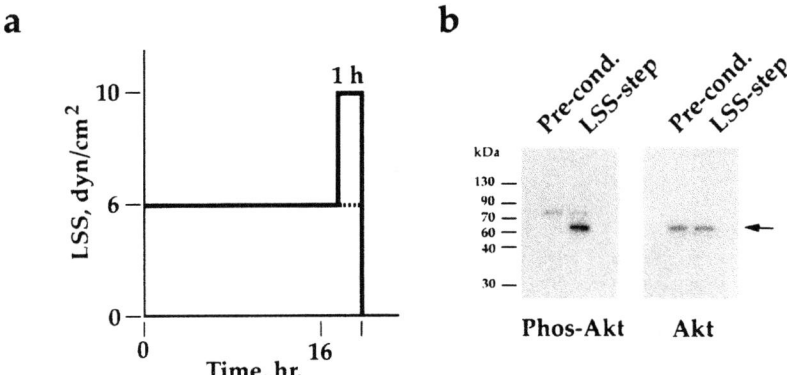

FIGURE 1. Increases in laminar shear stress result in augmentation of Akt phosphorylation. (**a**) Diagram of the *in vitro* pre-conditioning model that simulates changes in LSS that may occur under different physiological conditions. In this model, cells are exposed to LSS (6 dynes/cm^2) for 16 h, and then, the magnitude of LSS is instantaneously stepped to 10 dynes/cm^2 for an additional hour. As a control, following the pre-conditioning period, cells continue to be exposed for 1 h to 6 dynes/cm^2. (**b**) LSS pre-conditioned HUVEC were exposed (LSS-step), or not (Pre-cond.) to an increase in LSS. Cells were lysed, equal amounts of protein resolved by SDS/PAGE and western blotted with phospho-Akt (*left*) or anti-Akt (*right*) antibodies.

RESULTS AND DISCUSSION

To examine if exposure of human umbilical vein endothelial cells (HUVEC) to laminar shear stress (LSS) results in the phosphorylation and subsequent activation of Akt, we used a pre-conditioning model that simulates changes in laminar shear stress that may occur under different physiological conditions (i.e., exercise). In this model, cells are exposed to LSS (6 dynes/cm^2) for 16 h and then the magnitude of LSS is instantaneously stepped to 10 dynes/cm^2 for an additional hour. As a control, following the pre-conditioning period, cells continue to be exposed for 1 h to 6 dynes/cm^2 (FIG. 1a). As seen in FIGURE 1b, LSS preconditioning of HUVEC and subsequent increase in LSS results in the increase of Akt phosphorylation on serine 473 as compared to control cells (*left panel*). The total amount of cellular Akt does not change (*right panel*). This demonstrates that increases in LSS result in a concomitant increase in Akt phosphorylation.

To determine if the observed increase in Akt phosphorylation is dependent on the PI3-kinase signaling pathway, HUVEC were incubated with wortmannin (20 nM, a concentration known to specifically inhibit PI3K activity) for the last 30 min of the preconditioning period and then exposed to the increase in LSS. In the presence of wortmannin, the step-up in LSS no longer resulted in increased Akt phosphorylation (FIG. 2a, *right panel*). The total amount of cellular Akt does not change (FIG. 2a, *center panel*). Because phosphorylation of Akt augments its kinase activity, endogenous Akt kinase activity was assayed in Akt immunoprecipitates with the use of histone H2B as a substrate. A step change in LSS leads to increased Akt kinase activity and

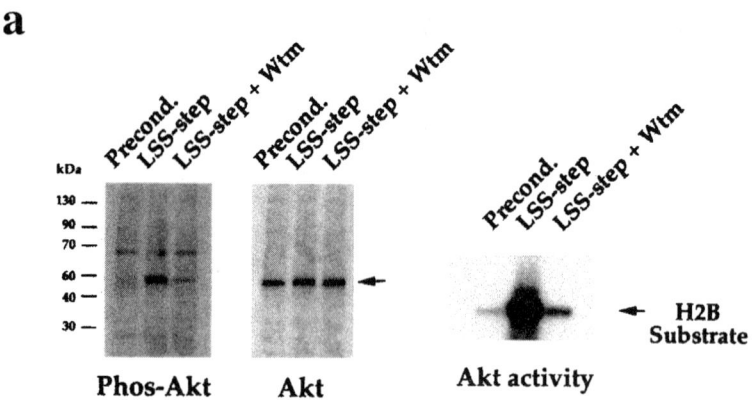

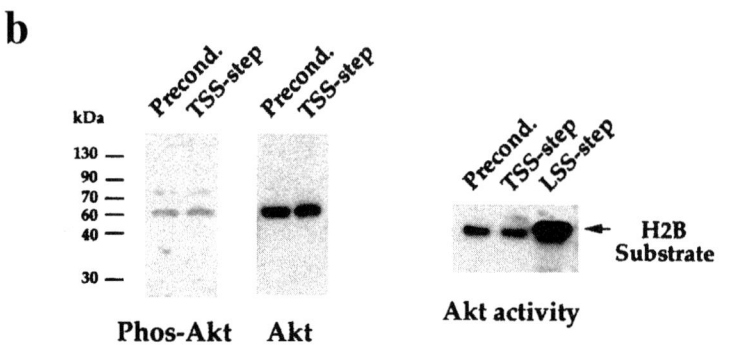

FIGURE 2. Differential activation of Akt by laminar versus turbulent shear stress. (**a**) Activation of Akt by LSS is PI3K dependent. LSS pre-conditioned HUVEC were exposed to an increase in LSS in the absence (LSS-step) or presence of wortmannin (LSS-step + Wtm). Cells were lysed, equal amounts of protein were resolved by SDS/PAGE and western blotted with phospho-Akt (*left*) and Akt (*center*) antibodies. In the right panel, cell lysates were precleared and endogenous Akt was immunoprecipitated with a polyclonal antibody specific for Akt. Immunocomplexes were collected with protein-A sepharose and used in an *in vitro* kinase assay using [γ-^{32}P]ATP and histone H2B as a substrate. Reaction products were resolved by SDS-PAGE, transferred to nitrocellulose filters and analyzed by autoradiography. (**b**) TSS does not increase the phosphorylation and activation of Akt. Pre-conditioned HUVEC were exposed to TSS (10 dynes/cm^2, TSS-step). Cell lysates were processed for phospho-Akt/Akt western blot analysis, and for the Akt *in vitro* kinase assay as described above.

this effect is inhibited by wortmannin (FIG 2a, *right panel*). Thus, phosphorylation and activation of Akt by increases in LSS are PI3-kinase–dependent.

Turbulent shear stress (TSS) may occur in large arteries under conditions of increased flow velocity and cardiac output.[11] Moreover, TSS induces vascular endothelial cell turnover *in vitro*.[12] Accordingly, we examined if HUVEC exposure to TSS resulted in a different pattern of activation of the Akt pathway than LSS. As seen in FIGURE 2b (*left and center panels*), exposure of LSS preconditioned HUVEC to TSS (10 dynes/cm^2) does not result in an increase of Akt phosphorylation nor a change in the total amount of Akt protein. Moreover, Akt kinase activity towards histone H2B does not increase under these conditions, as compared to the LSS step model (FIG. 2b, *right panel*). Thus, in contrast to LSS, exposure of HUVEC to TSS at an equivalent mean shear stress level does result in the phosphorylation and activation of Akt.

These findings reveal a mechanism by which distinct fluid mechanical stimuli (LSS versus TSS) can differentially activate a signal transduction cascade that leads to EC survival, and are consistent with the concept that local hemodynamic forces influence the focal nature of atherosclerosis via effects on survival and apoptosis of EC.

REFERENCES

1. ENGERMAN, R.L., D. PFAFFENBACH & M.D. DAVIS. 1967. Cell turnover of capillaries. Lab. Invest. **17:** 738–743.
2. HOBSON, B. & J. DENEKAMP. 1984. Endothelial proliferation in tumors and normal tissues: continuous labeling studies. Br. J. Cancer **49:** 405–413.
3. GIMBRONE, M.A., T. NAGEL & J.N. TOPPER. 1997. Biomechanical activation: an emerging paradigm in endothelial adhesion biology. J. Clin. Invest. **100:** S61–65.
4. GIMBRONE, M.A., N. RESNICK, T. NAGEL, L.M. KHACHIGIAN, T. COLLINS & J.N. TOPPER. 1997. Hemodynamics, endothelial gene expression and atherogenesis. Ann. N.Y. Acad. Sci. **811:** 1–10.
5. CAPLAN, B.A. & C.J. SCHWARTZ. 1973. Increased endothelial cell turnover in areas of *in vivo* evans blue uptake in the pig aorta. Atherosclerosis **17:** 401–417.
6. FRANKE, T.F., D.R. KAPLAN & L.C. CANTLEY. 1997. PI3K: Downstream AKT ion blocks apoptosis. Cell **88:** 435–437.
7. DATTA, S.R., H. DUDEK, X. TAO, S. MASTERS, H. FU, Y. GOTOH & M.E. GREENBERG. 1997. Akt phosphorylation of BAD couples survival signals to the cell-intrinsic death machinery Cell **91:** 231–241.
8. CARDONE, M.H., N. ROY, H.R. STENNICKE, G.S. SALVESEN, T.F. FRANKE, E. STANBRIDGE, S. FRISCH & J.C. REED. 1998. Regulation of cell death protease caspase-9 by phosphorylation. Science **282:** 1318–1321.
9. DIMMELER, S., J. HAENDELER, V. RIPPMAN, M. NEHLS & AM. ZEIHER. 1996. Shear stress inhibits apoptosis of human endothelial cells. FEBS Lett. **399:** 71–74.
10. DIMMELER, S., B. ASSMUS, C. HERMANN, J. HAENDELER & A.M. ZEIHER. 1998. Fluid shear stress stimulates phosphorylation of Akt in human endothelial cells. Circ. Res. **83:** 334–341.
11. KARINO, T., M. MOTOMIYA & H.L. GOLDSMITH. 1982. Biologic and Synthetic Vascular Protheses. Grune and Stratton. New York. pp.153–178.
12. DAVIES, P.F., A. REMUZZI, E.J. GORDON, C.F. DEWEY & M.A. GIMBRONE. 1986. Turbulent fluid shear stress induces vascular endothelial cell turnover *in vitro*. Proc. Natl. Acad. Sci. USA **83:** 2114–2117.

Mechanical Stress Modulates Glutathione Peroxidase Expression in Cultured Bovine Aortic Endothelial Cells

SAORI TAKESHITA, NOBUTAKA INOUE,[a] YOSHIYUKI RIKITAKE, SEINOSUKE KAWASHIMA, AND MITSUHIRO YOKOYAMA

The First Department of Internal Medicine, Kobe University School of Medicine, Kobe 650-0017, Japan

INTRODUCTION

Mechanical stress, such as shear stress and stretch force, has profound effects on vasculature and it can be a pathophysiological factor in cardiovascular diseases, such as atherosclerosis and hypertension. Pathological observations have shown that atherosclerosis occurs predominantly at low shear stress area, suggesting that laminar high shear stress has antiatherogenic property. Laminar shear stress has been reported to upregulate the expressions of Cu/Zn superoxide dismutase (SOD) and Mn SOD in endothelial cells.[1,2] Since oxidative stress plays a pivotal role in atherogenesis, the enhancement of SOD expression by laminar shear stress might be one of the mechanisms whereby high laminar shear stress has antiatherogenic property. SOD potently converses superoxide anion to H_2O_2, however, H_2O_2 has various atherogenic properties such as stimulatory effects on growth of smooth muscle cells and induction of adhesion molecules. H_2O_2 is reduced by glutathione peroxidase (GPx) and catalase to H_2O. GPx is a soluble selenoprotein in most tissues. Therefore, GPx plays an important role in cellular antioxidant defenses by reducing H_2O_2. In this study, we examine the effect of mechanical stress, such as shear stress and stretch force, on GPx expression in endothelial cells.

METHODS

Bovine aortic endothelial cells (BAECs) were seeded onto plastic rectangular tissue culture plates for shear stress experiments or laminin-coated deformable elastic dishes made of silicone for stretch force experiments. In the shear stress and stretch force experiments, 50 nM sodium selenite was added to the media. BAECs were exposed to steady laminar shear stress in a parallel-plate flow chamber as described previously.[3] In stretch experiments, the dishes were stretched by 10 or 20% in length along a single axis as described previously.[4] GPx mRNA expression was analyzed by Northern blotting with bovine GPx cDNA fragments amplified with RT-PCR from total RNA of

---

[a]Address for correspondence: Nobutaka Inoue, M.D., Ph.D., The First Department of Internal Medicine, Kobe University School of Medicine, 7-5-1 Kusunoki-cho, Chuo-ku, Kobe 650-0017, Japan. Voice: 81-78-382-5859; fax: 81-78-382-5846.
nobutaka@med.kobe-u.ac.jp

BAECs. GPx enzymatic activity was assayed as described previously.[5] Briefly, oxidized glutathione (GSSG) produced during GPx enzyme reaction was immediately reduced by NADPH and glutathione reductase. The rate of NADPH consumption was monitored as the rate of GSSG formation during GPx reaction. Cell homogenates of BAECs were incubated with a buffer containing 100 mM sodium phosphate (pH 7.0), 2 mM sodium azide, 2 mM GSH, 200 µM NADPH, 1 unit/ml of glutathione reductase, and 250 µM H_2O_2 at 25°C. The rate of decrease in absorption of NADPH was followed at 340 nm. The activity was calculated using an extinction coefficient for NADPH of 6.22 and expressed as milliunits (mU) per mg protein.

RESULTS

Selenium is required for GPx expression, since it is incorporated into selenoproteins by recognition of the stop codon UGA as a codon for selenocysteine. Therefore, the effect of selenium on GPx mRNA expression in BAECs was examined. Selenium enhanced GPx mRNA expression in BAECs in a dose-dependent manner (data not shown). The exposure of BAECs to steady laminar shear stress at 20 dynes/cm^2 resulted in a time-dependent increase in GPx mRNA levels. The increase of GPx mRNA levels appeared 8 h after application of shear stress and reached a peak level at 24 h to approximately 2.1-fold versus static control (FIG. 1A). FIGURE 1B shows the effect of shear force dependency on GPx expression. BAECs were exposed to low (5 dynes/cm^2) and high (20 dynes/cm^2) laminar shear stress for 24 hours. Levels of GPx mRNA were significantly increased by high shear stress, which appears to be at the physiological artery level, whereas no significant change occurred with low shear stress. As shown in FIGURE 2, the exposure of BAECs to steady laminar shear stress at 20 dynes/cm^2 for 24 h increased the enzymatic activity of GPx from 3.2 to 4.9 mU/mg protein. Next, the effect of stretch force on GPx mRNA expression was examined. The imposition of stretch force by stretching dishes by 10% and 20% did not enhance GPx expression, rather it tended to decrease expression (data not shown). It has been reported that shear stress enhances endothelial NO production via upregulation of the expression of endothelial NO synthase. Therefore, the involvement of NO in shear stress–induced GPx mRNA expression was examined using NOS inhibitor, L-NAME. L-NAME (1 mM) did not affect shear stress–induced GPx mRNA expression (data not shown).

DISCUSSION

The present study demonstrated that laminar shear stress upregulated GPx mRNA expression and its enzymatic activity in endothelial cells, whereas stretch force did not have any significant effect. In atherosclerotic vessels, the enhanced production of reactive oxygen species such as O_2^-, H_2O_2, and hydroxyl radical results in oxidative stress and further promotes atherosclerosis. H_2O_2 itself has various atherogenic properties. H_2O_2 is also reduced to hydroxyl radical, a potent prooxidant, in the presence of transitional metals by Fenton reaction. Since GPx is essential for the removing H_2O_2 and its product, hydroxyl radical, it plays a key antioxidant enzyme against oxidative stress. On the other hand, some oxidant species have been shown to inac-

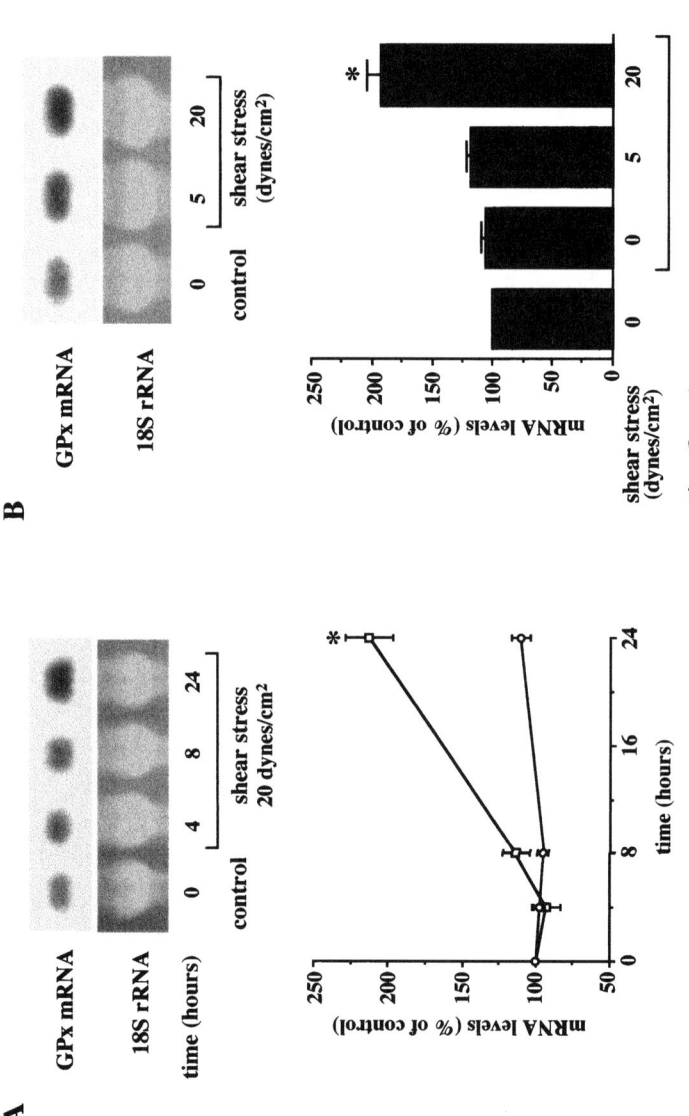

FIGURE 1. (A) Time course of GPx mRNA expression by laminar shear stress in BAECs. BAECs were exposed to laminar shear stress at 20 dynes/cm^2 for the indicated time periods, and Northern blot analysis was performed. (○) static control, (□) laminar shear stress. (B) Dependence on degrees of laminar shear stress on GPx mRNA expression in BAECs. BAECs were exposed to laminar shear stress at 0, 5, or 20 dynes/cm^2 for 24 hours, and Northern blot analysis was performed. Data represent the mean values ± S.E. of three independent experiments. *$p < 0.01$ versus control.

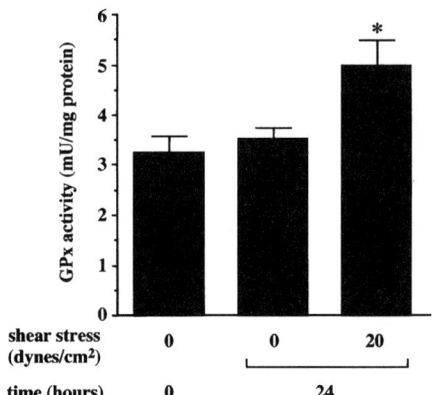

FIGURE 2. Effect of laminar shear stress on GPx enzymatic activity in BAECs. BAECs were exposed to laminar shear stress at 20 dynes/cm^2 for 24 h and GPx enzymatic activity was measured as described in *Methods*. Data represent the mean values ± S.E. of five independent experiments. *$p < 0.05$ versus control.

tivate GPx. Furthermore, recent study demonstrated that the GPx enzymatic activity in human atherosclerotic plaques was markedly reduced.[6] Therefore, physiological laminar flow might be necessary for maintaining antioxidant state in vessel walls. The present data suggest that the ability of laminar shear stress to induce the expression of GPx, a pivotal antioxidant enzyme against H_2O_2, might be an important mechanism whereby shear stress protects vascular cells against oxidative stress.

REFERENCES

1. INOUE, N., S. RAMASAMY, T. FUKAI, R.M. NEREM & D.G. HARRISON. 1996. Shear stress modulates expression of Cu/Zn superoxide dismutase in human aortic endothelial cells. Circ. Res. **79:** 32–37.
2. TOPPER, J.N., J. CAI, D. FALB & M.A. GIMBRONE. 1996. Identification of vascular endothelial genes differentially responsive to fluid mechanical stimuli: cyclooxygenase-2, manganese superoxide dismutase, and endothelial cell nitric oxide synthase are selectively up-regulated by steady laminar shear stress. Proc. Natl. Acad. Sci. USA **93:** 10417–10422.
3. LEVESQUE, M.J. & R.M. NEREM. 1985. The elongation and orientation of cultured endothelial cells in response to shear stress. J. Biomech. Eng. **107:** 341–347.
4. INOUE, N., S. KAWASHIMA, K. HIRATA, Y. RIKITAKE, S. TAKESHITA, W. YAMOCHI, H. AKITA & M. YOKOYAMA. 1998. Stretch force on vascular smooth muscle cells enhanced oxidation of LDL via superoxide production. Am. J. Physiol. **274:** H1928–1932.
5. PAGLIA, D.E. & W.N. VALENTINE. 1967. Studies on the quantitative and qualitative characterization of erythrocytes glutathione peroxidase. J. Lab. Clin. Med. **29:** 143–148.
6. LAPENNA, D., S. GIOIA, G. CIOFANI, A. MEZZETTI, S. UCCHINO, A.M. CALAFIORE, A.M. NAPOLITANO, C. ILIO & F. CUCCURULLO. 1998. Glutathione-related antioxidant defenses in human atherosclerotic plaques. Circulation **97:** 1930–1934.

Estrogen Receptor Deficiency Leads to Impaired Endothelial Nitric Oxide Production and Premature Coronary Arteriosclerosis

GABOR M. RUBANYI[a]

Gene Therapy and Genomics Research, Berlex Biosciences, Richmond, California 94804, USA

INTRODUCTION

Estrogen receptors (ER) are present in the blood vessel wall.[1,2] Their number is reduced in human atherosclerotic plaques,[3] but the pathophysiological importance of this finding is unknown. The availability of estrogen receptor–deficient mice (ERKO mice), in which the ERα gene was selectively disrupted,[4] and the identification of a male patient with mutation in both alleles of the ERα gene[5] allowed us, for the first time, to study whether the reduction or absence of functional ERα leads to pathophysiological consequences in the cardiovascular system.

ROLE OF ERα IN ENDOTHELIAL NITRIC OXIDE PRODUCTION IN MICE

Reduced endothelial nitric oxide (NO) production is documented in many cardiovascular diseases (e.g., hypertension and atherosclerosis) and has been suggested to contribute to these vascular pathological processes.[6]

Although previous studies showed that 17β-estradiol increased endothelial NO (EDNO) production in cultured cells,[7] and endothelium-dependent vasodilation in animals[8–10] and in humans,[11] the exact mechanism(s) of estrogen-induced upregulation of EDNO production is not known. In order to evaluate the role of functional ERα, we compared basal and stimulated EDNO production in thoracic aortas isolated from control and ERKO mice.[12]

Basal production of EDNO (estimated by endothelium-dependent contractions after inhibition of NO generation by N^G-L-nitro-arginine) was significantly greater in aortic rings isolated from control than from ERKO mice (FIG. 1). In contrast, acetylcholine-induced endothelium-dependent and nitroglycerin-induced endothelium-independent relaxations were similar in the two groups (not shown).[12]

The important observation of this study was that absence of functional ERα in ERKO mice leads to reduced basal EDNO production in aortic segments. This

---

[a]Address for correspondence: Gabor M. Rubanyi, M.D., Ph.D., Vice President and Head, Gene Therapy and Genomics Research, Berlex Biosciences, 15049 San Pablo Avenue, P. O. Box 4099, Richmond, CA 94804-0099; Voice: 510-262-7804; fax: 510-669-4750.

gabor_rubanyi@berlex.com

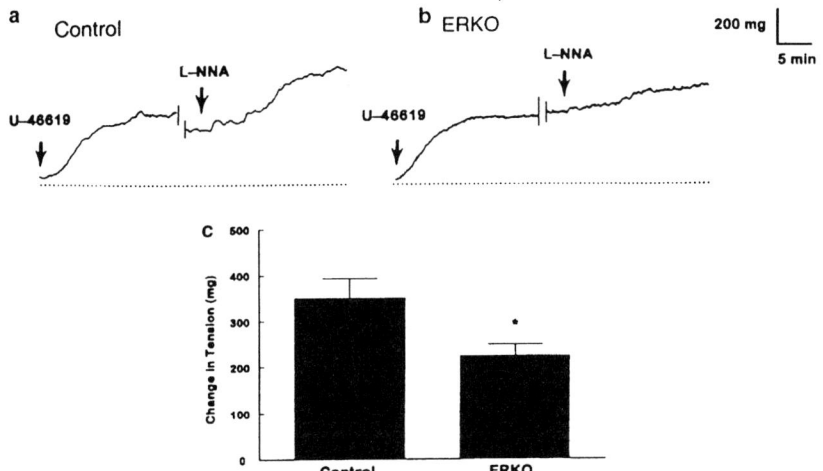

FIGURE 1. Decreased basal release of endothelial nitric oxide in aorta of ERKO mice. Comparison of endothelium-dependent facilitation of U-46619 (10^{-8} M)–induced contraction by N^G-L-nitro-arginine (L-NNA; 10^{-4} M) in aortic rings with endothelium isolated from control and ERKO mice: (**a**) original trace of a control aortic ring; (**b**) original trace of an ERKO aortic ring; (**c**) mean ± SEM of six experiments, expressed as percent facilitation of U-46619 contraction. *$p < 0.05$. (Reproduced with permission from Rubanyi et al.[12]).

change suggests that functional ERα in the vessel wall (presumably in endothelial cells) may play an important role in modulating endothelial EDNO production.

ENDOTHELIAL DYSFUNCTION AND PREMATURE CORONARY ARTERIOSCLEROSIS IN A MALE PATIENT WITH GENETIC MUTATION IN THE ESTROGEN RECEPTOR GENE

In order to test the hypothesis based on our observations in ERKO mice that absence of functional ERα causes endothelial dysfunction and, as a consequence, accelerated progression of arteriosclerosis in humans, we examined the only known living human subject (a 31-year-old man) with a documented disruptive mutation in both alleles of the ERα gene.[5] Laboratory analysis showed relatively low levels of total (130 mg/dl), LDL (97 mg/dl) and HDL (34 mg/dl) cholesterol and apo-AI (91.7 mg/dl); but normal levels of triglycerides (97 mg/dl) and probeta-1 HDL cholesterol (61 µg/ml).[14] Clinical examination of this patient revealed significant endothelial dysfunction in the brachial artery[13] and premature coronary arteriosclerosis.[14] High-frequency ultrasound examination of the brachial artery showed absence of detectable endothelium-dependent flow-induced vasodilation, despite the fact that the response of this artery to the endothelium-independent vasodilator, nitroglycerin and sublingual 17β-estradiol was normal (FIG. 2). In arteries of diameter 6 mm or less, the mean value for flow-mediated vasodilation has been reported to be $10 \pm 2\%$.[15] Flow-mediated vasodilation in peripheral conduit arteries has been shown to be mediated via release of NO from

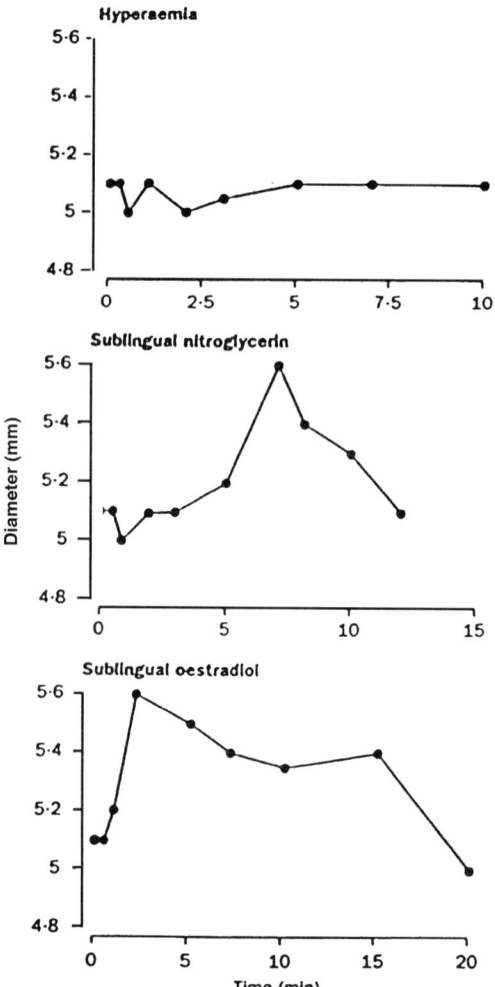

FIGURE 2. Diameter changes recorded from high-frequency ultrasound scans of the brachial artery. Endothelial dysfunction in a young male patient with a mutation in the ERα gene. The traces show no diameter change during reactive hyperemia (*top*), a 10% increase following administration of sublingual nitroglycerin (400 µg) (*middle*), and a 10% increase following administration of sublingual estradiol (2 mg) (*bottom*). (Reproduced with permission from Sudhir et al.[13]).

the endothelium.[16] The failure of such vasodilation in this patient is therefore likely to be due to impaired release of endothelial nitric oxide.

The patient also demonstrated evidence of premature coronary arteriosclerosis, as shown by calcium deposition (with a score of 47) in the left anterior descending coronary artery on electron beam computer tomography (EBCT).[14] EBCT calcium scores correlate well with angiographically documented coronary artery disease. A recent study showed that a coronary calcification score of greater than 100 predicted cardiovascular events in a cohort of 1,173 asymptomatic patients in a 19-month follow-up period.[17] By these criteria, this patient has an abnormal calcium score for his age.

Impaired endothelium-dependent vasorelaxation is a sign of vascular dysfunction and precedes angiographic evidence of atherosclerosis in human subjects with hypercholesterolemia.[18] However, in this patient, hypercholesterolemia is clearly not the cause of the lack of flow-dependent, NO-mediated vasodilation, or premature arteriosclerosis, because plasma concentrations of total and LDL cholesterol and the ratio of HDL/LDL cholesterol are well within normal range. These observations suggest that absence of functional ERα is a novel cardiovascular risk factor, which can lead to premature endothelial dysfunction and coronary arteriosclerosis.

ACKNOWLEDGMENTS

The studies reported here were performed in collaboration with Dr. Kenneth S. Korach (NIEHS, Research Triangle Park, NC) and Dr. Krishna Sudhir (UCSF, San Francisco, CA), whose valuable contribution is highly appreciated. I also wish to thank the following people for their active participation in the studies reviewed here: Dr. Wei Zheng (Amgen Corp., Thousand Oaks, CA), Dr. Geraldine Burton (Schering AG, Berlin), and Dr. Drew Sukovich, Dr. Katalin Kauser, and Ana D. Freay (Berlex Biosciences, Richmond, CA).

REFERENCES

1. COLBURN, P. & V. BOUNASSISI. 1978. Estrogen-binding sites in endothelial cell cultures. Science **201**: 817–819.
2. LIN, A.L. et al. 1982. Hormone receptors of the baboon cardiovascular system. Circ. Res. **50**: 610-616.
3. LOSORDO, D.W. et al. 1994. Variable expression of the estrogen receptor in normal and atherosclerotic coronary arteries of premenopausal women. Circulation **89**: 1501–1510.
4. LUBAHN, D.B. et al. 1993. Alteration of reproductive function but not prenatal sexual development after insertional disruption of the mouse estrogen gene. Proc. Natl. Acad. Sci. USA **90**: 11161–11166.
5. SMITH, E.P. et al. 1994. Estrogen resistance caused by a mutation in the estrogen-receptor gene in man. N. Engl. J. Med. **331**: 1056–1061.
6. RUBANYI, G.M. 1993. Role of endothelium in cardiovascular homeostasis and diseases. J. Cardiovasc. Pharmacol. **22**(Suppl. 4): S1–S13.
7. HISHIKAWA, K. et al. 1995. Upregulation of nitric oxide synthase by estradiol in human aortic endothelial cells. FEBS Lett. **360**: 291–293.
8. HAYASHI, T. et al. 1992. Basal release of nitric oxide from aortic rings is greater in female rabbits than in male rabbits: implications for atherosclerosis. Proc. Natl. Acad. Sci. USA **89**: 11259–11263.
9. KAUSER, K. & G.M. RUBANYI. 1994. Gender difference in bioassayable endothelium-derived nitric oxide release from isolated rat aortae. Am. J. Physiol. **267**: H2311–H2317.
10. KAUSER, K. & G.M. RUBANYI. 1995. Gender difference in endothelial dysfunction in the aorta of spontaneously hypertensive rats. Hypertension **25**: 517–523.

11. ROSSELLI, M. et al. 1995. Circulating nitric oxide (nitrate/nitrate) levels in postmenopausal woman substituted with 17β-estradiol and norethisterone acetate. A two year follow-up study. Hypertension **25:** 848–853.
12. RUBANYI, G.M. et al. 1997. Vascular estrogen receptors and endothelium-derived nitric oxide production in the mouse aorta: gender difference and effect of estrogen receptor gene disruption. J. Clin. Invest. **99:** 2429–2437.
13. SUDHIR, K. et al. 1997. Endothelial dysfunction associated with a disruptive mutation in the estrogen receptor gene. Lancet **349:** 1146–1147.
14. SUDHIR, K. et al. 1997. Premature coronary artery disease in a male patient with disruptive mutation in the estrogen receptor gene. Circulation **96:** 3774–3777.
15. CELEMAJER, D.S. et al. 1992. Non-invasive detection of endothelial dysfunction in children and adults at risk of atherosclerosis. Lancet **340:** 1111–1115.
16. JOANNIDES, R. et al. 1995. Nitric oxide is responsible for flow-dependent dilatation of human peripheral conduit arteries in vivo. Circulation **91:** 1314–1319.
17. ARAD, Y. et al. 1996. Predictive value of electron beam computed tomography of the coronary arteries: 19-month follow-up of 1173 asymptomatic subjects. Circulation **93:** 1951–1953.
18. DREXLER, H. & A.M. ZEIHER. 1991. Endothelial function in human coronary arteries in vivo. Focus on hypercholesterolemia. Hypertension **18** (4Suppl): I190–I199.

Differentiation-Induced Transmigration of HL60 Cells across Activated HUVEC Monolayer Involves E-selectin–Dependent Mechanism[a]

MASAYUKI YOSHIDA,[b,c] LEE-JUNG CHIEN,[d] YUKIO YASUKOCHI,[c] AND FUJIO NUMANO[d]

[c]*Department of Molecular Genetics, Medical Research Institute*
[d]*Department of Medicine, School of Medicine, Tokyo Medical and Dental University, Tokyo, Japan*

ABSTRACT: The leukocyte-endothelial adhesive interaction is one of the key mechanisms during inflammation. The human promyelocytic cell line HL60 has been used in a number of studies to characterize leukocyte-endothelial interactions, especially selectin-mediated adhesion. HL60 also has been used in studies to characterize the myeloid cell function during differentiation. In this study, we investigated the adhesive interactions of HL60 to vascular endothelium, either in its undifferentiated state or after dimethylsulfoxide-induced granulocytic differentiation. Granulocytic differentiation of HL60 cells significantly enhanced their transmigration across cytokine-activated (IL-1β 10 U/ml, 4 h) HUVEC monolayer. Interestingly, this enhanced transmigration of differentiated HL60 cells was inhibited by pretreatment of the monolayers with anti–E-selectin mAb as well as anti–ICAM-1 mAb or anti–VE-cadherin mAb, suggesting a potential role for E-selectin in transendothelial migration. Further study of this enhanced transmigration mechanism may elucidate the regulation of selectin-mediated leukocyte-endothelial interactions.

INTRODUCTION

The regulation of leukocyte-endothelial adhesive interactions plays an important role during inflammation and atherosclerosis.[1] In recent several years, numerous reports have revealed that several different groups of adhesion molecules are involved in leukocyte-endothelial interactions. E-selectin, a member of the selectin family of adhesion molecules, has been shown to participate in the initial phases of this process.[2] Several reports have suggested that oligosaccharide structures bearing sialic acid and fucose, such as sialyl-Lewis^x (sL^x) and sialyl-Lewis^a (sL^a), and similar sulfated oligosaccharide structures, are the ligands for selectins.[3]

---

[a]This work was supported by Grants-in-Aid for Scientific Research from the Ministry of Education, Science, Sports and Culture of Japan.
[b]Address for correspondence: Masayuki Yoshida, M.D., Department of Molecular Genetics, Medical Research Institute, Tokyo Medical and Dental University, 1-5-45, Yushima, Bunkyo-ku, Tokyo, 113 Japan. Voice: 81-3-5803-5827; fax: 81-3-5803-0242.
masamgen@mri.tmd.ac.jp

HL60, a maturation-arrested promyelocytic cell line, possesses a sL^x-bearing structure on the surface and has been utilized for the analysis of selectin-dependent leukocyte adhesion by many different groups. HL60 also has been used in numerous studies for the regulation of myeloid cell differentiation. Polar reagents, such as dimethyl sulfoxide (DMSO), can differentiate HL60 towards mature neutrophils and the concomitant regulation of the surface molecules has been well characterized.[4]

In this study, we investigated the adhesive interactions of HL60 cells with cytokine-activated HUVEC, during granulocytic differentiation induced by DMSO. Granulocytic differentiation of HL60 significantly induced transmigration across activated endothelial monolayer. Interestingly this induced transmigration is blocked by the pretreatment of anti–E-selectin mAb. Regulation of adhesive interactions to endothelium during granulocytic differentiation may have important implications for the mechanism of leukocyte-endothelial interactions. DMSO-treated HL60 cells could serve as a useful model for the understanding of selectin-dependent leukocyte adhesion to vascular endothelium.

METHODS

Endothelial Transmigration Assay

Human umbilical vein endothelial cells (HUVEC) were plated in fibronectin-coated Biocoat culture inserts (Becton-Dickinson, San Jose, CA). The monolayers were activated with IL-1β (10 U/ml, 4 h). HL60 cells, fluorescently labeled with BCECF-AM (Molecular Probes, Portland, OR) and 2×10^6 cells were added to each insert and incubated for 2 h at 37°C to allow transmigration of HL60 cells. The transmigrated HL60 cells in the lower chamber were collected and fluorescence intensity was measured by a fluorescent plate reader (Perceptive Biosystems, Framingham, MA). In some experiments, monolayers in the culture inserts were preincubated with indicated mAbs at 10 µg/ml for 20 min on ice before the transmigration assay. mAbs used in this study were: H18/7 (anti-human E-selectin),[5] Hu5/3 (anti-human ICAM-1),[6] BV6 (anti-human VE-cadherin obtained from Bioline Diagnostici, Giaveno, Italy), and K16/16 (non-binding control IgG).[6]

RESULTS AND DISCUSSION

Confluent monolayers of HUVEC on Biocoat membranes were activated for 4 h with 10 U/ml of IL-1β. Differentiation of HL60 cells was induced by incubation in the presence of 1% DMSO for 72 h. These cells were then fluorescently labeled with BCECF, resuspended in RPMI 1640 containing 1% FBS, and 2×10^6 cells were added to the upper wells of Biocoat chambers and incubated for 2 h at 37°C. The transmigrated cells from the bottom chamber then were collected and their fluorescence intensity was measured. As shown in FIGURE 1, differentiated HL60 cells (dHL60) exhibited a significantly higher level of transmigration across activated HUVEC, compared to undifferentiated HL60 cells (uHL60) (uHL60, 19.5 ± 2.1 relative fluorescent unit; dHL60, 32 ± 0.1; $p < 0.01$). We also demonstrated the effect of mAbs against endothelial adhesion molecules. Preincubation of HUVEC monolayers with

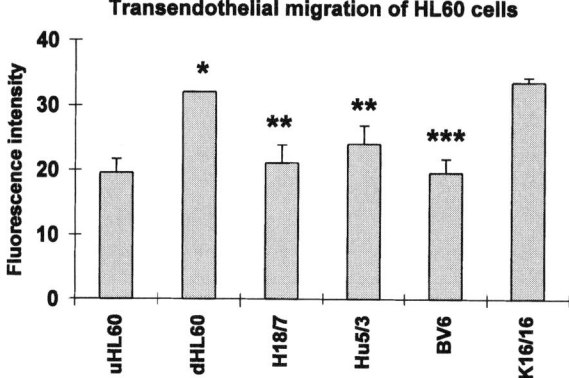

FIGURE 1. HL60 cells were incubated in the absence (uHL60, *open bar*) or presence (dHL60, *shaded bar*) of 1% DMSO for 72 h, fluorescently labeled, and added to activated HUVEC monolayer plated in Biocoat chambers. Transmigrated cells were collected from the bottom wells and fluorescence intensity was measured. *$p < 0.01$ versus uHL60. **$p < 0.05$ versus dHL60. ***$p < 0.01$ versus dHL60.

mAb against ICAM-1 (Hu5/3), and VE-cadherin (BV6) significantly reduced transmigration of dHL60 cells (Hu5/3, 24 ± 2.8, $p < 0.05$ versus dHL60; BV6, 19.5 ± 2.1, $p < 0.01$ versus dHL60). Interestingly, preincubation with mAb against E-selectin (H18/7) also reduced transmigration of dHL60 cells (H18/7, 21 ± 2.8, $p < 0.05$ versus dHL60). Preincubation with control mAb (K16/16) did not significantly change transmigration of dHL60 cells (33.5 ± 0.7).

Our observation suggested that differentiated HL60 cells exhibited an increased transmigration across activated HUVEC monolayers. We have recently reported that DMSO-induced differentiation of HL60 cells enhances their adhesion to activated endothelium via an E-selectin–dependent pathway.[7] As a biological consequence of adhesion, transmigration is a very important step in leukocyte-endothelial interactions. Numerous studies reported the importance of cell adhesion molecules, including PECAM-1, VE-cadherin, and integrins, in the transmigration process. In this study, we were able to document that differentiation of HL60 also induces transmigration across activated HUVEC monolayers. Moreover, we demonstrated that in addition to ICAM-1, VE-cadherin, and integrin, E-selectin is also involved in this transmigration process. So far, E-selectin is thought to play a role in the relatively early "rolling" phase of leukocyte-endothelial interactions. However, our results suggest a potential role for E-selectin in a later phase of leukocyte-endothelial interactions. Recent studies have revealed that E-selectin is important in the transition between rolling and stable arrest.[8] Our group recently reported the cytoskeletal interactions[5] and regulation of phosphorylation of E-selectin during leukocyte adhesion.[9] Based on these previous observations with E-selectin, though the precise mechanism of E-selectin participation in the transmigration of dHL60 is unclear, it is hypothesized that in the case of moderately differentiated DMSO-treated HL60 cells, E-selectin–dependent adhesion is required for consecutive transmigration to occur. Our finding of an enhanced transmigration of HL60 cells after differentiation to activated endothelium may provide a novel model for the study of E-selectin–dependent leukocyte adhesion(s).

REFERENCES

1. BUTCHER, E.C. 1991. Leukocyte-endothelial cell recognition; three (or more) steps to specificity and diversity. Cell **67:** 1033–1036
2. BEVILACQUA, M.P. & R.M. NELSON. 1993. Selectins. J. Clin. Invest. **91:** 379–387
3. ROSEN, S.D. & C.R. BERTOZZI. 1994. The selectins and their ligands. Curr. Opin. Cell. Biol. **6:** 663–673
4. COLLINS, S.J., F.W. RUSCENTTI, R.E. GALLAGHER & R.C. GALLO. 1978. Terminal differentiation of human promyelocytic leukemia cells induced by dimethyl sulfoxide and other polar compounds. Proc. Natl. Acad. Sci. USA **75:** 2458–2462.
5. YOSHIDA, M., W.F. WESTLIN, N. WANG, D.E. INGBER, A. ROSENZWEIG, N. RESNICK & M.A. GIMBRONE, JR. 1996. Leukocyte adhesion to vascular endothelium induces E-selectin linkage to the actin cytoskeleton. J. Cell Biol. **133:** 445–455.
6. LUSCINSKAS, F.W., M.I. CYBULSKY, J.M. KIELY, C.S. PECKINS, V.M. DAVIS & M.A. GIMBRONE, JR. 1991. Cytokine-activated human endothelial monolayers support enhanced neutrophil transmigration via a mechanism involving both endothelial-leukocytes adhesion molecule-1 (ELAM-1) and intercellular adhesion molecules (ICAM-1). J. Immunol. **146:** 1617–1625.
7. CHIEN, L.J. 1998. Granulocytic differentiation of HL60 cells enhances adhesive interactions to E-selectin J. Intern. Med. Taiwan **9:** 131–141
8. MILSTONE, D.S., D. FUKUMURA, R.C. PADGETT, P.E. O'DONNELL, V.M. DAVIS, O.J. BENAVIDEZ, W.L. MONSKY, R.J. MELDER, R.K. JAIN & M.A. GIMBRONE, JR. 1998. Mice lacking E-selectin show normal numbers of rolling leukocytes but reduced leukocyte stable arrest on cytokine-activated microvascular endothelium. Microcirculation **5:** 153–71
9. YOSHIDA, M., B.E. SZENTE, J.M. KIELY, A. ROSENZWEIG & M.A. GIMBRONE, JR. 1998. Phosphorylation of the cytoplasmic domain of E-selectin is regulated during leukocyte-endothelial adhesion. J. Immunol. **161:** 933–941.

Construction of Recombinant Adenoviral Vector of Annexin II

HIDETO ISHII,[a] MASAYUKI YOSHIDA,[b,c] KATHERINE A. HAJJAR,[d] YUKIO YASUKOCHI,[b] AND FUJIO NUMANO[a]

[a]*The Third Internal Medicine Department, School of Medicine, Tokyo Medical and Dental University, Tokyo, Japan*

[b]*Department of Molecular Genetics, Medical Research Institute, Tokyo Medical and Dental University, Tokyo, Japan*

[d]*Department of Pediatrics, Cornell University Medical College of New York, New York, New York, USA*

ABSTRACT: Annexin II is a member of the annexin family of calcium-dependent phospholipid binding proteins expressed in vascular endothelium. Recently this molecule was reported to play a role in control of fibrinolysis on the endothelial surface. To examine the role of annexin II in vascular endothelium critically, we developed a recombinant adenoviral vector containing the annexin II cDNA. A full-length annexin II cDNA was inserted into a shuttle vector, pAdRSV4, and co-transfected into 293 cells with a replication-deficient type 5 adenovirus, pJM17. Resulting plaques were isolated and checked for protein expression. The verified clone (AdRSV-ANII) was further analyzed. Characterization of this vector will facilitate the investigation of the mechanism of fibrinolysis on vascular endothelium.

INTRODUCTION

Annexin II, a calcium-dependent phospholipid binding protein with molecular weight of 30~40 kD, is a member of annexin family consisting of 13 members in mammalians.[1] It is implicated in the regulation of vesicular traffic[2] and endosome fusion[3] and is also known as a substrate for src type protein kinases.[4–6] Recently, annexin II has been identified as a co-receptor for t-PA and plasminogen and found to play an important role for fibrinolytic process on the endothelium.[7] To further investigate physiological function of this molecule on vascular endothelium, we constructed a recombinant adenoviral vector of annexin II and transduced with human umbilical vein endothelial cells (HUVEC). This vector will be a useful tool for the study of thrombolytic and fibrinolytic processes that take place on vascular endothelium.

[c]Address for correspondence: Masayuki Yoshida, M.D., Department of Molecular Genetics, Medical Research Institute, Tokyo Medical and Dental University, 1-5-45 Yushima Bldg. D-621, Bunkyo-ku, Tokyo 113-8510, Japan. Voice: 81-3-5803-5827; fax: 81-3-5803-0242.
masamgen@mri.tmd.ac.jp

METHOD

Cell Culture

The 293 cell line was obtained from the American Type Culture Collection (Rockville, MD) and cultured in DMEM supplemented with 10% FCS. Human umbilical vein endothelial cells (HUVEC) were cultured in RPMI-1640 supplemented with 20% FCS as previously described.[8] Murine anti–human annexin II was purchased from Zymed (South San Francisco, CA).

Construction of Recombinant Adenoviral Vector of Annexin II

Using the wild-type pCMV5–annexin II plasmid[7] as a template, polymerase chain reaction was carried out using 26-mer oligonucleotide forward and reverse primers and Taq polymerase. Primers (5′-GCGGCCGCAAAATGTCTACTGTTC-3′ and 5′-GTCGACTTCAGTCATCTCCACC AC-3′) corresponded, respectively, to bases 59–66 and 1053–1071 of the human annexin II cDNA and introduced a 5′ Not I restrict site and a 3′ Xho I restrict site. PCR product was digested with Not I and Xho I and the modified insert was purified from agarose gel slices using the QIAEX kit (Qiagen, Tokyo, Japan). The fragment was ligated in adenovirus shuttle vector PAdRSV4 (provided by Dr. David Dichek, University of California, San Francisco, CA) between RSV-LTR and SV40 poly A sequences. The resulting plasmid was cotransfected into 293 cells with PJM17 (provided by Dr. Frank C. Graham, McMaster University, Hamilton, Ont.) (FIG. 1). Plaques were isolated, propagated in 293 cells, and characterized for protein expression by Western blotting. A positive plaque was further purified to generate the recombinant adenovirus AdRSVAN-II. Large-scale production of adenovirus was carried out by two sequential CsCl gradient centrifugations and desalted by chromatography on PD-10 columns in storage buffer (10 mmol/l Tris, 1 mmol/l $MgCl_2$, 10% glycerol, pH = 7.4). AdRSVβ-gal (kindly pro-

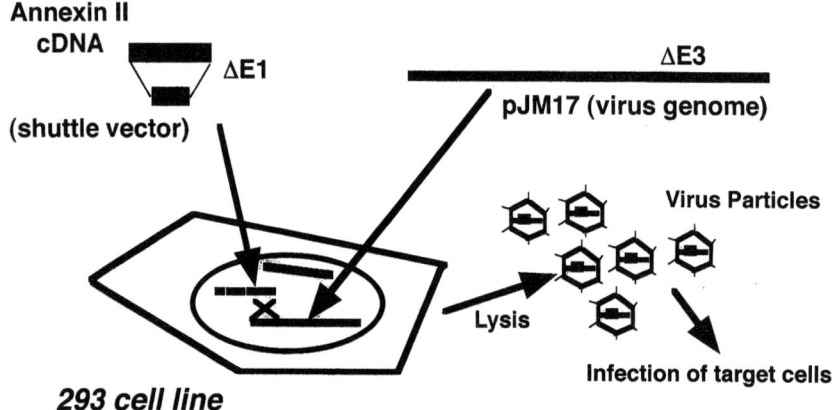

FIGURE 1. Construction of adenovirus vector containing annexin II.

vided by Dr. David Dichek), described in detail elsewhere,[9] carries a nuclear-targeted format of β-galactosidase and is structurally similar to AdRSVAN-II. Viral titer of purified stocks was determined by plaque assay in 293 cells as previously described. Several different viral stocks were used in this study. Stocks titer ranged from 10^9 to 10^{10} pfu/ml with particle-to-pfu ratio of approximately 10^2.

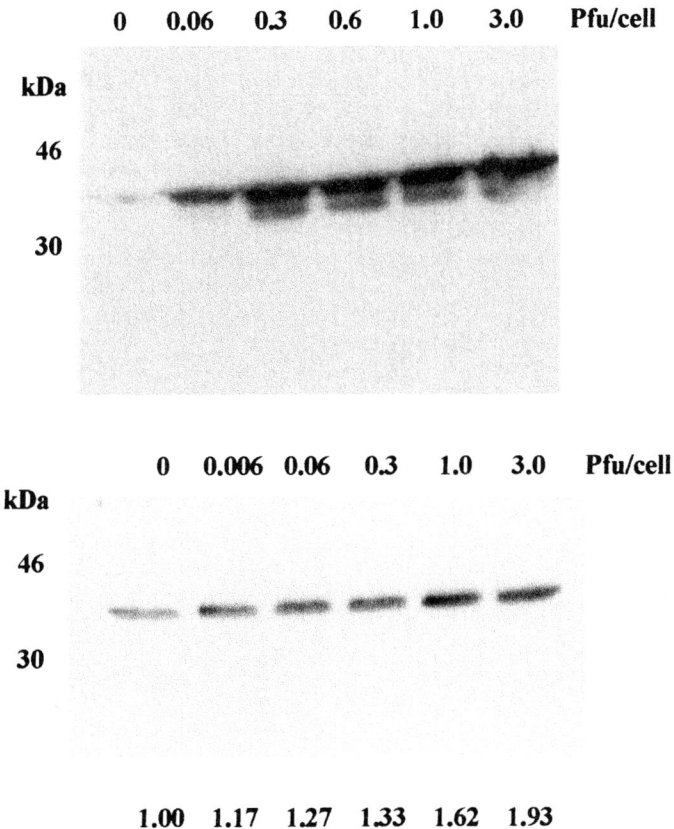

FIGURE 2. (A) Western blotting analysis of AdRSVAN-II–transduced 293 cells. The total cell lysates recovered from AdRSVAN-II–transduced 293 cells were subjected to 12.5% SDS-PAGE and Western blotting analysis was performed using an anti–annexin II mAb. (B) Western blotting analysis of AdRSVAN-II–transduced HUVEC. The total cell lysates recovered from AdRSVAN-II–transduced HUVEC were subjected to 12.5% SDS-PAGE and Western blotting analysis was performed using an anti–annexin II mAb. Infection of AdRSVAN-II successfully induced annexin II protein at the predicted molecular weight (36 kD). Numbers at the bottom of each lane represented relative density of the band compared to the control.

Infection of 293 Cells and HUVECs with Adenovirus Vectors

293 cells and HUVEC was plated in C-6 plates. Indicated amount of adenovirus was diluted in 0.5 ml of infection media (DMEM with 2% FCS; EBM with 2% FCS) incubated for 72 hours. The infected cells were then lysed with 0.5 ml of lysis buffer containing phosphatase inhibitors. The cell lysate was subjected to 12.5% SDS PAGE, transferred to a PVDF membrane, and Western blotting analysis was carried out using anti–human annexin II mAb as previously described.[8]

RESULTS AND DISCUSSION

Recombinant adenoviral vector of annexin II was constructed as described in FIGURE 1. Large-scale preparation of adenovirus yielded 10^9 to 10^{10} pfu/ml of recombinant annexin II adenovirus, AdRSVAN-II. As shown in FIGURE 2A, infection of AdRSVAN-II to 293 cells induced annexin II protein expression in 293 cells. To establish an overexpression model of annexin II in vascular endothelium, we infected AdRSVAN-II to HUVEC (FIG. 2B). Basal level of annexin II expression was observed in HUVEC without adenovirus infection. Infection of AdRSVAN-II enhanced annexin II protein expression in HUVEC. Densitometric analysis revealed that AdRSVAN-II infection induced almost twice as much annexin II as compared to uninfected HUVEC. AdRSVAN-II will be a useful tool for the investigation of annexin II and endothelial fibrinolysis process.

REFERENCES

1. WAISMAN, D.M. 1995. Annexin II tetramer: structure and function. Mol. Cell. Biochem. **149/150:** 301–322.
2. CREUTZ, C.E. 1992. The annexins and exocytosis. Science **258:** 924–931
3. EMANS, N., J.P. GORVEL, C. WALTER, V. GERKE, R. KELLNER, G. GRIFFITHS & J. GRUENBERG. 1993. Annexin II is a major component of fusogenic endosomal vesicules. J. Cell Biol. **120:** 1357–1369.
4. GLENNEY, J.R., JR. 1986. Two related but distinct forms of the M_r 36,000 tyrosine kinase substrate (calpactin) that interact with phospholipid and actin in a Ca^{2+}-dependent manner. Proc. Natl. Acad. Sci. USA **83:** 4258–4262.
5. GOULD, K.L., J.R. WOODGETT, C.M. ISACKE & T. HUNTER. 1986. The protein-tyrosine kinase substrate p36 is also a substrate for protein kinase C in vitro and in vivo. Mol. Cell. Biol. **6:** 2738–2744.
6. BRAMBILLA, R., R. ZIPPEL, E. STURANI, L. MORELLO, A. PERES & L. ALBERGHINA. 1991. Characterization of the tyrosine phosphorylation of calpactin I (annexin II) induced by platelet-derived growth factor. Biochem. J. **278:** 447–452.
7. HAJJAR, K.A., A.T. JACOVINA & J. CHACKO. 1994. An endothelial cell receptor for plasminogen/tissue plasminogen activator. J. Biol. Chem. **269:** 21191–21197.
8. YOSHIDA, M., W.F. WESTLIN, N. WANG, D.E. INGBER, A. ROSENZWEIG, N. RESNICK & M.A. GIMBRONE, JR. 1996. Leukocyte adhesion to vascular endothelium induces E-selectin linkage to actin cytoskeleton. J. Cell Biol. **133:** 445–455.
9. DONG, G., A. SCHULICK, M.B. DE YOUNG & D.A. DICHEK. 1996. Identification of a cis-acting sequence in the human PAI-1 gene that mediates TGF-1 responsiveness in endothelium in vivo. J. Biol. Chem. **271:** 29969–29977.

Effect of Leptin in Platelet and Endothelial Cells

Obesity and Arterial Thrombosis

IKURO MARUYAMA, MASANORI NAKATA, AND KAZUYO YAMAJI

Department of Laboratory and Molecular Medicine, Kagoshima University School of Medicine, Kagoshima, Japan

Obesity, especially visceral obesity, is one of the most important risk factor for "arterial" thrombosis, including ischemic heart disease. Several causative factors and pathomechanisms have been proposed for the high incidence of thromboembolism in obesity. They include hypertension, hyperlipidemia, and glucose intolerance/diabetes mellitus, which are often accompanied in obesity. These are, however, indirect causes for thrombosis. Increased tissue plasminogen activator (t-PA) inhibitor, type 1 (PAI-1) released from visceral fat is also proposed as a risk factor for thrombotic tendency in obesity.[1,2] However increased PAI-1 is not a risk factor of arterial thrombosis, but of a venous thrombosis. In this context, we have been investigating the pathomechanism of "arterial thrombosis" in obesity. Here we review the investigations of our recent work.

EFFECT OF LEPTIN ON PLATELET FUNCTION: LEPTIN POTENTIATES PLATELET FUNCTION THROUGH FUNCTIONAL RECEPTOR[3]

Leptin Induces Tyrosine Phosphorylation of Platelet Proteins

We investigated the effect of leptin on platelets. First we examined the expression of leptin receptor on platelets by immunoblotting. We demonstrated that OB-Rb, long form functional leptin receptor, is expressed in platelets by Western blotting using an anti–Ob-Rb polyclonal antibody (FIG. 1A). Next we examined the significance of the expression of functional leptin receptor in platelets. Leptin (50 ng/ml) induced phosphorylation of platelet proteins at the tyrosine residue as detected by analysis using PY20, an anti-phosphotyrosine monoclonal antibody (FIG. 1B). In the non-stimulated state, a protein with a molecular mass of ~60 kD was the main phosphoprotein. The stimulation of platelets by leptin induced tyrosine phosphorylation in a 60 kD protein band in a time-dependent manner. This phosphorylation appeared within 1 min and peaked at 3 min and later, other protein bands of ~190, 120, 80, and 70 kD were also phosphorylated. However, at the lower concentration of 10 ng/ml, leptin showed a much weaker effect, if any, on the tyrosine phosphorylation of proteins (FIG. 1C). At the concentration of 30 ng/ml, leptin had a weaker effect (data not shown). Thus leptin induced tyrosine phosphorylation of proteins in a concentration-dependent manner.

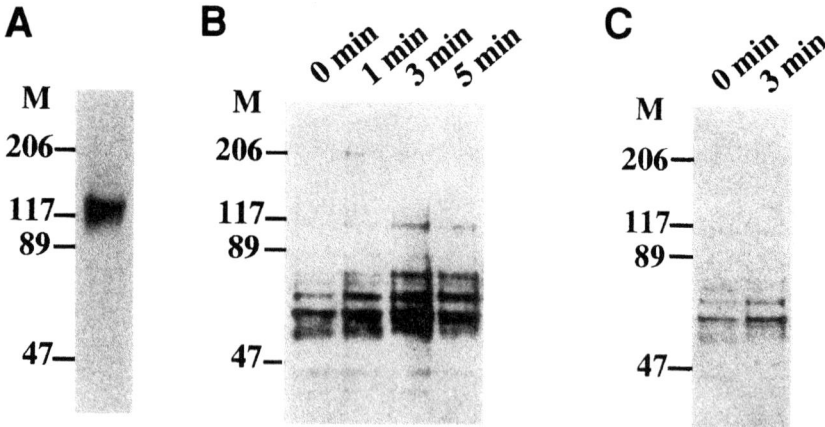

FIGURE 1. (**A**) Western blot analysis of Ob-Rb in human platelets showing expression of functional long form of the leptin receptor on the platelets. (**B**) and (**C**) Analyses of tyrosine phosphorylation induced by leptin at 50 (**B**) and 10 (**C**) ng/ml. After stimulation with leptin (50 ng/ml), total lysate was analyzed by Western blotting using anti-phosphotyrosine monoclonal antibody (PY20). In the nonstimulated state, a protein with a molecular mass of ~60 kD was the main phosphoprotein. The induction of tyrosine phosphorylation by leptin was time dependent.

Leptin Potentiates Platelet Aggregability

Next we examined the effects of leptin on the aggregation of human platelet. Neither leptin at concentrations <100 ng/ml (FIG. 2A) nor ADP at concentrations <2 µmol/l (FIG. 2B) affected platelet aggregability. Interestingly, the combination of leptin and ADP was effective: pretreatment with leptin at a concentration of 100 ng/ml for 5 min rendered platelets responsive to 2 µmol/l ADP, thereby causing aggregation (FIG. 2C). Thus, leptin and ADP at subthreshold concentrations acted synergistically. Pretreatment with leptin, even at the lower concentration of 30 ng/ml, moderately enhanced the platelet aggregation induced by 2 µmol/l ADP (FIG. 2C). At a concentration of 50 ng/ml, leptin markedly enhanced the platelet aggregation (FIG. 2C). At a concentration of 100 ng/ml, leptin produced a greater enhancement (FIG. 2C). Thus, the dose-response relationship for the effect of leptin on the tyrosine phosphorylation of proteins correlated with the effect of leptin on the platelet aggregation, suggesting that the tyrosine phosphorylation mediates the aggregation in response to leptin. Functional coupling of leptin-induced phosphorylation to potentiation of platelet aggregation was further supported by our observation that genistein, a tyrosine kinase inhibitor, blocked the ability of leptin to potentiate ADP-induced platelet aggregation (FIG. 3A). In addition, genistein inhibited the tyrosine phosphorylation of protein bands of ~120 kD (FIG. 3B). This finding suggested that the tyrosine phosphorylation mediates the potentiation of platelet aggregation in response to leptin.

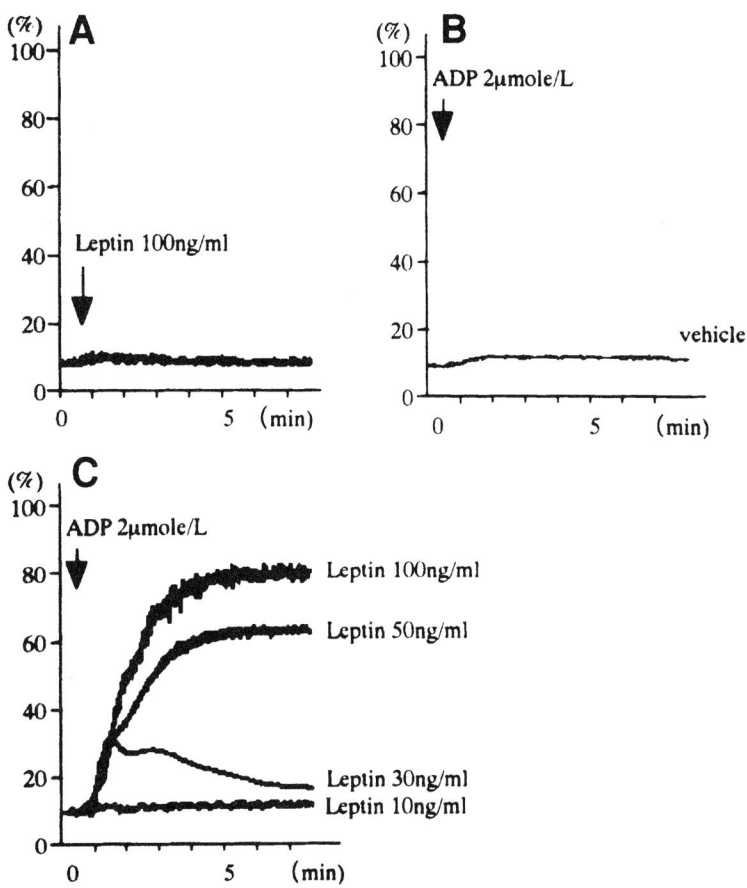

FIGURE 2. (**A**) and (**B**) Addition of 100 ng/ml leptin (**A**) and 2 µmol/l ADP (**B**) had no effect on the aggregation of human platelets. (**C**) The dose-dependent effects of leptin on ADP-induced aggregation. Pretreatment with leptin at the lower concentration of 30 ng/ml moderately enhanced ADP-induced platelet aggregation. Pretreatment with leptin at a concentration of 100 ng/ml resulted in greater enhancement.

Effect of Leptin on the Endothelial Cells

Next we investigated the effect of leptin on thrombomodulin (TM) expression. TM is an endothelial surface glycoprotein that converts thrombin from a procoagulant protease to an anticoagulant. It has been described that cell-surface TM is downregulated by exogenous and endogenous substances including endotoxin, interleukin-1 (IL-1), TNFα, oxidized LDL (OX-LDL), and advanced glycation endproducts (AGE). These may have a role in the thrombotic tendency found in endotoxemia, infection/inflammation, hyperlipidemia, and diabetes. Thus we investigated an effect of leptin on the

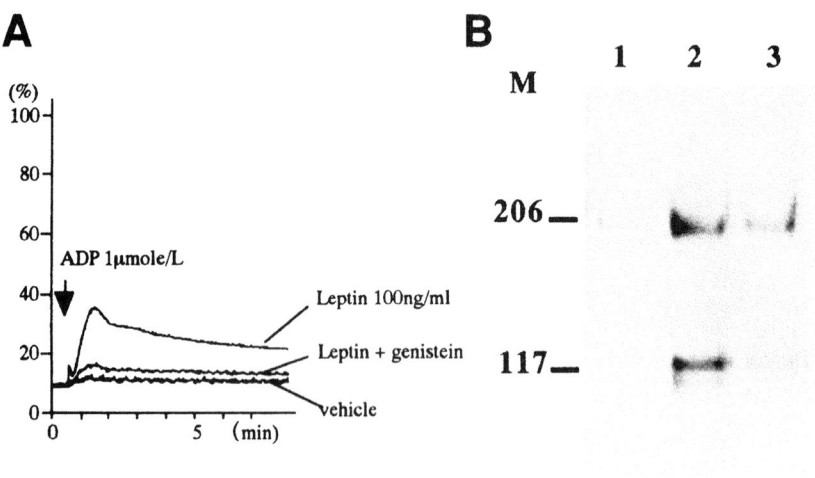

FIGURE 3. (**A**) Addition of 1 µmol/l ADP had no effect on the aggregation of human platelets. However, when pretreated with 100 ng/ml leptin for 5 min, 1 µmol/l ADP caused aggregation of platelets. When pretreatment was carried out with 100 ng/ml of leptin and 50 µmol/l genistein, the potentiation by leptin of ADP-induced aggregation was inhibited almost completely (the trace in **A** indicated by leptin + genistein). *Arrow* indicates the time of the addition of the agents. (**B**) Analyses of tyrosine phosphorylation induced by 100 ng/ml leptin with or without 50 µmol/l genistein by Western blot analysis using PY20. Vehicle control (lane 1), stimulation with 100 ng/ml leptin (lane 2), and 100 ng/ml leptin plus 50 µmol/ml genistein (lane 3).

expression of TM in the cultured human umbilical vein endothelial cells. We demonstrated that 50–100 ng/ml of leptin slightly decreased the cell-surface TM (up ~10%). However this effect of leptin was enhanced by the co-stimulation with OX-LDL or AGE (data not shown). This suggests that leptin may play one of a causative factor of thrombotic tendency in obese individuals.

SUMMARY

We demonstrated that leptin showed effects on both platelets and endothelial cells through its functional receptor. These effects are the vector to inducing thrombotic tendency. Leptin concentrations used in our experiments correspond to that of leptin in the circulation of obese individuals. Thus we suggest that increased leptin may act as a risk factor for thrombosis in obese individuals.

REFERENCES

1. FUNAHASHI, T. *et al.* 1999. Role of adipocytokines on the pathogenesis of atherosclerosis in visceral obesity. Intern. Med. **38:** 202–206.

2. MAVRI, A. *et al.* 1999. Impact of adipose tissue on plasma plasminogen activator inhibitor-1 in dieting obese women. Arterioscler. Thromb. Vasc. Biol. **19:** 1582–1587.
3. NAKATA, M. *et al.* 1999. Leptin promotes aggregation of human platelets via the long form of its receptor. Diabetes **48:** 426–429.

Cytokines and Soluble Cell Adhesion Molecules

Possible Markers of Inflammatory Response in Atherosclerosis

A.I. TEPLYAKOV,[a] E.V. PRYSCHEPOVA, N.G. KRUCHINSKY, AND T.I. CHEGEROVA

Research Institute for Ecopathology and Occupational Disease, Mogilev 212004, Belarus

INTRODUCTION

We hypothesize that cell-cell communication disturbance is an important pathogenetic mechanism in all steps of atherogenesis. The pathogenesis in most pathologic processes may be considered from a new point of view: as the result of disturbances of "habitual" cell-cell communications.[1] These "habitual" communications are made possible by four classes of mediators (messengers): cell adhesion molecules, extracellular matrix, cytokines, and protooncogens.[2]

The main goal of our research was the comparative analysis of cytokines, soluble cell adhesion molecule (sCAM) secretion after blood coagulation and high shear rate for studying the involvement of hemostasis in pathophysiology of atherosclerosis.

MATERIALS AND METHODS

The investigation studied 29 atherosclerotic patients. The original research technique has been developed. We based our study on the fact that thrombus generation and flow changes are adequate stimuli for fast cell inflammatory response.[3] The initial cytokines level [IL-1a, IL-1b, IL-6, IL-8, IL-10 (Immunotech, Prague)] and soluble cell adhesion molecules [sP- and sE-selectins, sICAM-1, sVCAM-1 (R&D, Abington Oxon, U.K.)] were established and their changes in response to coagulation and fibrinolysis (incubation of blood clot 6 h at 37°C) and to standardized viscosimetric flow using rotational viscosimeter (shear rate 100 1/sec, 60 sec at 37°C, samples incubation 6 h) were measured.

RESULTS

Measurement of initial cytokines concentration showed a high level of proinflammatory cytokines IL-1 (mainly IL-1b) and IL-6 (TABLE 1). In contrast IL-1a, the shear stress probe, induced excess secretion of IL-1b, dramatically exceeding the ini-

---

[a]Address for correspondence: A.I. Teplyakov, Vitebsky Ave, 70, Mogilev, 212004, Belarus. Voice/fax: 375-222-420-441.
niiepp@bcsmi.minsk.by

TABLE 1. Cytokines level, blood coagulation, and high shear stress in patients with atherosclerosis[a]

Cytokine (ng/ml)	Initial level	After shear stress (+ 6-h incubation)	After blood coagulation (+ 6-h incubation)
IL-1a	12.90 ± 6.72	62.09 ± 51.63*	51.68 ± 48.54*
IL-1b	55.28 ± 14.09	680.95 ± 589.97*	133.98 ± 132.68*,**
IL-6	65.16 ± 55.66	1610.81 ± 650.78*	847.55 ± 676.21*,**
IL-8	0	60.25 ± 42.75*	51.98 ± 44.46*
IL-10	0.81 ± 1.40	158.14 ± 112.62*	9.72 ± 4.78*,**
ET-1 (pg/ml)	15.88 ± 15.83	35.46 ± 11.49*	17.89 ± 15.16**

[a]Data are mean ± SD.
*Statistically significant in comparison to initial group.
**Statistically significant differences between responses to coagulation and high shear rate (t test).

TABLE 2. Concentration of sCAM in response to coagulation and high shear stress in patients with atherosclerosis

SCAM (ng/ml)	Initial level	After shear stress (+ 6-h incubation)	After blood coagulation (+ 6-h incubation)
sP-selectin	168.16 ± 127.62	589.67 ± 301.50*	118.54 ± 72.97*,**
sE-selectin	90.70 ± 47.93	80.87 ± 67.93*	91.85 ± 63.39
sICAM-1	515.65 ± 124.49	633.22 ± 105.63*	527.38 ± 137.83
sVCAM-1	1039.74 ± 528.87	1087.12 ± 300.13	1263.29 ± 239.91

*Statistically significant differences in comparison to initial means.
**Statistically significant differences between the both probes.

tial level and response to coagulation. A sharp increase of IL-6 in response to both probes was detected. However, its increase in response to shear activation exceeded the postcoagulation level. A similar tendency was observed for IL-10. Simultaneously, the IL-8 concentration changed in a manner similar to IL-1a with both probes.

Interestingly, ET-1 level increased in both probes (TABLE 2). The initial sCAMs concentration was unexpectedly high in all patients with atherosclerosis. The sE-selectin level after rheologic probes was statistically different from the initial level. The sP-selectin level after blood coagulation probes strongly increased. In contrast, after rheologic probes its concentration decreased significantly.

To reveal interrelationships between cytokines and sCAMs secretion we carried out the correlation analysis. This demonstrated the pleiotropy and regulatory manner of the processes. Initial IL-1b levels were closely related to ET-1 in coagulation and shear activation probes ($r = 0.61$ and 0.69, respectively, $p < 0.05$). Secretion of IL-1a and IL-1b correlated to other cytokines; IL-1b and IL-6 were closely correlated to IL-8 in both probes ($r = 0.83$ and 0.63, $N = 29$, $p < 0.02$). The initial sICAM-1 downregulated IL-1b, IL-8, and IL-10 secretion after viscosimetric flow ($r = -0.76$, -0.74 and -0.71, $p < 0.01$) and initial sVCAM-1 downregulated IL-1a and IL-8 secretion. Therefore, their levels after probes were closely related (for sVCAM-1 and IL-1a $r = -0.44$, $p < 0.05$ in rheologic probe and $r = -0.56$, $p < 0.02$ in coagulation probe). Similarly, the sICAM-1 decreased IL-10 secretion in coagulation probe. In contrast, the close negative correlation between initial sE-selectin concentrations and ET-1 in coagulation and viscosimetric probes was detected ($r = -0.9$ and $r = -0.89$, respectively, $p < 0.001$). At the same time, the initial sE-selectin level was downregulated by the IL-1a ($r = -0.39$, $p < 0.05$). The level of sP-selectin was positive correlated to IL-8 secretion after coagulation ($r = 0.46$, $p < 0.02$), to IL-1a level after shear stress ($r = 0.56$, $p < 0.01$) and initial IL-6 level ($r = 0.39$, $p < 0.05$).

CONCLUSIONS

(1) The increased levels of IL-1b, IL-6, sP- and sE-selectins, sICAM-1, and sVCAM-1, were found even without functional probes in patients with atherosclerosis. This serves as a convincing confirmation of the inflammatory nature of atherosclerosis.

(2) This is still hypothetical in that the pathophysiologic role of sCAM (in counterbalance to cell adhesion molecules expressed on the cell surface) consists of cytokine-secretion inhibition by possible blocking of the juxtacrine activating pathway. Therefore, obtained results suggest that the sCAM are cytokines themselves, because they have as their main features solubility, short-distant action, pleiotropy, and excessive synthesis.

(3) The VCAM-1 and ICAM-1 antagonists (monoclonal antibodies or non-antibodies origin) may be useful as antithrombotics and drugs and may be able to prevent ischemia-reperfusion injury.

REFERENCES

1. MARCUS, A.J., L.B. SAFIER, M.J. BROECKMAN et al. 1995. Thrombosis and inflammation as multicellular process: signficance of cell-cell interactions. Thromb. Haemost. **74:** 213–217.
2. NICOLA, N.A. 1994. Guidebook to Cytokines and Their Receptors. Oxford University Press. Oxford.
3. BEVILACQUA, M.P. & R.M. NELSON. 1993. Endothelial-leukocyte adhesion molecules in inflammation and methastasis. Thromb. Haemost. **70:** 152–154.

Inducible Expression of LOX-1, a Novel Receptor for Oxidized LDL, in Macrophages and Vascular Smooth Muscle Cells

NORIAKI KUME,[a] HIDEAKI MORIWAKI, HIROHARU KATAOKA, MANABU MINAMI, TAKATOSHI MURASE, TATSUYA SAWAMURA,[b] TOMOH MASAKI,[b] AND TORU KITA

Department of Geriatric Medicine, Graduate School of Medicine, Kyoto University, Kyoto, Japan

[b]*Department of Bioscience, National Cardiovascular Center Research Institute, Osaka, Japan*

ABSTRACT: Macrophages appear to take up oxidized low density lipoprotein (Ox-LDL) by multiple receptor-mediated pathways. This study, therefore, has been performed to determine if LOX-1, a novel receptor for Ox-LDL, which was identified in vascular endothelial cells, is also expressed in macrophages. Expression of LOX-1 can be induced after macrophage-like differentiation in human peripheral blood monocytes as well as THP-1 cells. Furthermore, expression of LOX-1 in macrophages is also upregulated by an inflammatory cytokine TNF-α, which was shown to be present in atherosclerotic arterial wall. Expression of this novel receptor LOX-1 may play an important role in Ox-LDL uptake and subsequent foam cell formation in macrophages.

INTRODUCTION

Accumulation of cholesterol-loaded foam cells derived from monocyte-macrophage lineage in the arterial intima appears to be a hallmark and key event of early atherogenesis. Several lines of evidence indicated that oxidative modification of low density lipoprotein (Ox-LDL) plays crucial roles in atherogenesis. Ox-LDL can be avidly taken up by macrophages by receptor-mediated endocytosis and can transform them into foam cells.[1,2] Several different molecules, such as class A macrophage scavenger receptors, MARCO, Fc-γRII, CD36, scavenger receptor class B type I (SR-BI), and CD68 (macrosialin),[3,4] have been identified as cell-surface receptors for atherogenic Ox-LDL. However, additional molecules may also be involved in Ox-LDL uptake and subsequent foam cell transformation in macrophages.

Recent studies in our laboratory have identified a novel class of Ox-LDL receptor, which has been designated lectin-like Ox-LDL receptor-1 (LOX-1) in vascular endothelial cells.[5] LOX-1 is a type II membrane glycoprotein with approximate molecular mass of 50 kD. LOX-1 can bind, be internalized, and proteolytically degrade

---

[a]Address for correspondence: Noriaki Kume, M.D., Ph.D., Department of Geriatric Medicine, Graduate School of Medicine, Kyoto University, 54 Kawahara-cho, Shogoin, Sakyo-ku, Kyoto 606-8507, Japan. Voice: 81-75-751-3465; fax: 81-75-751-3574.
nkume@kuhp.kyoto-u.ac.jp

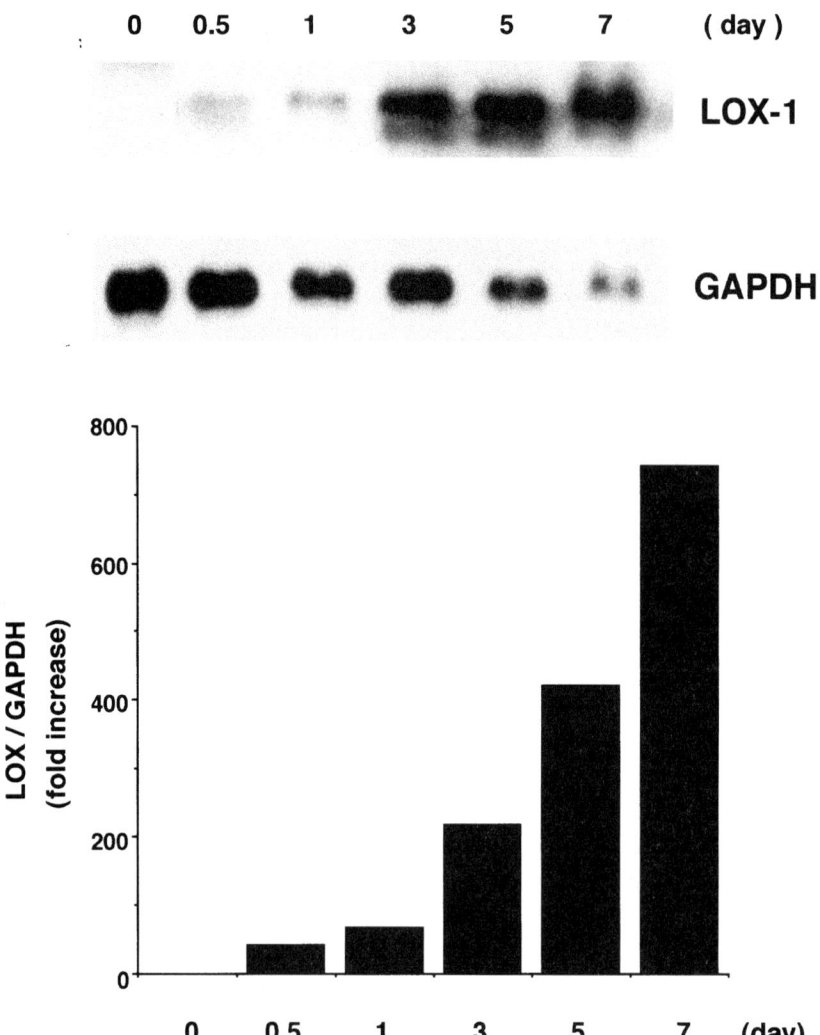

FIGURE 1. Expression of LOX-1 mRNA during differentiation of THP-1 cells by PMA. THP-1 cells were cultured in RPMI 1640 supplemented with 10% FBS in the presence of PMA. After incubation with 30 nM PMA for 12 h, 1, 3, 5, and 7 days, total RNA was isolated and subjected to Northern blot analysis.

Ox-LDL, but not significant amounts of acetylated LDL.[6] Expression of LOX-1 can be upregulated by TNF-α, PMA, and fluid shear stress, suggesting that LOX-1 expression *in vivo* in vascular endothelium may also be dynamically regulated by inflammatory and fluid mechanical stimuli.[7,8] In the present study, we explored whether LOX-1, a novel receptor for Ox-LDL identified in vascular endothelial cells, is also expressed in macrophages.

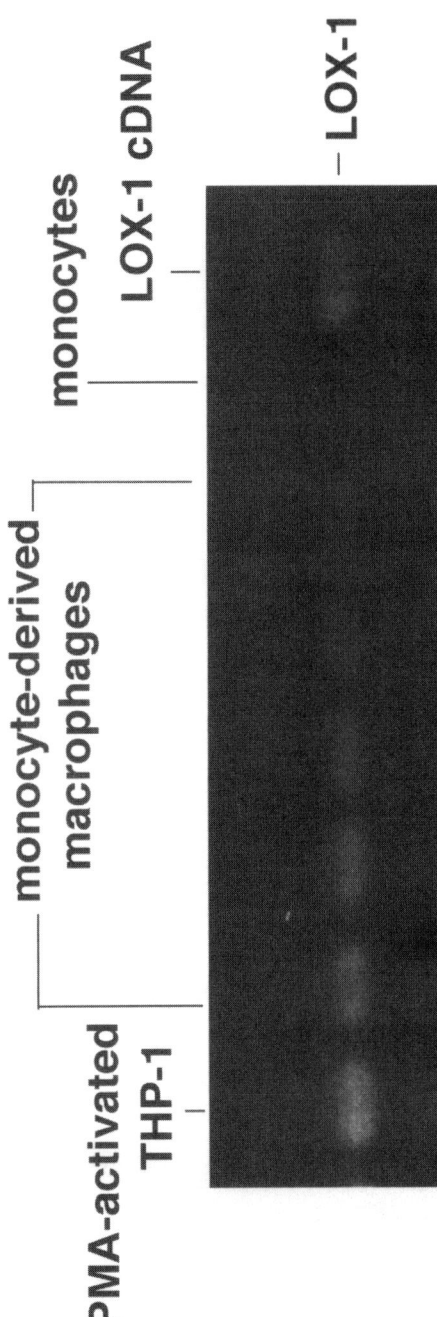

FIGURE 2. Expression of LOX-1 mRNA in human monocyte-derived macrophages. Human peripheral blood monocytes were cultured in RPMI 1640 containing 20% autologous serum for 10 days. Total cellular RNA was isolated and subsequently subjected to RT-PCR analysis.

RESULTS AND DISCUSSION

The human monocytic cell line, THP-1 cells, has been shown to be differentiated into macrophage-like cells after treatment with PMA. Therefore, THP-1 cells were treated with PMA (30 nM) for the indicated time periods, and Northern blotting was performed to evaluate LOX-1 mRNA expression. As shown in FIGURE 1, LOX-1 mRNA was not detectable in untreated THP-1 cells. In PMA-treated THP-1 cells, in contrast, LOX-1 mRNA expression was time-dependently induced. LOX-1 mRNA was detectable as early as 12 h after PMA treatment and remained expressed for at least 7 days (FIG. 1). With regard to the concentration dependency in PMA-induced LOX-1 expression, concentrations as low as 10 nM PMA can induce expression of LOX-1 mRNA after 3 days (data not shown). These results appear to be in parallel to the previous report, which showed time- and concentration-dependent induction of class A scavenger receptors in PMA-treated THP-1 cells. Immunocytochemistry using anti–LOX-1 antibody showed that THP-1 cells that have undergone macrophage-like differentiation by PMA treatment express LOX-1 as well as CD68, a macrophage marker (data not shown).

We further explored expression of LOX-1 mRNA in human monocyte-derived macrophages. Freshly isolated human peripheral blood monocytes were differentiated into macrophages after *in vitro* culture for 10 days, and RT-PCR analysis was performed. Although LOX-1 mRNA was not detectable in human monocytes, its expression was clearly detectable in human monocytes isolated from five different donors after macrophage-like differentiation in culture (FIG. 2).

In addition, murine peritoneal macrophages were harvested by peritoneal lavage, and expression of LOX-1 was evaluated. Expression of LOX-1 mRNA was detectable in murine peritoneal macrophages, and, furthermore, treatment with an inflammatory cytokine TNF-α significantly upregulated expression of LOX-1 mRNA in a time- and concentration-dependent manner (data not shown). We also examined LOX-1 expression in cultured vascular smooth muscle cells and found that LOX-1 expression can be induced by TNF-α, bacterial endotoxin, and PMA (data not shown). These results appear to be in parallel with our previous findings that LOX-1 expression can be upregulated by proinflammatory stimuli in cultured vascular endothelial cells.[7]

Uptake of Ox-LDL in macrophages and subsequent foam cell transformation appear to play key roles in atherogenesis. The present study provides evidence that LOX-1, a novel receptor for Ox-LDL originally identified in vascular endothelial cells, is also expressed in macrophages. Expression of LOX-1 in macrophages is also upregulated by an inflammatory cytokine, TNF-α. Interestingly, expression of class A scavenger receptors has been shown to be downregulated by TNF-α in macrophages. Since production of TNF-α in atherosclerotic lesions has been reported, LOX-1 may play more important roles in atherosclerotic lesions with inflammatory responses.

Our previous report has also shown that LOX-1 can support binding and engulfment of aged red blood cells and apoptotic cells.[9] LOX-1 in macrophages, therefore, may play important roles in the removal of these deteriorated cells.

In summary, this report provides evidence that LOX-1 is expressed in macrophages and upregulated by an inflammatory stimulus. Further studies related to pathophysiological roles of LOX-1 in macrophages and other cell types *in vivo* may add new insights into atherogenesis as well as inflammatory diseases.

REFERENCES

1. Ross, R. 1993. The pathogenesis of atherosclerosis: a perspective for the 1990s. Nature **362:** 801–809.
2. WITZTUM, J.L. & D. STEINBERG. 1991. Role of oxidized low density lipoprotein in atherogenesis. J. Clin. Invest. **88:** 1785–1792.
3. KRIEGER, M., S. ACTON, J. ASHKENAS, A. PEARSON, M. PENMAN & D. RESNICK. 1993. Molecular flypaper, host defense, and atherosclerosis. Structure, binding properties, and functions of macrophage scavenger receptors. J. Biol. Chem. **268:** 4569–4572.
4. RAMPRASAD, M. P., W. FISCHER, J.L. WITZTUM, G.R. SAMBRANO, O. QUEHENBERGER & D. STEINBERG. 1996. Cell surface expression of mouse macrosialin and human CD68 and their role as macrophage receptors for oxidized low density lipoprotein. Proc. Natl. Acad. Sci. USA **93:** 14833–14838.
5. SAWAMURA, T., N. KUME, T. AOYAMA, H. MORIWAKI, H. HOSHIKAWA, Y. AIBA, T. TANAKA, S.MIWA, Y. KATSURA, T. KITA & T. MASAKI. 1997. A novel receptor for oxidized low density lipoprotein. Nature **386:** 73–77.
6. MORIWAKI, H., N. KUME, T. SAWAMURA, T. AOYAMA, H. HOSHIKAWA, H. OCHI, E. NISHI, T. MASAKI & T. KITA. 1998. Ligand specificity of LOX-1, a novel endothelial receptor for oxidized low density lipoprotein. Arterioscler. Thromb. Vasc. Biol. **18:** 1541–1547.
7. KUME, N., T. MURASE, H. MORIWAKI, T. AOYAMA, T. SAWAMURA, T. MASAKI & T. KITA. 1998. Inducible expression of lectin-like oxidized low density lipoprotein receptor-1 in vascular endothelial cells. Circ. Res. **83:** 322–327.
8. MURASE, T., N. KUME, R. KORENAGA, J. ANDO, T. SAWAMURA, T. MASAKI & T. KITA. 1998. Fluid shear stress transcriptionally induces lectin-like oxidized low density lipoprotein receptor-1 in vascular endothelial cells. Circ. Res. **83:** 328–333.
9. OKA, K., T. SAWAMURA, K. KIKUTA, S. ITOKAWA, N. KUME, T. KITA & T. MASAKI. 1998. Lectin-like oxidized low density lipoprotein receptor 1 mediated phagocytosis of aged/apoptotic cells in endothelial cells. Proc. Natl. Acad. Sci. USA **95:** 9535–9540.

Expression of Lectin-like Oxidized LDL Receptor-1 in Human Atherosclerotic Lesions

HIROHARU KATAOKA, NORIAKI KUME,[a] MANABU MINAMI, HIDEAKI MORIWAKI, TATSUYA SAWAMURA,[b] TOMOH MASAKI,[b] AND TORU KITA

Department of Geriatric Medicine, Graduate School of Medicine, Kyoto University, Kyoto, Japan

[b]*Department of Bioscience, National Cardiovascular Center Research Institute, Osaka, Japan*

INTRODUCTION

Several lines of evidence suggest that Ox-LDL may play crucial roles in the pathogenesis of atherosclerosis.[1,2] Ox-LDL can modulate various endothelial functions relevant to atherogenesis and, furthermore uptake of Ox-LDL by macrophages and smooth muscle cells can transform these cells into foam cells. In macrophages, several molecules were identified as receptors for cellular uptake of acetylated LDL (Ac-LDL) and Ox-LDL.[3–6] In vascular endothelial cells, previous studies have suggested that endothelial uptake of Ox-LDL appears to depend on cell-surface receptors, which may be encoded by different genes from known receptors.[7] We have recently identified a novel receptor for Ox-LDL, designated C-type lectin-like Ox-LDL receptor-1 (LOX-1) in cultured bovine aortic endothelial cells.[8]

LOX-1 is a type II membrane protein that belongs to the C-type lectin family.[8] LOX-1 recognizes Ox-LDL, but not Ac-LDL.[9] Expression of LOX-1 can be induced by an inflammatory cytokine TNF-α[10] and fluid shear stress[11] in cultured vascular endothelial cells. These data indicate that LOX-1 expression is dynamically regulated by pathophysiological stimuli relevant to atherogenesis and inflammation. The relationship of this novel receptor for Ox-LDL to atherogenesis, however, has not yet been clarified.

In the present study, therefore, we have explored the expression of LOX-1 in atherosclerotic lesions of human carotid arteries.

MATERIALS AND METHODS

Tissue Sampling

Fresh frozen sections were prepared from human carotid endarterectomy specimens from 21 patients. These endarterectomy specimens contained both early ath-

---

[a]Address for correspondence: Noriaki Kume, M.D., Ph.D., Department of Geriatric Medicine, Graduate School of Medicine, Kyoto University, 54 Kawahara-cho, Shogoin, Sakyo-ku, Kyoto 606-8507, Japan. Voice: 81-75-751-3465; fax: 81-75-751-3574.

nkume@kuhp.kyoto-u.ac.jp

erosclerotic lesions distant from the center of the plaque and advanced lesions that consist of fibro-fatty plaques. Therefore, these specimens were divided into two pieces so that each piece contained either an early lesion with some endothelial infiltrates or an advanced atheromatous lesion. Fragments of human aortas without visible atherosclerotic lesions were obtained from two patients as normal controls.

RT-PCR Analysis

Total cellular RNA was isolated from eight endarterectomy samples and two aortic tissues. Total cellular RNA (250 ng) was reverse transcribed with random hexamer using Super Script (GIBCO). The transcribed cDNA was used for PCR amplification with specific primers for hLOX-1 and β-actin.

PCR amplification was carried out by 35 cycles of denaturation, annealing, and elongation with Taq DNA polymerase (New England Biolabs, Inc.). PCR products were analyzed by agarose gel electrophoresis and ethidium bromide staining.

Generation of Anti–LOX-1 Monoclonal Antibodies

Recombinant proteins corresponding to the extracellular domain of hLOX-1 were used as an antigen to immunize mice. Hybridomas were prepared by standard procedures and screened by enzyme-linked immunosorbent assay and immunoblot. An anti–bovine LOX-1 (bLOX-1) monoclonal antibody that crossreacts to hLOX-1 was used for double-label immunohistochemistry. The immunoreactivity and the specificity to hLOX-1 of these two monoclonal antibodies was confirmed by the cell-surface immunobinding to hLOX-1–transfected CHO cells.

Anti–human von Willebrand factor monoclonal antibody was purchased from DAKO; anti–human CD68 monoclonal antibody from DAKO; anti–human smooth muscle alpha actin monoclonal antibody from Zymed.

Single-Label Immunohistochemistry

An avidin-biotin complex (ABC) immunoperoxidase technique was employed as previously described.[13] In brief, after fixation with cold acetone, frozen sections were first incubated with 0.1% BSA-PBS containing 2% normal horse serum, and then with anti–hLOX-1 monoclonal antibody. The sections were then incubated with biotinylated secondary antibodies. Endogenous peroxidase activity was blocked by methanol containing 0.3% hydrogen peroxide, after which avidin-biotin peroxidase complexes (ABC Elite Kit, Vector Labs) were added. Antibody binding was visualized with 3,3′-diaminobenzidine tetrahydrochloride (Vector Labs), and then counterstained with Mayer's hematoxylin. Immunostaining with nonimmune mouse IgG (Zymed) served as negative controls.

Double-Label Immunohistochemistry

For double immunostaining, sections were first incubated with the anti–bLOX-1 monoclonal antibody and biotinylated anti–rat IgG, which was followed by incubation with an avidin-biotin peroxidase conjugate and 3,3′-diaminobenzidine tetrahydrochloride with nickel chloride (Vector Labs). They were subsequently incubated with primary antibodies for cell-type characterization, which was followed by alkaline phosphatase–labeled anti–mouse IgG and fast red alkaline phosphatase substrate solution (Vector Labs).

RESULTS AND DISCUSSION

Ox-LDL has been suggested to play crucial roles in the initiation and progression of atherosclerosis. Cellular uptake of Ox-LDL by macrophages and smooth muscle cells in the arterial intima appears to be involved in foam cell transformation and fatty streak formation.[2] In addition, endothelial activation elicited by Ox-LDL and its lipid constituents has been implicated in atherogenesis.[1,2] In this study, we provide evidence that LOX-1, a novel receptor for Ox-LDL, is expressed by luminal endothelial cells, neovascular endothelial cells, and nonendothelial cells in human atherosclerotic lesions. LOX-1 can potentially support Ox-LDL uptake in these cell types; therefore, LOX-1 expression in various stages of atherosclerotic lesions may play important roles in atherogenesis.

As illustrated in FIGURE 1, LOX-1 mRNA was expressed in atherosclerotic plaques. In unaffected aortas of humans, negligible amounts of LOX-1 mRNA were detectable. Luminal endothelial cells were positive for LOX-1 expression in most early atherosclerotic lesions with subendothelial infiltrates in human carotid arteries (FIG. 2C), although LOX-1 expression was not detectable in unaffected human aortic endothelium (FIG. 2A). These results indicate that LOX-1 expression is upregulated in human atherosclerotic lesions.

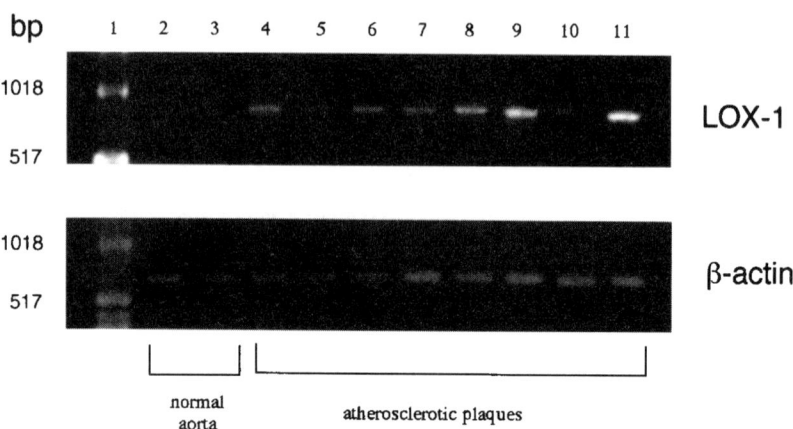

FIGURE 1. RT-PCR detection of LOX-1 mRNA in human atherosclerotic plaques. Total RNA (250 ng) from eight atherosclerotic plaques and two aortas was first reverse transcribed. cDNA fragments were amplified by a 35-cycle PCR with a set of primers for hLOX-1 (**A**) and β-actin (**B**). PCR products were visualized by ethidium bromide staining after agarose gel electrophoresis. Lane 1, DNA size marker; Lanes 2,3, normal aorta; Lane 4 through 11, atherosclerotic plaques.

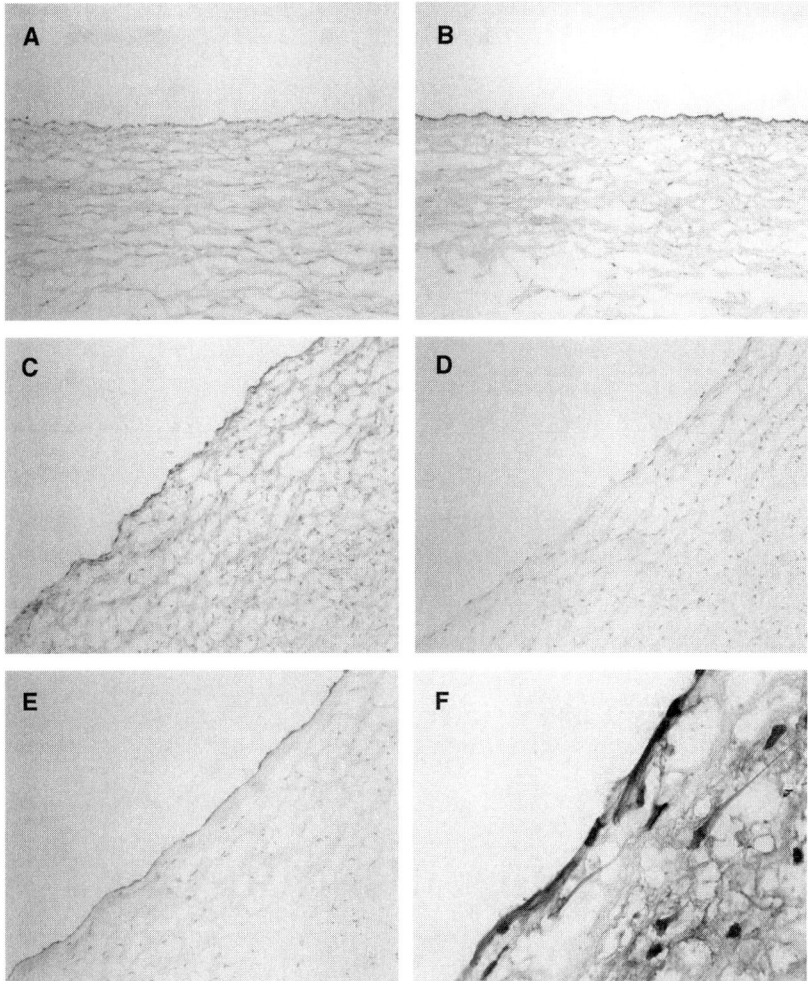

FIGURE 2. Immunohistostaining of human aorta without visible atherosclerotic changes (**A** and **B**) and early atherosclerotic lesions (**C–G**). (**A** and **B**) Cryostat serial sections of nonlesional aorta were stained with the anti–hLOX-1 monoclonal antibody (**A**, ×200) and the anti–von Willebrand factor antibody (**B**, ×200). LOX-1 was not expressed on luminal endothelial cells in nonlesional aorta (**A**). Serial sections showed uniform staining in the luminal surface of the aorta with the anti–von Willebrand factor antibody, indicating that intact endothelial linings were preserved (**B**). (**C–E**) Cryostat serial sections of early atherosclerotic lesions were stained with the anti–hLOX-1 monoclonal antibody (**C**, ×200), the anti–von Willebrand factor antibody (**E**, ×200) and nonimmune mouse IgG (**D**, ×200). LOX-1 was expressed on luminal endothelial cells in early atherosclerotic lesions with subendothelial infiltrates. Some nonendothelial cells in the intima were also positive for the anti–hLOX-1 monoclonal antibody. (**F**) Double immunohistostaining with the anti–LOX-1 antibody (*dark blue*) and the anti–von Willebrand factor antibody (*red*) of early atherosclerotic lesions (×1,000). LOX-1 expression on luminal endothelial cells was confirmed in early atherosclerotic lesions.

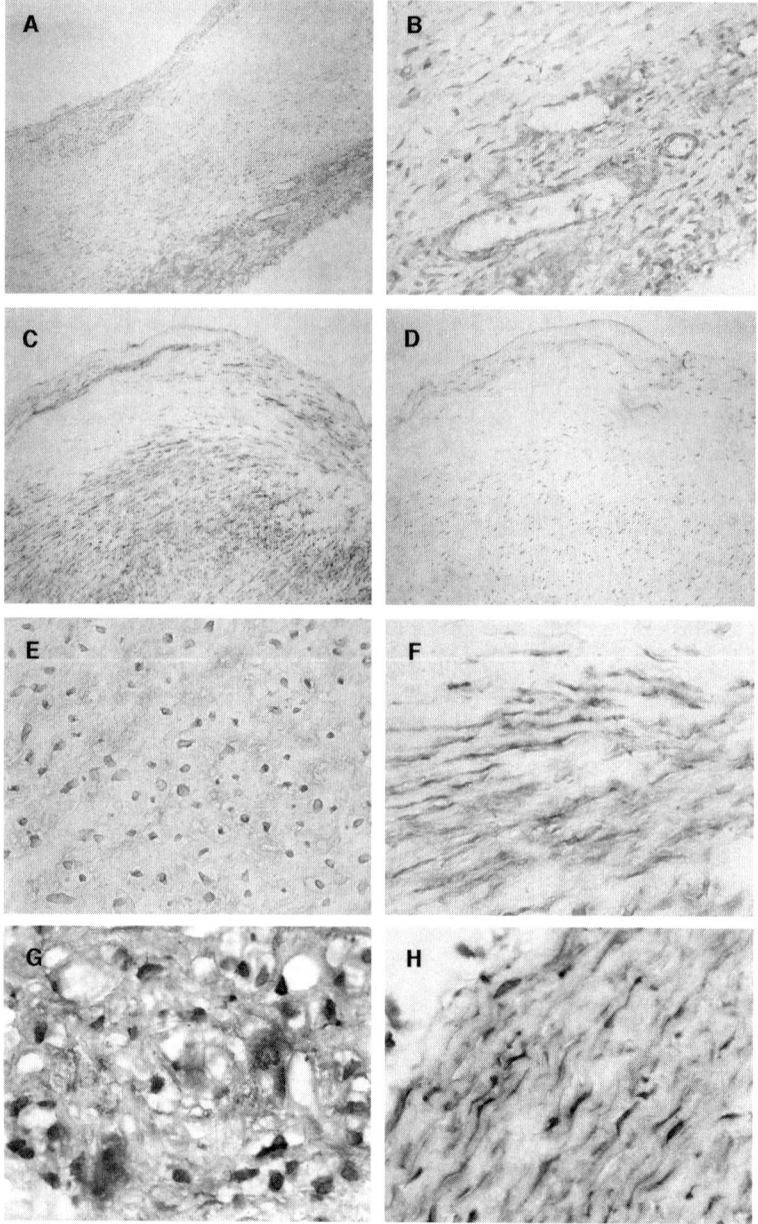

FIGURE 3. Immunohistostaining of advanced atherosclerotic lesions. (**A** and **B**) Sections were stained with anti–hLOX-1 monoclonal antibody. Intimal neovascular endothelium as well as intimal nonendothelial cells expressed hLOX-1. (**A**, ×100, **B**, ×400). (**C–F**) Cryostat serial sections of advanced atherosclerotic lesions were stained with the anti–

TABLE 1. Distribution of LOX-1 expression in the intima[a]

	Number of positive segments (%)		
	Arterial luminal endothelial cells	Intimal neovasculature	Intimal nonendothelial cells
Early lesions	15/21 (71.4%)	NA	21/21 (100%)
Advanced lesions	7/21 (33.3%)	10/18 (55.6%)	21/21 (100%)

[a]Early lesions indicate samples distant from the center of the plaques. Early lesions, which showed some subendothelial infiltrates, did not contain a lipid core or fibrous cap. Advanced lesions indicate samples that consisted of fibrofatty plaques. A total of 21 early lesions and 21 advanced lesions were examined in this study. Intimal neovasculature was not seen in any samples of early lesions. Of the segments with advanced lesions in this study, 18 of 21 (85.7%) had neovessel infiltration into the intima.

LOX-1 expression on luminal endothelial cells was confirmed by staining of an adjacent section with an anti–von Willebrand factor antibody (FIG. 2E) and double-label immunostaining (FIG. 2F) in early atherosclerotic lesions. In contrast, luminal endothelial cells in advanced atherosclerotic plaques were less frequently positive for LOX-1 expression. LOX-1 expression in association with arterial luminal endothelial cells was present in 71.4% of samples with early lesions and in 33.3% of samples with advanced lesions (TABLE 1). These results suggest that LOX-1 expression on luminal endothelial cells appears to be upregulated especially in the early stage of atherogenesis. LOX-1 has been shown to be upregulated by an inflammatory cytokine TNF-α,[10] phorbol ester,[10] and fluid shear stress[11] in cultured bovine aortic endothelial cells. Expression of LOX-1 *in vivo*, therefore, may also be upregulated in arterial endothelial cells by these humoral and hemodynamic factors.

In advanced atherosclerotic plaques, neovascular formation in the intima was frequently observed. In this study, 18 of 21 (85.7%) samples had infiltration of neovessels into the intima. In these microvascular endothelial cells, expression of LOX-1 was often observed (FIG. 3A and B). LOX-1 expression on endothelial cells of intimal neovasculature was present in 55.6% of advanced atherosclerotic plaques with intimal neovasculature (TABLE 1). Given the fact that LOX-1 is expressed on endo-

---

hLOX-1 monoclonal antibody (**C**, ×100) and nonimmune mouse IgG (**D**, ×100). LOX-1 was expressed by nonendothelial cells in the intima of advanced atherosclerotic lesions. Higher power view of **C** showed that LOX-1–positive subendothelial cells included round-shaped cells consistent with the morphology of macrophages (**E**, ×1,000) and spindle-shaped cells consistent with that of smooth muscle cells (**F**, ×1,000). (**G** and **H**) Double-label immunohistostaining with the anti–LOX-1 monoclonal antibody and antibodies for cell markers of advanced atherosclerotic lesions. Cell marker antibodies were visualized by an alkaline phosphatase method and appeared red, while the anti–bLOX-1 antibody was marked with an ABC-peroxidase technique and appeared dark blue. (**G**, ×1,000) Double immunohistostaining of the anti–hLOX-1 antibody (*dark blue*) and the anti–CD68 antibody (*red*). (**H**, ×1,000) Double immunohistostaining of the anti–hLOX-1 antibody (*dark blue*) and the anti–smooth muscle alpha actin antibody (*red*). LOX-1 was expressed by some macrophages (**G**) and smooth muscle cells (**H**) in advanced atherosclerotic intima.

thelium of intimal neovasculature, Ox-LDL uptake through LOX-1 in intimal neovascular endothelium may play an important role in endothelial activation in these microvessels.

In addition to vascular endothelium, cells consisting of neointima of advanced atherosclerotic plaques were also positive for LOX-1 expression (FIG. 3C–F). These LOX-1–positive nonendothelial cells were present in all the samples in this study (TABLE 1). Double-label immunohistochemistry confirmed that LOX-1 expression was observed in intimal smooth muscle cells and macrophages (FIG. 3G and H). CD3-positive T lymphocytes in the arterial intima did not show any significant staining with the anti–LOX-1 monoclonal antibody (data not shown).

Previous studies have demonstrated that MSR-A is expressed by macrophages accumulated in the intima of human atherosclerotic plaques[12] In contrast, MSR-A expression by smooth muscle cells in human atherosclerotic lesions has not been demonstrated,[12] although studies with hypercholesterolemic rabbits have shown that MSR-A is expressed by intimal smooth muscle cells.[13] Taken together, LOX-1, in addition to MSR-A, may play important roles in foam cell transformation of macrophages and smooth muscle cells. Especially in human atherosclerotic lesions, LOX-1 may play a major role in foam cell transformation of intimal smooth muscle cells. The present immunohistochemical study, for the first time, revealed that LOX-1 was also expressed by macrophages and smooth muscle cells *in vivo*, although this novel receptor for Ox-LDL was originally identified in cultured bovine aortic endothelial cells.[8] These results *in vivo* appear to be supported by the fact that LOX-1 is expressed on human and murine macrophages although expressed only weakly at best on circulatory monocytes.[14,15] LOX-1 expression in cultured vascular smooth muscle cells has also been shown (Kume and colleagues, manuscript submitted for publication).

In summary, the present study provides evidence that LOX-1 is expressed on luminal endothelial cells, especially in the early stage of atherogenesis, and on intimal neovascular endothelial cells. More importantly, LOX-1 was highly expressed by macrophages and smooth muscle cells accumulated into the intima of human carotid atherosclerotic plaques. Further studies related to regulatory mechanisms of LOX-1 expression in various cell types, as well as pathophysiological consequences of Ox-LDL uptake through this novel Ox-LDL receptor, may provide new insights into the pathogenesis of atherosclerosis.

REFERENCES

1. GIMBRONE, M.A. JR., M.I. CYBULSKY, N. KUME, T. COLLINS & N. RESNICK. 1995. Vascular endothelium: an integrator of pathophysiological stimuli in atherogenesis. Ann. N.Y. Acad. Sci. **748:** 122–132.
2. ROSS, R. 1993. The pathogenesis of atherosclerosis: a perspective for the 1990's. Nature **362:** 801–809.
3. KODAMA, T., M. FREEMAN, L. ROHRER, J. ZABRECKY, P. MATSUDAIRA & M. KRIEGER. 1990. Type I macrophage scavenger receptor contains alpha-helical and collagen-like coiled coils. Nature **343:** 531–535.
4. ENDEMANN, G., L.W. STANTON, K.S. MADDEN, C.M. BRYANT, R.T. WHITE & A.A. PROTTER. 1993. CD36 is a receptor for oxidized low density lipoprotein. J. Biol. Chem. **268:** 11811–11816.
5. ACTON, S.L., P.E. SCHERER, H.F. LODISH & M. KRIEGER. 1994. Expression cloning of SR-BI, a CD36-related class B scavenger receptor. J. Biol. Chem. **269:** 21003–21009.

6. RAMPRASAD, M.P., W. FISCHER, J.L. WITZTUM, G.R. SAMBRANO, O. QUEHENBERGER & D. STEINBERG. 1995. The 94- to 97-kDa mouse macrophage membrane protein that recognizes oxidized low density lipoprotein and phosphatidylserine-rich liposomes is identical to macrosialin, the mouse homologue of human CD68. Proc. Natl. Acad. Sci. USA **92:** 9580–9584.
7. KRIEGER, M., S. ACTON, J. ASHKENAS, A. PEARSON, M. PENMAN & D. RESNICK. 1993. Molecular flypaper, host defence, and atherosclerosis. Structure, binding properties, and functions of macrophage scavenger receptors. J. Biol. Chem. **268:** 4569–4572.
8. SAWAMURA, T., N. KUME, T. AOYAMA, H. MORIWAKI, Y. AIBA, T. TANAKA, S. MIWA, Y. KATSURA, T. KITA & T. MASAKI. 1997. A novel receptor for oxidized low-density lipoprotein. Nature **386:** 73–77.
9. MORIWAKI, H., N. KUME, T. SAWAMURA, T. AOYAMA, H. HOSHIKAWA, H. OCHI, E. NISHI, T. MASAKI & T. KITA. 1998. Ligand specificity of LOX-1, a novel endothelial receptor for oxidized low density lipoprotein. Arterioscler. Thromb. Vasc. Biol. **18:** 1541–1547.
10. KUME, N., T. MURASE, H. MORIWAKI, T. AOYAMA, T. SAWAMURA, T. MASAKI & T. KITA. 1998. Inducible expression of lectin-like oxidized LDL receptor-1 in vascular endothelial cells. Circ. Res. **83:** 322–327.
11. MURASE, T., N. KUME, R. KORENAGA, J. ANDO, T. SAWAMURA, T. MASAKI & T. KITA. 1998. Fluid shear stress transcriptionally induces lectin-liKe oxidized LDL receptor-1 in vascular endothelial cells. Circ. Res. **83:** 328–333.
12. YLA-HERTTUALA, S., M.E. ROSENFELD, S. PARTHASARATHY, E. SIGAL, T. SARKIOJA, J.L. WITZTUM & D. STEINBERG. 1991. Gene expression in macrophage-rich human atherosclerotic lesions: 15-lipoxygenase and acetyl low density lipoprotein receptor messenger RNA colocalize with oxidation specific lipid-protein adducts. J. Clin. Invest. **87:** 1146–1152.
13. LI, H., M.W. FREEMAN & P. LIBBY. 1995. Regulation of smooth muscLE cell scavenger receptor expression in vivo by atherogenic diets and in vitro by cytokines. J. Clin. Invest. **95:** 122–133.
14. MORIWAKI, H., N. KUME, H. KATAOKA, T. MURASE, E. NISHI, T. SAWAMURA, T. MASAKI & T. KITA. 1998. Expression of lectin-like oxidized low density lipoprotein receptor-1 in human and murine macrophages. Upregulated expression by TNF-α. FEBS Lett. **440:** 29–32.
15. YOSHIDA, H., N. KONDRATENKO, S. GREEN, D. STEINBERG & P. QUEHENBERGER. 1998. Identification of the lectin-like receptor for oxidized low-density lipoprotein in human macrophages and its potential role as a scavenger receptor. Biochem. J. **334:** 9–13.

Chylomicron Remnant Induces Apoptosis in Vascular Endothelial Cells

SATORU KAWASAKI, TAKAHIRO TANIGUCHI,[a] YOSHIO FUJIOKA,[b]
AKIHIRO TAKAHASHI, TOMOSABURO TAKAHASHI, KOJI DOMOTO,
MASAKO TAGUCHI, YUICHI ISHIKAWA,[c] AND MITSUHIRO YOKOYAMA

First Department of Internal Medicine and [c]The Faculty of Health Science, Kobe University School of Medicine, Kobe,650-0017, Japan

[b]The First Department of Internal Medicine, Hyogo College of Medicine, Nishinomiya, 663-8501, Japan

INTRODUCTION

Chylomicron remnant (CR) is a cholesterol- and apoE-enriched particle derived from the lipolytic processing of intestinal chylomicron, and has been regarded as an atherogenic lipoprotein in postprandial hyperlipidemia.[1,2] However, little is known about the mechanisms through which CR promotes atherosclerosis. Recent studies suggest that remnant lipoproteins induce vascular endothelial dysfunction assessed by measuring endothelium-dependent vasorelaxation.[3] Endothelial injury and dysfunction induced by atherogenic lipoprotein are believed to play pivotal roles in atherogenesis. Apoptosis in endothelial cell is considered to be involved in this process.[4,5] This hypothesis is supported by the findings that proatherosclerotic factors, such as oxidized low density lipoprotein (LDL), reactive oxygen species, and inflammatory cytokines, have all been shown to induce apoptosis of vascular endothelial cells.[6,7]

We postulated that CR may promote atherosclerosis by inducing apoptosis in vascular endothelial cells. To examine our hypothesis, we isolated CR and investigated whether CR induces apoptosis in vascular endothelial cells *in vitro*.

METHODS

Preparation of CR

Chylomicron was isolated by ultracentrifugation from lymph that was collected from gastrostomized SD rats fed egg solution for 48 h. The functional hepatectomy, which consisted of the ligation of mesenteric arteries, celiac artery, and portal vein and the resection of the entire digestive tract, was performed as previously described.[8] These hepatectomized rats were injected with chylomicron and exsanguinated after 3 hours. Finally, CR was isolated from the plasma of these hepatectomized rats by ultracentrifugation.

---

[a]Address for correspondence: Takahiro Taniguchi, M.D., The First Department of Internal Medicine, Kobe University School of Medicine, 7-5-1, Kusunoki-cho, Chuo-ku, Kobe, 650-0017, Japan. Voice: 81-78-382-5846; fax: 81-78-382-5859.

taniguch@med.kobe-u.ac.jp

Cell Culture

Cultured human umbilical vein endothelial cells (HUVEC) were isolated by collagenase digestion and grown in RPMI 1640 medium with 20% (vol/vol) heat-inactivated fatal calf serum and endothelial cell growth factor on gelatin-coated dishes. Bovine aortic endothelial cells (BAEC) were grown in DMEM with 10% (vol/vol) heat-inactivated fetal calf serum.

Cell Viability Assay

HUVECs cultured at 1×10^4 cells per well of 96-well plates were treated at 37°C for indicated periods of time with CR or in RPMI 1640 medium supplemented with 1% heat-inactivated fetal calf serum. At the end of each incubation, the viable cells were measured with WST-1 reagent (Boeringher Mannheim) according to the manufacturer's procedure.

Analysis for Apoptotic cells

Confluent BAECs were incubated for 24 h with CR in serum-free DMEM. 90% confluent HUVEC were also incubated for 24 h with CR in RPMI 1640 medium supplemented with 1% heat-inactivated fetal calf serum. Cells were fixed and stained by the TdT-mediated dUTP nick end labeling (TUNEL) procedure using biotin-dUTP or FITC-dUTP, and subsequently observed by microscopy. At 6 h incubation, annexin-V binding to cell membrane and cell membrane integrity were assessed by flow cytometry using FITC–annexin-V and propidium iodide.

Immunoblot Analysis

HUVECs were treated for 16 h with CR (10 µg protein/ml) in RPMI 1640 supplemented with 1% heat-inactivated fetal calf serum. Protein from cell lysates was subjected to SDS-PAGE on 10% gels, and p12 and p20 active subunits of human CPP32 were detected by Western blotting using enhanced chemiluminescence.

RESULTS AND DISCUSSION

First, we analyzed apoproteins and lipid compositions of isolated CR. Analysis of the apoprotein content of CR by SDS-PAGE revealed that apoE content of CR was markedly increased compared to that of chylomicron (data not shown). It is well known that the acquisition of apoE is the most obvious change in protein composition during the conversion of chylomicron to CR. We observed that the cholesterol-triglyceride ratio was remarkably increased in CR by 17-fold compared to chylomicron (data not shown). These data verified that isolated CR was a cholesterol- and apoE-enriched particle caused by lipolysis and cholesterol transfer from HDL. In standard experiment, we used CR at the concentration of 10 µg protein/ml, which is supposed to be the physiological plasma concentration of CR based on the fact that remnant-like particle (RLP) cholesterol used in clinical diagnosis is within 5 mg cholesterol/dl in normal subjects.

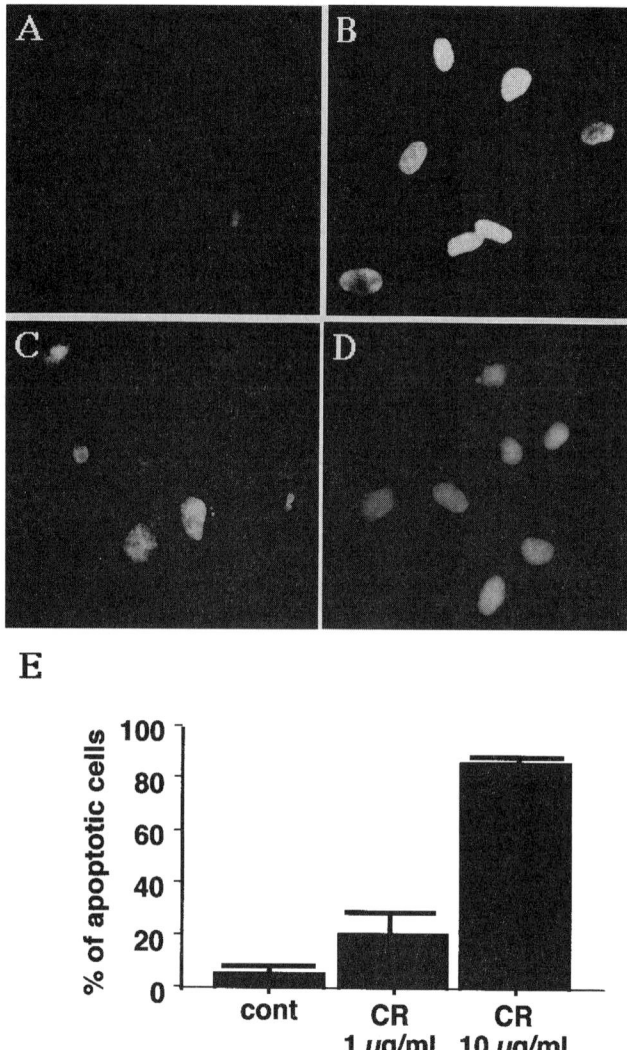

FIGURE 1. (A–D) Induction of apoptosis in HUVEC by chylomicron remnant analyzed by FITC-labeled TUNEL staining. 90% confluent HUVEC were either untreated (**A**), or treated with DNase for 30 min before the TUNEL staining (**B**), or treated with 100 μg protein/ml oxidized LDL (**D**) or 10 μg protein/ml chylomicron remnant (**C**) in RPMI 1640 supplemented with 1% heat-inactivated fetal calf serum. After 24-h incubation, cells were stained by the TUNEL procedure using FITC-conjugated dUTP, and subsequently observed by fluorescence microscopy. (**E**) Induction of apoptosis in BAEC by CR analyzed by TUNEL staining. Confluent BAECs were incubated for 24 h with CR in serum-free DMEM. Cells were fixed and stained by TUNEL procedure. The proportion of TUNEL-positive cells is expressed as the number of TUNEL-positive cells percent cells. The results are representative of three different preparations of CR.

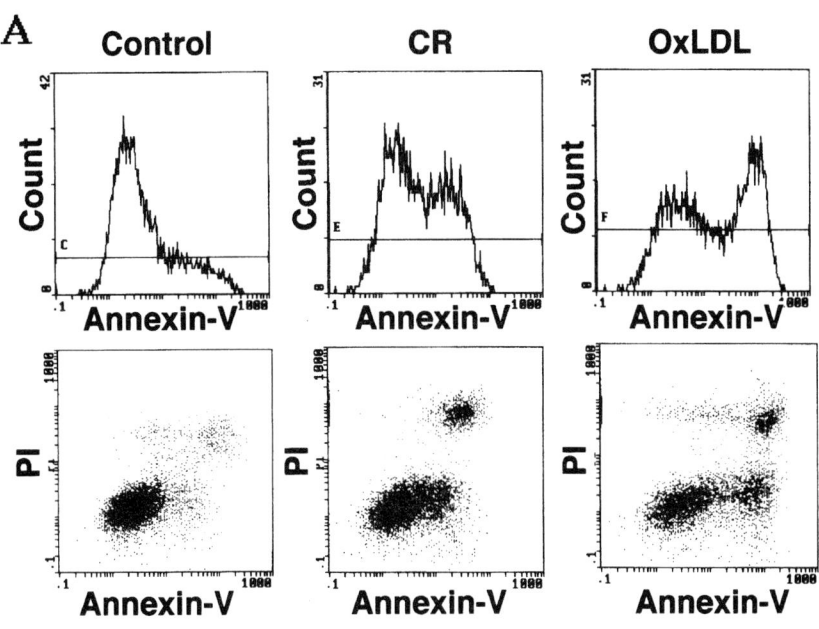

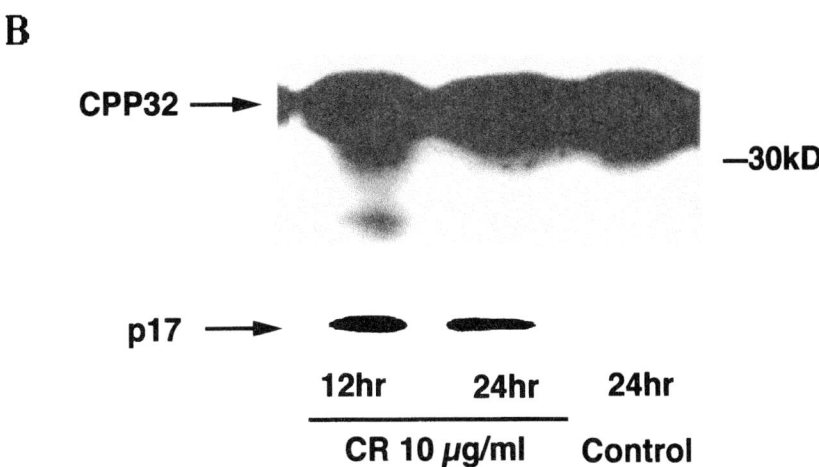

FIGURE 2. (**A**) Flow cytometry analysis of annexin-V binding to cell membrane, which is one of characteristics of early apoptotic cells. After incubation of HUVEC, as described in the legend of *Figure 1*, for 6 h. The results are representative of three different preparations of chylomicron remnants. (**B**) Activation of CPP32 by CR in HUVEC. HUVEC were treated for indicated times with CR (10 μg protein/ml) in RPMI 1640 supplemented with 1%

Next, we examined the effect of CR on cell viability of HUVEC and BAEC by WST-1 assay. WST-1 assay demonstrated that CR reduced the number of viable cells in a dose- and time-dependent manner. In contrast chylomicron did not affect the cell viability at the concentration of chylomicron containing the equal amount of triglyceride to that of CR (data not shown).

To evaluate apoptosis, we quantified apoptotic cells by TUNEL staining. After 24 h treatment of HUVEC with CR at the concentration of 10 µg protein/ml, the number of TUNEL-positive cells were significantly increased compared to that of control cultures (FIG. 1A and C), and condensed or fragmented nuclei, i.e., characteristics of apoptotic cells, were identified among CR-treated HUVEC. Similar observations were revealed in oxidized LDL-treated HUVEC (FIG. 1D). After 24 h treatment of BAEC with CR at the concentration of 1 µg protein/ml, the number of TUNEL-positive cells were significantly increased compared to that of control cultures. When CR was used at 10 µg protein/ml, the proportion of TUNEL-positive cells reached almost 80% (FIG. 1E). To further investigate the effect of CR on endothelial cells, we analyzed the population of HUVECs with increased annexin-V binding to cell membrane, which is one of the characteristics of early apoptotic cells. As shown in FIGURE 2A, FACScan analysis demonstrated that CR increased the population of HUVECs with increased annexin-V binding to cell membrane at 6 h treatment. This population maintained a low staining with propidium iodide, which is indicative of membrane integrity (FIG. 2A). Therefore, this result revealed that CR caused early apoptotic change on HUVEC at 6-h incubation. Since it has been shown that apoptosis can be induced by the members of ICE-like proteases including CPP32/Caspase-3, and that oxidized LDL induces apoptosis of human endothelial cells by activation of CPP32-like proteases, we examined the effect of CR on CPP32 activation.[9,10] Western blot analysis showed that CR induced the proteolytic cleavage of CPP32 into its active subunit p17 in HUVEC (FIG. 2B).

In conclusion, our data demonstrates that CR causes endothelial injury by induction of apoptosis and suggests that CPP32 activation could be involved in this process. We propose that this effect of CR may contribute to its atherogenicity.

REFERENCES

1. ZILVERSMIT, D.B. 1979. Atherogenesis: a postprandial phenomenon. Circulation **60:** 473–485.
2. KARPE, F & A. HAMSTEN. 1995. Postprandial lipoprotein metabolism and atherosclerosis. Curr. Opin. Lipidol. **6:** 123–129.
3. KUGIYAMA, K. 1998. Association of remnant lipoprotein levels with impairment of endothelium-dependent vasomotor function in human coronary arteries. Circulation **97:** 2519–2526.
4. FRENCH, J.E. 1996. Atherosclerosis in relation to the structure and function of the arterial intima, with special reference to the endothelium. Int. Rev. Exp. Pathol. **5:** 253.
5. ROSS, R. 1993. The pathogenesis of atherosclerosis: a perspective for the 1990s. Nature **362:** 801.

---

heat-inactivated fetal calf serum. Protein from cell lysates was subjected to SDS-PAGE on 10% gels, and p12 and p20 active subunits of human CPP32 were detected by Western blot analysis. The results are representative of three experiments.

6. ZHAO, B. *et al.* 1995. Endothelial cells injured by oxidized low density lipoproteins. Am. J. Hematol. **49:** 250–252.
7. HAENDELER, J., A.M. ZEIHER & S. DIMMELER. 1996. Vitamins C and E prevent lipopolysaccharide-induced apoptosis in human endothelial cells by modulation of Bcl-2 and Bax. Eur. J. Pharmacol. **317:** 407–411.
8. COOPER, A.D. & P.Y.S. YU. 1978. Rates of removal and degradation of chylomicron remnants by isolated perfused rat liver. J. Lipid Res. **19:** 635–643.
9. ENARI, M. *et al.* 1996. Sequential activation of ICE-like and CPP32-like proteases during Fas-mediated apoptosis. Nature **380:** 723–726.
10. DIMMELER, S. *et al.* 1997. Oxidized low-density lipoprotein induces apoptosis of human endothelial cells by activation of CPP32-like proteases. Circulation **95:** 1760–1763.

Granulocyte Macrophage Colony-Stimulating Factor Plays a Priming Role in Murine Macrophage Growth Induced by Oxidized Low Density Lipoprotein

AKIRA MIYAZAKI,[a] TAKESHI BIWA,[a,b] HIDEKI HAKAMATA,[a] MASAKAZU SAKAI,[b] YUICHIRO SAKAMOTO,[a] KYU KYU MAUNG,[a] MEHTAP YUKSEL,[a] AND SEIKOH HORIUCHI[a,c]

[a]*Department of Biochemistry and* [b]*Department of Metabolic Medicine, Kumamoto University School of Medicine, Kumamoto 860-0811, Japan*

INTRODUCTION

One of the characteristic events in the atherosclerotic lesion is the proliferation of cellular components. It is generally accepted that smooth muscle cells migrated from media into intima proliferate in the atherosclerotic lesions. It was recently demonstrated, however, that macrophages also proliferate in the early stage of atherosclerotic lesions.[1]

Using an *in vitro* culture system, we have shown that macrophages obtained from mouse,[2–5] rat,[6] and human[7] are able to proliferate upon incubation with oxidized LDL (Ox-LDL). It then becomes clear that the specific uptake of lysophosphatidylcholine (lyso-PC) of Ox-LDL through the macrophage scavenger receptor type A-I/A-II (MSR-AI/AII) is essential for Ox-LDL–induced macrophage proliferation.[3,5,7] The activation of protein kinase C (PKC) was also shown to be involved in this phenomenon.[8] These *in vitro* observations strongly suggest that Ox-LDL acts as a growth factor for macrophage *in vivo*. The present study was undertaken to elucidate the molecular cascade(s) leading to Ox-LDL–induced macrophage proliferation. The results indicate that Ox-LDL–mediated release of granulocyte macrophage colony-stimulating factor (GM-CSF) from macrophages may play an important role in macrophage proliferation.

MATERIALS AND METHODS

Cell Culture

Murine peritoneal macrophages were collected from male DDY mice with 8 ml ice-cold PBS and suspended in RPMI 1640 supplemented with 10% heat-inactivated

[c]Address for correspondence: Seikoh Horiuchi, M.D., Ph.D., Professor and Chairman, Department of Biochemistry, Kumamoto University School of Medicine, 2-2-1 Honjo, Kumamoto 860-0811, Japan. Fax: 81-96-364-6940; Voice: 81-96-373-5068.
horiuchi@gpo.kumamoto-u.ac.jp

newborn calf serum. Cell suspensions were dispersed in each well and incubated for 90 min for adherence.

Determination of Macrophage Proliferation

The macrophage monolayers (5×10^4 cells/well in 24-well tissue culture plates) were cultured with 1 ml of RPMI 1640 medium in the presence of the lipoproteins to be tested. After a 5-day incubation, [^{3}H]thymidine incorporation assay was performed as described previously.[9] The number of adhered cells were counted at day 7.[9]

GM-CSF Analyses

Cells were incubated with Ox-LDL for various periods followed by extraction of total RNA with TRIzol. The levels of GM-CSF mRNA expression were determined by Northern blotting as well as RT-PCR as described.[9] The concentration of GM-CSF in the medium was determined by an ELISA kit purchased from Amersham.[9]

RESULTS AND DISCUSSION

Effect of Medium Exchange on Ox-LDL–Induced Macrophage Proliferation

To test whether a soluble factor secreted from macrophages is involved in Ox-LDL–induced macrophage growth, we examined the effect of medium exchange on macrophage proliferation. Incubation of macrophages with 20 µg/ml of Ox-LDL for 5 days without medium exchange resulted in a significant [^{3}H]thymidine incorporation. However, when macrophages were incubated with Ox-LDL for 5 days, replacing the medium at day 1 or 2 by fresh medium containing the same concentration of Ox-LDL, [^{3}H]thymidine incorporation was markedly reduced by 75% or 60%, respectively.[9] In contrast, replacement of the medium at day 3 or 4 did not affect [^{3}H]thymidine incorporation. Cell-counting assay showed a consistent result, suggesting that a soluble factor(s) released from macrophages by Ox-LDL into the medium during day 1 to 2 may be involved in the induction of macrophage proliferation by Ox-LDL.

An Anti–GM-CSF Antibody Suppresses Ox-LDL–Induced Macrophage Proliferation

We next examined the effects of neutralizing antibodies against four cytokines, such as GM-CSF, M-CSF, IL-3, and IL-5, on Ox-LDL–induced macrophage proliferation. The anti–GM-CSF antibody significantly suppressed [^{3}H]thymidine incorporation by 80%, whereas the other antibodies had no effect (FIG. 1). The cell-counting assay also showed a consistent result, suggesting the involvement of GM-CSF in Ox-LDL–induced macrophage proliferation.

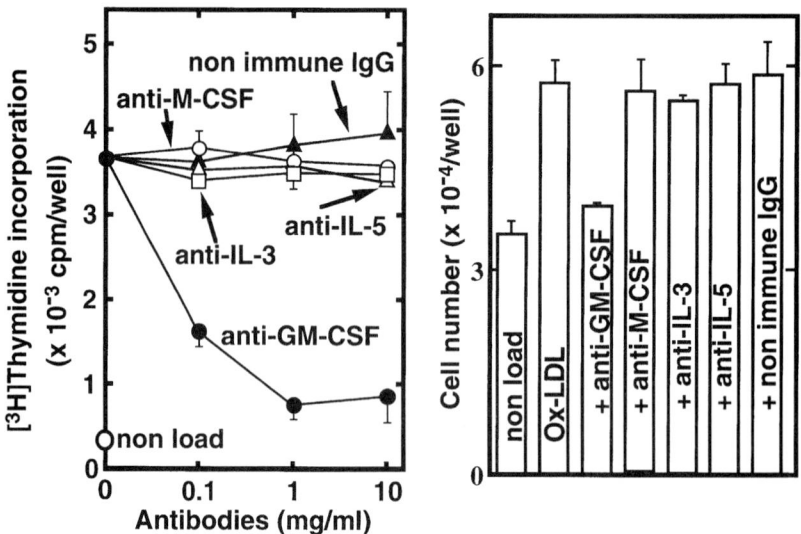

FIGURE 1. Anti–GM-CSF antibody inhibits Ox-LDL–induced macrophage growth. Mouse macrophages (5×10^4 cells/well) were incubated with 20 μg/ml of Ox-LDL in the absence or presence of various antibodies against cytokines such as GM-CSF, M-CSF, IL-3, and IL-5. Macrophage proliferation was determined by [^{3}H]thymidine incorporation (*left*) or by cell counting (*right*).

Ox-LDL Induces GM-CSF Expression in Macrophages

We also examined whether Ox-LDL could induce mRNA expression of GM-CSF. Time course studies by RT-PCR showed that a 368 bp band of GM-CSF appeared at 30 min and reached a peak at 1 h when cells were incubated with Ox-LDL. Northern blot analysis also showed induction of GM-CSF mRNA by Ox-LDL.[9]

In the next step, we determined whether Ox-LDL could induce GM-CSF secretion into the medium from macrophages. The concentrations of GM-CSF in the medium increased by addition of Ox-LDL and reached a peak level at 4 h, followed by a time-dependent decrease to basal level at 24 hours.[9] Thus, the increase in GM-CSF mRNA by Ox-LDL is linked to the subsequent release of GM-CSF protein into the medium. Taken into consideration with the inhibitory effect of an anti–GM-CSF antibody on Ox-LDL–induced macrophage proliferation, Ox-LDL–induced macrophage growth was mediated by GM-CSF released from macrophages in an autocrine or paracrine manner.

Mechanism of GM-CSF Induction in Macrophages by Ox-LDL

To elucidate the involvement of lyso-PC in induction of GM-CSF by Ox-LDL, we examined the effect of phospholipase A_2 (PLA_2)–treated acetyl-LDL on GM-CSF secretion. Upon treatment with PLA_2, 75% of the total PC in acetyl-LDL was converted to lyso-PC and a significant growth-promoting activity appeared. Although untreated acetyl-LDL did not increase GM-CSF concentration in the medium, PLA_2-treated acetyl-LDL significantly induced GM-CSF secretion.[9] Secretion of GM-CSF by PLA_2-treated acetyl-LDL was less than half of Ox-LDL, suggesting that some other components in Ox-LDL are also involved in GM-CSF production in macrophages.

To characterize the role of MSR-AI/AII, Ox-LDL–induced GM-CSF secretion from macrophages obtained from MSR-AI/AII-knockout mice was compared with those from their wild-type littermates. The level of GM-CSF release induced by Ox-LDL from MSR (–) macrophages was reduced by 75% as compared with that from MSR (+) macrophages.[9] It is therefore likely that MSR-mediated endocytosis of lyso-PC (or some other components) also plays a crucial role in Ox-LDL–induced GM-CSF production.

To evaluate the role of PKC in GM-CSF production, we tested the effect of calphostin C, a PKC inhibitor, on Ox-LDL–induced GM-CSF release. Ox-LDL–induced GM-CSF release was effectively inhibited by calphostin C in a dose-dependent manner,[9] suggesting the involvement of PKC activation in Ox-LDL–induced GM-CSF production.

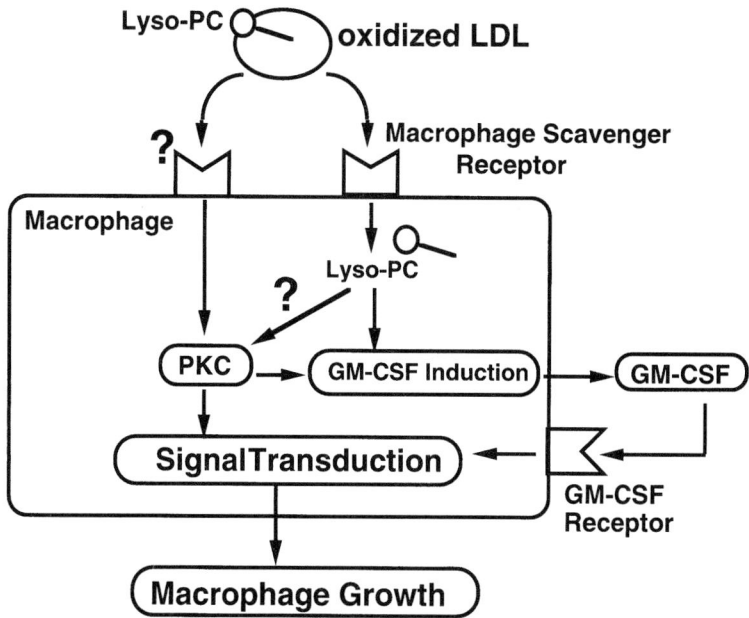

FIGURE 2. The possible mechanism of macrophage growth by Ox-LDL. Endocytic uptake lyso-PC (or some other components) in Ox-LDL through macrophage scavenger receptors induces PKC activation. This PKC activation induces mRNA expression of GM-CSF and its secretion. Secreted GM-CSF acts on macrophages in an autocrine or paracrine fashion and induces macrophage proliferation. It is possible that another receptor for Ox-LDL and a cytokine(s) other than GM-CSF are also involved in Ox-LDL–induced macrophage growth.

CONCLUSIONS

The possible mechanism of macrophage growth by Ox-LDL is summarized in FIGURE 2. Endocytic uptake of mitogenic components in Ox-LDL including lyso-PC through MSR induces PKC activation followed by GM-CSF expression and secretion. Secreted GM-CSF acts on macrophages in an autocrine or paracrine fashion and induces macrophage growth. It is also suggested that a soluble factor(s) other than GM-CSF or another receptor for Ox-LDL is involved in Ox-LDL–induced macrophage proliferation.

REFERENCES

1. SAKAI, M. et al. 1997. Role of macrophage scavenger receptor for internalization of lysophosphatidylcholine in oxidized low density lipoprotein-induced macrophage growth. Ann. N.Y. Acad. Sci. **811:** 378–384.
2. YUI, S. et al. 1993. Induction of murine macrophage growth by modified LDLs. Arterioscler. Thromb. **13:** 331–337.
3. SAKAI, M. et al. 1994. Lysophosphatidylcholine plays an essential role in the mitogenic effect of oxidized low density lipoprotein on murine macrophages. J. Biol. Chem. **269:** 31430–31435.
4. SAKAI, M. et al. 1997. HMG-CoA inhibitors suppress macrophage growth induced by oxidized low density lipoprotein. Atherosclerosis **133:** 51–59.
5. SAKAI, M. et al. 1996. The scavenger receptor serves as a route for internalization of lysophosphatidylcholine in oxidized low density lipoprotein-induced macrophage proliferation. J. Biol. Chem. **271:** 27346–27352.
6. SATO, Y. et al. 1996. Lipoprotein (a) induces cell growth in rat peritoneal macrophages through inhibition of transforming growth factor-β activation. Atherosclerosis **125:** 15–26.
7. SAKAI, M. et al. 1996. Lysophosphatidylcholine potentiates the mitogenic activity of modified LDL for human monocyte-derived macrophages. Arterioscler. Thromb. Vasc. Biol. **16:** 600–605.
8. MATSUMURA, T. et al. 1997. Two intracellular signaling pathways for activation of protein kinase C are involved in oxidized low-density lipoprotein-induced macrophage growth. Arterioscler. Thromb. Vasc. Biol. **17:** 3013–3020.
9. BIWA, T. et al. 1998. Induction of murine macrophage growth by oxidized low density lipoprotein is mediated by granulocyte macrophage colony-stimulating factor. J. Biol. Chem. **273:** 28305–28313.

Transgenic Rabbits Expressing Human Apolipoprotein(a) as a Useful Model for the Study of Lipoprotein(a)[a]

JIANGLIN FAN,[b] MIREILLE CHALLAH, HIROAKI SHIMOYAMADA, AND TERUO WATANABE

Department of Pathology, Institute of Basic Medical Sciences, University of Tsukuba, Tsukuba, Japan

INTRODUCTION

The lipoprotein(a) [Lp(a)] particle closely resembles low-density lipoprotein (LDL) in both lipid composition and the presence of apolipoprotein B-100 (apoB-100). Lp(a) is distinguished from LDL by the presence of an additional protein component designated as apolipoprotein (a) [apo(a)], which is complexed to apoB-100 by disulfide linkage.[1] A number of studies,[2,3] but not all,[4,5] have shown that elevated plasma Lp(a) constitutes an independent risk factor for coronary heart disease and restenosis. However, the study of human Lp(a) has been hampered due to the lack of appropriate animal models since apo(a) is found only in primates and humans. In addition, human apo(a) in transgenic mice can not bind to murine apoB to form Lp(a) particles.[6] To create a new, relatively large-animal model for the study of the biological functions of Lp(a), we developed a transgenic rabbit model that expresses human apo(a) in the plasma.[7]

EXPERIMENTAL PROCEDURES AND RESULTS

For the pronuclear microinjection, we used two human apo(a) transgenic constructs that consisted of the full-length human apo(a) cDNA fragment containing 17 copies of kringle 4 repeats under the control of either the mouse transferrin promoter (pTfHa17) or the human apoAI promoter (pAIHa17),[6,8] which were kindly provided by Dr. M.R. Lawn. Among 93 pups analyzed by Southern blot analysis, we obtained 11 transgenic rabbits. However, only three TfHa17 transgenic rabbit founders exhibited detectable apo(a) in the plasma as shown in Western blot analysis (FIG. 1). These three transgenic rabbit founders expressed human apo(a) in their plasma at ~1.8

---

[a]This work was supported by Grants-in-Aid for scientific research from the Ministry of Education, Science, and Culture of Japan, Ono Medical Foundation, Japan, Uehara Memorial Foundation, Japan, Japan Heart Foundation, Japan, Tokyo Biochemical Research Foundation, Ichiro Kanehara Foundation, Takeda Medical Research Foundation, and Japan Society for the Promotion of Sciences (JSPS-RFTF96I00202).

[b]Address for correspondence: Jianglin Fan, M.D., Ph.D., Department of Pathology, Institute of Basic Medical Sciences, University of Tsukuba, Tsukuba 305-8575, Japan. Voice: 81-298-53-3165; fax: 81-298-53-3262.
j-lfan@md.tsukuba.ac.jp

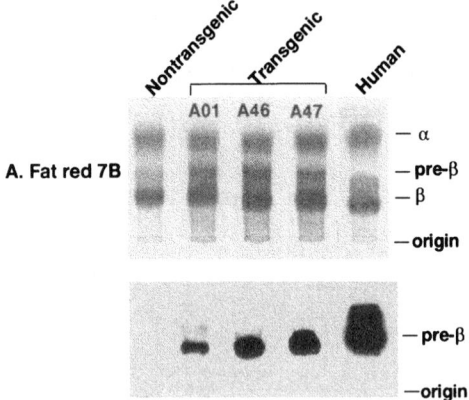

FIGURE 1. Agarose gel electrophoresis of the plasma from human apo(a) transgenic rabbits. Plasma (2 μl) was electrophoresed on a 1% agarose gel; the gels were either stained for neutral lipids with Fat red 7B (**A**) or used for Western blotting probed with anti–human apo(a) mAb (**B**). Lanes 1, plasma from nontransgenic rabbit; lanes 2–4, plasma from three independent transgenic rabbit founders (A01, A46, A47); lane 5, plasma from a normolipidemic human subject.

(A01 line), ~3.4 (A46 line), and ~4.5 mg/dl (A47 line) as quantitated by apo(a)-specific ELISA. Human apo(a) in the founder transgenic rabbit plasma was located in the pre-β position, with a similar mobility to that of human plasma apo(a) (FIG. 1). In human populations, the apo(a) concentration in the plasma ranges from 0.1~100 mg/dl, with the distribution skewed to lower concentrations.[1] The plasma level (~4.5 mg/dl) of apo(a) in the transgenic rabbits is equivalent to a relatively low level of apo(a) in humans. By Northern blot analysis, we found that the human apo(a) mRNA was expressed mainly in the liver and slightly in the kidney of transgenic rabbits. To study whether human apo(a) can bind to rabbit apoB to form Lp(a) complex, we analyzed transgenic rabbit plasma Lp(a) by Western blot analysis.[6] We found that human apo(a) in transgenic rabbit was variously associated with rabbit apoB although some amounts of apo(a) existed in a free form in the plasma (FIG. 2). Under nonreducing conditions, the apo(a)/apoB complex in transgenic rabbit plasma existed as a large molecular weight form similar to human Lp(a) (FIG. 2). This complex was dissociated under reducing conditions, suggesting that Lp(a) complex in transgenic rabbits are bound by disulfate linkage. Lp(a)-like particle formation in transgenic rabbit plasma was further indicated by the colocalization of apo(a) with apoB at the pre-β position within the same density fractions. The efficient assembly of Lp(a) particles in transgenic rabbits is consistent with a recent report by others.[9] Thus, the human apo(a) transgenic rabbits provide a useful animal model for the study of human Lp(a). By crossbreeding human apo(a) transgenic rabbits with WHHL rabbits, which have defective LDL receptor (LDLr) functions, we were able to study whether LDLr is involved in the catabolism of Lp(a). We found that in het-

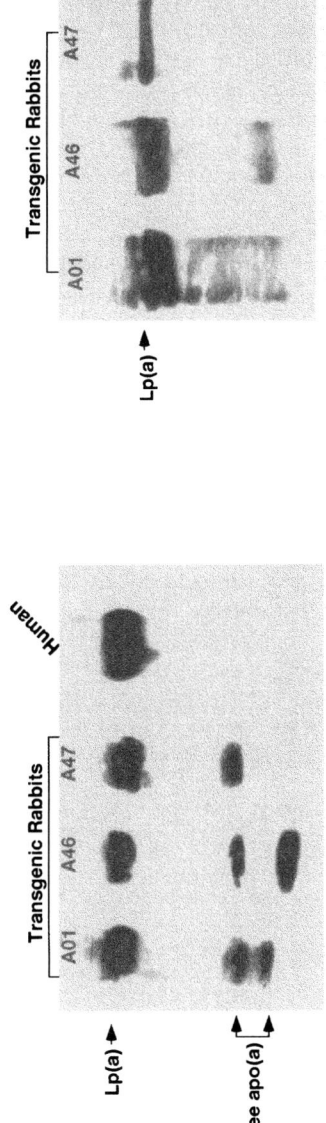

FIGURE 2. Immunoblotting analysis of transgenic rabbit plasma apo(a). Aliquots of plasma from three transgenic founder rabbits were separated by either 3.5% nondenaturing polyacrylamide gel electrophoresis (**A**) or 3.5% SDS-PAGE (**B**) under nonreducing conditions. After electrophoretic transfer, the proteins were immunoblotted using an anti–human apo(a) mAb. Human plasma was used as a control.

erozygous WHHL transgenic rabbits (apo(a)+/0/LDLr–/+), pre-β lipoproteins were markedly increased accompanied by a twofold increase in the plasma Lp(a) compared with apo(a)+/0 rabbits with normal LDLr function. Since hepatic production of apo(a) in apo(a) transgenic WHHL rabbits was unchanged, absence of a functional LDLr results in a reduced catabolism of plasma Lp(a) in human apo(a) transgenic WHHL rabbits.[10] This result is consistent with the study by Liu and colleagues who demonstrated that in WHHL rabbits, there is a delayed catabolism of injected ^{125}I-labeled human Lp(a) compared to normal rabbits.[11] In addition to providing important insights into Lp(a) assembly and apo(a) expression, several unique features of transgenic rabbits may make them a good model for the study of Lp(a) and atherosclerosis.[12] In this respect, we fed five transgenic rabbits (A01 line) and eight nontransgenic littermate rabbits a diet containing 0.3% cholesterol for 16 weeks. Transgenic rabbits showed similarly elevated cholesterol levels response to a cholesterol-diet compared with nontransgenic rabbits. However, human apo(a) transgenic rabbits showed more extensive atherosclerotic lesions than nontransgenic rabbits in the aorta and coronary artery (Fan and colleagues, unpublished data). In addition, we have found that apo(a) and apoB are colocalized in atherosclerotic lesions in the aorta and coronary arteries of the transgenic rabbits fed on a cholesterol-rich diet, suggesting that Lp(a) may confer proatherogenic effects in the setting of a cholesterol-rich diet in transgenic rabbits.

CONCLUSIONS

An Lp(a) transgenic rabbit model was established. Human apo(a) in transgenic rabbits showed an efficient assembly of Lp(a) through the disulfate linkage.

On a cholesterol-rich diet, Lp(a) transgenic rabbits showed more extensive lesion development in the aorta and coronary artery than those of nontransgenic rabbits. This transgenic model should provide a useful model for the study of Lp(a) functions and its role in atherosclerosis.

REFERENCES

1. UTERMANN, G. 1989. The mysteries of lipoprotein(a). Science **246:** 904–910.
2. SCANU, A.M., R.M. LAWN & K. BERG. 1991. Lipoprotein(a) and atherosclerosis. Ann. Intern. Med. **115:** 209–218.
3. MAHER, V.M. & B.G. BROWN. 1995. Lipoprotein (a) and coronary heart disease. Curr. Opin. Lipid. **6:** 229–235.
4. JAUHIAINEN, M., P. KOSKINEN, C. EHNHOLM, M.H. FRICK, M. MANTTARI, V. MANNINEN & J.K. HUTTUNEN. 1991. Lipoprotein (a) and coronary heart disease risk: a nested case-control study of the Helsinki Heart Study participants. Atherosclerosis **89:** 59–67.
5. RIDKER, P.M., C.H. HENNEKENS & M.J. STAMPFER. 1993. A prospective study of lipoprotein(a) and the risk of myocardial infarction. J. Am. Med. Assoc. **270:** 2195-2199.
6. CHIESA, G., H.H. HOBBS, M.L. KOSCHINSKY, R.M. LAWN, S.D. MAIKA & R.E. HAMMER. 1992. Reconstitution of lipoprotein(a) by infusion of human low density lipoprotein into transgenic mice expressing human apolipoprotein(a). J. Biol. Chem. **267:** 24369–24374.
7. FAN, J., M. ARAKI, L. WU, M. CHALLAH, H. SHIMOYAMADA, M.R. LAWN, H. KAKUTA, H. SHIKAMA & T. WATANABE. 1999. Assembly of lipoprotein (a) in transgenic rab-

bits expressing human apolipoprotein (a). Biochem. Biophys. Res. Commun. **255:** 639–644.
8. BOONMARK, N. W., X.J. LOU, Z.J. YANG, K. SCHWARTZ, J.L. ZHANG, E.M. RUBIN & R.M. LAWN. 1997. Modification of apolipoprotein(a) lysine binding site reduces atherosclerosis in transgenic mice. J. Clin. Invest. **100:** 558–564.
9. ROUY, D., N. DUVERGER, S.D. LIN, F. EMMANUEL, L.M. HOUDEBINE, P. DENEFLE, C. VIGLIETTA, E. GONG, E.M. RUBIN & S.D. HUGHES. 1998. Apolipoprotein(a) yeast artificial chromosome transgenic rabbits. Lipoprotein(a) assembly with human and rabbit apolipoprotein B. J. Biol. Chem. **273:** 1247–1251.
10. FAN, J. *et al.* 2000. Defect of the LDL receptor in WHHL transgenic rabbits leads to a marked accumulation of plasma lipoprotein(a). J. Lipid Res. In press.
11. LIU, R., K. SAKU, G.M. KOSTNER, K. HIRATA, B. ZHANG, M. SHIOMI & K. ARAKAWA. 1993. In vivo kinetics of lipoprotein (a) in homozygous Watanabe heritable hyperlipidaemic rabbits. Eur. J. Clin. Invest. **23:** 561–565.
12. FAN, J., M. CHALLAH & T. WATANABE. 1999. Transgenic rabbit model for biomedical research. Pathol. Intl. **49:** 583–594.

The Role of Remnant Lipoproteins in Atherosclerosis

AKIO KAWAKAMI,[a] AKIRA TANAKA, TAKAMITSU NAKANO,[b]
KATSUYUKI NAKAJIMA,[b] AND FUJIO NUMANO

Third Department of Internal Medicine, Tokyo Medical and Dental University,
1-5-45 Yushima, Bunkyo-ku, Tokyo 113-8519 Japan

[b]Japan Immunoresearch Laboratories, 351-1 Nishiyokote-cho, Takasaki,
Gumma 370-0021 Japan

INTRODUCTION

In recent years, attention has been focused on the relationship between atherosclerosis and triglyceride-rich lipoproteins (TRL), in particular, remnant lipoproteins produced by hydrolysis of chylomicron and VLDL.[1–7] Some of the foam cells found in the fatty streak and fibrous plaques are considered to originate from vascular smooth muscle cells (SMC), which migrate from the media to the intima.[8,9] Regarding the contribution of SMC to atherosclerosis, we investigated the effect of remnant-like particles (RLP) and oxidized RLP on SMC proliferation *in vitro*.

RLP were separated from human plasma in postprandial state using an immunoaffinity gel containing anti–human apo A-I and anti–human apo B-100 monoclonal antibodies.[10,11] The particles in the RLP fraction consist of chylomicron (CM) remnants and very low density lipoprotein (VLDL) remnants.[10,11]

MATERIALS AND METHODS

Four patients with hypertriglyceridemia were selected for the present study. None of the patients was given antioxidants, lipid-lowering agents, or insulin injection. Blood was taken at two hours after their usual meal. VLDL (defined as lipoproteins that float in the ultracentrifuge at a density of 1.006 g/ml) was isolated from serum.

Immunoaffinity gel (RLP-C Kit, JIMRO, Takasaki, Japan) contained 5 mg each of anti–apo B 100 and anti–apo A-I IgG antibody coupled with 1 ml of CNBr-Sepharose 4B gel. RLP was separated from VLDL using the immunoseparation technique; briefly, immunoaffinity gel was added at 300 µl per 5 µl of VLDL and was left standing for 15 min after gentle shaking for 60 min at room temperature. Within the immunoaffinity gel, nascent VLDL particles containing apo B-100 adsorb to anti–apo B 100 IgG antibody, while nascent chylomicrons containing apo A-I adsorb to anti–apo A-I IgG antibody. The supernatant (unbound fraction) was recovered as

---

[a]Address for correspondence: Dr. Akio Kawakami, Third Department of Internal Medicine, Tokyo Medical and Dental University, 1-5-45 Yushima, Bunkyo-ku, Tokyo 113-8519 Japan. Voice: 81-3-5803 5231; fax: 81-3-5803-0133.
akio-ka@mx6.mesh.ne.jp

RLP.[10,11] The lipoprotein particles in the RLP fraction are rich in particles containing apo E, apo B-48, and apo B-100 with multiple molecules of apo E that have not been recognized by the anti–apo B-100 antibody.[10,11] RLP primarily represent VLDL remnants and chylomicron remnants.

VLDL and RLP were diluted to 200 µg protein/ml with PBS[12] and then oxidized by incubating with 5 µM Cu^{2+} for 24 h at 37°C in a CO_2 incubator to obtain oxidized VLDL (oxVLDL) and oxidized RLP (oxRLP). Lipid peroxide levels were determined as thiobarbituric acid reactive substances (TBARS) before and after oxidation.[13] TBARS values were expressed as nmol/mg protein.

Porcine coronary artery smooth muscle cells were seeded in 96-well plates at a concentration of 3×10^3/well. Then, 100 µl of Dulbecco's modified Eagle's medium (DMEM) containing 10% fetal bovine serum, 100 IU/ml penicillin, and 100 µg/ml streptomycin (GIBCO BRL, Scotland) was added to each well and the plates were cultured for 48 h at 37°C in a CO_2 incubator.

The medium in each well was replaced with 100 µl of DMEM containing a 10% volume of VLDL, oxVLDL, RLP, or oxRLP at a concentration of 20 µg protein/ml. After starting the incubation with lipoproteins, the cells were counted at 0, 24, 48, 72, and 96 h by the WST-1 method using a cell-counting kit (Wako, Japan).[14] The proliferation index (PI) with each lipoprotein was calculated as the ratio of the number of SMC at an indicated time to the cell count at time 0 (taken as 1).

Data are analyzed using analysis of variance (ANOVA). Results are expressed as the mean ± S.E.M.

RESULTS

TBARS values were 2.27 ± 0.41, 24.7 ± 1.54, 6.01 ± 0.94, 7.46 ± 0.65 for PBS, VLDL, oxVLDL, RLP, and oxRLP, respectively (FIG. 1). TBARS value showed a marked increase of about 10-fold upon incubation of VLDL with Cu^{2+}. TBARS also showed an increase of about 1.2-fold upon incubation of RLP with Cu^{2+}. These results indicated that RLP was more resistant to oxidation by Cu^{2+} than VLDL. However, RLP showed a significantly higher TBARS value than VLDL before oxidation, indicating that there were greater lipid peroxides present in native RLP than in VLDL.

The SMC proliferation assay was performed using lipoprotein preparations. The sum of PI values at 24, 48, 72, and 96 h (ΣPI) was compared to assess the enhancement of SMC proliferation by each lipoprotein fraction. ΣPI were 1.83 ± 0.85, 1.95 ± 0.70, 2.75 ± 0.52, 3.30 ± 0.65, and 3.55 ± 0.46 after incubation with PBS, VLDL, oxVLDL, RLP, and oxRLP, respectively (FIG. 2). Incubation with VLDL caused no significant difference of ΣPI compared with PBS. However, ΣPI was significantly higher with RLP compared with VLDL. The results indicated that RLP significantly enhance SMC proliferation *in vitro*.

ΣPI of oxidized lipoproteins (oxVLDL and oxRLP) was compared with the native VLDL or RLP. Incubation with oxVLDL showed a significantly higher ΣPI than with VLDL. oxRLP also showed a higher ΣPI than RLP, but the difference was not statistically significant. Native VLDL showed little enhancement of SMC proliferation. However, when VLDL was oxidized, it appeared to significantly enhance SMC proliferation. In contrast, RLP did not show a greater proliferative effect upon oxidation, but native RLP had about the same proliferative effect as oxidized VLDL.

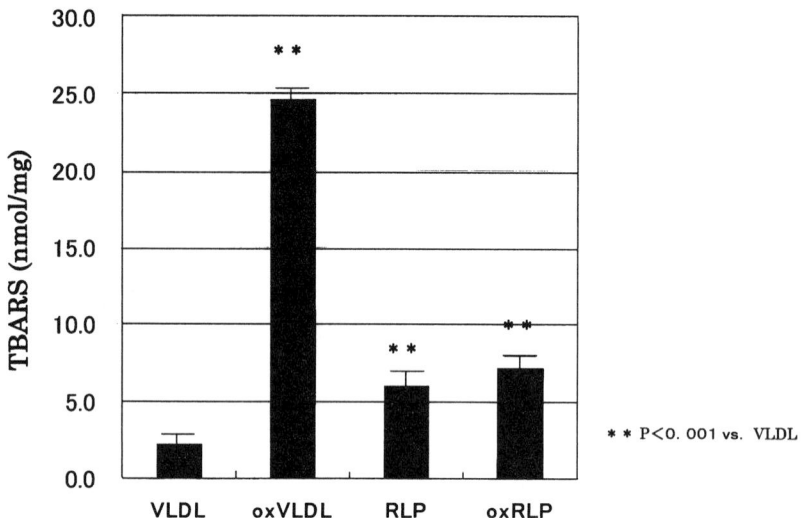

FIGURE 1. Effects of oxidative modification on thiobarbituric acid reactive substances (TBARS) of VLDL and RLP. Oxidation was performed by incubating VLDL and RLP at a concentration of 200 µg protein/ml with PBS containing 5 µM $CuSO_4$ for 24 hours. Values are mean ± S.E.M. for TBARS of each lipoprotein. **$p < 0.001$ versus VLDL.

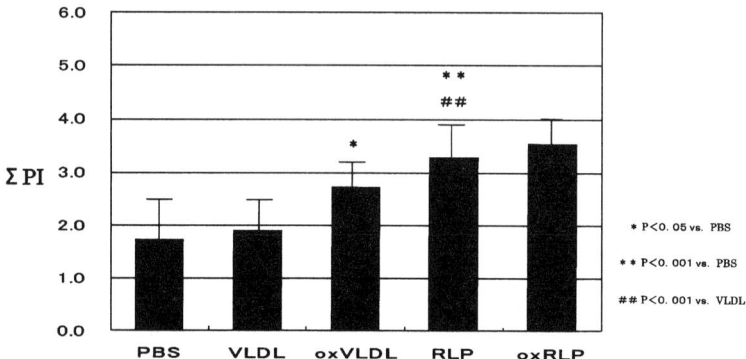

FIGURE 2. Comparison of various lipoprotein preparations to enhance SMC proliferation. Values are mean ± S.E.M. for total PI at 24, 48, 72, and 96 hours (ΣPI) for each lipoprotein preparation and PBS. **$p < 0.001$ versus PBS. ##$p < 0.001$ versus VLDL. +$p < 0.05$ versus oxVLDL.

DISCUSSION

To date, the relationship between atherosclerosis and serum lipids has been studied mainly with respect to LDL or oxidized LDL.[15–17] However, many studies have reported elevation of TRL in patients with coronary artery disease without marked hypercholesterolemia.[1–3] It has also been shown that postprandial hypertriglyceridemia could be a coronary risk factor.[4]

The present study showed that RLP significantly enhanced SMC proliferation *in vitro*, indicating that remnant lipoproteins may promote atherosclerosis by stimulating SMC proliferation. Since VLDL did not enhance SMC proliferation, the proliferative effect of RLP is considered to be an intrinsic property. When oxidized, VLDL also had a significant proliferative effect, which is reported here for the first time. Remnants are supposed to be taken up by macrophages, vascular wall cells, and other cells that express the scavenger receptor or remnant receptors, thus promoting atherosclerosis.[18,19]

In the present study, we examined whether oxidative modification of TRL, such as VLDL and RLP, influences their ability to enhance SMC proliferation as is seen with LDL.[17] SMC proliferation was markedly enhanced when VLDL was oxidized. However, this was not true for RLP, and RLP showed much smaller changes in TBARS values after oxidation with Cu^{2+} compared with VLDL.

Although the TBARS level of RLP was higher than that of VLDL, the following results suggested that the proliferative effect of RLP did not necessarily depend on the lipid peroxides content. (1) Even if not oxidized, RLP caused the same or greater enhancement of SMC proliferation compared with oxVLDL. (2) Oxidation of RLP did not significantly increase SMC proliferation compared to native RLP.

In conclusion, the results of the present study indicate that remnant lipoproteins directly enhance SMC proliferation and, therefore, may promote atherosclerosis. RLP exert SMC proliferative effects even if they are not oxidized, which is in a striking contrast to LDL and VLDL.

REFERENCES

1. SIMONS, L.A., T. DWYER, J. SIMONS, L. BERNSTEIN, P. MOCK, N.S. POONIA, S. BALASUBRAMANIAM, D. BARON, J. BRANSON, J. MORGAN & P. ROY. 1987. Chylomicrons and chylomicron remnants in coronary artery disease: a case control study. Atherosclerosis **65:** 181–189.
2. GROOT, P.H.E., W.A.H.J. VAN STIPHOUT, X.H. KRAUSS, H. JANSEN, A. VAN TOL, E. VAN RAMHORST, S. CHIN-ON, A. HOFMAN, S.R. CRESSWELL & L. HAVEKES. 1991. Postprandial lipoprotein metabolism in normolipidemic men with and without coronary artery disease. Arterioscler. Thromb. **11:** 653–662.
3. PATSCH, J.R., G. MEISENBOCK, T. HOPFERWEISER, V. E. MUHLBERGER, KNAPP, J.K. DUNN, A.M. GOTTO & W. PATSCH. 1992. Relation of triglyceride metabolism and coronary artery disease: studies in the postprandial state. Arterioscler. Thromb. **12:** 1336–1345.
4. KARPE, F., G. STEINER, K. UFFELMAN, T. OLIVECRONA & A. HAMSTEN. 1994. Postprandial lipoproteins and progression of coronary atherosclerosis. Atherosclerosis **106:** 83–97.
5. RAPP, J.H., A. LESPINE, R.L. HAMILTON, N. COLYVAS, A.H. CHAUMETON, J. TWEEDIE-HARDMAN, L. KOTITE, S.T. KUNITAKE, R.J. HARVEL & J.P. KANE. 1994. Triglyceride-rich lipoproteins isolated by selected-affinity anti-apolipoprotein B immunosorption from human atherosclerotic plaque. Arterioscler. Thromb. **14:** 1767–1774.

6. ZILVERSMIT, D.B. 1995. Atherogenic nature of triglycerides, postprandial lipidemia, and triglyceride-rich remnant lipoproteins. Clin. Chem. **41:** 153–158.
7. TANAKA, A, N. TOMIE, T. NAKANO, K. NAKAJIMA, K. YUI, M. TAMURA & F. NUMANO. 1998. Measurement of postprandial remnant-like particles (RLPs) following a fat-loading test. Clin. Chim. Acta **275:** 43–52
8. FAGGIOTTO, A. & R. ROSS. 1984. Studies of hypercholesterolemia in the non human primates. II. Fatty streak conversion to fibrous plaque. Arteriosclerosis **4:** 25–34.
9. SCHWARTZ, S.M., G.R. CAMPBELL & J.H. CAMPBELL. 1986. Replication of smooth muscle cells in vascular disease. Circ. Res. **58:** 427–444.
10. CAMPOS, E., K. NAKAJIMA, A. TANAKA & R.J. HAVEL. 1992. Properties of an apolipoprotein E-enriched fraction of triglyceride-rich lipoproteins isolated from human blood plasma with a monoclonal antibody to apolipoprotein B-100. J. Lipid Res. **33:** 369–380.
11. NAKAJIMA, K., T. SAITO, A. TAMURA, T. SUZUKI, T. NAKANO, M. ADACHI, A. TANAKA & N. TADA. 1993. A new assay method for the quantification of cholesterol in remnant like lipoproteins in human serum using monoclonal anti apo B-100 and apo A-I immunoaffinity mixed gels. Clin. Chim. Acta **223:** 53–71.
12. LOWRY, O.H., N.J. ROSEBROUGH, A.L. FARR & R.J. RANDALL. 1951. Protein measurement with the Folin phenol reagent. J. Biol. Chem. **193:** 265–275.
13. MIHARA, M. & M. UCHIYAMA. 1978. Determination of malondialdehyde precursor in tissues by thiobarbituric acid test. Anal. Biochem. **86:** 271–278.
14. ISHIYAMA, M., M. SHIGA, K. SASAMOTO, M. MIZOGUCHI & H. PIN-GANG. 1993. A new sulfonated tetrazolium salt that produces a highly water-soluble formazan dye. Chem. Pharm. Bull. **41:** 1118–1122.
15. HENRIKSEN, T., E.M. MAHONEY & D. STEINBERG. 1981. Enhanced macrophage degradation of low density lipoprotein previously incubated with cultured endothelial cells: recognition by receptors for acetylated low density lipoproteins. Proc. Natl. Acad. Sci. USA **78:** 6499–6503.
16. WITZTUM, J.L. & D. STEINBERG. 1991. Role of oxidized low density lipoprotein in atherogenesis. J. Clin. Invest. **88:** 1785–1792.
17. CHATTERJEE, S. & N. GHOSH. 1996. Oxidized low density lipoprotein stimulates aortic smooth muscle cell proliferation. Glycobiology **6:** 303–311.
18. TOMONO, M., S. KAWAZU & N. KATO. 1994. Uptake of remnant like particles (RLP) in diabetic patients from mouse peritoneal macrophages. J. Atheroscl. Thromb. **1:** 98–102.
19. WHITMAN, S.C., D.B. MILLER, B.M. WOLFE, R.A. HEGELE & M.W. HUFF. 1997. Uptake of type III hypertriglyceridemic VLDL by Macrophages is enhanced by oxidation, especially after remnant formation. Arterioscler. Thromb. Vasc. Biol. **17:** 1707–1715.

Enhanced Expression of Osteopontin by High Glucose

Involvement of Osteopontin in Diabetic Macroangiopathy[a]

MINORU TAKEMOTO,[b,c] KOUTARO YOKOTE,[c] MASASHI YAMAZAKI,[d] AMY L. RIDALL,[e,f] WILLIAM T. BUTLER,[e] TARO MATSUMOTO,[c] KEN TAMURA,[c] YASUSHI SAITO,[c] AND SEIJIRO MORI[c]

[c]Second Department of Internal Medicine and [d]Department of Orthopedics, School of Medicine, Chiba University, 1-8-1 Inohana, Chuou-ku, Chiba 260-0856, Japan

[e]Departments of Basic Science and [f]Prosthodontics, Dental Branch, University of Texas Houston-Health Science Center, Houston, Texas 77030, USA

ABSTRACT: Atherosclerotic vascular disease is a major complication of diabetic patients. Osteopontin has recently been implicated in the development of atherosclerosis. In the present study, we have investigated the effects of high glucose on expression of osteopontin in cultured rat aortic smooth muscle cells. High concentrations of glucose increased osteopontin secretion from the cells, and the increased secretion was completely inhibited by an inhibitor of protein kinase C, GF109203X. Northern blot analysis confirmed the enhanced effect of glucose on expression of osteopontin mRNA. Promoter activity of osteopontin, measured using the osteopontin promoter/luciferase expression vector system, was increased by high glucose, and the enhanced effect was completely inhibited by GF109203X. Glucosamine also increased the promoter activity of osteopontin. Azaserine, an inhibitor of glutamine:fructose-6-phosphate amidotransferase, the key enzyme of the hexosamine pathway, profoundly inhibited high glucose–mediated increase in the promoter activity. Taken together, these data indicate that high glucose enhances the expression of osteopontin at the transcriptional level possibly through the activation of protein kinase C as well as the hexosamine pathway. Our results suggest that osteopontin could play a role in the development of diabetic vascular complications.

INTRODUCTION

Diabetic patients are prone to atherosclerotic vascular diseases such as ischemic heart disease and arteriosclerosis obliterance.[1,2] It is also known that diabetic vascular lesions tend to undergo restenosis after angioplasty and often display linear-type

---

[a]This work was supported by grants from the Ministry of Education, Science, Sports and Culture of Japan (Nos. 10163204 and 10044239) and from Japan Foundation of Cardiovascular Research. K.Y. is a Research Fellow of the Japan Society for the Promotion Science.

[b]Address for correspondence: Minoru Takemoto, Second Department of Internal Medicine, School of Medicine, Chiba University, 1-8-1 Inohana, Chuou-ku, Chiba 260-0856, Japan. Voice: 81-43-226-2089; fax: 81-43-226-2095.
mtakemo@intmed02.m.chiba-u.ac.jp

calcification.[3,4] However, the reason for the accelerated atherogenesis in diabetes mellitus has not been fully understood.

Several proteins have been shown to be highly expressed in calcified atheromatous plaques,[5] among which is osteopontin (OPN). OPN was originally purified from bone,[6] and has been independently identified by different laboratories in different tissues, namely, the loop of Henle and the distal convoluted tubes in kidney, blood vessels, inner ear, epithelial cells of the gallbladder, urinary tract, gastrointestinal tract, and mammary gland (reviewed in Refs. 7 and 8). OPN is a negatively charged glycosylated phosphoprotein with a 32,000 molecular weight backbone. It has an E-F hand-like Ca^{2+} binding site and an RGD cell adhesion sequence common to many integrin ligands.[9] Overexpression of OPN was found in several physiological as well as pathological conditions including immunological disorders,[10] neoplastic transformation,[11] progression of metastasis,[12] formation of urinary stones,[13] and wound healing.[14]

It was reported that OPN stimulated migration of rat and bovine vascular smooth muscle cells (SMC) via its action through integrin β3.[15,16] Furthermore, OPN was found to potently enhance platelet-derived growth factor–induced proliferation of cultured human arterial SMC.[17] Neutralizing antibodies directed against OPN inhibited rat carotid neointimal thickening after endothelial denudation.[18] These reports have suggested the involvement of OPN, in addition to its possible contribution to calcification process, in the development of atherosclerosis especially in the process of intimal thickening. Indeed, it was also reported that high levels of OPN mRNA and protein were detectable in the rat and human aorta and carotid arteries during neointima formation[19–21] and that selective αvβ3 integrin blockade potently limited neointimal hyperplasia and lumen stenosis following deep coronary arterial stent injury.[22]

The present study was undertaken to gain more insight into the mechanism of the development of diabetic vascular complications. We demonstrate that incubation of cultured rat aortic SMC in the medium containing higher concentrations of glucose increases the expression of OPN at the transcriptional level possibly through the activation of protein kinase C as well as the hexosamine pathway. Our data, together with previous reports suggesting the involvement of OPN in atherogenesis, imply that OPN plays a causative role in the accelerated atherogenesis in diabetes mellitus.

METHODS AND RESULTS

High Glucose Enhances OPN Secretion through the Activation of Protein Kinase C in Cultured SMC

We first examined the effect of high glucose on OPN secretion by cultured rat aortic SMC. The cells were incubated in the culture medium containing either 5.5 mM, 25 mM glucose, or 25 mM glucose in the presence of the protein kinase C inhibitor, GF109203X, for five days. The medium was exchanged every two days. On the fifth day, the medium was replaced with serum-free medium and was collected after 48 h of incubation. The conditioned medium was subjected to Western blotting with the anti-OPN antibody. As shown in FIGURE 1A, 66 kD multiple bands, which most likely represent heterogeneously phosphorylated OPN molecules,[6] were detected in each lane. Treatment of the cells with high concentration of glucose (25 mM) dra-

A

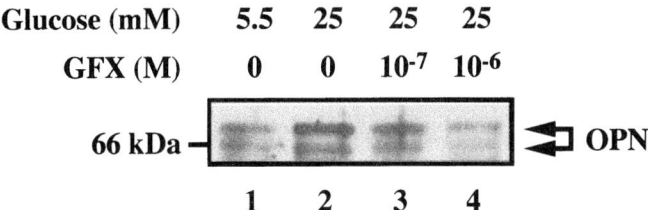

B

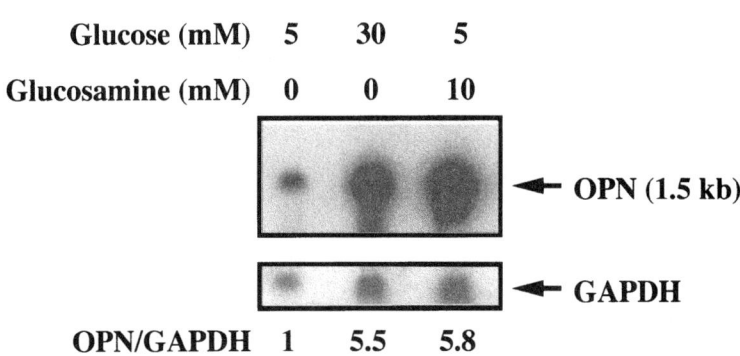

FIGURE 1. (A) Effect of high glucose on OPN secretion by cultured rat aortic SMC. The cells were incubated in the culture medium containing either 5.5 mM glucose, 25 mM glucose, or 25 mM glucose with the indicated concentrations of GF109203X (GFX) for 5 days. Thereafter the medium was replaced with serum-free medium and was collected after 48 h of incubation. OPN was semipurified from the conditioned medium using DE52 anion exchanger gel as described[33] and subjected to SDS-10% PAGE. The materials were transferred to a nitrocellulose membrane. The membrane was immunoblotted with the anti-OPN antibody. Sites of antibody binding were visualized using the ECL Western blotting detection system (Amersham). No significant differences were found in the number of the cells for each condition counted after removal of the conditioned medium. (B) Effects of high glucose and glucosamine on OPN transcript level in cultured rat aortic SMC. The cells were incubated in the culture medium containing 5 mM or 30 mM glucose, or 5 mM glucose and 10 mM glucosamine, for five days. After incubation, total RNA was isolated and Northern hybridization was performed essentially as described[34] using ^{32}P-labeled rat OPN cDNA probe or rat glyceraldehyde-3-phosphate dehydrogenase (GAPDH) cDNA probe, and signals were detected by autoradiography.

matically increased the intensity of the OPN bands (lane 2). In contrast, treatment with 25 mM D-mannitol, providing an equivalent osmolarity as 25 mM glucose, did not change the intensity of the bands (data not shown), suggesting that the observed enhanced effect on OPN secretion is specific to glucose. It was also found that GF109203X dose-dependently inhibited high glucose–mediated increase in the intensity of the OPN bands (FIG. 1A, lanes 3 and 4). These data indicate that high glucose enhances OPN secretion possibly through the activation of protein kinase C in cultured rat aortic SMC.

High Glucose Enhances the Expression of OPN at the Transcriptional Level in Cultured SMC

Next, we examined the effect of high glucose on the transcriptional level of OPN in cultured rat aortic SMC by Northern blotting. The cells were incubated in the culture medium containing 5 mM or 30 mM glucose for five days. The medium was exchanged every two days. On the fifth day, total RNA was isolated and subjected to Northern blotting using the OPN cDNA probe. As shown in FIGURE 1B, a 1.5 kb band, which represents the OPN mRNA, was detected in each lane and relative ratios of OPN density and GAPDH density were determined. Treatment of the cells with 30 mM glucose increased the intensity of the OPN band by approximately 5.5-fold. These data indicate that high glucose increases the transcript level of OPN in cultured rat aortic SMC.

We then examined the effect of high glucose on OPN promoter activity in cultured rat aortic SMC using the OPN promoter/luciferase expression vector system. The cells were transfected with the OPN promoter/luciferase construct. The transfected cells were incubated in various concentrations of glucose with or without the protein kinase C inhibitor, GF109203X, or incubated in 50 mM L-glucose or 50 mM D-mannitol for 24 h. After incubation, luciferase activity of the cell lysates was measured. As shown in FIGURE 2A, the luciferase activity was stimulated with the increased concentrations of glucose and reached the maximal level at 30–50 mM glucose. Treatment with GF109203X dose-dependently inhibited high glucose–mediated increase in the luciferase activity, as expected. Again, it was confirmed that treatment with either 50 mM L-glucose or 50 mM D-mannitol did not appreciably change the luciferase activity. These data indicate that high glucose–stimulated expression of OPN is mediated at the transcriptional level and is possibly dependent on the activation of protein kinase C.

High Glucose–Stimulated Transcription of OPN Is also Mediated by the Hexosamine Pathway

Recently, several reports have suggested that the end product of the hexosamine biosynthetic pathway, UDP-N-acetylglucosamine, mediates some of high glucose–induced biological responses.[23–25] Therefore, we also examined the effect of glucosamine on luciferase activity of the OPN promoter/luciferase construct–transfected cells. As shown in FIGURE 2B, glucosamine dose-dependently increased the luciferase activity. Furthermore, treatment of the cells with azaserine, an inhibitor of glutamine:fructose-6-phosphate amidotransferase, the key enzyme of the hexosamine pathway,[23] profoundly inhibited high glucose–mediated increase in the lu-

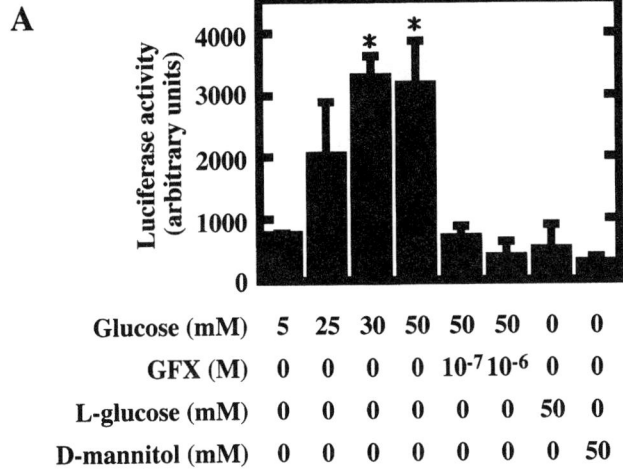

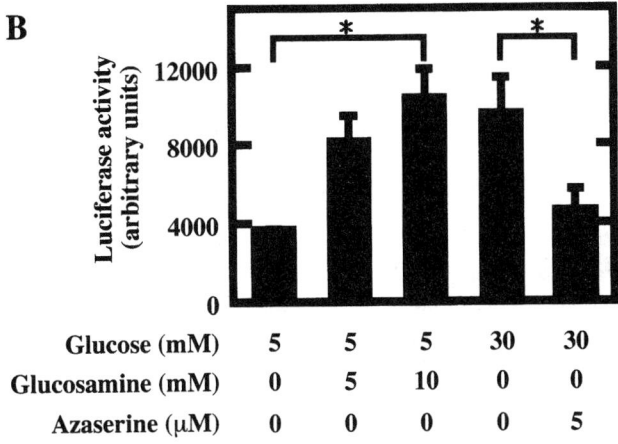

FIGURE 2. (**A**) Effect of high glucose on luciferase activity of the OPN promoter/luciferase construct–transfected cells. Cultured rat aortic SMC were transfected with the OPN promoter/luciferase construct containing a 2.0-kb promoter region of the OPN gene upstream of the luciferase reporter.[32] Twenty-four hours after transfection, the cells were deprived of serum, and incubated in the indicated concentrations of glucose with or without GF109203X (GFX), or in 50 mM L-glucose or 50 mM D-mannitol for 24 h. After incubation, the cells were harvested and the luciferase activity of the cell lysate was measured. Representative results of three independent experiments are presented. Bars represent mean ± SD. *$p < 0.01$ versus 5 mM glucose. (**B**) Effect of glucosamine on luciferase activity of the OPN promoter/luciferase construct–transfected cells. The cells were cultured in 5 mM or 30 mM glucose with or without the indicated concentrations of glucosamine or azaserine for 24 h. *$p < 0.05$.

ciferase activity. As shown in FIGURE 1B, glucosamine-induced increase of OPN at the transcriptional level was confirmed by Northern blotting; treatment of cultured rat aortic SMC with 10 mM glucosamine increased the OPN mRNA by approximately 5.8-fold. We also found that glucosamine potently increased the secretion of OPN in cultured rat aortic SMC (data not shown). These data suggest the involvement of the hexosamine pathway, in addition to the protein kinase C–dependent pathway, in high glucose–stimulated transcription of OPN.

DISCUSSION

Our present study demonstrates that incubation of cultured rat aortic SMC in the medium containing higher concentrations of glucose increases the expression of OPN at the transcriptional level, possibly through the activation of protein kinase C as well as the hexosamine pathway. The results, together with the previous reports[14–21] suggesting the involvement of OPN in atherogenesis, imply that OPN plays a causative role in the accelerated atherogenesis in diabetes mellitus.

The activation of protein kinase C by high concentrations of glucose has been proposed as a mechanism for the development of diabetic vascular complications.[26,27] High glucose stimulates *de novo* synthesis of diacylglycerol from glycolytic intermediates[28,29] and the increased intracellular diacylglycerol activates protein kinase C, which is involved in a variety of cellular functions, such as the signaling process of growth factors and cytokines, thus leading to cellular responses and gene expressions.[30] Our present finding that high glucose–induced OPN expression is mediated possibly by protein kinase C–dependent pathway further supports the notion that the pathway plays an important role in the development of atherosclerotic vascular disease in diabetes mellitus. It has also been reported that 12-*O*-tetradecanoylphorbol 13-acetate–stimulated transcription of the OPN gene apparently occurs via a protein kinase C/mitogen–activated protein kinase–dependent mechanism,[31] suggesting that the activation of protein kinase C is a common mechanism mediating the expression of OPN under various extracellular stimuli.

It has been reported that high glucose activates protein kinase C after incubation for 3–5 days with aortic SMC and endothelial cells in a confluent state.[26] In our assay system, however, high glucose stimulated the OPN promoter activity within 24 h, suggesting the existence of another pathway besides the protein kinase C pathway in mediating high glucose–induced activation of the OPN promoter. In the present study, we have found that the hexosamine pathway also seems to be involved in the activation process. Although precise mechanism(s) responsible for glucosamine-induced upregulation of gene transcription are not known at present, McClain and colleagues[24] have identified a 130 base pair glucosamine response element of the transforming growth factor-α promoter that includes three potential binding sites for the transcription factor Sp1. Indeed, the OPN promoter region used in the present study also contains a possible Sp1 binding site,[32] but its functional role remains to be elucidated.

ACKNOWLEDGMENTS

We thank Dr. Yohko U. Katagiri (Department of Pathology, National Children's Medical Research Center, Japan) and Prof. Toshimitu Uede (Section of Immmunopathology, Institute of Immunological Science, Hokkaido University, Japan) for helpful discussion.

REFERENCES

1. AMERICAN DIABETES ASSOCIATION. 1989. Diabetes Care **12:** 573–579.
2. ANDERSEN, J.L. *et al.* 1996. Diabetes **45:** S91–S94.
3. VAN BELLE, E. *et al.* 1997. Circulation **96:** 1454–1460.
4. KORNOWSKI, R. *et al.* 1997. Circulation **95:** 1366–1369.
5. SHANAHAN, C.M. *et al.* 1994. J. Clin. Invest. **93:** 2393–2402.
6. FRANZEN, A. & D. HEINEGARD. 1985. Biochem. J. **232:** 715–724.
7. RODAN, G.A. *et al.* 1995. Ann. N.Y. Acad. Sci. **760:** 1–5.
8. BUTLER, W.T. *et al.* 1989. Connect. Tissue Res. **23:** 123–136.
9. DENHARDT, D.T. & X. GUO. 1993. FASEB J. **7:** 1475–1482.
10. CANTOR, H. *et al.* 1995. Ann. N.Y. Acad. Sci. **760:** 143–150.
11. SENGER, D.R. *et al.* 1989. Anticancer Res. **9:** 1291–1300.
12. CRAIG, A.M. *et al.* 1990. Int. J. Cancer **46:** 133–137.
13. KOHRI, K. *et al.* 1993. J. Biol. Chem. **268:** 15180–15184.
14. LIAW, L. *et al.* 1998. J. Clin. Invest. **101:** 1468–1478.
15. LIAW, L. *et al.* 1994. Circ. Res. **74:** 214–224.
16. YUE, T. L. *et al.* 1994. Exp. Cell Res. **214:** 459–464.
17. PANDA, D. *et al.* 1997. Proc. Natl. Acad. Sci. USA **94:** 9308–9313
18. LIAW, L. *et al.* 1997. Arterioscler. Thromb. Vasc. Biol. **17:** 188–193.
19. GIACHELLI, G.M. *et al.* 1993. J. Clin. Invest. **92:** 1686–1696.
20. IKEDA, T. *et al.* 1993. J. Clin. Invest. **92:** 2814–2820.
21. LIAW, L. *et al.* 1995. J. Clin. Invest. **95:** 713–724.
22. SRIVATSA, S.S. *et al.* 1997. Cardiovasc. Res. **36:** 408–428.
23. MARSHALL, S. *et al.* 1991. J. Biol. Chem. **266:** 4706–4712.
24. MCCLAIN, D.A. *et al.* 1992. Proc. Natl. Acad. Sci. USA **89:** 8150–8154.
25. KOLM-LITTY, V. *et al.* 1998. J. Clin. Invest. **101:** 160–169.
26. LEE, T.S. *et al.* 1989. Proc. Natl. Acad. Sci. USA **86:** 5141–5145.
27. CRAVEN, P.A. & F.R. DERUBERTIS. 1989. J. Clin. Invest. **83:** 1667–1675.
28. AYO, S.H. *et al.* 1991. Am. J. Physiol. **261:** F571–F577.
29. CRAVEN, P.A. *et al.* 1990. Diabetes **39:** 667–674.
30. KOYA, D. *et al.* 1998. Diabetes **47:** 859–866.
31. ATKINS, K.B. *et al.* 1997. Arch. Biochem. Biophys. **343:** 157–163.
32. RIDALL, A.L. *et al.* 1995. Ann. N.Y. Acad. Sci. **760:** 59–66.
33. KATAGIRI, Y. *et al.* 1995. Ann. N.Y. Acad. Sci. **760:** 371–374.
34. TAMURA, K. *et al.* 1998. Biochem. Biophys. Res. Commun. **251:** 677–680.

The Second Nationwide Study of Atherosclerosis in Infants, Children, and Young Adults in Japan

Comparison with the First Study Carried Out 13 Years Ago[a]

MASAMI IMAKITA,[b] CHIKAO YUTANI,[b,c] ISAMU SAKURAI,[d]
AKINOBU SUMIYOSHI,[e] TERUO WATANABE,[f] MASAKO MITSUMATA,[g]
YOSHIAKI KUSUMI,[d] SHOICHI KATAYAMA,[h] MASAYUKI MANO,[i]
SHUNROKU BABA,[j] TOSHIFUMI MANNAMI,[j] KATSUO SUEISHI,[k]
AND KENZO TANAKA[l]

[b]*Department of Pathology, National Cardiovascular Center, Osaka, Japan*

[d]*Department of Pathology, Nihon University, School of Medicine*

[e]*Department of Pathology, Miyazaki Medical College*

[f]*Department of Pathology, University of Tsukuba, School of Medicine*

[g]*Department of Pathology, Yamanashi Medical University*

[h]*Department of Pathology, Kure National Hospital*

[i]*Department of Pathology, Osaka Medical Center for Cancer and Cardiovascular Disease, Osaka, Japan*

[j]*Department of Epidemiology, National Cardiovascular Center, Osaka, Japan*

[k]*Department of Pathology, Faculty of Medicine, Kyushu University*

[l]*Fukuoka Dental College*

It has been become obvious that death from coronary heart disease and cerebral infarction is increasing as the Japanese life-style is westernized. We have carried out the second nation-wide cooperative study to determine the extent and the prevalence of atherosclerosis in present generations in Japanese to improve our knowledge of the natural history of atherosclerosis in Japanese infants, children, and young adults and to determine its association with the risk factors for coronary heart disease.

---

[a]This work was supported by the Research Grant for Cardiovascular Disease (7C-1 and 10C-7) from the Ministry of Health and Welfare, Japan.

[b]Address for correspondence: Masami Imakita, M.D., Department of Pathology, National Cardiovascular Center, 5-7-1 Fujishirodai, Suita, Osaka 565-8456, Japan. Voice: 06-6833-5012, fax: 06-6872-7486.
mimakita@hsp.ncvc.go.jp

[c]Address for correspondence: Chikao Yutani, M.D., Ph.D., Department of Pathology, National Cardiovascular Center, 5-7-1 Fujishirodai, Suita, Osaka 565-8456, Japan. Voice: 06-6833-5012, fax: 06-6872-8100.
cyutani@hsp.ncvc.go.jp

MATERIALS AND METHODS

We collected aortas and coronary arteries from the patients who had been autopsied between January 1991 and December 1995 in 67 hospitals in Japan and ranged in age from 1 month to 39 years. Quantitative assessment of the atherosclerotic lesions of the arteries was performed by the point-counting method. We evaluated each point of the arteries indicated by a dot on the transparent plastic sheet, as having no atherosclerotic lesions (N) or three different types of atherosclerotic lesions: fatty streaks (F), fibrous plaques (P), and complicated lesions (C). The scores such as SI [(surface involvement) = $(F + P + C)/(N + F + P + C) \times 100$] and AI [(Atherosclerotic index) = $(F + P \times 10 + C \times 100)/(N + F + P + C)$] were calculated and utilized as indices of extent and severity of atherosclerosis of each artery. Clinical information including sex, age at death, geographical residence, underlying diseases, blood pressure, serum cholesterol, serum triglyceride, uric acid, and platelet count were obtained from autopsy and clinical records. Also, the results of our study were compared with those of the first study, which was performed between January 1978 and December 1982.[1]

RESULTS

TABLE 1 shows the number of the patients and the means of SI and AI of aorta and coronary arteries in each sex-age group. In aortas, the means of SI and AI of aortas increased with age in both sexes. The means of SI in males were lower in the third and the fourth decade of the second study and the third decades of the first study than those in females of each study. The means of AI in males were lower in the fourth decade of the current study and the second and third decades of the first study than those in females of each study. However, differences were not statistically significant. Fatty streaks increased with age in both sexes, compared to the preceding decade except for that in the fourth decade. In the fourth decade, fatty streaks still occupied approximately 90% of the lesions, but fibrous plaques rather than fatty streak showed a rapid increase. Complicated lesions showed an increase with age, but the extent was slight, compared with other lesions. The tendency for the progression of the extent of atherosclerotic lesions appeared to be similar between the first and second studies. The means of those scores did not show significant difference among these four groups.

In coronary arteries, the means of SI and AI in males showed a rapid increase from the second decade to the fourth decade. Those means in males were significantly greater in the third and fourth decades of the second study and the fourth decade of the first study than those in females. Fatty streaks were predominant lesions. However, raised lesions occupied a larger proportion in third and fourth decades than was observed in the aorta. There was a significant difference in the means of SI and AI among the four groups. The means of the SIF, SIP SI(P + C), SI and AI in the fourth decade of both studies and the SIP and the SI(P + C) in the third decades of the second study were significantly greater than those in females. Also, the means of SIP, SI(P + C) and SI in the third and fourth decades of males and that of AI in the fourth decade of males showed the significant difference between the second and first studies.

TABLE 1. Atherosclerosis of aortas and coronary arteries (means of SI and AI)

	Aorta					Coronary artery				
	0	1–9	10–19	20–29	30–39	0	1–9	10–19	20–29	30–39
Males										
1991–1995										
Patients (N)	68	81	91	140	185	72	76	82	152	207
Fatty streaks	0.930	6.157	23.916	25.829	25.518	0.208	0.463	4.528	7.153	8.176
Plaques	0.047	0.037	0.668	2.427	4.064	0.000	0.039	0.399	2.094	4.339
Complicated	0.000	0.000	0.000	0.039	0.187	0.000	0.000	0.000	0.000	0.355
Total	0.976	6.194	24.585	28.295	24.768	0.208	0.502	4.926	9.247	12.871
AI	0.0140	0.0653	0.3060	0.5397	0.8485	0.0021	0.0085	0.0852	0.2809	0.8709
1978–1982										
Patients (N)	155	246	195	242	482	52	147	156	204	389
Fatty streaks	2.787	7.072	20.738	28.720	28.846	0.000	0.614	2.217	4.829	7.032
Plaques	0.023	0.143	0.699	1.227	4.034	0.000	0.000	0.268	0.667	2.550
Complicated	0.000	0.000	0.011	0.009	0.173	0.000	0.000	0.004	0.000	0.048
Total	2.810	7.215	21.448	29.956	33.053	0.000	0.614	2.490	5.496	9.629
AI	0.0302	0.0850	0.2881	0.4187	0.8647	0.0000	0.0061	0.0530	0.1151	0.3729
Females										
1991–1995										
Patients (N)	63	54	49	79	133	59	59	49	82	136
Fatty streaks	0.702	4.907	21.224	29.220	27.879	0.161	0.524	3.491	4.823	5.615
Plaques	0.000	0.051	0.652	1.236	3.774	0.000	0.000	0.132	0.216	1.713
Complicated	0.000	0.000	0.000	0.000	0.273	0.000	0.000	0.000	0.000	0.000
Total	0.702	4.958	21.876	30.456	31.925	0.161	0.524	3.623	5.040	7.327
AI	0.0070	0.0542	0.2774	0.4158	0.9291	0.0016	0.0052	0.0481	0.0699	0.2274
1978–1982										
Patients (N)	161	174	136	191	330	36	95	106	174	255
Fatty streaks	3.060	5.701	22.202	30.875	29.105	0.000	0.317	2.596	4.752	4.848
Plaques	0.000	0.190	0.478	1.635	3.174	0.000	0.000	0.214	0.683	0.610
Complicated	0.000	0.000	0.028	0.115	0.110	0.000	0.000	0.000	0.052	0.109
Total	3.060	5.891	22.708	32.625	32.389	0.000	0.317	2.810	5.486	5.567
AI	0.0306	0.0760	0.2982	0.5876	0.7182	0.0000	0.0032	0.0473	0.1674	0.2182

Simple correlation coefficients between various scores of atherosclerosis and the risk factors in the second study are summarized in TABLE 2. Age and systolic blood pressure significantly correlated with each value of SI and AI of aorta and coronary

TABLE 2. Simple correlation coefficients between selected measures of risk factors and indexes of atherosclerosis of aorta and coronary artery[a]

Aorta						Coronary artery					
SI		SIPC		AI		SI		SIPC		AI	
AGE	0.572*	AGE	0.308*	AGE	0.302*	AGE	0.383*	SBP	0.346*	SBP	0.271*
Chol	0.244*	DBP	0.127	SBP	0.258*	SBP	0.193*	DBP	0.224*	DBP	0.163*
SBP	0.210*	SBP	0.122	DBP	0.176*	DBP	0.138	AGE	0.223*	AGE	0.151*
DBP	0.163*	Chol	0.084	Chol	0.093	Chol	0.071	Chol	–0.001	UA	0.025
Trig	0.082	PLT	0.023	PLT	0.024	Trig	0.046	UA	0.004	Trig	0.011
PLT	–0.47	UA	–0.002	UA	–0.009	UA	0.023	Trig	0.004	Chol	–0.035
UA	–0.58	Trig	–0.056	Trig	–0.024	PLT	–0.90	PLT	–0.075	PLT	–0.037

[a]Abbreviations: SI, surface involvement; SIPC, surface involvement of plaque and complicated lesion; AI, atherosclerotic index; Chol, serum cholesterol (mg/dl); SBP, systolic blood pressure (mm Hg); DBP, diastolic blood pressure (mm Hg); Trig, triglyceride (mg/dl); UA, uric acid (mg/dl); PLT, platelet count (per mm^3).
*Significant correlation ($p < 0.05$).

arteries and the value of SI(P + C) of coronary artery. Diastolic blood pressure significantly correlated with each value of SI and AI of aorta and SI(P + C) and AI of coronary artery. Also, serum cholesterol significantly correlated with the value of SI of aorta. On the other hand, triglyceride, uric acid, and platelet counts showed no significant correlation.

In the stepwise multiple regression analysis, SIF, SIP, SIC, SI, SI(P + C), and AI of aortas and coronary arteries were studied as dependent variables. Sex (female: 1, male: 2), age, systolic blood pressure, and serum cholesterol could be used as independent variables. The value of SI of the aorta significantly correlated with serum cholesterol and age, whereas that of AI of the aorta significantly correlated with systolic blood pressure and age. This result was explained by the observations that serum cholesterol was a stronger factor for progression of fatty streaks (SIF) and that systolic blood pressure was a stronger factor for progression of complicated lesion (SIC), because AI values are much more influenced by the extent of complicated lesion. Age was the strong factor for SIP, SI(P + C), SI, and AI. In coronary arteries, systolic blood pressure and age were significant factors for SI, and systolic blood pressure for AI. Systolic blood pressure was the strongest factor for SIP, SIC, SI(P + C), SI, and AI. Serum cholesterol was not the strong factor.

DISCUSSION

It is generally considered that the Japanese have less severe atherosclerosis of the aorta and coronary arteries than do Caucasians. Ishii and colleagues compared the extent of atherosclerotic lesions in 25–44 year old men in Tokyo and New Orleans by age and cause of death. The coronary arteries and abdominal aorta of black and white men from New Orleans showed significantly more extensive involvement with raised lesions than those of men from Tokyo in this age group.[2] However, the first study conducted by K. Tanaka had findings quite similar to the findings from the study of atherosclerosis in the United States, a multi-institutional study known as PDAY (Pathobiological Determinants of Atherosclerosis in Youth).[3] Furthermore, it has been become obvious that death from coronary heart disease and cerebral infarction is increasing as the Japanese life-style is westernized. Therefore, we carried out the second nation-wide cooperative study and determined the extent and the prevalence of atherosclerosis in present generations in Japanese.

The results of this study were compared with those of the first study. Although the method and materials used in both studies were basically similar, the standardization of grading procedure between the pathologists in the first and second studies was impossible. However, one of pathologists (C.Y.) in this study had been the member of the first study and could show us the three different types of atherosclerotic lesions according to the definition in the first study. Before starting the quantitative assessment of the atherosclerotic lesions of the arteries, all the assigned pathologists reaffirmed the definition of three different types of atherosclerotic lesions on representative samples of aortas and coronary arteries. Therefore, it was assumed that there would not be great difference in the quantitative assessment of the atherosclerotic lesions between the first and second studies.

The extent of the coronary atherosclerosis in male of the second study was significantly more severe than those in other groups in the third and fourth decades. From the view point of sex differences in atherosclerosis, it is generally considered that coronary atherosclerosis is more severe in males. Strong and colleagues stated that raised lesions (fibrous plaques and complicated lesion) in coronary arteries are more extensive in white males than in white females.[4] As regarding the marked progression in males between the first and second studies, the data from Japanese national surveys on circulatory disorders showed that systolic blood pressure was decreasing constantly among 1971, 1980, and 1990 surveys in both males and females and that serum cholesterol was increasing rapidly in both men and women between 1980 and 1990.[5] However, the means of systolic blood pressure and serum cholesterol in males whose coronary arteries were evaluated in the second study did not show significant difference, although relatively large numbers of data were missing.

REFERENCE

1. TANAKA, K., J. MASUDA, T. IMAMURA et al. 1988. A nation-wide study of atherosclerosis in infants, children and young adults in Japan. Atherosclerosis **72:** 143–156.
2. ISHII, T., W.P. NEWMAN, M.A. GUZMAN et al. 1986. Coronary and aortic atherosclerosis in young men from Tokyo and New Orleans. Lab. Invest. **54;** 561–565.
3. STRONG, J.P., G.T. MALCOM, M.C. OALMANN et al. 1995. Environmental and genetic risk factors in early human atherogenesis: Lessons from the PDAY study. Pathology Intl. **45:** 403–408.
4. STRONG, J.P., C. RESTREPO & M. GUZMAN. 1978. Coronary and aortic atherosclerosis in New Orleans. II. Comparison of lesions by age, sex, and race. Lab. Invest. **39:** 364–369.
5. SAKATA, K. & D.R. LABARTHE. 1996. Changes in cardiovascular disease risk factors in three Japanese national surveys 1971–1990. J. Epidemiol. **6:** 93–107.

Gene Therapy for Cardiovascular Disease Using Hepatocyte Growth Factor

RYUICHI MORISHITA,[a-c] MOTOKUNI AOKI,[b] SHIGEFUMI NAKAMURA,[b] JITSUO HIGAKI,[b] YASUFUMI KANEDA,[c] AND TOSHIO OGIHARA[b]

[b]*Department of Geriatric Medicine and* [c]*Division of Gene Therapy Science, Osaka University Medical School, Suita 565, Japan*

ENDOTHELIUM AS AN IDEAL TARGET FOR GENE THERAPY TO TREAT CARDIOVASCULAR DISEASE

The concept of the local control of vascular function by locally synthesized compounds has been recently described. Locally synthesized growth factors may play a major role in the regulation of both vascular tone and structure. These local systems appear to be independently regulated by regional factors and may play important physiologic and pathophysiologic roles. On the other hand, endothelial cells are known to secrete various vasoactive substances. Recently, it has been hypothesized that endothelial cells may also modulate vascular growth, because many anti-proliferative factors, such as nitric oxide (NO) and vascular natriuretic peptides, are secreted from endothelial cells. Thus, multiple endothelium-derived substances (PGI_2, NO, CNP) also have profound influences on vascular smooth muscle function. Indeed, co-culture of endothelial cells with vascular smooth muscle cells (VSMC) resulted in a significant decrease in DNA synthesis of VSMC.[1] Therefore, following vascular injury (by denuding endothelial cells), locally synthesized cytokines and growth factors contribute to the development of neointimal lesions. Alternatively, it is apparent that dysfunction of endothelial cells may promote abnormal vascular growth, such as in atherosclerosis. The growth of VSMC is controlled by a balance of growth inhibitors and growth promoters and, in the normal adult vessel, this balance results in a very low rate of growth of smooth muscle. However, following vascular injury by either mechanical or biochemical means, this balance is shifted such that proliferation of smooth muscle cells occurs, due to lack of endothelial cells. Given the importance of endothelial cells, we hypothesized that rapid regeneration of endothelial cells, not accompanied by VSMC growth, may have therapeutic potential in prevention of abnormal vascular growth, such as neointimal formation after angioplasty. From this viewpoint, we have focused on hepatocyte growth factor (HGF) as a candidate (FIG. 1).

---

[a]Address for correspondence: Ryuichi Morishita, M.D., Ph.D., Associate Professor, Division of Gene Therapy Science, Osaka University Medical School, Suita 565, Japan. Voice: 81-6-6879-3902; fax: 81-6-6879-3909.
morishit@geriat.med.osaka-u.ac.jp

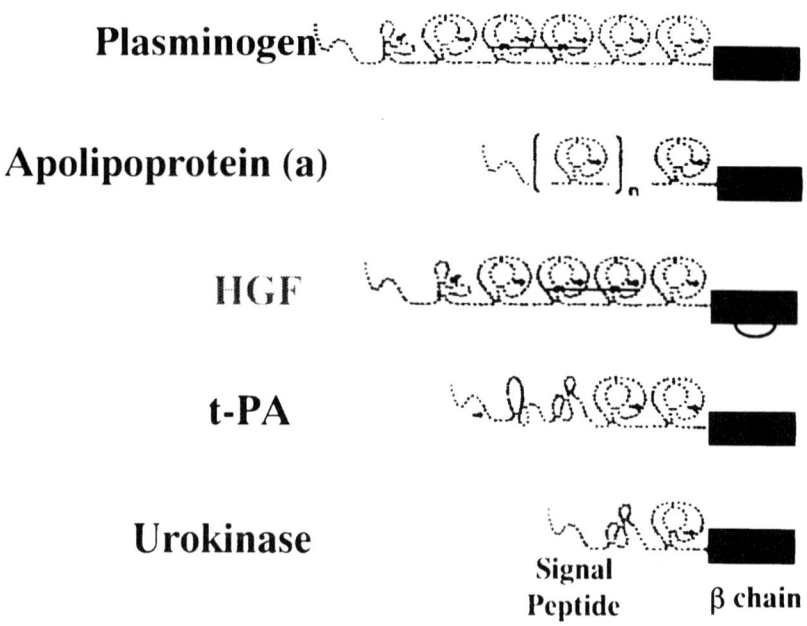

FIGURE 1. Structure of HGF. Hepatocyte growth factor is "Heart and vessels Growth Factor."

HGF AS AN ENDOTHELIUM-SPECIFIC GROWTH FACTOR

HGF is a mesenchyme-derived pleiotropic factor that regulates cell growth, cell motility, and morphogenesis of various types of cells. It is thus considered a humoral mediator of epithelial-mesenchymal interactions responsible for morphogenic tissue interactions during embryonic development and organogenesis.[2] In addition to the classical concept, we found that HGF stimulated DNA synthesis in a dose-dependent manner.[1,2] Of importance, DNA synthesis stimulated by HGF was significantly greater than that stimulated by bFGF or VEGF, demonstrating that HGF was most potent in stimulating endothelial cell growth.[1,2] In contrast, HGF or VEGF did not stimulate DNA synthesis in VSMC, whereas the addition of exogenous bFGF resulted in a significant increase in DNA synthesis.[1] Overall, HGF has the characteristics of an endothelium-specific growth factor the same as VEGF secreted from VSMC, and to act on endothelial cells. Interestingly, the presence of HGF mRNA was detected in human and rat aortic endothelial cells, VSMC, and cardiac myocytes by RT-PCR.[3] The presence of c-met RNA was also detected in human and rat endothelial cells and VSMC. Of importance, the existence of a local HGF system (HGF and c-met) was also confirmed in the aorta of rat and human *in vivo*.[3] In addition to the *in vitro* evidence, HGF mRNA was readily detected in heart, kidney, and blood vessels *in vivo* of WKY (Wistar-Kyoto rats) and SHR (spontaneously hypertensive rats).[4]

Of interest, HGF could abrogate the decrease in DNA synthesis and cell death of endothelial cells mediated by serum-free treatment.[5] HGF should be classed as a new member of the growth factors with anti–cell death actions. More importantly, we demonstrated that high D-glucose, but not mannitol and L-glucose, induced aortic endothelial cell death and L-glucose, induced aortic endothelial cell death, probably apoptosis, which was attenuated by addition of rHGF, and stimulated VSMC growth.[6,7] The mechanisms by which HGF prevented endothelial cell death mediated by these conditions are still unclear. HGF is known to stimulate phosphatidylinositol-3′-kinase (PI3K), protein tyrosine phosphatase 2, phospholipase C-r, pp60[c-src], and grb2/hSos1. Moreover, HGF also stimulated the rho- and ras-mediated signal transduction pathway, resulting in an increase in actin fibers. The activation of these signal transduction pathways suggests that HGF will act to prevent cell death.

Since the local HGF system is expected to have a role in the pathogenesis of cardiovascular disease, we focused on the interaction of TGF-β and angiotensin (Ang) II with the HGF system. A marked reduction of local HGF production by TGF-β and

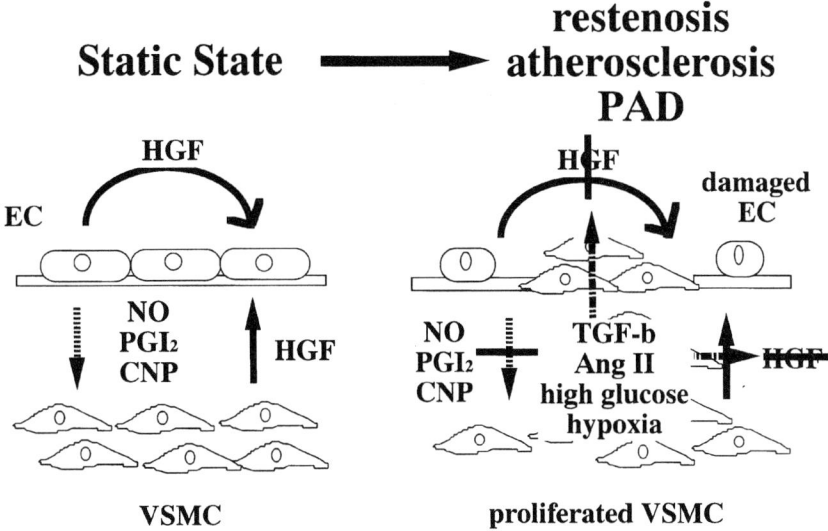

FIGURE 2. Hypothesis in the role of HGF in the maintenance of the vascular structure. In static state, HGF secreted from VSMC and endothelial cells may maintain the vascular structure in an autocrine-paracrine manner, whereas endothelial cells may inhibit VSMC growth through the production of anti-proliferative substances (NO, PGI$_2$, CNP, etc.) as a biological barrier. In contrast, in injured vessels, such as in atherosclerosis, the impairment of endothelial cells may have occurred through the downregulation of local HGF production by TGF-β, Ang II, high D-glucose, and/or hypoxia. Therefore, the proliferation of VSMC may be accelerated by the loss of anti-proliferative substances.

Ang II treatment was observed in endothelial cells and VSMC.[8] The promoter region of HGF gene contains various binding sites for transcription factors, e.g., interleukin 6 response elements, a TGF-β inhibitory element, and a cAMP-responsive element. Probably, TGF-β inhibits HGF production through a TGF-β inhibitory element at the transcriptional level. On the other hand, exogenous addition of recombinant rat HGF stimulated local human HGF release into the culture medium both in human endothelial cells and human VSMC.[9] This phenomenon provides the interesting hypothesis that HGF itself regulates local HGF production by autoloop-positive feedback and works in an autocrine-paracrine manner (FIG. 2). The break of this autocrine-loop, which maintains endothelial cell growth, by TGF-β and Ang II may result in the abnormal growth of VSMC and cardiac myocytes. The suppression of local HGF production also occurred in more physiological conditions. Local HGF production in endothelial cells and VSMC was markedly suppressed by high D-glucose, due to increased TGF-β.[6] These results suggest that decreased local HGF production may promote the progression of arteriosclerotic vascular changes in diabetes mellitus. Prostaglandin (PG) E, PGI_2 analogue, and cilostazol, which are well known to improve peripheral arterial disease in patients with DM, attenuated endothelial cell death induced by high D-glucose through the stimulation of local HGF production.[7] Increased vascular HGF production by these agents may contribute to the usefulness of PGI_2 analogue and cilostazol in the treatment of peripheral arterial disease, such as arteriosclerosis obliterans (ASO), observed in diabetes mellitus.

POTENTIAL GENE THERAPY FOR RESTENOSIS AFTER ANGIOPLASTY BY HGF

What is the importance of this local synthesis of HGF? Although the expression of HGF in the vasculature is orders of magnitude lower than that observed in the liver, due to the limited extracellular volume within the vessel wall, low expression of HGF may result in high extracellular levels of the cytokine. Moreover, the ability of the local tissues to respond to changes in the local environment allows the rapid regulation of local function. To pursue these questions, we have examined the consequences of HGF expression in vascular cells in cell culture. Overexpression of HGF resulted in a significant increase in endothelial cell number.[9] Interestingly, this mitogenic effect was significantly stronger than that of rHGF at concentrations of 100 ng/ml. Our data showed a marked increase in rat immunoreactive HGF in cells transfected with human HGF vector. HGF may exert auto-looped positive feedback on HGF production, consistent with findings that rHGF upregulated endogenous HGF production in VSMC. We have successfully reported gene therapy for restenosis after angioplasty using transgenes and ODN-based technology.[10–12] However, none of these strategies has been reported to induce regeneration of endothelial cells. As mentioned earlier, endothelial cells can secrete biological substances to inhibit VSMC growth and vasodilating factors. Therefore, it is logical that rapid regeneration of endothelial cells has potential therapeutic value against VSMC proliferation (in restenosis after angioplasty). The stimulatory action of HGF gene transfer could also be observed in co-culture using human cells to investigate its potential therapeutic value in human vascular diseases. In the co-culture system with human VSMC transfected with HGF vector, the cell growth of quiescent non-transfected human endothelial cells was significantly increased. These results demonstrated that endothelial cells and VSMC directly transfected with HGF expression vector exhibited increases in cell growth of endothelial cells in an autocrine/paracrine manner.

In addition, we investigated *in vivo* gene transfer of human HGF that is downregulated in injured vessels. Transfection of human HGF gene into balloon-injured rat carotid artery resulted in significant inhibition of neointimal formation up to at least 8 weeks after transfection, accompanied by detection of human immunoreactive HGF. Induction of re-endothelialization induced by overexpression of human HGF gene transfer into balloon-injured vessels is supported by several lines of evidence. (1) Administration of HGF vector, but not control vector, markedly inhibited neointimal formation, accompanied by a significant increase in vascular human and rat HGF concentrations. (2) Planimetric analysis demonstrated a significant increase in re-endothelialized area in arteries transfected with human HGF vector. (3) Induction of NO content in balloon-injured vessels transfected with human HGF vector was observed in accordance with the recovery of endothelial vasodilator properties in response to acetylcholine. As endogenous HGF expression in balloon-injured vessels was significantly decreased as compared to normal vessels, the present study demonstrated the successful inhibition of neointimal formation by transfection of human HGF gene as "cytokine supplement therapy" in a rat balloon-injury model.

GENE THERAPY FOR ISCHEMIC DISEASE BY HGF

As described above, we and others have reported that HGF exclusively stimulated the growth of endothelial cells without replication of VSMC, thereby indicating it to be a potential angiogenic growth factor. Unexpectedly, the mitogenic activity of HGF is more potent than that of VEGF in human aortic endothelial cells.[1,2] Therefore, we reasoned that HGF might be a potential therapeutic angiogenic growth factor, in addition to VEGF. Interestingly, vascular HGF concentration in the diseased segments of blood vessels from patients with peripheral arterial disease was significantly decreased as compared to that in disease-free segments of blood vessels from the same patients as control vessel.[13] Downregulation of the vascular HGF system may be related to the pathogenesis of peripheral arterial disease. The decrease in local HGF production in the vessels of patients with ASO was due to TGF-β or hypoxia, which are strong suppressors of vascular HGF *in vitro* as well as *in vivo*.[14] Given the significant decrease in endogenous HGF production in the ischemic limb, we hypothesized that administration of recombinant HGF into the ischemic limb might result in a beneficial effect in hypoxia. Therefore, rHGF was intra-arterially administered via the internal iliac artery of rabbits in which the femoral artery was excised to induce unilateral hind-limb ischemia. Of importance, administration of rHGF into the ischemic limb on day 10 and 12 after surgery produced significant augmentation of collateral vessel development as assessed by angiography on day 30 in the ischemia model ($p < 0.01$). Serial angiograms revealed progressive linear extension of collateral arteries from the origin stem artery to the distal point of the reconstituted parent vessel in HGF-treated animals. Moreover, we evaluated a single administration of rHGF in the ischemia model and found that it also caused a significant increase in angiographic score as compared to vehicle-treated rabbits.[13] The feasibility of a novel therapeutic strategy using angiogenic growth factors by expediting and/or augmenting collateral artery development has recently entered the realm of treatment of ischemic diseases. Indeed, the clinical utility of gene therapy using VEGF gene has been recently reported for the treatment of critical limb ischemia.[15] Thus, we also tested the feasibility of gene therapy of intramuscular injection of HGF gene into rat hind-limb ischemic model. Transfection of HGF gene stimulated the collateral formation and increased blood flow, and its degree was significantly greater than that by administration of rHGF. Currently, we submitted the clinical protocol to treat the patients with peripheral arterial disease by HGF gene transfer. In the presence of decreased endogenous HGF, administration of rHGF or HGF gene transfer induced therapeutic angiogenesis in the ischemic hind-limb, as potential "cytokine supplement therapy" for peripheral arterial disease (FIG. 3).

Alternatively, *in vivo* transfer of HGF gene may salvage myocardial infarction as gene therapy. Expectedly, in myocardium transfected with HGF vector, a significant increase in PCNA-positive endothelial cells could be observed, while few PCNA-positive endothelial cells were detected in control-vector transfected and untreated myocardium. The number of vessels around the injection sites of hearts transfected with HGF gene was significantly increased as compared to control vector or vehicle ($p < 0.01$). Angiogenic activity induced by transfection of HGF vector was also confirmed by the activation of a transcription factor, ets, that is essential for angiogenesis, assessed by the immunohistochemistry and gel mobility shift assay. Furthermore, we studied the pathophysiological role of HGF in the myocardial infarction model. Endogenous HGF concentration was significantly decreased in infarcted hearts. Moreover, transfection of human HGF into the infarcted hearts also

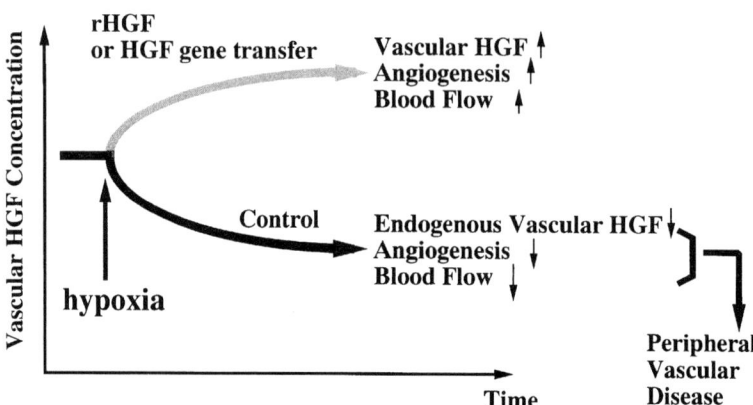

FIGURE 3. Schema of HGF supplement therapy for peripheral arterial disease. In the vessels of patients with peripheral arterial disease, endogenous HGF was downregulated by hypoxia, thereby attenuating angiogenesis in response to hypoxia. Total limb blood flow may be decreased in peripheral arterial disease. Correction of the insufficient supply of vascular HGF by administration of rHGF might enhance angiogenesis, resulting in a significant increase in blood flow to prevent critical limb ischemia.

TABLE 1. Potential utility of HGF therapy in cardiovascular disease

Disease	Targets
ASO/Buerger	Angiogenesis
Myocardial infarction	Angiogenesis, anti-fibrosis
Chronic heart failure	Angiogenesis, anti-fibrosis
Restenosis	Re-endothelialization
Cardiomyopathy	Anti-fibrosis

resulted in a significant increase in vessels number ($p < 0.01$). Overall, we provide direct *in vivo* evidence for angiogenesis induced by transfection of human HGF gene in rat non-infarcted and infarcted myocardium. Continuous local production of HGF resulting from the transgene may be considered as a novel therapeutic angiogenesis strategy for myocardial infarction.

IS HGF A POTENTIAL THERAPEUTIC GROWTH FACTOR?

Overall, we showed that HGF is a novel member of endothelium-specific growth factors that stimulated re-endothelialization and angiogenesis. Features of HGF in cardiovascular disease is summarized in TABLE 1. We speculated that HGF might be a therapeutic growth factor for the treatment of cardiovascular diseases, e.g., restenosis after angioplasty, peripheral arterial disease, and myocardial infarction.

REFERENCES

1. NAKAMURA, Y. *et al.* 1996. Hepatocyte growth factor (HGF) is a novel member of endothelium-specific growth factors: additive stimulatory effect of HGF with basic fibroblast growth factor, but not vascular endothelial growth factor. J. Hypertens. **14:** 1067–1072.
2. NAKAMURA, Y. *et al.* 1996. A vascular modulator, hepatocyte growth factor, is associated with systolic pressure. Hypertension **28:** 409–413.
3. NAKAMURA, Y. *et al.* 1995. Expression of local hepatocyte growth factor system in vascular tissues. Biochem. Biophys. Res. Commun. **215:** 483–488.
4. NAKANO, N. *et al.* 1997. Role of angiotensin II in the regulation of a novel vascular modulator, hepatocyte growth factor, in experimental hypertensive rats. Hypertension **30:** 1448–1454.
5. YO, Y. *et al.* 1998. Actions of hepatocyte growth factor as a local modulator in the kidney: potential role in pathogenesis of renal disease. Kid. Int. **53:** 50–58.
6. MORISHITA, R. *et al.* 1997. Potential role of endothelium-specific growth factor, hepatocyte growth factor, on endothelial damage in diabetes mellitus. Diabetes **46:** 138–142.
7. MORISHITA, R. *et al.* 1997. Role of hepatocyte growth factor in endothelial regulation: Prevention of high D-glucose-induced endothelial cell death by prostaglandins and phosphodiesterase type 3 inhibitor. Diabetologia **40:** 1053–1061.
8. NAKANO, N. *et al.* 1998. Negative regulation of local hepatocyte growth factor (HGF) expression by angiotensin II and transforming growth factor-β in blood vessels: potential role of HGF in cardiovascular disease. Hypertension **32:** 444–451.
9. HAYASHI, S. *et al.* 1996. Autocrine-paracrine effects of over-expression of hepatocyte growth factor gene on growth of endothelial cells. Biochem. Biophys. Res. Commun. **220:** 539–545.

10. MORISHITA, R. *et al.* 1993. Single intraluminal delivery of antisense cdc 2 kinase and PCNA oligonucleotides results in chronic inhibition of neointimal hyperplasia. Proc. Natl. Acad. Sci. USA **90:** 8474–8479.
11. VON DER LEYEN, H.E. *et al.* 1995. Gene therapy inhibiting neointimal vascular lesion: in vivo transfer of endothelial-cell nitric oxide synthase gene. Proc. Natl. Acad. Sci. USA **92:** 1137–1141.
12. MORISHITA, R. *et al.* 1995. A novel molecular strategy using cis element "decoy" of E2F binding site inhibits smooth muscle proliferation in vivo. Proc. Natl. Acad. Sci. USA **92:** 5855-5859.
13. MORISHITA, R. *et al.* 1999. Therapeutic angiogenesis induced by human recombinant hepatocyte growth factor in rabbit hind limb ischemia model as "cytokine supplement therapy." Hypertension **33:** 1379–1384.
14. HAYASHI, S. *et al.* 1999. Potential role of hepatocyte growth factor, a novel angiogenic growth factor, in peripheral arterial disease: down-regulation of HGF in response to hypoxia in vascular cells. Circulation **100:** II 301–308.
15. BAUMGARTNER, I. *et al.* 1998. Constitutive expression of phVEGF165 after intramuscular gene transfer promotes collateral vessel development in patients with critical limb ischemia. Circulation **97:** 1114–112311.

Index of Contributors

Abe, H., 134–139
Abe, M., 201–207
Abedin, J., 163–172
Acharya, S.S., 265–271
Aikawa, M., 140–152
Amano, J., 77–83
Anderson, K.R., 230–240, 294–297
Aoki, M., 369–376
Arai, H., 95–102
Arai, T., 103–112

Baba, S., 364–368
Berceli, S.A., 153–162
Berra, E., 187–200
Biwa, T., 342–346
Blangero, J., 1–7
Bruce, C., 103–112
Butler, W.T., 357–363

Campbell, G.R., 224–229
Campbell, J.H., 224–229
Carmeliet, P., 249–264
Carragher, N.O., 39–52
Challah, M., 347–351
Chegerova, T.I., 320–322
Chien, L.-J., 307–310
Clowes, A.W., 153–162
Collen, D., 249–264

Ding, H.A., 288–293
Doi, T., 163–172
Domoto, K., 283–287, 336–341

Efendy, J.L., 224–229
Eriksson, P., 27–38

Fan, J., 84–94, 347–351
Fayad, Z.A., 173–186
Febbraio, M., 128–133

Fluiter, K., 113–127
Fujioka, Y., 336–341
Fujisawa, K., 272–282
Fuster, V., 173–186

Garcia-Cardeña, G., 230–240, 294–297
Garcia-Zepeda, E.A., 288–293
Gerszten, R.E., 288–293
Gimbrone, M.A., Jr., xi–xii, 230–240, 288–293, 294–297
Gothié, E., 187–200

Hajjar, D.P., 128–133
Hajjar, K.A., 265–271, 311–314
Hakamata, H., 342–346
Hamsten, A., 27–38
Han, C.-L., 224–229
Han, J., 128–133
Hansson, G.K., 53–64
Henney, A.M., 27–38
Herijgers, N., 113–127
Higaki, J., 8–16, 369–376
Higashide, T., 163–172
Hixson, J.E., 1–7
Horiuchi, H., 95–102
Horiuchi, S., 342–346

Imakita, N., 364–368
Inoue, N., 241–248, 298–301
Ishii, H., 311–314
Ishii, K., 95–102
Ishikawa, Y., 283–287, 336–341
Isobe, M., 77–83
Ito, M., 201–207
Iwasa, S., 84–94

Jiang, X.-C., 103–112
Jormsjö, S., 27–38
Jukema, J.W., 17–26

Kakuta, T., 65–76
Kaneda, Y., 77–83, 369–376
Kanno, S., 201–207
Kastelein, J.J.P., 17–26
Kataoka, H., 95–102, 323–327, 328–335
Katayama, S., 364–368
Kato, I., 163–172
Katsuya, T., 8–16
Kawakami, A., 352–356
Kawasaki, K., 163–172
Kawasaki, S., 283–287, 336–341
Kawashima, S., 241–248, 298–301
Kishi, Y., 65–76
Kita, T., 95–102, 323–327, 328–335
Kobayashi, Y., 65–76
Kowase, K., 214–223
Koyama, H., 39–52
Kruchinsky, N.G., 320–322
Kume, N., 95–102, 323–327, 328–335
Kurabayashi, M., 214–223
Kusumi, Y., 364–368

Libby, P., 140–152
Lim, Y.-C., 288–293
Loskutoff, D.J., 272–282
Luscinskas, F.W., 288–293
Luster, A.D., 288–293

Mannami, T., 364–368
Mano, M., 364–368
Maruyama, I., 315–319
Masaki, T., 323–327, 328–335
Matsumoto, T., 357–363
Maung, K.K., 342–346
Mauri, L., 294–297
Migita, H., 163–172
Milanini, J., 187–200
Minami, M., 95–102, 323–327, 328–335
Mitsumata, M., 364–368
Miyazaki, A., 342–346
Mori, S., 357–363
Morishita, R., 77–83, 369–376
Morita, I., 208–213
Moriwaki, H., 95–102, 323–327, 328–335
Murase, T., 323–327
Murota, S.-I., 208–213

Nagai, R., 214–223
Nagel, T., 230–240
Nakajima, K., 352–356
Nakamura, S., 369–376
Nakano, T., 352–356
Nakata, M., 315–319
Nicholson, A.C., 128–133
Nion, S., 113–127
Numano, F., xiii, 65–76, 307–310, 311–314, 352–356

Oda, N., 201–207
Ogihara, T., 8–16, 369–376
Ohkawara, M., 65–76
Okamoto, H., 163–172
Okuda, M., 283–287
Onodera, M., 208–213

Pagès, G., 187–200
Paulsson, G., 53–64
Pouysségur, J., 187–200
Pryschepova, E.V., 320–322

Raines, E.W., 39–52
Richard, D.E., 187–200
Ridall, A.L., 357–363
Rikitake, Y., 298–301
Rosenzweig, A., 288–293
Rubanyi, G.M., 302–306

Saito, Y., 357–363
Sakai, M., 342–346
Sakamoto, Y., 342–346
Sakurai, I., 364–368
Sakurai, S., 163–172
Samad, F., 272–282
Sato, Y., 201–207
Sawamura, T., 323–327, 328–335

Segawa, Y., 163–172
Shibuya, M., 201–207
Shimoyamada, H., 347–351
Shitara, K., 201–207
Silver, D.L., 103–112
Silverstein, R.L., 128–133
Sueishi, K., 364–368
Sumiyoshi, A., 364–368
Suzuki, J.-I., 77–83

Taguchi, M., 283–287, 336–341
Takahashi, A., 283–287, 336–341
Takahashi, T., 283–287, 336–341
Takasawa, S., 163–172
Takemoto, M., 357–363
Takeshita, S., 298–301
Tall, A.R., 103–112
Tamura, K., 357–363
Tanaka, A., 65–76, 352–356
Tanaka, K., 364–368
Tanaka, N., 163–172
Taniguchi, T., 283–287, 336–341
Teplyakov, A.I., 320–322
Topper, J.N., 230–240
Törnquist, E., 53–64
Tsuji, H., 163–172

Unoki, H., 84–94, 163–172

Van Berkel, T.J.C., 113–127
van Eck, M., 113–127

Viñals, F., 187–200

Wakatsuki, Y., 95–103
Wang, H., 163–172
Watanabe, T., 84–94, 347–351, 364–368
Whatling, C., 27–38
Wu, P.-S., 163–172

Yamada, N., 134–139
Yamagishi, S.-I., 163–172
Yamaji, K., 315–319
Yamamoto, H., 163–172
Yamamoto, Y., 163–172
Yamazaki, M., 357–363
Yasukochi, Y., 307–310, 311–314
Ye, S., 27–38
Yokode, M., 95–103
Yokote, K., 357–363
Yokoyama, M., 241–248, 283–287, 298–301, 336–341
Yonekura, H., 163–172
Yoshida, M., 288–293, 307–310, 311–314
Yuksel, M., 342–346
Yutani, C., 364–368

Zenda, T., 163–172
Zhang, B., 27–38
Zhou, X., 53–64

UNIVERSITY LIBRARY

have